Sexually Transmitted Diseases

Ioannis Mylonas

Sexually Transmitted Diseases

A Guide for Gynecologists and Obstetricians

Springer

Ioannis Mylonas
Obstetrics, Gynecology and Infectious Diseases
Athens, Greece

ISBN 978-3-031-78203-9 ISBN 978-3-031-78204-6 (eBook)
https://doi.org/10.1007/978-3-031-78204-6

Based on the book by Mylonas I (2025) Sexuell übertragbare Erkrankungen: Ein Leitfaden für Frauenärztinnen und Frauenärzte. 2nd edition, Springer Verlag Heidelberg.

This Springer imprint is published by the registered company Springer Nature Switzerland AG
The registered company address is: Gewerbestrasse 11, 6330 Cham, Switzerland

Preface

Dear Readers,

Sexually transmitted diseases (STDs) have been documented throughout history and have exerted a profound influence on medical practice, particularly within gynecology and obstetrics. Reproductive anatomy and function are directly affected by these infections, obstetric and perinatal outcomes are consequently determined by their presence, and innovations in diagnostics, therapeutics, vaccination, and public-health practice have been driven by their burden.

The mid-twentieth century introduction of penicillin transformed the management of bacterial STDs. Syphilis and gonorrhea became reliably treatable, and reductions in complications—neurosyphilis, pelvic inflammatory disease, and infertility—were observed, decreasing overall public-health burden. Substantial improvements in clinical skills and laboratory techniques have been achieved. History taking, appropriate specimen collection, and implementation of nucleic acid amplification tests and other molecular diagnostics have been refined, and evidence-based therapeutic algorithms have been established.

Despite these advances, STDs remain a major global health challenge. Political, social, and economic shifts—coupled with increased global mobility—have contributed to rising incidence and changing epidemiologic patterns of many infections. Health disparities persist: insufficient sexual health education, limited access to prevention programs (including screening and vaccination), underfunded public health infrastructures, and constrained clinical services in low-resource settings impede timely diagnosis and treatment. Antimicrobial resistance has further complicated management: *N. gonorrhoeae* and other pathogens have acquired multidrug resistance mechanisms, reducing the efficacy of previously reliable regimens and necessitating continual revision of therapeutic guidelines. Viral infections such as human immunodeficiency virus (HIV) and human papillomavirus (HPV) retain epidemic or endemic significance in many regions despite progress in antiretroviral therapy and vaccination. From a clinical perspective, sexually transmitted diseases must be understood as more than isolated symptoms, diagnostic findings, or individual therapeutic measures. They have significant consequences for reproductive health, including impaired fertility, increased risk of adverse pregnancy outcomes (such as miscarriage, preterm birth, and neonatal infections), and the potential for congenital disorders. Effective management therefore necessitates a comprehensive approach that integrates obstetric considerations, partner evaluation and treatment, and interventions aimed at preventing vertical transmission.

In many high-income countries, the responsibility for STD management has increasingly shifted to specialized sexual health clinics or infectious disease units. However, workforce shortages—particularly in rural and underserved regions—and varying levels of clinical expertise are reshaping the distribution of care responsibilities. As a result, it is crucial that general practitioners, gynecologists, obstetricians, midwives, and nursing personnel maintain thorough practice-oriented knowledge of prevalent and clinically significant STDs. Essential competencies include accurate recognition of clinical presentations; appropriate utilization of laboratory diagnostics, such as nucleic acid amplification tests, serology, and culture when indicated; adherence to evidence-based treatment protocols with correct durations; application of contact tracing principles; implementation of vaccination programs (e.g., human papillomavirus and hepatitis B vaccines); and delivery of individualized prevention counseling based on patient risk profiles.

Comprehensive care for individuals affected by STDs extends beyond biomedical treatment. Proficient communication skills, patient-centered counseling, strict confidentiality, and cultural sensitivity are vital to establishing trust and enhancing adherence to prevention and therapeutic regimens. Clinicians frequently address psychosocial issues, support informed reproductive decision-making, and coordinate multidisciplinary care when complications arise. Furthermore, ethical responsibilities—such as partner notification and public health reporting—must be carefully balanced with respect for patient autonomy and privacy.

This volume has been structured and authored to meet the practical needs of gynecologists, obstetricians, infectious disease specialists, dermatologists, urologists, primary care providers, and adolescent medicine clinicians involved in the management of sexually transmitted infections in females across a wide range of clinical environments—including referral centers, community practices, and rural settings. The focus is on delivering concise, evidence-based recommendations integrated with pragmatic, logical management strategies that can be tailored to different resource levels. Key topics include pathogen-specific clinical manifestations, current diagnostic algorithms, treatment protocols aligned with standards, prevention measures such as vaccination and screening programs, management of pregnancy-related complications, and effective communication techniques encompassing partner notification and counseling.

The completion of this work was made possible by the invaluable support of many colleagues and contributors. Special thanks are due to Mrs. A. Born, Mr. S. Eickhoff, and Mrs. D. Kraplow at Springer Publishing for their unwavering dedication throughout the project. Responsibility for the layout rested solely with Misses E. Kayalvizhi, P. Sathishkumar, and D. Vijayakandeepan (Straive, a service provider to Springer Nature).

I am also deeply grateful to the patients who have entrusted me with their care over the past two decades. Being involved in pivotal moments of another person's life is both a profound responsibility and an honor.

Diagnosing and treating illness extends far beyond adherence to guidelines, financial considerations, prestige, or authority. Above all, it embodies the deeply human aspect of medicine, revealing its essential dimension rooted in empathy, compassion, and respect for individual dignity. This experience continually reminds me of the vital importance of humanism in modern medical practice—the need to see patients not merely as cases or conditions but as whole persons with unique stories and needs. The clinician's encounter with suffering, hope, and healing highlights the intricate balance of scientific knowledge, empathy, and ethical commitment that forms the foundation of medical care. This text honors the narratives shared by patients and acknowledges the extraordinary resilience, courage, dignity, and vulnerability they have exhibited throughout their healthcare experiences.

Athens (Greece), Munich (Germany)
and Vancouver (Canada)

Ioannis Mylonas

About the Book

Using this book

- It is recommended that readers initially obtain an overview of the different sections. Each section is arranged in alphabetical order, facilitating rapid reference.
- For each disease, a list of treatment options is provided, enabling physicians to select the most appropriate option according to the patient's individual circumstances. Occasionally, older treatments that have previously proven successful are also listed.
- This book includes a list of common medicines with proven efficacy. However, certain medications may only be available in select countries. In such instances, it is recommended that the treating physician contact the local pharmacy if there is any uncertainty regarding the availability of a drug.

Sexually transmitted disease (STD) or sexually transmitted infection (STI)?
In clinical practice and patient communication, the term "sexually transmitted disease" (STD) is often preferred over "sexually transmitted infection" (STI) for several important reasons. First, "disease" clearly emphasizes symptomatic illness, which patients are more likely to understand. The word "infection" can sometimes imply a subclinical or laboratory-only finding, leading to confusion among patients who may equate infection with harmless colonization or carriage.

Second, most clinical guidelines and treatment protocols are based on the presence of symptoms or visible signs rather than asymptomatic infections detected through screening. Using "STD" reinforces the focus on diagnosing and managing manifest illness, aligning terminology with symptom-based clinical decision-making.

Third, public health surveillance and statutory notification systems have traditionally used the term "STD." Maintaining this consistency helps avoid discrepancies between clinical records, epidemiological data, and public health reporting, ensuring clear communication across these domains.

While the term "disease" can carry stigma, many patients find "STD" to be a more concrete concept that highlights the necessity for treatment and partner notification. Conversely, the more abstract term "infection" may lead some individuals to underestimate their personal risk or delay seeking care.

Finally, decades of public health education campaigns have used “STD,” making it a familiar and accessible term across diverse populations and varying levels of health literacy. This shared vocabulary enhances effective communication between healthcare providers and patients.

In summary, although “STI” is microbiologically precise and includes asymptomatic infections, “STD” remains the more practical and patient-centered term in many clinical, public health, and educational contexts. Therefore, the term STD has been used throughout this book.

Medications and Treatment

- Some medications may not be available in the patient's country of residence, though they may be accessible in other jurisdictions.
- The local pharmaceutical market is often subject to fluctuations, which can lead to shortages. It is meanwhile not uncommon for essential medicines to be in limited supply and to have to be sourced from abroad.
- Discrepancies may arise due to varying dosage recommendations for a given medication. For example, metronidazole is commonly prescribed at 400 mg in some countries, despite studies suggesting a higher dosage may be more effective.
- There is mounting concern in numerous countries about the increasing prevalence of drug shortages affecting a diverse range of essential medications.
- Supply constraints affect not only rare drugs but also common ones, such as penicillins, cephalosporins, and antivirals. These are due to global supply chains, geopolitical tensions, and a lack of stockpiles. In many cases, physicians can no longer prescribe the appropriate medicine; instead, they switch to the one available in their country. This situation is particularly prevalent outside metropolitan areas and leads to compromised patient care. Ultimately, the physician's sole recourse before prescribing an anti-infective drug is to verify its availability with the pharmacy.

Final Remarks

- Despite rigorous efforts to ensure accuracy, errors may still occur. Therefore, it is strongly advised that prescribing physicians verify the dosage of any unfamiliar medication prior to prescribing it. This can be accomplished by consulting the registration data or reviewing the package insert.
- Given the significant shortage of certain drugs, it is essential to assess the availability of the prescribed medication. However, due to structural limitations within specific healthcare systems, this may not always be feasible in a timely manner. To mitigate this issue, healthcare professionals are encouraged to consult their local pharmacy in advance to confirm the availability of the prescribed medication.
- This book is designed to serve as a valuable resource in the diagnosis and treatment of sexually transmitted diseases. Nevertheless, the ultimate therapeutic decisions rest with the attending physician, who must exercise clinical judgment to act in the best interests of each individual patient.

Contents

About the Author

Ioannis Mylonas After completing his studies at the Technological Educational Institute of Athens in Greece, the University of Rostock in Germany, Brown University in the USA, and the University of Melbourne in Australia, Prof. Dr. med. Dr. h.c. Ioannis Mylonas commenced his training in gynecology and obstetrics at the Women's Clinic of the University of Rostock. In 2002, he was awarded his doctorate from the Medical Faculty of the University of Rostock with the highest honors, receiving the Joachim Jungius Prize. Upon completion of his specialist training, he obtained his habilitation at the Ludwig Maximilian University of Munich in 2008. By 2012, he had been appointed as a Professor at the Ludwig Maximilian University of Munich through an expedited process. In March 2014, he became one of the youngest physicians and gynecologists in both Greece and Germany to be conferred an honorary doctorate (Dr. h.c.) by Democrite University in Greece.

Prof. Dr. med. Dr. h.c. I. Mylonas has authored over 300 scientific articles published in national and international journals. Additionally, he has contributed more than 100 articles to textbooks and clinical guidelines within the fields of gynecology, obstetrics, and infectious diseases. His scientific contributions include authoring and co-editing six books.

Prof. Dr. med. Dr. h.c. Ioannis Mylonas was a member of numerous national and international societies and has participated in various guideline commissions. He also served as an expert reviewer for national and international journals and institutions.

"Τὰ μικρὰ μὴ φροντίζων, τὰ μεγάλα ζημιώσῃ"

"By not caring for small things, you will suffer great losses."

Menander (342–291 BC)

Ἀρετή τέχνη ἐστίν, ἣ διὰ μελέτης καὶ ἐθισμοῦ κτάται. Οὐ γὰρ ὀρθῶς πράττομεν διὰ τὸ ἔχειν ἀρετήν ἢ ἀριστείαν, ἀλλὰ ἔχομεν αὐτὰ διὰ τὸ ὀρθῶς πράττειν. Ἐσμέν, ὅπερ πολλάκις ποιοῦμεν. Ἀρετή οὖν οὐκ ἐνέργεια, ἀλλὰ ἕξις ἐστίν.

"Virtue is an art that is acquired through practice and habit. We do not act rightly because we have virtue or excellence, but we rather have them because we have acted rightly. We are what we repeatedly do. Excellence, then, is not an act, but a habit."

Aristoteles (384–322 BC)

Part I

Background

1 Historical Excursion: Sexually Transmitted Diseases in Gynecology and Obstetrics

Abstract

Sexually transmitted diseases (STD) have significantly impacted the field of gynecology and obstetrics throughout history. Venereal diseases such as gonorrhea and chancroid were prevalent in ancient Roman baths, while syphilis, introduced to Europe in the fifteenth century via Columbus's voyages, spread widely and affected various social strata, including the clergy and nobility. Notably, the herpes simplex virus was identified by Hippocrates, and later recognized by Emperor Tiberius for its transmissibility. Obstetrics faced historical challenges, particularly in areas of hygiene and societal regard, until the introduction of antiseptic handwashing drastically reduced puerperal fever mortality. Advances such as the identification of the distinct nature of gonorrhea and syphilis and the introduction of modern microbiological techniques have improved medical understanding and treatment. Recent developments like the discovery of HIV/AIDS and the role of HPV in cervical cancer have underscored the evolving landscape of STDs. Today's global health challenges, including multidrug-resistant pathogens and pandemics like COVID–19, necessitate comprehensive infectious disease education in medical training for optimal patient care.

1.1 Background

Historically, venereal diseases and puerperal fever held significant relevance in gynecology. The Old Testament references venereal diseases acquired by some Jewish individuals from Moabite women during their exodus to the Promised Land, a consequence of ritual prostitution. Similar forms of temple prostitution were present in ancient Babylonia. Evidence indicates that gonorrhea and chancroid were prevalent in Roman baths, which functioned as brothels.

I. Mylonas, *Sexually Transmitted Diseases*,
https://doi.org/10.1007/978-3-031-78204-6_1

Conversely, obstetrics was once met with considerable disdain as a medical specialty. Obstetric departments were often located in the older, dilapidated sections of hospitals, characterized by unsatisfactory hygiene conditions. The majority of patients were from economically disadvantaged backgrounds.

1.2 Sexually Transmitted Diseases and Their History

1.2.1 Romeo and Juliet: Can Kissing Be Dangerous?

Hippocrates (460 BC–circa 370 BC) was the first to recognize the genital manifestation of the herpes simplex virus as symptomatic of a disseminating vesicular disease. The transmissibility of this disease was acknowledged as early as Roman antiquity, with **Emperor Tiberius** (42 BC–37 AD) prohibiting kissing at public ceremonies after observing the spread of cold sores. Throughout Europe in the sixteenth and seventeenth centuries, herpes labialis emerged as a widespread condition, with the transmission of the virus through kissing gaining significant notoriety, as famously depicted in William Shakespeare's tragedy *Romeo and Juliet*.

In 1736, **Jean Astruc** (1684–1766) identified genital herpes as an independent disease, moving beyond the prior belief that genital blisters were variants of gonorrhea or syphilis. Dermatologist **Paul Gerson Unna** (1850–1929) noted in 1883 the frequent co-occurrence of genital herpes alongside other venereal diseases. The herpes simplex virus (HSV) was first isolated and characterized by **Howard B. Slavin** (1928–2008) and **Elisabeth Gavett** (1945–2014) in 1946. However, differentiation between the two distinct virus strains was not accomplished until the 1960s by **André J. Nahmias** (1936–2020) and **Karl Eduard Schneweis** (1883–1965).

1.2.2 Syphilis and World Politics

The etiology of syphilis has long been a subject of debate. The dominant hypothesis suggests that syphilis was introduced to Europe in 1493, brought by soldiers and sailors who accompanied **Christopher Columbus** (1451–1506). Prior to this period, there are no substantial recorded mentions of the disease in European literature. The transmission of this venereal disease from the southern Spanish port city of Palos, where Columbus set sail, can be traced through the Guadalquivir River to Seville and Barcelona. French King **Charles VIII**, who invaded Naples in 1494, had a considerable number of Spanish auxiliaries in his mercenary forces, further propagating the disease across Italy and eventually throughout Europe (1495), India (1498), and even into China (1505) through Spanish soldiers infected in Spain.

Syphilis was known by various names, including "large pox," "lues venereum" (venereal disease), "morbus gallicus" (French disease), and "Italian, Spanish, German, or Polish disease," though the prevailing term remained syphilis. **Hieronymus Fracastorius** (1478–1553) is credited with coining the term "syphilis" in his poem *Syphilis Sive Morbus Gallicus* around 1530, which likely references a mythical shepherd named Syphilus.

The infectious disease proliferated rapidly and indiscriminately across all social strata, including the clergy and nobility. The association of syphilis with increased risk of premature births and stillbirths profoundly influenced historical and political contexts. Individuals during the Baroque and Rococo periods often concealed facial stigmata attributed to syphilis (roseoles). Wearing wigs and applying face powder to disguise skin lesions and hair loss also became fashionable during this time. While syphilis was dismissed as trivial at royal courts and nobility, it carried significant social stigma among the general populace and sex workers, often leading to social ostracization.

During that period, syphilis and gonorrhea were mistakenly perceived as one disease. This misconception was corrected in 1838 by Parisian physician **Philippe Ricord** (1800–1889), who demonstrated their distinct clinical presentations through what are now considered unethical human experiments. Ricord was also the first to classify syphilis into three stages: primary, secondary, and tertiary. **Giovanni Lancisi** (1654–1720) and **Herman Boerhaave** (1668–1738) were among the first to link syphilis with cardiovascular disease, while **Alfred Fournier** (1832–1914) recognized the syphilitic origins of neurosyphilis. **Paul Diday** (1812–1894) and **Jonathan Hutchinson** (1828–1913) made substantial contributions to understanding congenital infections.

In 1905, **Fritz Schaudinn** (1871–1906) and **Erich Hoffmann** (1868–1959) successfully identified the pathogen responsible for syphilis in the fluid from secondary syphilitic lesions. Japan's **Hideyo Noguchi** (1876–1928) achieved the first microbiological detection of the pathogen in 1911, and 2 years later identified the link between *Treponema pallidum* infection, progressive paralysis, and tabes dorsalis by detecting treponemes in brain and bone marrow samples. **August von Wassermann** (1866–1925) developed a serum reaction for syphilis in 1906, establishing serological testing for the disease. At that time, treatments primarily included mercury, organic arsenic compounds, and bismuth. In 1943, penicillin was successfully administered to the first four patients with syphilis, and more than 50 years later, it still remains the treatment of choice.

1.2.3 Self-Experimentation and Gonorrhea

The earliest descriptions of gonorrhea are found in the Old Testament and fragmented writings of **Aretaios**, a Greek physician of the Hippocratic school from the first century AD. Gonorrhea and syphilis were collectively classified as "venereal disease," implying a shared etiology. In 1767, Scottish surgeon and anatomist **John Hunter** (1728–1793) (Fig. 1.1) attempted to demonstrate the commonality of these two diseases through a sensational self-experiment; he inoculated himself with pus from a patient diagnosed with gonorrhea. Unfortunately, the patient also harbored syphilis, leading Hunter to incorrectly conclude that he had shown a common origin for both diseases.

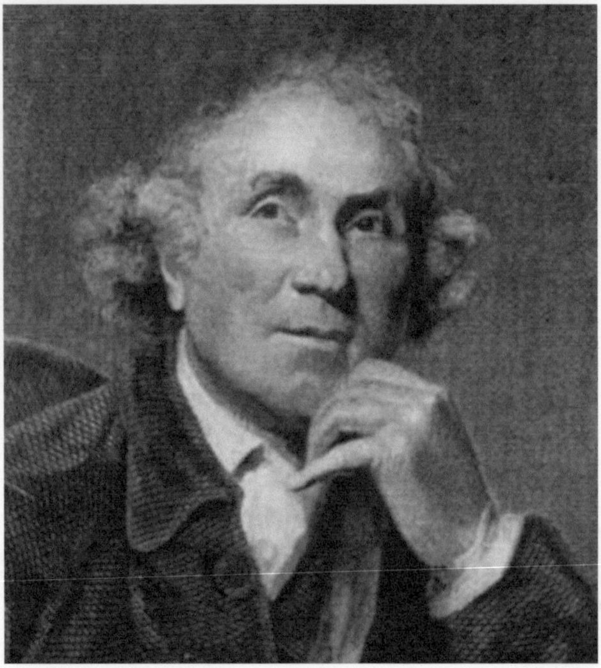

Fig. 1.1 John Hunter (1728–1793) (Seiler 2009)

Philippe Ricord (1800–1889) made an outstanding advancement in 1867 by establishing that gonorrhea is a separate and distinct disease. In 1879, Breslau dermatologist **Albert Neisser** (1855–1916) identified gonococci as the causative agent of gonorrhea, thus resolving the longstanding debate regarding the common origin of syphilis and gonorrhea. Gynecologist and obstetrician **Ernst Bumm** (1858–1925) was the first to culture these pathogens on media, linking them to gonoblennorrhea in newborns. In 1884, **Karl Sigmund Franz Credé** (1819–1892) initiated the practice of instilling a 1% silver nitrate solution into the eyes of newborns at birth to prevent gonoblennorrhea—an intervention maintained in midwifery regulations until 1987.

1.2.4 Ignorance, Arrogance, and Intrigue: The History of Puerperal Fever

The history of puerperal fever is riddled with episodes of ignorance and arrogance. In 1847, **Ignaz Semmelweis** (1818–1865) (Fig. 1.2), an assistant physician at the first obstetrics department of the General Hospital in Vienna, mandated that doctors and students wash their hands with a 4% chlorinated lime solution. The directive was issued in response to the enigmatic demise of a forensic pathologist colleague, who fell victim to blood poisoning following an injury incurred during a cadaver

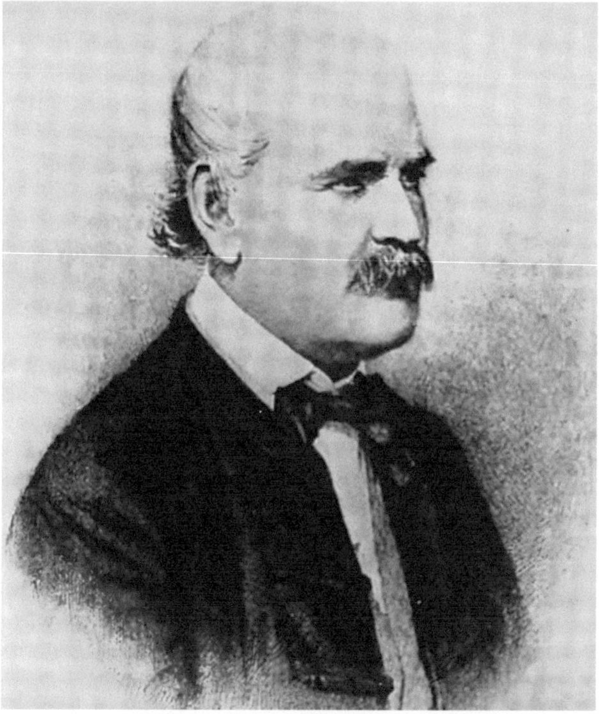

Fig. 1.2 Ignaz Philipp Semmelweis (1818–1865) (Boutellier and Heinzen 2014)

dissection. Notably, medical students conducting dissections also examined recently delivered women following these cadaveric studies. The incidence of puerperal fever was significantly lower in sections attended only by prospective midwives, who had no contact with cadavers, highlighting the impact of Semmelweis's intervention, which reduced maternal mortality from 12.2% to 1.9% within 3 months.

Despite the importance of Semmelweis's intervention, it remained unrecognized for an extended period. Aspersions cast by students and the medical community toward Semmelweis's findings were frequent, resulting in significant professional backlash. His proposal for a commission to evaluate these findings was met with rejection at the ministerial level by Prof. Dr. Klein, the hospital director. Following professional isolation, Semmelweis relocated to Pest, Hungary, within 5 days of his appointment due to the opposition he faced and later became a full professor of obstetrics at that university in 1855.

In July 1865, Semmelweis was involuntarily admitted to the Döbling mental asylum near Vienna by three medical colleagues, without a formal diagnosis. Two weeks after his institutionalization, he died from blood poisoning, reportedly due to physical altercations with staff members at the facility. Alternative accounts suggest he was brutally killed by orderlies. Interestingly, his medical records cite "cerebral palsy" as the cause of death. Notably, a marked shift in Semmelweis's mental state is documented from 1850 to 1865, aligning with a similar change in the tone of his writings on puerperal fever. This has led to discussions about the possibility of *Treponema pallidum* infection affecting his mental health.

Following Semmelweis's death, the introduction of carbolic acid-impregnated wound dressings by **Joseph Baron Lister** (1827–1912) in 1867 marked a paradigm shift in surgical practice, resulting in decreased surgical and patient mortality. Lister's research further contributed to the establishment of aseptic and antiseptic principles in medical practice, a response to Semmelweis's findings. **Robert Koch** (1843–1910) and **Louis Pasteur** (1822–1895) subsequently elucidated the microbial basis of infectious diseases, with Pasteur demonstrating the ability of heat to eliminate pathogens, advancing sterilization techniques for medical instruments.

The term "Semmelweis reflex," coined by **Robert Anton Wilson** (1932–2007), persists in English language usage, describing the immediate dismissal of information or scientific findings without thorough investigation or verification, frequently culminating in punitive responses rather than recognition.

1.2.5 "Fishy Smell" in Gynecology

In 1954, gynecologist **Herman Lawrence Gardner** (1912–1982), in collaboration with bacteriologist **James W. Dukes**, published a significant paper, "Haemophilus vaginalis Vaginitis: A Newly Defined Specific Infection Previously Classified 'Non-specific' Vaginitis." The authors identified a gram-negative rod, which they named *Haemophilus vaginalis*, in 141 of 1181 examined women (12%). Gardner and Dukes sought to validate the four Henle–Koch postulates. While they did not demonstrate complete compliance with each postulate, they achieved partial validation.

Following the introduction of Fluor vaginalis into the vagina of 15 healthy female volunteers with "Haemophilus vaginalis vaginitis," 11 of the 15 participants developed symptoms characteristic of bacterial vaginosis, such as a fishy-smelling discharge, vaginal epithelial redness, and, in some cases, irritation. This research by Gardner and Dukes ignited further inquiry into vaginal infections, emphasizing the significance of anaerobic vaginal flora and its implications for gynecological conditions. Additionally, insights gained about the association between vaginal infections and premature birth are highly relevant to contemporary clinical practice. In honor of Gardner's contributions, *Gardnerella* became the designated genus for this significant bacterium associated with bacterial vaginosis.

1.2.6 The Problems Persist

The emergence and development of the human immunodeficiency virus (HIV) and acquired immune deficiency syndrome (AIDS) have been mired in numerous theories and misconceptions. In 1981, immunologist **Michael Gottlieb** reported cases of four homosexual patients suffering from atypical *Pneumocystis carinii* pneumonia, a condition associated with severe immunodeficiency. This prompted investigations into the infection's etiology, leading to the proposal of an infectious cause and subsequent research into risk factors and the disease's origins.

HIV was first identified in 1983 by **Luc Montagnier** (1932–2022) and **Françoise Barré-Sinoussi** (1947–) at the Institut Pasteur in Paris. Their discovery earned them the Nobel Prize for Medicine in 2008. However, uncertainty regarding the origin of HIV persisted for years. In May 2005, research elucidated that HIV likely originated in African monkeys, with certain samples from wild chimpanzees exhibiting antibodies against the Simian Immunodeficiency Virus (the equivalent in apes). Notably, 12 of these samples shared a high degree of similarity with HIV–1 in humans. Nevertheless, chimpanzees are not considered the original source of HIV; these apes were likely infected by other primate species. The exact mechanism by which the virus transferred to humans remains elusive. The earliest confirmed case of HIV infection, based on blood samples, originated in the Congo in 1959. Estimates suggest that HIV spread to Haiti around 1966 before making its way to the United States.

Currently, the global prevalence of HIV infection poses alarming public health and economic challenges, particularly in developing countries where vaccination and treatment options remain deficient. In obstetrics, the emergence of HIV has catalyzed research efforts. Since the mid-1980s, various research groups have dedicated themselves to lowering transmission rates to newborns. Through rigorous research and combination therapy, the risk of maternal-to-child transmission has been reduced to approximately 1.5%. Additionally, vaginal delivery has become feasible in educated patients when viral load is undetectable (below the detection threshold of 50 to <20 viral copies/μl).

1.2.7 HPV Infection: From Infectious Disease to Oncology

Harald zur Hausen (1936–2023), who was awarded the Nobel Prize in 2008, is to be commended for his research on herpes viruses, which led to the identification of human papillomaviruses (HPV) and the subsequent demonstration of their role as the causative agents of cervical cancer in women. Zur Hausen faced considerable resistance to his findings, including skepticism from gynecologists and cytologists. However, the development of two commercially available vaccines has enabled the reduction of cervical carcinoma precursors through the vaccination of girls who have not yet been infected with HPV. Epidemiologists in the United Kingdom have projected a nearly 60% reduction in cervical cancer among the vaccinated population by 2025, provided consistent vaccination efforts are maintained. Unfortunately, this significant benefit may not be realized in many countries, as less than 30% of girls aged 12–17 are currently in many developed countries vaccinated, largely due to widespread vaccination fatigue.

1.2.8 Zika Virus and the 2016 Olympic Games in Rio de Janeiro, Brazil

The Zika virus, first discovered in Uganda in 1947, has garnered global attention in recent years due to its potential effects on pregnant women and newborns. Particularly since 2016, when the virus was recognized as both a sexually transmitted disease and one transmitted by mosquitoes, it has increasingly become a focal point in gynecology and obstetrics. The potential for significant adverse outcomes in infants born to mothers infected with the Zika virus, including microcephaly and other neurological complications, has prompted efforts to control transmission and develop preventive measures. The threat posed by the Zika virus came to the forefront just before the 2016 Olympic Games in Rio de Janeiro, leading to intensified efforts to contain the disease. To date, no therapeutic options or vaccines are available.

1.3 Personalities and Sexually Transmitted Infections

Sexually transmitted diseases have significantly impacted human history over the past few centuries. Many prominent figures from the aristocracy, politics, and the arts were afflicted with syphilis, while gonorrhea and chancroid also played important cultural and political roles. A multitude of kings, monarchs, politicians, and generals contracted infections that influenced their actions and decisions.

1.3.1 Monarchs, Politicians, Military, and Church Representatives

One prominent example is **King Henry VIII** (1491–1557) of England, who is believed to have suffered from syphilis. The assumption is based on the presence of pronounced ulcers on both thighs that persisted throughout his life. Despite numerous therapies, none proved efficacious, and the ulcers worsened, eventually extending to the bone. When the pain became unbearable, hundreds of individuals were executed for minor offenses; it is estimated that Henry VIII executed approximately 3% of the English population. The leg ulcers that afflicted him likely contributed to a greater number of deaths than those attributed to Richard of Burgundy's ingrown toenail. Henry VIII's multiple marriages were associated with a higher incidence of premature births and stillbirths. His first wife, **Catherine of Aragon**, bore five children, all of whom died either at birth or shortly thereafter, leaving only one daughter to survive.

As he lacked a male heir, Henry sought a divorce from his wife, but Pope **Clement VII** refused to annul the marriage. Consequently, Henry VIII separated from the Roman Church and established the Anglican Church, appointing himself its head. In February 1533, he married his second wife, the young **Anne Boleyn**, and on September 7, 1533, **Princess Elizabeth**, who would later become **Queen Elizabeth I** (1533–1603), was born. It has been suggested that Elizabeth may not have been Henry's biological child. Subsequent pregnancies of Anne resulted in miscarriages, and she was eventually executed in the Tower of London on charges of adultery. **Jane Seymour**, who married Henry in May 1536, bore him a son, the future King **Edward VI**. However, Henry's subsequent marriages resulted in no further children, likely due to his progressive syphilitic illness.

Ivan the Terrible (1530–1584) is another significant historical character linked to syphilis. After the death of his first wife, **Anastasia Romanovna Zakharjina**, Ivan contracted the disease, leading to a drastic transformation in his personality. His reign was marked by violent outbursts, including the murder of thousands and even the killing of his own son.

Giacomo Casanova (1725–1798) (Fig. 1.3), the famous lover, was not exempt from the consequences of venereal disease. It is suggested that he contracted syphilis during his life, along with four cases of gonorrhea, five instances of soft chancre, and one episode of genital herpes, likely spending a substantial portion of his life managing these afflictions.

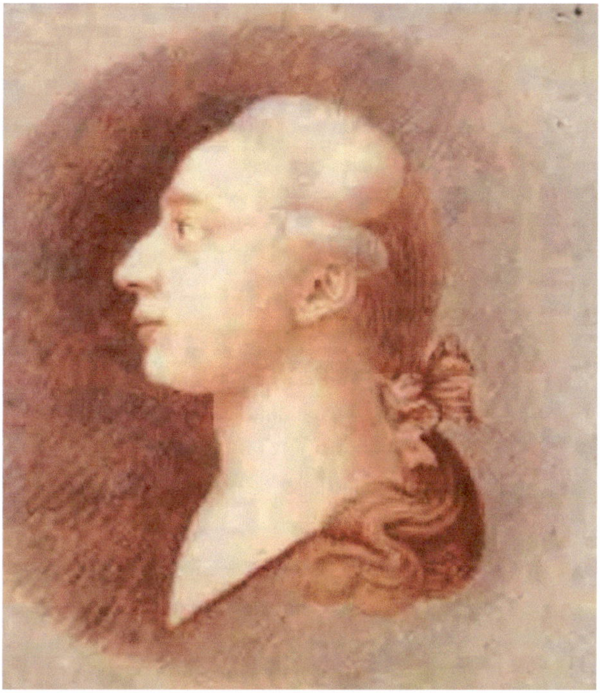

Fig. 1.3 Giacomo Casanova (1725–1798), portrait by Francesco Casanova, circa 1750 (Hatzinger and Hatzinger 2009)

Catherine II of Russia, known as **Catherine the Great** (1729–1796), ruled for 30 years following the violent death of her husband. Her son, **Paul I** (1754–1801), exhibited obvious indicators of syphilis at a young age, contributing to Catherine's pronounced "venerophobia." In St. Petersburg, she established the first hospital for venereal diseases, providing 50 beds. Various myths and facts surround her sexual life; due to fears of syphilis, her paramours were evaluated by a committee of six women before acceptance.

Napoleon Bonaparte (1769–1821) contracted gonorrhea as a young lieutenant in Paris, leading to a protracted recovery and potential complications such as painful urethral strictures. He also suffered from scabies for an extended period and is believed to have contracted syphilis following his escape from Elba.

Lord Cardigan (1797–1868) (James Thomas Brudenell, seventh Earl of Cardigan) commanded the "Charge of the Light Brigade" during the Crimean War, an infamous attack known for its high casualties. It is speculated that Lord Cardigan suffered from chronic orchitis related to gonorrhea, which may have led to his less vigorous charge into battle, preserving his life.

Sexually transmitted diseases were not uncommon among clergy prior to the institution of celibacy. Evidence suggests that three popes—**Alexander VI** (1431–1503), **Julius II** (1441–1513), and **Leo X** (1475–1521)—were infected with syphilis. **Cardinal Richelieu** (1585–1642), a central figure in seventeenth-century French politics, is also thought to have suffered from a venereal disease, as indicated by a significant anal abscess and urinary retention.

1.3.2 Philosophers

Instances of sexually transmitted diseases were less common among philosophers, likely due to their self-image as superior beings, making them less susceptible to the influence of women. The most prominent philosophers who suffered from syphilis include **Friedrich Nietzsche** (1844–1900) and **Arthur Schopenhauer** (1788–1860) (Fig. 1.4). Nietzsche contracted the disease in 1865 at a brothel he described as the "sole venue for sexual intercourse." His medical history records severe symptoms, including syphilitic meningitis and general paralysis, but he remarkably continued to produce significant works during this period. Schopenhauer also contracted syphilis as a student and endured prolonged and painful mercury treatments, likely contributing to his disdain for women.

1.3.3 Writers, Composers, and Visual Artists

Writers and poets represent the occupational group with the highest prevalence of sexually transmitted diseases. **François Villon** (1431–ca. 1463) is often regarded as the most significant poet of Late Middle Ages France, likely suffering from soft

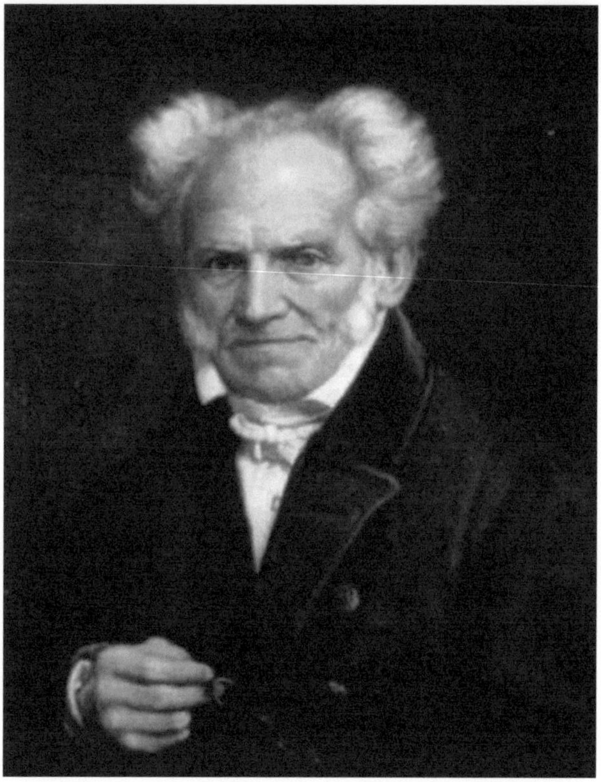

Fig. 1.4 Arthur Schopenhauer (1788–1860) (Vormbaum and Bohlander 2014)

chancre and genital warts, along with complete hair loss potentially caused by syphilis. He engaged in various criminal activities, leading to multiple death sentences and eventual exile from Paris.

At the age of 24, **Heinrich Heine** (1797–1856) began experiencing severe headaches, which are often the first signs of syphilis. By 1840, he suffered from facial nerve palsy, which progressively worsened and ultimately led to his withdrawal from public life. A number of other distinguished figures, including **Vincent van Gogh** (1853–1890) (Fig. 1.5), **Claude Monet** (1840–1926), and **Paul Gauguin** (1848–1903), also suffered from syphilis. **Oscar Wilde** (1854–1900), **Fyodor Dostoyevsky** (1821–1881), and **Robert Schumann** (1810–1856) were similarly afflicted. **Franz Schubert** (1797–1828) contracted syphilis at age 24 and received standard mercury treatments but ultimately died young from tuberculosis. The possibility that **Ludwig van Beethoven** (1770–1827) and **Wolfgang Amadeus Mozart** (1756–1791) suffered from syphilis remains a subject of ongoing debate among histrorians.

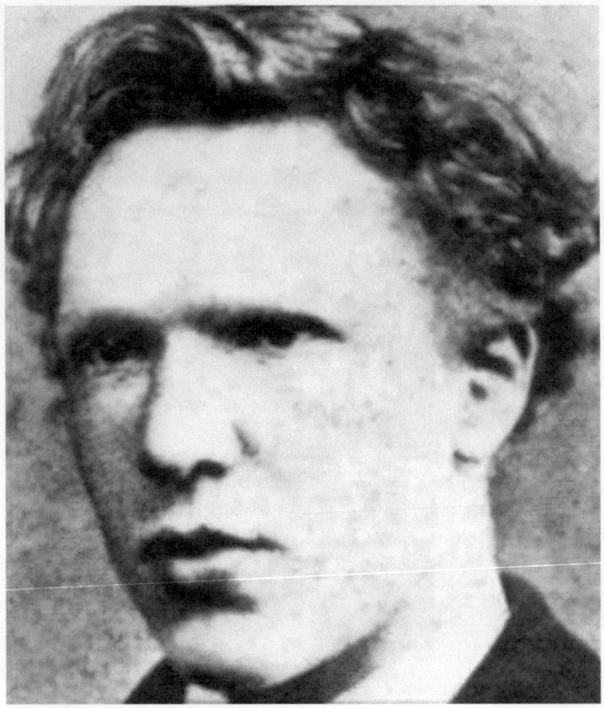

Fig. 1.5 Vincent van Gogh (1853–1890), photograph from 1871 (Allen 2014)

1.4 The Significance of Infectious Diseases

Infectious diseases have played a crucial role in the history of science. Important personalities such as **Louis Pasteur**, **Joseph Lister**, **Simon Flexner** (1863–1946), **Shibasaburo Kitasato** (1853–1931), and **Kiyoshi Shiga** (1871–1957) made groundbreaking contributions. Also significant are **Rudolf Virchow** (1821–1902) (Fig. 1.6), **Emil von Behring** (1854–1917; who died at 63 from general paralysis caused by syphilis), **Paul Ehrlich** (1854–1914), **Gerhard Domagk** (1895–1964), and **Robert Koch** (1843–1910) (Fig. 1.7), four of whom received the Nobel Prize.

Robert Koch, considered the pioneer of modern bacteriology, formulated the contagions doctrine emphasizing infectious disease causation through pathogenic germs. His principles, known as the Henle–Koch postulates, remain fundamental to understanding infectious diseases today.

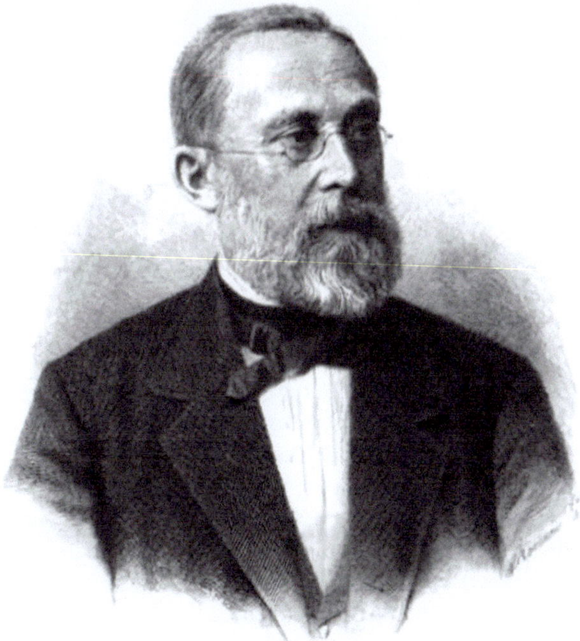

Fig. 1.6 Rudolf Virchow (1821–1902) (Harms 2008)

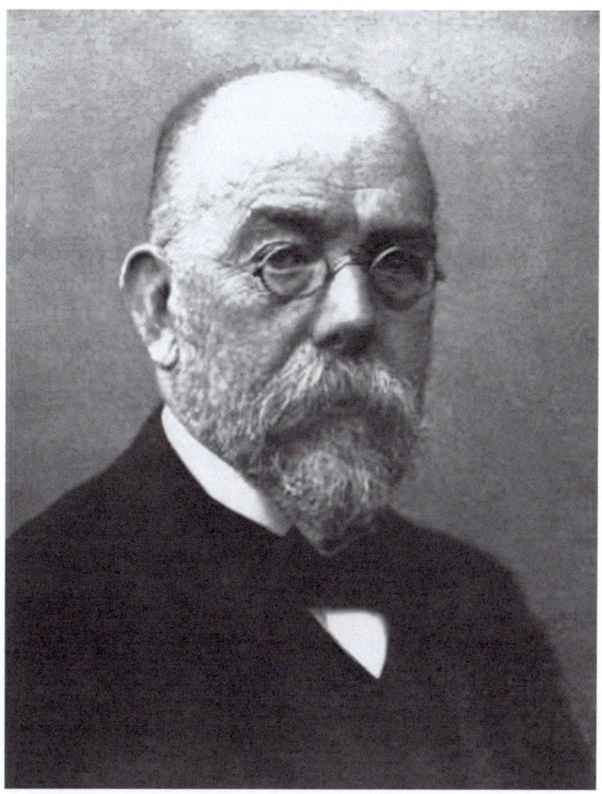

Fig. 1.7 Robert Koch (1843–1910) (© picture alliance/dpa)

The Henle–Koch postulates state:

- The specific causative agent must be present in high concentrations in all organisms afflicted with the disease and absent in healthy organisms.
- The causative agent must be isolated from a diseased organism and cultured in pure form.
- The cultured causative agent should induce disease when introduced into a healthy organism.
- The causative agent must be re-isolated from the experimentally infected host and identified as identical to the original specific causative agent.

Significant advancements in the treatment of infectious diseases have also been achieved over the past centuries. **Sir Alexander Fleming** (1881–1955) transformed medical treatment with his discovery of penicillin in 1928, marking the beginning of the antibiotic era. Similarly, **Paul Ehrlich**'s research on selective toxicity and "magic bullets" enabled targeted chemotherapy. The contributions of **Florence Nightingale** (1820–1910) during the Crimean War (1853–1856) significantly advanced nursing as a profession and highlighted the critical role of sanitation and hygiene in preventing infections.

Gerhard Domagk's experience with the Nobel Prize was marked by significant political decisions in Nazi Germany. He was awarded the 1939 Nobel Prize in Physiology/Medicine for his discovery of the antibacterial effects of prontosil, which paved the way for the development of the first effective antibiotics. However, Domagk was unable to accept the honor because of Nazi policies that prohibited German nationals from receiving Nobel Prizes—a decree issued by Adolf Hitler in 1937 in retaliation for Carl von Ossietzky's Nobel Peace Prize win in 1935. When Domagk learned of his award in October 1939, he was arrested by the Gestapo and detained for a week, during which he was coerced into formally declining the prize. He was released only after demonstrating his loyalty to National Socialism. It was not until after World War II and the fall of the Nazi regime that he was able to receive his Nobel Prize medal and diploma in 1947; however, he did not receive the monetary portion of the prize, as it had already been returned to the Nobel Foundation due to the delay.

1.5 Outlook

Infectious diseases play a significant role in gynecology and obstetrics, yet they are often inadequately addressed in medical education and training across several countries. As infectious diseases regain prominence, exemplified by the rise of multidrug-resistant pathogens and the global pandemic caused by SARS-CoV-2, the current deficiencies in medical education are concerning and may ultimately impact the quality of patient care. It is crucial for medical professionals to receive comprehensive education and training in infectious diseases to effectively treat and prevent them. In light of the evolving landscape of infectious diseases, healthcare providers must remain informed and proficient, ensuring optimal care for their patients. By prioritizing or incorporating infectious disease education into undergraduate and graduate training programs, healthcare professionals can better meet the challenges posed by multidrug-resistant infections and emerging global pandemics.

What Are Sexually Transmitted Diseases?

2

Abstract

Sexually transmitted diseases (STD) are of significant epidemiological and clinical importance. The predominant mode of transmission for these diseases is unprotected sexual intercourse, which can have complex and severe health effects. In addition to heightening the risk of other STDs, such as Human Immunodeficiency Virus (HIV), they may lead to serious complications, including infections of the genital tract and pregnancy-related issues. The most prevalent STDs include chlamydia, gonorrhea, syphilis, and trichomoniasis. According to estimates by the World Health Organization (WHO), approximately one million new cases of STDs are reported daily, with approximately 376 million new cases documented in 2016. It is critical that effective prevention measures are implemented, regular testing is ensured, and early diagnosis and treatment are facilitated to combat the spread of STDs.

2.1 Background

Approximately 54.75 million people die each year worldwide. The World Health Organization reported that in 2021, there were 68 million deaths globally. Recent epidemiological data indicate that infectious diseases account for a significant portion of global mortality, with approximately 14.7 million deaths annually. This figure constitutes about 26.1% of all deaths worldwide, illustrating the substantial impact infectious diseases have on global health. Infectious diseases significantly impact morbidity, as evidenced by the burden measured in disability-adjusted life years (DALYs). In 2019, 85 pathogens collectively accounted for 704 million DALYs globally, representing 28% of all DALYs across all causes.

Almost every third death is attributable to infection.

Transmission occurs through unprotected sexual intercourse during vaginal, oral, and anal contact. Even with the use of prophylactic measures, such as condoms, the risk of infection cannot be entirely mitigated.

I. Mylonas, *Sexually Transmitted Diseases*,
https://doi.org/10.1007/978-3-031-78204-6_2

Sexually transmitted diseases can affect individuals of any gender, socio-economic status, and age. However, young and sexually active individuals are particularly impacted.

2.2 Definitions

The term "sexually transmitted infections" (STI) has replaced the older terms "venereal diseases" and "venereal infections." In clinical practice and patient communication, "sexually transmitted disease" (STD) is often preferred over STI because:

- "Disease" more clearly signals symptomatic illness to patients, whereas "infection" may be interpreted as subclinical colonization.
- Clinical management algorithms and many guidelines are based on signs and symptoms rather than screening-detected asymptomatic infections.
- Public health surveillance and statutory reporting have historically used "STD," so consistent terminology reduces discrepancies across clinical, epidemiologic, and reporting contexts.
- Widespread public health messaging has made "STD" familiar to diverse populations

While the term "disease" can carry some stigma, many patients find it clearer and helpful because it highlights the need for treatment and partner notification. Clinicians should choose their wording based on the situation, patient preference, and communication goals.

STDs are of substantial epidemiological and clinical significance and are associated with considerable global medical burden; more than 40 pathogenic microorganisms—including bacteria, viruses, and parasites—are known to be transmitted via sexual contact.

Clinical manifestations of STDs can vary significantly and may include conditions such as urethritis, cervicitis, genital ulcers, warts, HIV, or hepatitis. A notable challenge is that these infections frequently present asymptomatically, resulting in undetected transmission to sexual partners. Untreated STDs can lead to considerable complications, including epididymitis, infections of the female genital tract, and complications during pregnancy. The diagnosis of STDs relies on clinical findings, age, gender, sexual history, and epidemiological data, underscoring the necessity for reliable diagnoses and targeted treatments. Advances in diagnostics and therapies have emerged, including effective treatments for *Mycoplasma genitalium* infections.

STDs constitute a heterogeneous group of infections, all of which share the common characteristic of being primarily or secondarily transmissible via sexual intercourse.

2.3 Subdivision

Given that STDs and their causative pathogens encompass a broader spectrum of infections beyond the four "classic" types (syphilis, gonorrhea, chancroid, and lymphogranuloma venereum; see Table 2.1), a practical division into three categories is proposed for clarity:

- **"Classic" STDs:**
  - Syphilis.

Table 2.1 Alphabetical listing of sexually transmitted diseases (STDs)

Disease/infection	Causes	See chapter
Amoebae	*Entamoeba histolytica*	Section 22.4.1
Bacterial vaginosis	*Gardnerella vaginalis*, *Mobiluncus* spp., and others	Chapter 35
Campylobacter	*Campylobacter jejuni*, *Campylobacter coli*	Section 22.2.1
Chancroid (soft chancre, ulcus molle)	*Haemophilus ducreyi*	Chapter 13
Chlamydia trachomatis	*Chlamydia trachomatis*	Chapter 17
Condylomata acuminata	Human papillomavirus (HPV)	Chapter 18
Cytomegaly	Cytomegalovirus (CMV)	Chapter 29
Endemic syphilis (bejel)	*Treponema pallidum* subsp. *endemicum*	Section 26.4.1.2
Genital herpes (HSV)	Herpes simplex virus type 1 and type 2	Chapter 20
Giardiasis	*Giardia lamblia*	Section 22.5.2
Gonorrhea	*Neisseria gonorrhoeae*	Chapter 14
Granuloma inguinale	*Klebsiella granulomatis*	Chapter 19
Hepatitis A	Hepatitis A virus (HAV)	Section 22.3.1
Hepatitis B	Hepatitis B virus (HBV)	Chapter 30
Hepatitis C	Hepatitis C virus (HCV)	Chapter 31
Hepatitis D	Hepatitis D virus (HDV)	Chapter 30
Hepatitis E	Hepatitis E virus (HEV)	Section 22.3.2
HIV/AIDS	Human immunodeficiency virus (HIV)	Chapter 32
Human T-cell lymphotropic virus (HTLV)	Human T-cell lymphotropic virus	Chapter 33
Intestinal pathogens	Various bacterial, viral, and parasitic pathogens	Chapter 22
Lymphogranuloma venereum (LGV)	Chlamydia trachomatis serovars L1, L2, L3	Chapter 15
Molluscum contagiosum	Molluscum contagiosum virus	Chapter 25
Monkeypox (mpox)	Monkeypox virus	Chapter 24
Mycoplasma genitalium	*Mycoplasma genitalium*	Chapter 21
Non-venereal treponematoses	*Treponema* species	Chapter 26
Pinta	*Treponema carateum*	Section 26.4.1.3
Pubic lice (crabs)	*Pthirus pubis*	Chapter 27
Salmonella	*Salmonella enterica*	Section 22.2.2
Scabies	*Sarcoptes scabiei*	Chapter 28
Shigella	*Shigella* species	Section 22.2.3
Syphilis (lues)	*Treponema pallidum*	Chapter 16
Trichomoniasis	*Trichomonas vaginalis*	Chapter 23
Vulvovaginal candidosis	*Candida albicans*	Chapter 36
Yaws	*Treponema pallidum* subsp. *pertenue*	Section 26.4.1.1
Yersinia	*Yersinia enterocolitica*, *Yersinia pseudotuberculosis*	Section 22.3.4
Zika virus (ZIKV)	Zika virus	Chapter 34

- Gonorrhea.
- Chancroid.
- Lymphogranuloma venereum.
- **Other STDs:**
  - Those transmitted via sexual intercourse.
  - Those transmitted through intimate contact during intercourse.
- **STDs involving other organs and systemic spread.**
  - i.e., Hepatitis B and C, HIV, Zika virus,
  - Sexually transmitted intestinal infections.

Emerging evidence suggests that additional pathogens may also be sexually transmitted, though conclusive evidence remains limited. As these pathogens hold significant relevance for gynecology and obstetrics, they are discussed further within the context of bacterial vaginosis and vulvovaginal candidosis. In English-speaking countries, these infections are typically classified as STDs. However, such classification is less common for example in Europe, primarily due to their elevated prevalence in the absence of a prior sexual encounter.

2.4 How Prevalent Are Sexually Transmitted Infections?

The most prevalent STDs include chlamydia, gonorrhea, syphilis, and trichomoniasis (Table 2.2).

Global assessments indicate:

- The WHO estimates approximately one million new cases of STDs occur daily worldwide.
- In 2016, an estimated 376 million new cases of the four treatable STDs (chlamydia, gonorrhea, syphilis, trichomoniasis) were reported.
- The incidence of new infections in 2016 was approximately 5% higher than in 2012.
- Additionally, the WHO estimates hundreds of millions of people contract herpes or human papillomavirus (HPV) annually.

Table 2.2 Global estimated incidence of sexually transmitted infections in millions (WHO)

Illness	2012	2016	2020
Chlamydia	89–95	129	-[a]
Genital herpes (HSV-2)	30–50	490	-[a]
Gonorrhea	60–70	87	82
HIV (UNAIDS)	5,3	1,7	1,3
Human papillomaviruses (HPV)	75–90	290 (women)	-[a]
Syphilis	5,6	6	7,1
Trichomoniasis	170	156	156

[a]No estimates

Specific estimates for individual infections are as follows:

- Trichomoniasis accounts for a significant portion of STDs, representing over 40% of cases. In 2016, there were an estimated 156 million new infections annually, with the current estimate being 174 million new cases.
- The WHO estimates 127 million new cases of chlamydia occur globally each year.
- It is estimated that 70–80% of sexually active individuals will be infected with HPV at some point in their lifetime. Approximately 70% of cases resolve within 1 year post-infection, while 90% are eliminated within 2 years.

2.5 Risk Factors

Various behavioral, biological, and socioeconomic determinants have been shown to facilitate the transmission and acquisition of sexually transmitted diseases (STDs). The principal risk factors are described below.

- **Age (15–30 years):** Individuals aged 15–30 years, particularly adolescents and young adults, are at increased risk. Higher rates of partner change, more frequent sexual activity, lower uptake of preventive services, and inconsistent barrier-method use are commonly observed in this cohort; additionally, cervical ectopy in younger females confers increased mucosal susceptibility to some pathogens.
- **Frequent Partner Change and Multiple Concurrent Partnerships:** A history of multiple or recently acquired sexual partners increases the cumulative probability of exposure to an infected contact. Concurrent partnerships amplify transmission chains within sexual networks and accelerate spread in affected populations.
- **Group Sexual Activities:** Participation in group sex raises exposure frequency and network connectivity, thereby increasing the likelihood of encountering an infected partner and facilitating rapid pathogen dissemination.
- **Unprotected Sexual Intercourse and High-Risk Practices:** Vaginal or anal intercourse without barrier protection is a major determinant of STD transmission. Practices that disrupt mucosal integrity (anal intercourse, traumatic intercourse, and genital piercing) increase per-act transmission probabilities. The presence of a concomitant STD may further enhance susceptibility to other infections, including HIV.
- **Ulcerative Genital Infections:** Ulcerative STDs (e.g., syphilis and primary genital herpes) cause mucocutaneous breaches that facilitate HIV entry; epidemiologic studies have demonstrated several-fold increases in HIV acquisition risk in the presence of genital ulcers.
- **Limited Access to Counseling, Screening, and Treatment:** Inadequate availability of diagnostic testing, sexual-health counseling, and timely therapy allows asymptomatic infections to persist and be transmitted, undermining control efforts.

- **Substance Use and Injection Drug Use:** Alcohol and noninjecting recreational drug use impair judgment and increase the likelihood of unprotected or coercive sexual encounters. Sharing of injection equipment transmits bloodborne pathogens (HIV, HBV, and HCV) directly.
- **Socioeconomic Disadvantage and Structural Barriers:** Poverty, low educational attainment, unstable housing, and restricted healthcare access are associated with higher STD incidence due to reduced prevention uptake, delayed presentation, and limited treatment availability.
- **Stigmatization and Social Isolation:** Stigma related to sexual infections discourages disclosure, testing, and care-seeking, thereby increasing the duration of untreated infectiousness and onward transmission.

Additional behaviors and contextual factors—such as travel to high-prevalence regions, sexual contact with partners from high-prevalence groups, engagement in commercial or transactional sex, and a history of sexual violence—further increase acquisition risk (Table 2.3).

Prevention and control should be multifaceted and tailored to individual and population-level determinants. Recommended interventions include consistent and correct condom use, routine targeted screening based on risk and local epidemiology, accessible counseling and diagnostic services, vaccination (human papillomavirus and hepatitis B), harm-reduction programs for people who inject drugs, partner notification and treatment, and structural measures to reduce socioeconomic and access barriers. Patient-centered discussions that address stigma and promote health literacy are essential to improve uptake of preventive measures and timely treatment.

In the care and treatment of patients with STDs, individuals are often categorized by risk groups and factors. However, sexual experimentation during adolescence is a normal part of growth and hormonal development.

A significant portion of risk factors signifies a transformation in sexual behaviors over the past 50 years. Certain infectious diseases, such as HIV, syphilis, and hepatitis C, are concentrated within specific demographic groups. However, the majority of pathogens are widely distributed and can more likely be seen in sexually active populations, including HPV, chlamydia, trichomoniasis, and genital herpes. Furthermore, some infections can facilitate or contribute to the development of malignancies (e.g., hepatitis B, HPV, HIV).

A considerable challenge inherent to many STDs is that infections frequently progress asymptomatically or with minimal symptoms in adults, potentially resulting in a lack of medical intervention.

Table 2.3 Identified risk factors for acquisition of sexually transmitted infections

Risk factor	Rationale/Clinical relevance
Young age (15–30 years)	Higher rates of new sexual partnerships, inconsistent condom use, and lower uptake of sexual-health services; biologic susceptibility (immature cervical ectopy) further increases vulnerability to mucosal infection
Multiple or recent partners (≥1 new partner or >2 partners in the past year)	Cumulative probability of exposure to an infected partner rises with partner number and recency; recent partner change is an independent predictor of incident infection
Sexual contact with a partner known or suspected to have an STD	Direct exposure to an infected individual markedly elevates transmission probability; untreated partners perpetuate transmission chains and reinfection risk
Sexual contact with unfamiliar partners	Unknown sexual and medical histories reduce the ability to assess risk; encounters are more likely to be casual, brief, and occur without barrier protection
Unprotected intercourse and high-risk practices (anal sex and traumatic sex)	Absence of condoms allows direct mucosal exposure; anal intercourse and practices causing mucosal disruption confer higher per-act transmission probabilities for many pathogens
Prior history of STD	Indicates persistent behavioral risk or biological sequelae (e.g., epithelial disruption); prior infection is associated with increased susceptibility and risk of reinfection
Inconsistent or nonuse of condoms	Condoms substantially reduce transmission of many STDs; inconsistent use is a leading modifiable determinant of incident infection
Use of hormonal or intrauterine contraception without condom use	These methods prevent pregnancy but do not protect against STDs; perceived protection may reduce condom use, increasing exposure when new or high-risk partners are involved
Low socioeconomic status and limited access to healthcare	Financial, educational, and structural barriers reduce access to prevention (vaccination and condoms), screening, timely diagnosis, and effective treatment, resulting in higher prevalence and delayed care
Substance use—injection and non-injection	Injection drug use transmits bloodborne pathogens via shared equipment (HIV, HBV, and HCV); alcohol and noninjecting drug intoxication impair judgment, lower condom negotiation, and increase likelihood of high-risk sexual encounters
Travel to endemic areas/ sexual activity while abroad	Exposure to pathogens with elevated regional prevalence, unfamiliar sexual networks, and reduced access to routine prevention or care increase acquisition risk
Sexual contact with partners from high-prevalence groups	Partnerships with individuals from populations that have higher STD prevalence (e.g., commercial sex workers, people who inject drugs, and certain MSM networks) increase probability of encountering infections
Commercial sex work and transactional sex	High partner turnover, economic pressures limiting condom negotiation, and stigma or legal barriers to healthcare facilitate transmission and impede prevention and treatment
Unsafe abortion or inadequate obstetric/ gynecologic care	Nonsterile procedures, retained products, or mucosal injury can precipitate local infection and increase susceptibility to subsequent genital pathogens; limited postprocedural care worsens outcomes
Sexual assault	Forced intercourse often causes genital trauma and immediate exposure to pathogens; survivors may face barriers to prompt prophylaxis, testing, and treatment, increasing risk of acquisition and sequelae
Severe mental illness or cognitive impairment	Impaired judgment, reduced capacity for risk assessment, difficulties in accessing services, and lower adherence to prevention strategies increase vulnerability to STDs and reduce engagement with care

2.6 Infection and Pregnancy

The transmission of various sexually transmitted pathogens before or during birth can result in both systemic and local infections in the unborn or newborn child. Such infections can lead to a range of adverse outcomes, including:

- **Miscarriage:** Associated with pathogens such as syphilis.
- **Premature Birth:** Linked to infections such as chlamydia and *Trichomonas vaginalis*.
- **Direct Infection of the Fetus or Newborn:** This can lead to malformations and long-term complications associated with infections like syphilis, cytomegalovirus (CMV), herpes simplex virus (HSV), and hepatitis B virus (HBV).

For instance, approximately one million pregnancies worldwide are adversely impacted by maternal syphilis annually. The prevalence of severe complications is significant: Untreated or late-treated syphilis during pregnancy results in adverse birth outcomes in 50–80% of cases, including stillbirths, premature births, low birth weight, and congenital infections in newborns. According to the most recent estimates by the World Health Organization (WHO), this results in over 200,000 stillbirths and neonatal deaths each year—a figure that is significantly higher than the number of cases reported for other neonatal infections, including HIV with approximately 540,000 cases per year and tetanus with around 300,000 cases per year.

From a medical perspective, the prevention, diagnosis, and treatment of STDs constitute a cross-sectoral area of action encompassing both medical and political dimensions due to their significant effects on health and individual life planning.

2.7 Complications of STD

Complications caused by sexually transmitted diseases (STD) can significantly impact individual health and quality of life. Below are several examples of these complications, organized by specific STDs:

Bacterial Vaginosis (BV): Although not classified strictly as a sexually transmitted infection, bacterial vaginosis represents a dysbiosis of the vaginal microbiota characterized by depletion of lactobacilli and overgrowth of anaerobic bacteria, such as *Gardnerella vaginalis*. BV increases susceptibility to STDs, including HIV, chlamydia, and gonorrhea by disrupting mucosal defenses. It is also associated with adverse pregnancy outcomes, such as preterm birth, premature rupture of membranes, and postpartum endometritis. Treatment with appropriate antibiotics reduces symptoms, but recurrence is common.

Chlamydia: *Chlamydia trachomatis* infection is a common sexually transmitted bacterial disease. If left untreated, it can ascend the female reproductive tract, resulting in pelvic inflammatory disease (PID), characterized by inflammation of the uterus, fallopian tubes, and adjacent pelvic structures. PID can cause chronic pelvic pain due to scarring and adhesions, and importantly, it significantly increases the risk of infertility by damaging the fallopian tubes. Moreover, inflammation and tubal scarring predispose affected women to ectopic pregnancy, where a fertilized egg implants outside the uterine cavity, posing a life-threatening emergency. Early diagnosis and treatment are essential to prevent these serious reproductive sequelae.

Gonorrhea: *Neisseria gonorrhoeae* infection shares clinical similarities with chlamydia but may be more aggressive in causing upper genital tract infections. Untreated gonorrhea can lead to PID in women, resulting in complications such as chronic pelvic pain and tubal infertility. In men, persistent urethritis may lead to epididymitis and potential infertility. Disseminated gonococcal infection (DGI) occurs when bacteria invade the bloodstream, manifesting as arthritis-dermatitis syndrome with migratory polyarthritis, tenosynovitis, and characteristic pustular or vesiculopustular skin lesions. DGI requires urgent systemic antibiotic therapy to prevent severe complications.

Hepatitis B and C: Hepatitis B virus (HBV) and hepatitis C virus (HCV) are bloodborne pathogens transmissible sexually as well as via percutaneous exposure. Chronic infection with HBV or HCV can lead to progressive liver fibrosis culminating in cirrhosis, liver failure, and hepatocellular carcinoma (HCC). Both viruses are associated with extrahepatic manifestations; HBV may cause polyarteritis nodosa and membranous nephropathy, while HCV is linked to mixed cryoglobulinemia, renal disease, and dermatologic conditions such as lichen planus. Early diagnosis and antiviral therapy improve long-term outcomes.

Herpes Simplex Virus (HSV): HSV infection is characterized by recurrent episodes of painful genital ulcerations caused predominantly by HSV type 2 (and increasingly HSV type 1). After initial infection, HSV establishes latency in sensory ganglia with periodic reactivation. Recurrent outbreaks can result in significant morbidity, including pain and psychosocial impact. Furthermore, active genital herpes lesions disrupt mucosal barriers, substantially increasing the risk of HIV acquisition and transmission. Antiviral suppressive therapy can reduce outbreak frequency and viral shedding.

Human Immunodeficiency Virus (HIV): HIV infection gradually depletes CD4+ T lymphocytes, resulting in profound immunodeficiency characteristic of acquired immunodeficiency syndrome (AIDS). Untreated HIV predisposes individuals to opportunistic infections (e.g., pneumocystis pneumonia and cryptococcal meningitis) and malignancies (e.g., Kaposi sarcoma and non-Hodgkin lymphoma). Neurological complications include HIV-associated neurocognitive disorders ranging from mild cognitive impairment to severe dementia, as well as peripheral neuropathies causing pain and sensory deficits. Antiretroviral therapy has transformed HIV into a manageable chronic condition but requires lifelong adherence.

Human Papillomavirus (HPV): Certain oncogenic HPV genotypes (notably types 16 and 18) are causally associated with cervical cancer, the fourth most common cancer among women globally. Persistent infection with high-risk HPV types leads to cervical intraepithelial neoplasia and invasive carcinoma if untreated. HPV is also implicated in other anogenital cancers, such as anal, vulvar, vaginal, penile, and oropharyngeal malignancies. Additionally, low-risk HPV types cause genital warts—benign exophytic lesions that may cause discomfort, bleeding, or psychological distress. Prophylactic HPV vaccination has significantly reduced the incidence of HPV-related diseases.

Syphilis: *Treponema pallidum* infection progresses through several stages if untreated. Late-stage syphilis can involve the central nervous system, causing neurosyphilis with symptoms ranging from headaches and cognitive dysfunction to stroke and tabes dorsalis. Cardiovascular syphilis primarily affects the aorta, leading to aortitis, aneurysm formation, and valvular insufficiency. Congenital syphilis results from transplacental transmission during pregnancy and can cause miscarriage, stillbirth, intrauterine growth restriction, low birth weight, and a spectrum of malformations, including bone deformities, rash, hepatosplenomegaly, and neurological impairment in the neonate. Prevention relies on early maternal screening and treatment.

Trichomoniasis: Trichomonas vaginalis infection is a common protozoal sexually transmitted disease that often causes vaginal discharge and irritation in women but is frequently asymptomatic in men. The inflammatory response induced by trichomoniasis increases genital mucosal susceptibility to HIV acquisition and transmission. In pregnancy, trichomoniasis is linked to adverse outcomes, including premature rupture of membranes (PROM), preterm delivery, and low birth weight infants. Screening and timely treatment during pregnancy are recommended to mitigate these risks.

Complications from STDs can be serious and sometimes life-threatening. Regular screening and prompt treatment of STDs are vital to minimize these risks and protect overall health.

2.8 Prevention

The prevention of sexually transmitted diseases (STDs) encompasses a wide range of evidence-based measures to minimize risk factors and sustainably reduce the risk of infection. The implementation of many prevention strategies often proves challenging in practice.

2.8.1 Core Strategies for STD Prevention

- Use of condoms

  Condoms should be used correctly and consistently during vaginal, anal, and oral sex to significantly reduce the risk of transmission of numerous STDs.

  Latex condoms form an effective barrier against even the smallest pathogens.

  The protective effect varies depending on the infection:

  HIV: 80–90% reduction in risk

  Bacterial infections such as gonorrhea and chlamydia: 50–80% reduction

  Infections through skin-to-skin contact (e.g., genital herpes, HPV, and syphilis): lower but significant protective effect

  Epidemiological studies indicate that condoms are 71–77% effective in heterosexual HIV-discordant couples and about 70% effective in MSM (men who have sex with men).
- Regular testing

  Early detection and treatment are crucial, especially for high-risk groups.

  At least one HIV test is recommended for all sexually active individuals between the ages of 13 and 64.

  Annual testing for gonorrhea and chlamydia is recommended for sexually active women under the age of 25 and for women over the age of 25 with risk factors.

  Pregnancy tests include syphilis, HIV, and hepatitis B and C at the beginning of pregnancy; if there are risk factors, chlamydia and gonorrhea should also be tested.

  MSM should be tested for syphilis, chlamydia, and gonorrhea at least once a year; more frequent testing (every 3–6 months) is advisable if they have multiple or anonymous partners.

  The frequency of testing should be tailored to the individual; if partners change frequently, testing every 3 months or monthly may be advisable.
- Education and information

  Comprehensive education about transmission routes, symptoms, and prevention options is essential for reducing risk.

  Evidence-based education programs lead to an average risk reduction of about 4% (relative risk reduction of 23%).

  Effective programs teach condom use skills and promote communication and negotiation skills, each of which leads to a risk reduction of about 30%.

  Reducing the frequency of sexual intercourse or the number of sexual partners can reduce the risks by 28–36%.

  School-based programs show significant success in delaying the age of first sexual intercourse, reducing the number of sexual partners, and increasing condom use.

- Vaccinations
  - Vaccinations are a highly effective preventive measure against certain STDs.
  - HPV vaccination protects uninfected young women against HPV types 16/18 with an efficacy of 91–100%.
  - Protection against cervical intraepithelial neoplasia grade 2+ (CIN2+) is 92.9–97.4%.
  - It is 100% effective against external anogenital lesions caused by HPV types 6/11/16/18.
  - Hepatitis B vaccination is recommended worldwide and has led to a significant decline in the disease in countries with high immunization rates.
- Pre-exposure prophylaxis (PrEP) and post-exposure prophylaxis (PEP)

  PrEP significantly reduces the risk of HIV infection in people at increased risk: daily use reduces the risk through sexual intercourse by approximately 99%.

  A risk reduction of at least 74% is achieved in injecting drug users.

  Studies show a risk reduction of up to 86% under real-world conditions.

  Doxycycline as PEP (Doxy-PEP) is effective against bacterial STIs when taken within 72 h of unprotected sex: 55–60% reduction in the risk of gonorrhea, as well as a reduction in the risk of chlamydia and syphilis.
- Safer sex practices

  In addition to condom use, safer sex includes other behaviors to minimize risk: reducing the number of sexual partners, maintaining monogamous relationships, open communication about sexual health, and regular health checkups.

  Interventions to reduce the frequency of sexual intercourse or the number of partners reduce STD incidence by 5–7% (relative reduction of 28–36%).

2.8.2 Innovative Prevention Approaches

- Expedited partner therapy (EPT)

  EPT enables the treatment of sexual partners without prior medical examination in order to interrupt chains of infection.

  Repeat infections are reduced by 20–29% with EPT.

  Higher treatment rates among partners are achieved compared to standard notification.

  EPT is particularly recommended for male partners of women with chlamydia or gonorrhea.
- Mobile health applications (mHealth)

  Apps provide information on STDs, prevention, and testing options, as well as features, such as skin detection via photo or video.

  Peer support platforms promote risk reduction strategies and are valued by users.
- Home test kits

  FDA-approved home test kits enable reliable testing for common STDs such as HIV, chlamydia, and gonorrhea in the privacy of one's own home.

The market is growing rapidly and is estimated to exceed US$800 million by 2030.

Reliability varies depending on the type of test; false negative results may occur, especially during the incubation period.

- Telemedicine

  Telemedicine services allow consultation, diagnosis, and treatment without visiting a clinic.

  Point-of-care testing devices provide rapid results on site.

  These technologies improve care and reduce transmission, especially in resource-poor regions.

2.8.3 Prevention Programs and Their Effectiveness

- Evidence-based interventions
  - Meta-analyses show a significant reduction in STD incidence through comprehensive prevention programs, with a relative reduction of up to 17%.
  - Programs with intensive group counseling (>120 min of contact time) show stronger effects.
  - Less intensive measures also increase condom use and effectively reduce the number of partners.
- Cost-effectiveness
  - Intervention studies such as "Safe in the City" demonstrate cost-effective reductions in new infections in hospital settings.
  - The net cost per case prevented was approximately $75 in the baseline scenario.
- Social media and campaigns
  - Social media are used as platforms for STD prevention messages (e.g., hashtags #STIweek, #SaferSexGamePlan).
  - Campaigns such as "Prepare Before You're There" promote safe sexual practices and provide information about local testing options.

Effective implementation of preventive measures can help minimize the risk of STD infection and promote overall sexual health. Nevertheless, access to specialized personnel, healthcare facilities, or governmental and non-governmental organizations is often necessary. Unfortunately, such resources can be lacking in low-resource settings or inadequately funded in more affluent countries.

Key Points

- Infections remain a significant cause of morbidity and mortality in the twenty-first century, responsible for approximately 17.3 million deaths annually attributed to infectious diseases.
- One-third of all deaths worldwide can be traced back to infections.
- Sexually transmitted diseases (STD) hold considerable epidemiological and clinical significance and often manifest as conditions such as urethritis, cervicitis, and genital ulcers. An important challenge in STD management is the often asymptomatic nature of these diseases, which can facilitate the unwanted spread of pathogens.
- Diseases can be categorized into two groups: classic sexually transmitted diseases and other infections transmitted through sexual activity or intimate contact. There is also emerging evidence of sexual transmission of previously unclassified pathogens.
- It is estimated that approximately one million new cases of STDs occur globally each day. Among the most prevalent are chlamydia, gonorrhea, syphilis, and trichomoniasis, the incidence of which is rising in Europe.
- Chlamydia and HPV are particularly common in developed countries. HIV, syphilis, and hepatitis B are mandatory reportable diseases in many countries.
- Adolescents and young adults are especially vulnerable to contracting STDs, frequently due to unprotected sexual intercourse and multiple partner changes. Socioeconomic factors and drug abuse can further increase this risk.
- STDs during pregnancy may lead to premature births, miscarriages, and infections in the fetus, highlighting the critical need for preventive measures and early diagnosis.
- Effective prevention strategies include the consistent use of condoms, regular testing, and education about transmission routes. Vaccinations, safe sex practices, and government-supported prevention programs are also essential for minimizing the spread of STDs.

Clinical Considerations and Practical Procedure

3

Abstract

The diagnosis and management of sexually transmitted diseases (STDs) pose a significant challenge. Consequently, a symptom-oriented and structured approach is of paramount importance. The utilization of clinical syndromes offers several advantages, including early disease detection, the development of effective treatment strategies, and the ability to make prognoses. Nevertheless, the use of syndromes also carries certain risks, such as potential generalization and stigmatization. A comprehensive sexual history is invaluable. In addition to clinical examination, laboratory analyses, imaging procedures, and histological examinations are employed to facilitate precise diagnosis. The treatment plan is contingent upon the underlying cause and may be either curative or palliative. Furthermore, the provision of aftercare, particularly in the form of information and treatment for sexual partners, is of significant importance. In summary, the care of patients with STDs requires an empathetic, respectful, and objective approach.

3.1 Background

The diagnosis of a sexually transmitted disease (STD) represents a significant challenge for the treating physician. Although many of these diseases manifest primarily in the genital area, some STDs present a range of often uncharacteristic symptoms, complicating rapid diagnosis.

Suspicion of Sexual Transmitted Disease:

- **Among younger individuals.**
- **During acute onset.**
- **If sexual contact is mentioned spontaneously as a possible cause.**
- **If similar episodes of the disease have occurred in the past.**

I. Mylonas, *Sexually Transmitted Diseases*,
https://doi.org/10.1007/978-3-031-78204-6_3

3.2 Clinical Syndromes

Clinical syndromes are groups of symptoms and signs that occur together and indicate a specific disease or condition (Table 3.1). They represent specific manifestations of pathological processes within the body. A syndrome might be precipitated by various factors, including genetic predisposition, infection, or environmental influences. These syndrome diagnoses play a pivotal role in medical practice, as they facilitate the development of a diagnostic and therapeutic plan based on observed symptom constellations.

Table 3.1 Clinical syndromes and their possible pathogens

Syndrome	Symptoms and signs	Associated micro organisms
Arthritis-dermatitis syndrome	– Joint and skin manifestations in a sexually active adult – Single indurated ulcer with a clean base, rolled borders, painless; rash on trunk, palms, soles, genitals – Bilateral inguinal lymphadenopathy	– *N. gonorrhoeae* – *C. trachomatis*
Cervicitis	– Abnormal vaginal discharge – Bleeding after intercourse – Cervical mucopus or friability – Petechiae or erosions on the cervix	– *Neisseria gonorrhoeae* – *Chlamydia trachomatis* – *Trichomonas vaginalis* – *Mycoplasma genitalium* – Herpes simplex virus
Enteritis	– Diarrhea and abdominal cramping – Possible fecal leukocytes; positive O and P	– Shigella sp., Salmonella sp., Campylobacter sp., Cryptosporidium, Microsporidium, Isospora, *Mycobacterium avium intracellulare*
Epididymitis/orchitis	– Swelling and pain in the scrotum/testes – Edema, erythema, or tenderness of the testes and epididymis	– *Neisseria gonorrhoeae* – *Chlamydia trachomatis* – Streptococcus sp. – Anaerobic bacteria
Genital ulcer disease	– Single or multiple ulcers or erosions – Diffuse rash – Possible systemic symptoms – Single or multiple erosions – Bilateral inguinal or femoral lymphadenopathy	– Herpes simplex virus – *T. pallidum* – *H. ducreyi* – LGV strains of *Chlamydia trachomatis*
Pelvic inflammatory disease (pid)	– Abnormal vaginal discharge – Lower abdominal pain – Bleeding between periods – Dyspareunia – Cervical motion tenderness: Pain experienced during manipulation of the cervix – Cervicitis: signs such as purulent or mucopurulent discharge, cervical friability, and erythema	– *Neisseria gonorrhoeae* – *Chlamydia trachomatis*

(continued)

Table 3.1 (continued)

Syndrome	Symptoms and signs	Associated micro organisms
Proctitis	– Pus or blood in stools – Tenesmus – Anorectal pain – Possible constipation – Erythema of rectal tissue – Purulent discharge – Erosions or ulcers	– *Neisseria gonorrhoeae* – *Chlamydia trachomatis* – *Trichomonas vaginalis* – Herpes simplex virus
Proctocolitis	– Proctitis symptoms plus diarrhea and abdominal cramping – Similar to proctitis, possibly with fecal leukocytes	– Campylobacter sp., Shigella sp., *Entamoeba histolytica*, LGV serovars of *Chlamydia trachomatis*, CMV (in severely immunosuppressed patients)
Reactive arthritis	– Previous or concurrent infection with eye, skin, genitourinary, gastrointestinal, and/or joint symptoms – Tenosynovitis, polyarthritis, or dermatitis; urethritis or cervicitis	– Enteric pathogens
Urethritis	– Discharge – Dysuria – Itching at the urethral opening – Mucoid, mucopurulent, or purulent discharge – Enlarged inguinal or femoral lymph nodes	– *Neisseria gonorrhoeae* – *Chlamydia trachomatis* – M*ycoplasma genitalium*
Vaginitis/ colpitis	– Abnormal vaginal discharge – Unusual odor – Vaginal irritation – Vaginal itching – Dysuria – Altered vaginal pH – Vaginal erythema	– *Trichomonas vaginalis* – *Candida albicans* and other Candida species – *Gardnerella vaginalis* – Anaerobic bacteria

Advantages:

- **Early Detection and Diagnosis**: Identification of a syndrome often leads to rapid diagnosis, especially for complex or rare diseases characterized by unique symptom combinations. This enables prompt treatment in resource-limited settings, bypassing the need for additional laboratory diagnostic procedures.
- **Treatment Strategies**: Identification of specific syndromes allows for the development of tailored treatment options, addressing the unique symptoms and challenges associated with each syndrome, reflecting the current acceptance of clinical guidelines.
- **Prognosis**: Some syndromes have well-documented courses, enabling predictable disease progression and providing adequate care and advice to patients.
- **Research and Development**: Classification of syndromes aids research by providing defined patient groups with similar symptoms and causes, facilitating focused and efficient investigation.

- **Education and Awareness-Raising**: Recognition and nomenclature of syndromes enhance awareness and understanding.
- **Education and Training**:
  - **Practice-Oriented Learning**: Focusing on real clinical symptoms allows for the application of knowledge in real-world contexts.
  - **Enhancing Diagnostic Abilities**: Recognizing and interpreting clinical symptoms enhances observational and judgmental skills.
  - **Differential Diagnostic Considerations**: Working with syndromes facilitates the consideration of different causes and the development of differential diagnoses.
  - **Adaptability to New Developments**: A profound understanding of symptoms enables professionals to address novel or infrequent clinical scenarios by discerning and interpreting patterns.
  - **Enhancing Patient Safety**: Well-founded symptom training can reduce misdiagnosis, thereby enhancing patient safety.

Disadvantages:

- **Generalization**: Diagnosis based on a group of symptoms can overlook individual differences in symptom severity or underlying causes.
- **Diagnostic Uncertainty**: Undefined diagnostic criteria for certain syndromes can lead to uncertainty or diagnostic delays, hindering timely and appropriate treatment.
- **Stigmatization**: Specific syndrome diagnoses can stigmatize affected individuals, negatively impacting self-image and social interactions, and potentially leading to discrimination.
- **Impact on Treatment**: Focusing on syndrome symptoms may overlook other unrelated health issues.
- **Misdiagnosis**: Disproportionate focus on syndromes can lead to overlooking rare or atypical symptoms of different clinical pictures.
- **Restriction of Research**: Narrowing the perspective through syndrome classification can hinder research into diseases outside these defined parameters.
- **Psychological Impact**: Syndrome diagnoses can cause anxiety, stress, and uncertainty, especially in genetic or lifelong conditions. Classifying patients into specific syndromes can deteriorate the doctor-patient relationship.
- **Education and Training**:
  - **Simplification**: Clinical syndrome use can oversimplify complex clinical pictures, leading to an incomplete understanding.
  - **Lack of Flexibility**: Rigid categorization impedes flexible thinking required for diagnosing unusual or multiple coexisting conditions.
  - **Outdated Information**: Educational materials may become outdated due to constant medical science evolution.
  - **Dependence on Doctrine**: Excessive reliance on known syndrome characteristics can stifle critical thinking and differential diagnostic skills.
- **Variable Interpretations**: Inconsistent interpretations of clinical syndromes can result in diagnostic variances.
- **Neglect of Psychosocial Factors**: Focusing on the clinical picture may neglect the psychosocial aspects of patient care.

The reliance on broad clinical syndromes in modern medical practice can have detrimental consequences, particularly in the fields of infectious diseases and gynecology. For example, the nonspecific diagnosis of a “flu-like illness” often leads to the overlooking of more specific and potentially serious viral infections, such as influenza or respiratory syncytial virus (RSV). This generalization may result in delayed or inappropriate management, negatively affecting patient outcomes. Additionally, economic pressures within healthcare systems frequently encourage minimizing diagnostic testing, which can compound these issues.

In cases of vaginal discharge, clinical evaluation commonly focuses solely on the three most prevalent infectious causes—bacterial vaginosis, trichomoniasis, and vulvovaginal candidiasis—while other important etiologies are often neglected. This selective approach frequently leads to an overdiagnosis of vulvovaginal candidiasis, resulting in inappropriate treatment and potential persistence or transmission of undiagnosed infections. Such oversimplification delays targeted therapy and may contribute to ongoing morbidity and spread within the community.

Similarly, in gynecology, the broad clinical syndrome of pelvic inflammatory disease (PID) or salpingitis is frequently attributed primarily to *Chlamydia trachomatis* infection. However, this perspective neglects the polymicrobial nature of PID, where gram-positive cocci (e.g., streptococci), gram-negative rods (e.g., *Escherichia coli*), and anaerobic bacteria (e.g., Bacteroides species) commonly play significant pathogenic roles. Current clinical guidelines tend to emphasize treatment targeting chlamydial and gonococcal infections, potentially overlooking other causative organisms that require different therapeutic approaches.

These examples underscore the critical importance of precise diagnostic evaluation rather than relying on generalized clinical syndromes. Accurate identification of the underlying pathogens enables timely, targeted therapy, improves patient outcomes, and helps prevent further transmission. Optimizing diagnostic strategies and avoiding overgeneralization are essential steps toward effective and individualized patient care in infectious diseases and gynecology.

The diagnosis and treatment of infectious clinical syndromes necessitate a nuanced and individualized medical approach.

3.3 Medical History

3.3.1 Symptom-Oriented Approach

The medical history is focused on the patient’s subjective complaints that led to the visit to the doctor. Vaginal discharge is undoubtedly the most common reason for a visit to a gynecologist. Nevertheless, other frequent triggers include discomfort

Table 3.2 Characterization of the leading symptoms

Category	Details
Localization	– Location, radiation, and spread of the complaints
Quality	– Burning, stinging, pulling, or colicky
Intensity	– Progressive or decreasing intensity
Temporal occurrence	– Acute onset
	– Chronic condition
	– Frequency
"Trigger"	– Unprotected sexual intercourse
	– New sexual partner
	– Sexual intercourse practices
Clinical course	– Improvement or worsening of the symptoms
	– Chronic condition
	– Taking medication (including nonprescription medication)
Accompanying symptoms	– Fever, nausea, vomiting, etc.
Previous diagnostics	– Previous visits to the doctor for the same or similar symptoms and the resulting diagnostic or therapeutic measures

when urinating, unclear lower abdominal discomfort, and itching and burning in the genital area.

If the primary symptoms occur alongside sexual intercourse, a sexually transmitted disease should be considered as a possible diagnosis.

In the case of pregnancy, vaginal bleeding or increased vaginal discharge, as well as concerns about the unborn child, are the most common reasons for an acute presentation at the doctor's office or clinic. A structured approach should be employed when obtaining the medical history. At the outset, a comprehensive anamnestic characterization of the symptoms should be conducted (Table 3.2).

In cases of suspected STDs, it is essential to ask about vaginal discharge and vulvar symptoms. If the patient also presents with systemic symptoms, it is important to inquire about rectal discharge, conjunctivitis, arthritis, and any genital or generalized skin rashes (exanthema and enanthema).

General Gynecological and Obstetric Anamnesis

- Pre-existing conditions and their treatment.
- Medication history.
- Operations.
- Sexual anamnesis and previous sexual diseases.
- Number and course of pregnancies.
- Menstrual history.
- Preliminary gynecological examinations and previous cytological smears.
- Contraceptive measures (e.g., oral contraceptives or hormone replacement therapy).

It is also essential to obtain detailed information regarding the patient's obstetric and gynecological history. This includes the number and outcomes of previous pregnancies, menstrual cycle characteristics (such as regularity, duration, and any abnormalities), and findings from prior gynecological examinations. Additionally, documentation of current contraceptive methods—such as oral contraceptives or other forms of birth control—is important for comprehensive care planning.

A thorough medication history must be collected, encompassing all prescribed and over-the-counter drugs. Particular attention should be given to previous treatments with anti-infective agents, including details on the specific medications used, dosages, duration of therapy, and clinical indications. Assessing adherence to prescribed regimens is crucial; the clinician should inquire about the patient's regularity in taking medications and explore any barriers to compliance. Understanding reasons for non-adherence—such as adverse effects like nausea, diarrhea, or other tolerability issues—is vital to optimizing treatment outcomes and tailoring future therapeutic strategies.

3.3.2 Sexual Anamnesis

Conducting a thorough and effective sexual anamnesis demands a careful balance of sensitivity, privacy, and clear communication. The process should begin with establishing rapport and assuring the patient of strict confidentiality, which fosters trust and openness. It is advisable to introduce more personal or intimate questions gradually, reserving them for later in the consultation once the patient feels comfortable and understands the clinical purpose behind these inquiries (Table 3.3).

A comprehensive sexual history should include detailed information about the patient's current and previous sexual partners, including the number and gender of partners, as well as the nature, frequency, and context of sexual activities. Exploring the types of sexual practices—such as vaginal, anal, and oral intercourse—is essential to determine appropriate anatomical sites for testing and to tailor counseling efforts effectively.

Table 3.3 Key questions regarding sexual history

Topic	Example of sensitively phrased questions	Purpose/notes
Timing of Exposure	When did you have the sexual contact that you associate with your current symptoms? When was your last sexual encounter?	To narrow down the incubation period; prioritize diagnostic tests (e.g., NAAT and serology)
	Have you experienced any recent symptoms following sexual contact?	To correlate exposure with symptom onset and guide further evaluation
Type of Sexual Contact	Was the sexual contact vaginal, oral, and/or anal?	To determine anatomical sites for testing (urethra, cervix, rectum, and oropharynx) and assess risk of different pathogens

(continued)

Table 3.3 (continued)

Topic	Example of sensitively phrased questions	Purpose/notes
	Do you or your partners engage in any specific sexual practices that we should be aware of to guide testing?	To tailor diagnostic approach and counseling based on sexual behaviors
Current and Recent Partners	With whom have you had sexual contact in the past weeks/months? (Partner role: steady partner/spouse/casual acquaintance/unknown)	To map sexual networks for contact tracing and risk assessment
	How often do you have sexual contact with these partners?	To assess frequency of exposure and infection risk
Relationship Status and Dynamics	Do you have a steady partner? How long have you been together? Are there any concerns in the relationship (e.g., violence)?	To assess exposure risks, psychosocial support needs, and necessary protective measures; observe mandatory reporting if violence is disclosed
	Have there been any recent changes in your relationship status or sexual activity?	To identify new risks or changes in exposure
Sexual Orientation and Partner Gender	With which gender(s) have you had sexual contacts? (male/female/both/other)	Relevant for identifying differential risk profiles and providing targeted counseling
	Are you comfortable discussing your sexual orientation and preferences?	To ensure an open, nonjudgmental environment for accurate history-taking
Travel and Contacts Abroad	Have you or your partner recently traveled abroad? Were there any sexual contacts during this time?	To consider endemic pathogens and regional antimicrobial resistance patterns
	Which countries or regions have you visited recently?	To tailor risk assessment for region-specific infections
Number of Sexual Partners	How many sexual partners have you had in the last 2–3 months? In the past year? (If needed, provide a detailed chronology over the last 3–24 months)	To quantify exposure risk and inform screening intervals
	Have you engaged in concurrent partnerships or overlapping sexual relationships?	To assess complex exposure networks and transmission dynamics
Condom Use	Do you use condoms? If yes: always/sometimes/never—with which sexual practices?	To assess protective behaviors and provide appropriate education and prevention advice
	What barriers or challenges do you face in using condoms consistently?	To identify obstacles to safer sex practices and address them in counseling

(continued)

Table 3.3 (continued)

Topic	Example of sensitively phrased questions	Purpose/notes
Previous STDs and Treatment	Have you previously had a sexually transmitted infection? If yes: which one(s), when, and how were they treated?	Important for assessing risk of reinfection, partner treatment needs, and guiding therapy choices
	Did you complete the full course of treatment during your last infection?	To evaluate treatment adherence and potential for persistent infection
Substance Use and IV Drug History	Do you consume alcohol or drugs? If yes: which substances and how often? Do you inject drugs intravenously, and is equipment shared?	To identify additional infection risks (e.g., bloodborne pathogens) and determine vaccination and counseling needs
	Do substance use behaviors impact your sexual activity or decision-making?	To assess risk behaviors linked to substance use
Tattoos/Piercings	Do you have tattoos or piercings? When were they done, and under what conditions (e.g., sterile instruments)?	To evaluate nosocomial or procedure-related infection risks
	Have you ever experienced complications after tattoos or piercings?	To identify possible previous exposures to bloodborne infections
Social and Notification Aspects	Would you like assistance with notifying partners? Are there any legal or mandatory reporting issues to discuss?	To plan partner notification, comply with legal reporting requirements (e.g., Infection Protection Act), and initiate protective measures
	Do you have concerns about confidentiality or stigma related to partner notification?	To address patient concerns and support informed decision-making
Psychosocial and Support Needs	Do you require psychosocial support, pregnancy counseling, or protective accommodation?	To ensure comprehensive care, patient empowerment, and safety
	Are there any mental health or social factors affecting your well-being that you would like support with?	To identify broader support needs that may impact health outcomes

Equally important is assessing the use of protective measures during sexual activity. Clinicians should inquire about condom usage patterns, including consistency and correctness, and discuss other preventive strategies such as pre-exposure prophylaxis (PrEP) for HIV where indicated. The conversation should also address partner notification practices, emphasizing the importance of informing current and past partners to facilitate timely testing and treatment, thereby limiting further transmission.

Throughout the anamnesis, it is critical to maintain a nonjudgmental, empathetic, and supportive approach. This encourages honest disclosure, improves risk assessment accuracy, and strengthens the foundation for effective prevention and management of sexually transmitted infections. Tailoring communication to the patient's cultural background, language proficiency, and health literacy further enhances engagement and outcomes.

Subject Possible Questions

Alcohol and Drug Use

Do you consume alcohol? Do you use drugs? If so, which substances and how frequently?

If you use intravenous drugs, have you shared needles or other paraphernalia with anyone?

If so, when was the last time this occurred?

Have you ever received treatment for substance use? If so, what was the outcome?

Tattoos or Piercings

Do you have any tattoos or piercings? If yes, when were they done, and under what conditions (e.g., sterile equipment)?

Have you ever had any complications from your tattoos or piercings (e.g., infection, allergic reaction)?

Overall Health

Do you have any other health conditions that may impact sexual health (e.g., diabetes, immune disorders)?

Are you currently taking any medications that could affect your sexual function or health?

Recommendations for Conducting a Sexual Anamnesis: Relevant Radiological Examinations

Radiological imaging plays an important role in the assessment, diagnosis, and management of complications arising from sexually transmitted diseases (STDs). Appropriate imaging modalities should be selected based on clinical presentation, suspected pathology, and patient factors.

- **Ultrasound:** Ultrasound is a first-line, non-invasive imaging modality essential for evaluating pelvic inflammatory disease (PID), a common complication of untreated STDs, such as *Chlamydia trachomatis* and *Neisseria gonorrhoeae* infections. It allows visualization of pelvic

(continued)

structures to detect fluid collections, tubo-ovarian abscesses, and signs of inflammation or adhesions. In pregnant patients, ultrasound is invaluable for assessing fetal well-being and identifying complications related to maternal STDs, including congenital infections and placental abnormalities.

- **Magnetic Resonance Imaging (MRI):** MRI offers superior soft tissue contrast resolution and is useful for evaluating complex pelvic pain or masses when ultrasound findings are inconclusive. It is particularly beneficial in identifying and characterizing abscesses related to severe PID. MRI also plays a critical role in assessing central nervous system involvement in STDs such as neurosyphilis, where it can detect meningovascular changes, infarcts, or cranial nerve involvement.
- **Computed Tomography (CT) Scan:** CT imaging is indicated in cases where detailed cross-sectional visualization of pelvic or abdominal structures is required. It effectively identifies complications such as pelvic or peritoneal abscesses secondary to PID. CT scans are also instrumental in evaluating hepatobiliary manifestations related to viral hepatitis or liver abscesses associated with systemic infections. Additionally, CT can assess inguinal or pelvic lymphadenopathy often seen in conditions like lymphogranuloma venereum or non-gonococcal urethritis.

Specific Sexually Transmitted Diseases and Associated Radiological Findings

- **Gonorrhea and Chlamydia:** Transvaginal or transabdominal ultrasound may reveal thickened, fluid-filled fallopian tubes (hydrosalpinx), enlarged ovaries, free pelvic fluid, or abscess formation indicative of PID. These findings guide timely intervention to prevent permanent reproductive damage.
- **Human Immunodeficiency Virus (HIV):** Advanced HIV/AIDS patients are prone to opportunistic infections requiring imaging evaluation. Chest CT may detect pneumocystis pneumonia (PCP), while brain MRI assesses central nervous system infections, such as toxoplasmosis or progressive multifocal leukoencephalopathy. Imaging is also used to evaluate HIV-associated malignancies, including non-Hodgkin lymphoma.
- **Syphilis:** In neurosyphilis, MRI and CT can demonstrate meningeal enhancement, infarcts due to meningovascular involvement, or cranial nerve pathology. CT angiography may identify cardiovascular complications like aortitis or aortic aneurysms in tertiary syphilis.

(continued)

- **Herpes Simplex Virus (HSV):** MRI is the preferred modality for evaluating HSV encephalitis and neurological sequelae. Although genital lesions are primarily diagnosed clinically, pelvic ultrasound may assist in visualizing deep soft tissue involvement when suspected.
- **Human Papillomavirus (HPV):** Standard imaging is not routinely employed in HPV diagnosis; however, colposcopy combined with biopsy remains the gold standard for detecting cervical intraepithelial neoplasia (CIN) and invasive cervical cancer. Imaging-guided biopsies may be utilized for lesion characterization in selected cases.

Specific STDs and Associated Radiological Findings

- **Gonorrhea and Chlamydia: Ultrasound**
  - May reveal thickened fallopian tubes, enlarged ovaries, or the presence of pelvic fluid associated with PID.
  - Can identify complications, such as abscesses or peritonitis if they develop.
  - Human Immunodeficiency Virus (HIV): CT or MRI
  - Imaging may be warranted for opportunistic infections, such as pneumocystis pneumonia (PCP) or central nervous system infections in advanced HIV/AIDS cases.
  - Non-Hodgkin lymphoma, a malignancy often associated with HIV, may also be evaluated using imaging studies.
- **Syphilis: MRI/CT**
  - In cases of neurosyphilis, imaging of the brain may show alterations, including meningovascular changes or involvement of cranial nerves.
  - CT scans may reveal cardiovascular complications such as aortitis in patients with tertiary syphilis.
- **Herpes Simplex Virus (HSV): MRI**
  - Useful for assessing encephalitis or neurological complications stemming from HSV infection.
  - While pelvic ultrasound can visualize genital lesions, these are primarily diagnosed through clinical examination.
- **Human Papillomavirus (HPV): Colposcopy with Imaging**
  - Although standard imaging is not used for HPV, imaging-guided biopsies may be utilized to evaluate suspicious lesions for cervical intraepithelial neoplasia (CIN) or invasive cervical cancer.

By systematically addressing these components, the sexual anamnesis can be conducted comprehensively, ensuring that all relevant facets of the patient's sexual health are thoroughly evaluated. It is imperative to use neutral, nonjudgmental language throughout the interview, fostering an environment of trust and openness. Attention should also be given to the patient's verbal and nonverbal cues to gauge understanding and comfort.

Equally important is the meticulous documentation of all information obtained during the anamnesis. Accurate and detailed records facilitate appropriate follow-up care, enable continuity between healthcare providers, and support tailored counseling interventions. This comprehensive approach promotes effective risk assessment, diagnosis, and management of sexually transmitted infections and other sexual health concerns.

In the case of STDs, it is advisable to take the medical history in private, as the presence of the partner may be stressful and counterproductive for the patient.

If the sexual partner is not present during the clinical examination or declines evaluation, it is essential to obtain a detailed symptom history from the patient regarding any signs or symptoms their partner may be experiencing. This information can provide critical clues to the partner's potential infection status and guide clinical decision-making for both diagnosis and treatment.

The clinician should inquire about a broad range of symptoms, including but not limited to:

- Urethral Discharge: Ask if the partner has noticed any abnormal urethral discharge, noting its color, consistency, and quantity. Such discharge may indicate urethritis caused by infections like chlamydia or gonorrhea.
- Dysuria: Determine whether the partner has experienced burning, stinging, or pain during urination, which often accompanies urethral or urinary tract infections.
- Genital Itching or Irritation: Inquire about any itching, redness, or discomfort in the genital area that could suggest infestations (e.g., pubic lice and scabies), fungal infections, or dermatitis.
- Rashes or Ulcerations: Ask if any rashes, sores, ulcers, blisters, or vesicular lesions have been observed on the partner's external genitalia. These may represent syphilitic chancres, herpes simplex virus lesions, molluscum contagiosum, or other dermatologic conditions.
- Testicular or Scrotal Pain and Swelling: Assess whether the partner has reported pain, heaviness, swelling, or tenderness in the testicles or scrotum, which can be indicative of epididymo-orchitis often associated with bacterial STDs.

- Penile or Genital Lesions: Query about lumps, bumps, warts, or other growths on the penis or genital skin that may suggest human papillomavirus (HPV) infection or other conditions.
- Foul Odor: Ask if there has been any unusual or foul-smelling genital discharge or odor, which can be a sign of bacterial vaginosis in female partners or certain bacterial infections in males.
- Pain During Intercourse (Dyspareunia): Inquire whether the partner experiences pain during sexual activity, which may signal underlying infections or inflammation.
- Systemic Symptoms: Ask if the partner has had fever, malaise, swollen lymph nodes (inguinal or generalized), night sweats, or unexplained weight loss—symptoms that could indicate systemic involvement, such as disseminated gonococcal infection or secondary syphilis.
- Urinary Frequency or Urgency: Determine if the partner has experienced increased frequency or urgency of urination, which can accompany urethritis or urinary tract infections.
- Discomfort or Burning After Ejaculation: Ask if there is any pain or burning sensation following ejaculation, a symptom that may suggest prostatitis or urethritis.

Collecting this comprehensive symptom history regarding the sexual partner—even when obtained secondhand—broadens the diagnostic perspective and aids in risk stratification. It facilitates timely partner notification and testing and supports appropriate empirical treatment decisions. This approach enhances infection control efforts and helps prevent ongoing transmission within sexual networks.

Although gynecologists are traditionally focused on the treatment of women, in certain cases, it may be necessary to extend the evaluation to the sexual partner. This approach is particularly beneficial in cases where the patient's symptoms are non-specific and there is a high suspicion of a sexually transmitted disease.

3.4 Diagnosis

A comprehensive medical history can provide valuable insight into the potential presence of infectious diseases. In particular, inquiring about similar illnesses in the surrounding area can be insightful. Additionally, the travel history and vaccination status can provide information about various infectious agents. Subsequently, a physical examination is conducted, yielding further crucial insights. Laboratory tests such as blood counts and specific antibody tests are often essential for diagnosing infectious diseases. In certain instances, imaging procedures, such as X-rays or ultrasound, may be employed to facilitate precise diagnosis. A systematic diagnostic approach is of paramount importance.

3.4.1 Clinical Manifestation

The respective symptoms and clinical findings provide initial indications of a sexually transmitted infection. These specific symptoms and findings suggest the possibility of an infection transmitted through sexual intercourse. These signs should be taken seriously initiate appropriate diagnostic measures.

3.4.2 Clinical Examination

The initial indications of an infection are often skin efflorescences in the external genital area.

In the event that significant symptoms are reported in the absence of clinical findings, venereophobia should be considered as a potential diagnosis of exclusion.

Patients with suspected STDs should undergo a clinical examination using the following methods:

- **Inspection and Palpation**: Inspection and palpation of the anal and genital areas are essential components of the clinical examination. Initial indications of an infection often manifest as efflorescence in these regions.
- **Vaginal Speculum Examination**: A vaginal speculum examination may be conducted to thoroughly assess the vagina and cervix. This examination aids in evaluating discharge, identifying morphological changes, and collecting microbiological smears or tissue biopsies. The use of split specula (i.e., Doyen specula, Kristeller specula) is recommended to optimize this examination.
- **Bimanual and Sonographic Gynecological Examination**: A bimanual and sonographic gynecological examination allows for the assessment of lower abdominal complaints.
- **Proctoscopy**: In the event of rectal complaints, a proctoscopy can be performed or arranged as needed.
- **Additional Tests**: Further tests may be conducted based on the patient's medical history and presenting complaints. For example, a comprehensive skin assessment may be warranted.
- **Examination of the Partner**: Inspection and palpation of the external male genitalia may, in certain instances, provide insights into the etiology of the female sexual partner's symptoms.

By systematically conducting these examinations, a comprehensive assessment can be achieved, facilitating accurate diagnosis and appropriate treatment planning.

3.4.3 Clinical Chemistry Laboratory

For diagnosis and evaluation of infectious diseases, a standardized panel of clinical-chemical laboratory parameters is employed to quantify systemic inflammatory responses and to detect organ-specific involvement.

Hematologic Parameters

A complete blood count with differential remains a fundamental diagnostic tool. Leukocytosis (>10,000/μL) with a left shift (increased bands/immature neutrophils) is typical of acute bacterial infection. Characteristic hematologic patterns include:

- Bacterial infections: leukocytosis, neutrophilia, left shift
- Viral infections: relative or absolute lymphocytosis with normal or decreased total leukocyte count
- Allergic or parasitic processes: eosinophilia
- Chronic inflammatory states: monocytosis

Acute-Phase Proteins

- C-reactive protein (CRP) is a hepatic pentraxin induced by interleukin-6 (IL-6). CRP begins to rise 4–6 h after inflammatory stimulus, peaks at approximately 48 h, and may increase 10- to 100-fold above the reference (<0.5 mg/dL). Representative ranges:
  - Mild elevation (10–40 mg/L): viral infections, low-grade inflammation, pregnancy
  - Moderate to marked elevation (40–200 mg/L): bacterial infections, pneumonia, sepsis
  - Relatively low elevation (<50 mg/L): parasitic infections
- Procalcitonin (PCT) provides greater specificity for bacterial infection than CRP because interferon-γ produced during viral infections suppresses PCT synthesis. Suggested interpretation thresholds:
  - <0.25 ng/mL: viral infection or localized bacterial infection unlikely to be systemic
  - 0.25–0.5 ng/mL: possible bacterial infection
  - ≥0.5 ng/mL: probable bacterial infection or sepsis
  - ≥2 ng/mL: severe bacterial infection or overt sepsis
- Interleukin-6 (IL-6) is an early proinflammatory cytokine that rises prior to CRP and is particularly useful in obstetric and neonatal indications. IL-6 measurement in amniotic fluid is highly sensitive for intrauterine infection and chorioamnionitis. In suspected amniotic infection syndrome, IL-6 discriminates inflammatory from noninflammatory processes. Rapid point-of-care assays yield results within ~20 min; an amniotic fluid cutoff of ~745 pg/mL has been associated with sensitivity ≈93% and specificity ≈91% for intrauterine inflammation. However, optimal cutoffs ranging from 1389.82 pg/mL to 2500–3500 pg/mL have been reported depending on the study population and methodology. A maternal serum IL-6 ≥19.5 pg/mL has been proposed as a noninvasive predictor of histologic chorioamnionitis in preterm prelabor rupture of membranes. In pregnancy-associated sepsis, IL-6 has demonstrated superior diagnostic performance compared with traditional markers (reported AUROC ≈0.94 in pregnant

women, 0.91 in children, and 0.86 in neonates). IL-6 increases within 1–2 h after infection onset, whereas CRP and PCT generally peak at 24–48 h.

Organ-Specific Markers

Selected laboratory tests indicate specific organ involvement and guide targeted evaluation.

Liver: Elevations of alanine aminotransferase (ALT) and aspartate aminotransferase (AST) are indicative of hepatocellular injury and should prompt evaluation for etiologies, such as viral hepatitis or pyogenic liver abscess. In contrast, increased alkaline phosphatase (ALP) and gamma-glutamyl transferase (γ-GT) predominantly reflect cholestatic injury or biliary obstruction, as seen in cholangitis or obstructive choledocholithiasis. Measurement of total and fractionated bilirubin quantifies conjugated and unconjugated hyperbilirubinemia and helps differentiate hepatocellular dysfunction from cholestasis; marked hyperbilirubinemia supports significant hepatic injury or obstructive pathology.

Kidney: Serum creatinine and blood urea nitrogen (BUN) are primary markers of renal function; rising concentrations indicate decreased glomerular filtration and may reflect acute tubular injury, immune-mediated nephritis, or sepsis-associated acute kidney injury. Urinalysis provides complementary information: Persistent proteinuria and hematuria support involvement of the glomerulus (e.g., glomerulonephritis), whereas pyuria or bacteriuria suggests lower urinary tract infection. Correlation of serum indices with urinalysis findings and clinical context is required to distinguish pre-renal, intrinsic renal, and post-renal causes and to guide further diagnostic and therapeutic steps.

Additional Inflammatory Indices

- Erythrocyte sedimentation rate (ESR) rises more slowly than CRP but remains elevated for longer intervals; it remains valuable for monitoring chronic inflammatory conditions despite lower utility for acute diagnosis. Clinical contexts in which ESR is informative include:
  - Infective Endocarditis: Persistent ESR elevation (>60 mm/h) supports diagnosis and therapeutic monitoring over 4–6 weeks.
  - Tuberculosis: Moderate to marked ESR elevation (≈30 to 80 mm/h) used for follow-up; persistent elevation may indicate complications.
  - Osteomyelitis: Elevated ESR accompanies prolonged antimicrobial therapy, particularly in chronic disease.
  - Sarcoidosis: ESR correlates with disease activity and response to therapy.
  - Septic arthritis and Spondylodiscitis: Elevated ESR aids diagnosis and longitudinal assessment.

A combined evaluation of hematologic indices, acute-phase reactants, organ-specific markers, and microbiological results, interpreted in the clinical context, optimizes diagnostic accuracy and supports evidence-based therapeutic decision-making. Serial measurements and trends are emphasized over single values for assessment of disease trajectory and treatment response.

3.4.4 Wet Mount Microscopy—Phase-Contrast Microscopy

3.4.4.1 Preparation of a Native Vaginal Secretion

- **Preparation and Collection**: A native vaginal secretion preparation should be prepared for microscopic examination. Secretions are collected from the anterior vaginal wall using a speculum. The collected vaginal secretion is placed on a microscope slide with a drop of physiological saline solution and observed under a microscope at 400× magnification. It is recommended to use a phase-contrast microscope, as this method provides more vivid images.
- **Application Method**: To obtain accurate results, it is essential to apply a minimal amount of material to the slide to avoid cell overlap. In addition to the saline solution preparation, the native specimen can be stained with a 0.1% methylene blue solution. It should be noted that the use of methylene blue, Gram, or Papanicolaou stains does not yield superior outcomes compared to the saline solution preparation.
- **Amine Test (Whiff Test)**: In cases of suspected bacterial vaginosis, an amine test (also known as Whiff Test) can be conducted. A drop of potassium hydroxide solution is placed on the slide. The presence of an unpleasant fishy odor indicates a positive test result, suggesting the presence of bacterial vaginosis.
- **Potassium Hydroxide (KOH) Preparation**: For vulvar preparations, a 10–15% potassium hydroxide solution can be used to dissolve horny scales, enhancing the identification of yeasts. However, this technique is not suitable for use with vaginal secretions (see Whiff Test).

3.4.4.2 Interpretation of the Native Vaginal Secretion Preparation

When examining the native preparation, it is essential to pay close attention to the following aspects:

- **Clean** Lactobacilli Flora: Does the sample exhibit a clean Lactobacilli flora (Figs. 3.1 and 3.2)?
- **Disturbed** Microbial Flora: Is there evidence of disturbed microbial flora?
- **Leukocyte Increase:** Is there an increase in leukocytes?
- **Clue Cells**: The presence of clue cells must also be considered.
- **Fungal Elements**: Are pseudohyphae, pseudomycelia, or germ cells (blastospores) present?
- **Trichomonas**: It is important to ascertain whether trichomonads are present.

The number of leukocytes per visual field provides insight into the nature of the process, whether inflammatory or noninflammatory. A urethral or cervical sample with a high leukocyte count is always classified as highly suspicious of infection. In the diagnosis of bacterial vaginosis, the detection of clue cells plays a decisive role. Additionally, the characteristic pear-shaped structures of trichomonads can be observed and dissolved by the addition of potassium hydroxide. The identification of pseudohyphae, pseudomycelia, or sprout cells is indicative of candidosis.

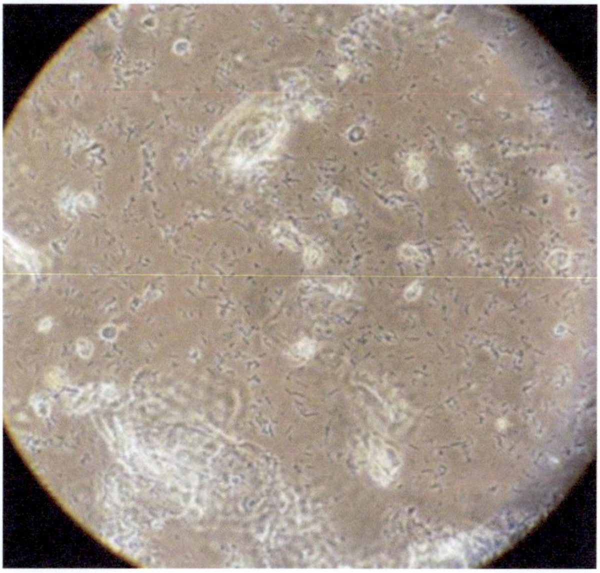

Fig. 3.1 Lactobacilli flora (magnification ×100). Numerous lactobacilli are discernible even at low magnification (Mylonas 2016)

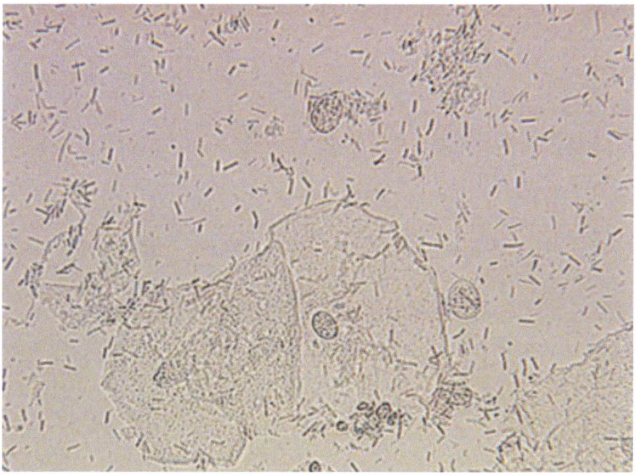

Fig. 3.2 Lactobacilli flora (magnification ×250) (Mylonas 2013, 2016)

For microbiological examination, it is crucial to prepare a Gram preparation for the laboratory. This can provide important information about the composition of the microbial flora and the degree of purity. However, the phase-contrast microscopic assessment of the native preparation is highly subjective. Deficiencies in the training of microscopic diagnostics have led to the development of standardized criteria for the fixed Gram preparation. The number of lactobacilli, gram-negative and gram-labile rods, and curved mobile rods is assessed at 1000x magnification using the Nugent score.

Although the Nugent score allows for more objective assessment of vaginal secretions, this method is rarely employed in most countries due to the time and resources required. This method also has methodological weaknesses, particularly regarding the significance of the "intermediate" finding.

3.4.5 Microbiological Tests

3.4.5.1 Indirect Microbiological Detection (Serological Testing)

Indirect microbiological detection refers to the identification and quantification of pathogen-specific antibodies in patient serum, thereby providing evidence of the host immune response to infection rather than direct pathogen isolation. This approach is particularly useful in diagnosing viral infections, slow-growing microorganisms, and pathogens that are challenging to culture in vitro. Serological testing enables detection of both acute and past infections by measuring different immunoglobulin classes: Immunoglobulin M (IgM) antibodies generally indicate recent or ongoing infection, whereas Immunoglobulin G (IgG) antibodies reflect prior exposure or chronic infection.

Qualitative serological assays determine the presence or absence of specific antibodies and are commonly employed as screening tools. Quantitative serological tests measure antibody titers, reflecting antibody concentration in serum, which can inform on the stage and intensity of the immune response. Interpretation of serological results requires consideration of several clinical factors, including the timing of specimen collection relative to symptom onset, potential cross-reactivity with related pathogens (serological cross-reactivity), and the patient's immunological status (e.g., immunosuppression). Confirmation with direct detection methods (e.g., PCR and culture) is often necessary to differentiate active infection from past exposure, especially when clinical decisions depend on accurate diagnosis.

3.4.5.2 Direct Microbiological Detection

Direct microbiological detection comprises various methodologies aimed at identifying the causative microorganisms themselves rather than relying on host immune markers.

Microscopic Examination

In gynecological and obstetric practice, phase-contrast microscopy of fresh specimens is a fundamental diagnostic tool that allows visualization of unstained biological structures such as bacteria, fungi, protozoa, and cellular alterations indicative of infection. This technique exploits differences in refractive indices among cellular components to generate high-contrast images without staining, enabling rapid evaluation at the bedside. Phase-contrast microscopy is a cost-effective and immediate method that facilitates detection of motile pathogens (e.g., *Trichomonas vaginalis*), assessment of specimen adequacy, and preliminary diagnosis to guide further testing or treatment.

Microbiological Cultivation and Antimicrobial Susceptibility Testing

Conventional culture methods remain indispensable for isolating viable pathogens and enabling detailed phenotypic characterization. Bacterial culture is routinely performed on selective and differential media under standardized incubation conditions; however, viral culture requires specialized cell lines and laboratory expertise, often limiting its routine use due to technical complexity and prolonged turnaround time.

The critical advantage of culture lies in obtaining pure isolates for species-level identification and comprehensive antimicrobial susceptibility testing (AST). AST employs standardized protocols—such as disk diffusion (Kirby-Bauer), broth microdilution, and agar dilution—to determine minimum inhibitory concentrations (MICs). These data inform clinicians on effective antimicrobial agents, optimizing therapeutic regimens amid rising antimicrobial resistance.

Point-of-Care Diagnostics

Point-of-care diagnostics (POC) are laboratory medical tests that are performed at the site of patient care and that yield actionable results within minutes. The temporal and spatial gap between specimen collection and result reporting is therefore substantially reduced. In gynecology and obstetrics, POC systems permit immediate diagnosis of STD, such as *Chlamydia trachomatis*, *Neisseria gonorrhoeae*, *Treponema pallidum*, and *Trichomonas vaginalis*, enabling initiation of therapy during the same patient encounter.

Modern POC systems are based on diverse detection technologies. Lateral-flow immunoassays (LFIA) rely on antigen–antibody reactions and produce rapid visual results by means of color development on test strips. These chromatographic methods use capillary flow and typically report results within 5–30 min. Microfluidic platforms integrate sample preparation, reaction and detection on miniaturized chips and demonstrate substantially higher analytical sensitivity than conventional lateral-flow tests. Molecular genetic approaches, for example, cartridge-based polymerase chain reaction (PCR) systems, achieve sensitivity comparable to laboratory nucleic acid amplification tests (NAATs) without extensive sample processing. Additional novel detection modalities include time-resolved fluorescence spectroscopy (TRF) with lanthanoid labels, which provide greater sensitivity than conventional fluorescence assays, as well as enzymatic, amperometric, and ion-selective electrode techniques.

Optimal POC system development is guided by the WHO ASSURED criteria (Affordable, Sensitive, Specific, User-friendly, Rapid and robust, Equipment-free, Delivered to those who need them). Multiplex assays enable simultaneous detection of multiple pathogens from a single specimen, a feature of particular relevance for common coinfections. Despite these advantages, POC implementation requires rigorous quality-assurance processes, appropriately trained personnel, and robust information-technology integration.

Matrix-Assisted Laser Desorption/Ionization Time-of-Flight Mass Spectrometry (MALDI-TOF MS)

MALDI-TOF MS technology has revolutionized microbial identification by enabling rapid, precise, and cost-efficient species-level identification of bacteria, yeasts, and certain filamentous fungi directly from culture isolates. Following minimal sample preparation involving protein extraction or direct smear application, microbial ribosomal proteins are ionized by laser desorption and their mass-to charge ratios detected. The resulting spectral fingerprint is matched against extensive reference databases to yield identification within minutes.

This method significantly reduces turnaround time compared to traditional biochemical assays and decreases per-sample costs after initial instrument acquisition. Its high-throughput capacity suits busy clinical microbiology laboratories, and continuous expansion of spectral libraries enhances detection capabilities for emerging or rare pathogens.

Molecular Biological Techniques

Molecular diagnostics have transformed pathogen detection through nucleic acid-based technologies, encompassing polymerase chain reaction (PCR), real-time quantitative PCR (qPCR), nucleic acid amplification tests (NAATs), and next-generation sequencing (NGS). These methods deliver rapid, sensitive, and specific detection of microbial DNA or RNA.

PCR and NAATs utilize primers or probes designed for target-specific amplification of minute quantities of microbial nucleic acids, allowing identification of non-cultivable or anatomically inaccessible organisms. Quantitative real-time PCR measures fluorescence signals proportional to template concentration, enabling:

- Monitoring viral load in chronic infections, such as HIV and hepatitis B or C, guiding therapy adjustments and prognosis.
- Assessing treatment efficacy by tracking reductions in pathogen nucleic acid levels.
- Evaluating disease severity, as higher initial nucleic acid loads often correlate with more severe clinical presentations.

Recent advances include extraction-free PCR protocols that bypass conventional nucleic acid purification by employing direct lysis reagents, thereby reducing assay turnaround time from approximately 2 h to 25–45 min without compromising sensitivity or specificity. These streamlined assays are effective across bacterial, fungal, and viral targets, facilitating rapid point-of care testing and high-throughput laboratory workflows.

Multiplex NAAT platforms enable simultaneous amplification and detection of multiple pathogens within a single reaction mixture. Syndromic panels targeting respiratory, gastrointestinal, and sexually transmitted infections enhance diagnostic efficiency by providing comprehensive pathogen profiles from a single clinical specimen. This approach is critical in conditions with overlapping symptomatology caused by diverse microorganisms.

Beyond targeted amplification, next-generation sequencing provides unbiased, high-throughput analysis of microbial communities (metagenomics) and pathogen genomes directly from clinical samples. Clinical applications include:

- Identification of rare or novel pathogens not detectable by conventional assays
- Detection of antimicrobial resistance genes to predict resistance phenotypes
- Outbreak investigation and strain typing through whole-genome comparisons

Emerging molecular techniques such as digital droplet PCR (ddPCR) partition samples into thousands of micro-reactions to achieve absolute quantification without reliance on standard curves, enhancing sensitivity and reproducibility for low-abundance targets.

Integration of molecular diagnostics with conventional microscopy, culture, and MALDI-TOF MS ensures a comprehensive diagnostic strategy that maximizes pathogen detection accuracy, accelerates result delivery, and informs targeted antimicrobial therapy in gynecology and obstetrics clinical practice.

3.4.6 Radiological Examinations

Imaging procedures such as sonography, X-ray, or computed tomography can aid in the localization of foci of infection.

Radiological examinations are generally not the primary diagnostic tools for STD, as most of these diseases are diagnosed through clinical evaluation and laboratory tests, including cultures, serological tests, and nucleic acid amplification tests. However, imaging studies can be useful in evaluating specific complications associated with STDs or in ambiguous clinical presentations. The following outlines relevant radiological examinations for STDs:

- **Relevant Radiological Examinations**.
  - **Ultrasound**.
    - Ultrasound is a vital tool for assessing pelvic inflammatory disease (PID), a common complication of untreated STDs, particularly caused by chlamydia and gonorrhea.
    - It can help visualize fluid collections, abscess formation, or signs indicative of tubo-ovarian abscesses.
    - In pregnant patients, ultrasound can evaluate fetal health and detect complications arising from STDs, such as congenital infections.
  - **Magnetic Resonance Imaging (MRI)**.
    - MRI is valuable for evaluating complicated pelvic pain or masses resulting from STDs.
    - It is particularly beneficial in diagnosing abscesses associated with severe PID when ultrasound findings are inconclusive.
    - Additionally, MRI can assess potential complications of STDs, such as lesions in the central nervous system resulting from neurosyphilis.

- **Computed Tomography (CT) Scan**.
  - CT imaging may be indicated for diagnosing complications of STDs, including PID or the presence of abscesses in the pelvic or peritoneal regions.
  - It can also reveal hepatobiliary complications associated with hepatitis or liver abscesses linked to STDs.
  - CT scans are useful for evaluating inguinal or pelvic lymphadenopathy, which may arise from various STDs, particularly in cases of nongonococcal urethritis or lymphogranuloma venereum.

- **Specific STDs and Associated Radiological Findings**.
  - **Gonorrhea and Chlamydia:** Ultrasound
    - May reveal thickened fallopian tubes, enlarged ovaries, or the presence of pelvic fluid associated with PID.
    - Can identify complications such as abscesses or peritonitis if they develop.
  - **Human Immunodeficiency Virus (HIV):** CT or MRI
    - Imaging may be warranted for opportunistic infections, such as pneumocystis pneumonia (PCP) or central nervous system infections in advanced HIV/AIDS cases.
    - Non-Hodgkin lymphoma, a malignancy often associated with HIV, may also be evaluated using imaging studies.
  - **Syphilis:** MRI/CT
    - In cases of neurosyphilis, imaging of the brain may show alterations, including meningovascular changes or involvement of cranial nerves.
    - CT scans may reveal cardiovascular complications such as aortitis in patients with tertiary syphilis.
  - **Herpes Simplex Virus (HSV):** MRI
    - Useful for assessing encephalitis or neurological complications stemming from HSV infection.
    - While pelvic ultrasound can visualize genital lesions, these are primarily diagnosed through clinical examination.
  - **Human Papillomavirus (HPV):** Colposcopy with Imaging
    - Although standard imaging is not used for HPV, imaging-guided biopsies may be utilized to evaluate suspicious lesions for cervical intraepithelial neoplasia (CIN) or invasive cervical cancer.

Radiological examinations play a supporting role in the evaluation of STDs, primarily aiding in the assessment of complications or cases with unclear diagnoses. The choice of imaging modality will depend on the suspected complications and the patient's clinical presentation. Laboratory tests remain the cornerstone of STD diagnosis and management.

3.4.7 Pathology

Biopsies can be taken to identify characteristic inflammatory reactions in the tissue and to detect the pathogen directly using specific antibodies. However, this is not always achievable for many microbiological agents.

3.5 Treatment

3.5.1 General

Treatment can be curative for infections caused by bacteria, fungi, or parasites. In the case of viral infections, only palliative or suppressive therapy is often possible. Patients should be informed of the necessary dosage and duration of intake. It is crucial to adhere to the recommended dosage and duration of medication, even if symptoms subside earlier than expected. Similarly, medication should not be discontinued without authorization due to side effects or shared with a sexual partner.

Patients must be informed of the potential side effects of various medications and the resulting behavior. If vomiting occurs within 1 h of taking the medication, the patient must be instructed to take the medication again.

Individuals diagnosed with a bacterial STD or trichomoniasis should refrain from unprotected sexual intercourse for 7 days following the conclusion of their treatment regimen.

In the event of suspected noncompliance, a single dose of a carefully chosen medication is preferable.

3.5.2 Challenges of Selecting the Right Drug for STD Treatment

The selection of an appropriate medication for treating STD involves several complex challenges that healthcare providers must consider to achieve optimal patient outcomes (Table 3.4). These challenges include:

Table 3.4 Challenges of selecting the right drug for STD treatment

Parameters	Description
Diversity of STDs	– Various types of STDs (bacterial, viral, parasitic) require differing therapeutic approaches – Unique treatment protocols and resistance patterns for each infection – Co-infections may necessitate combination therapy
Variability in clinical presentation	– Symptoms range from asymptomatic to severe – Delays in diagnosis complicate treatment decisions – Accurate diagnostic tools are not always available

(continued)

Table 3.4 (continued)

Parameters	Description
Antimicrobial resistance	– Resistance in pathogens like *Neisseria gonorrhoeae* complicates treatment – Local resistance patterns require ongoing surveillance – Treatment adjustments based on resistance trends can lead to inconsistencies
Pharmacokinetics and pharmacodynamics	– Drug absorption, distribution, metabolism, and excretion are crucial for efficacy – Pharmacokinetic variables affect dosing schedules and adherence – Complex regimens may overwhelm patients, impacting success
Individual patient factors	– Factors such as age, gender, immune status, allergies, and comorbidities influence therapy selection – Special considerations for pregnant and immunocompromised individuals – Comprehensive medical history evaluation is essential
Adverse effects and tolerability	– Side effects can impact compliance significantly – Common effects include gastrointestinal disturbances and allergic reactions – Providers must balance treatment risks and benefits while communicating with patients
Cost and accessibility	– Medication costs can be a barrier, especially for uninsured patients – Newer therapies may be financially prohibitive – Clinical efficacy must be balanced with affordability
Guideline variability	– Clinical practice guidelines vary among organizations/countries and evolve with new research – Variability can cause confusion and inconsistency – Continuous education about guidelines is necessary for effective implementation
Psychosocial considerations	– Emotional impact of diagnosis can hinder adherence – Patients may face stigma, anxiety, or isolation – Addressing psychosocial factors alongside medical management improves outcomes
Patient education and awareness	– Patients need clear information about their condition and the importance of adherence – Misinformation can lead to neglecting treatment regimens – Proper education empowers patients and encourages active participation in health management
Cultural and social factors	– Cultural perceptions affect patient behavior and willingness to seek help – Stigma may deter discussion of sexual health or pursuit of treatment – Addressing cultural barriers is crucial for improved outcomes
Impact of public health initiatives	– Public health policies shape treatment practices and testing accessibility – Effective initiatives promote awareness and timely intervention – Inadequate initiatives may result in underdiagnosis or delayed treatment

(continued)

Table 3.4 (continued)

Parameters	Description
Follow-up and recurrence management	– Regular follow-up is vital for managing recurrences effectively – Patients should be encouraged to attend follow-up visits for comprehensive care – Structured follow-up plans aid in adherence to treatment protocols
Regulatory and legal considerations	– Providers must navigate legal aspects of medication prescribing carefully – Compliance with local guidelines is crucial for safety – Understanding the legal context aids informed decision-making about treatment options
Emerging treatments and technologies	– The treatment landscape continuously evolves with new protocols – Integration of new therapies poses practical challenges – Continuous evaluation of new treatments' safety, efficacy, and cost-effectiveness is essential

The various challenges involved in choosing the right drug for STD treatment require a comprehensive, patient-centered approach. Overcoming these barriers necessitates collaboration between patients and healthcare providers, along with ongoing education and awareness initiatives.

By focusing on individualized care, informed decision-making, and understanding the broader context of public health, clinicians can improve treatment adherence, patient outcomes, and overall public health in the management of STDs. Continuous evaluation and adaptation to emerging trends and challenges will be essential for effective and equitable STD care.

3.6 Aftercare

Sexual partners of patients with an STD should be informed, diagnosed, and treated. The period and the partners to be informed should be determined according to the medical history and the incubation period of the pathogen (Table 3.5). It is the responsibility of the patient to inform their sexual partners about the disease.

In the absence of a sexual partner during the specified period, the individual's most recent sexual partner should be informed, tested, and treated. If all sexual partners have tested negative within the specified period, the last sexual partner should be informed, tested, and treated.

Informing the sexual partner is crucial as part of secondary prevention. The testing and treatment of the partner can prevent both the reinfection of the patient and

Table 3.5 Duration of infection and notification of sexual partners

Infection	Recommended period	Information
Chancroid	14 days	Sex partner
Chlamydia trachomatis	2–3 months	Sexual partner, newborn
Cmv (cytomegalovirus)	Now and in the future	Sex partner?
Genital herpes	Current and future partners	Sexual partner, newborn
Gonorrhea	2–3 months	Sexual partner, newborn
Hepatitis B	Variable	Sexual partners, newborns, own children, people in the same household
Hepatitis C	Variable	Sexual partners, newborns, own children, people in the same household
HIV	Variable (individual factors)	Sexual partner, newborn, own children
Hpv (human papillomavirus)	Current and future partners	Sex partner
Latent syphilis	One year	Sexual partner, newborn
Lymphogranuloma venereum	2–3 months	Sexual partner, newborn
Monkeypox	Now	Sex partner
Pid (pelvic inflammatory disease)	2–3 months	Sex partner
Primary syphilis	2–3 months	Sexual partner, newborn
Pubic lice	Now	Sex partner
Secondary syphilis	6 months	Sexual partner, newborn
Trichomoniasis	Now	Sex partner
Urethritis	2–3 months	Sex partner
Zika virus	Now	Sex partner

the further infection of other individuals. Detailed advice on viable avoidance strategies for STD is also available.

It is important to consider the potential psychosocial barriers the affected patient may face in informing their sexual partner.

Concerns may include fear of losing the partner, fear of domestic violence, fear of contacting an unknown sexual partner, or fear of legal consequences. Once these concerns are identified, an optimal solution should be sought, including informing the partner directly by the attending physician.

The consistent use of condoms can significantly reduce the spread of sexually transmitted diseases. Educating children and young people about sexuality, sexually transmitted infections, and sexual hygiene is crucial.

3.7 Practical Suggestions

- **Definition and Transmission**: STDs are characterized by their primary mode of transmission-sexual intercourse.
- **Diverse Symptoms and Effects**: STDs exhibit a wide range of symptoms and physical effects, varying from localized, asymptomatic conditions to severe, systemic, acute, and chronic ailments.
- **Stigma and Communication**: The stigma surrounding STDs can inhibit open discourse and essential preventive measures, resulting in suboptimal communication, misinformation, and increased risk of further transmission. Both patients and physicians often avoid the topic out of shame, which affects the quality of care.
- **Role of Healthcare Professionals**: Healthcare professionals have an opportunity to educate patients and modify behaviors. Open, honest discussions about STDs should be conducted with empathy for the psychosocial effects on patients. It is crucial to convey the opportunities for personal development and behavior change through preventative measures.

Equaliy in Care: All patients must be treated with equal respect and care, regardless of various personal attributes. Healthcare professionals have the responsibility to provide unbiased advice and support.

- **Evidence-Based Diagnosis and Treatment**: Diagnosis and treatment of STDs must be based on sound medical knowledge and objective evidence to provide the best possible care.
- **Extragenital Signs and Holistic Examination**: Extragenital signs and symptoms, such as rashes, fever, and swollen lymph nodes, may indicate STDs. Gynecologists must examine other body areas to identify these signs.

Focus on Medical Indicators: Evaluations should focus on medical indicators, excluding emotional or existential aspects to facilitate accurate diagnosis and adequate treatment

- **Vaccination Status**: Conversations about vaccination status should be incorporated into sexual health counseling to address immediate and future health issues.
- **Collaboration and Avoiding Embarrassment**: A collaborative approach avoiding embarrassment ensures effective treatment plans. The patient's well-being and full recovery should be prioritized over the physician's wisdom or skill.

- **Cost-Effectiveness Considerations**: While important, cost-effectiveness should not be overemphasized. The focus should be on delivering optimal patient care.
- **Public Health and Private Actions**: STDs represent the intersection of public health and private actions. Thus, prevention, early detection, and treatment must be topics of public discourse and private conversations between physicians and patients.

Combining Expertise and Empathy: Providing optimal care for patients with STDs requires profound medical knowledge, clinical expertise, and empathy.

Key Points

- Sexually transmitted diseases (STDs) are suspected in younger people with acute onset, indication of sexual contact, and previous similar clinical pictures.
- It is possible to transfer several STDs at the same time.
- The identification, classification, and utilization of clinical syndromes offer various benefits, including early detection, development of treatment strategies, prognosis, research and development, as well as education and awareness raising.
- However, there are also disadvantages to this approach, including the potential for generalization, diagnostic uncertainty, stigmatization, and a focus on symptoms.
- A symptom-oriented approach to characterizing the main symptoms and a detailed gynecological and sexual history are of paramount importance.
- Diagnosis is based on the clinical picture and clinical examination, which are then supplemented by laboratory tests such as microbiology, clinical chemistry, imaging, and pathology.
- The treatment is curative for bacteria, fungi, and parasites, while it is palliative or suppressive for viruses.
- It is of the utmost importance to educate patients and ensure their compliance.
- In addition to the aforementioned treatment, post-treatment care includes the provision of information and treatment for sexual partners, as well as the promotion of prevention through the use of condoms.
- It is of the utmost importance to promote an understanding of the uniqueness of STDs, to cultivate an empathetic and respectful approach, and to focus on medical facts rather than prejudices.

Part II

Clinical Syndromes

Vulvitis and Vaginitis

4

Abstract

Vulvitis and vaginitis are inflammatory conditions of the vulva or vagina that frequently present with symptoms such as pruritus, burning, edema, erythema, and increased discharge. The etiology of these conditions is multifactorial, including infections (such as candidosis), allergies, inadequate hygiene, or dermatoses. A comprehensive medical history and thorough examination are essential for accurate diagnosis, enabling appropriate treatment initiation according to the underlying cause. Emphasis should be placed on correctly diagnosing infections and considering the management of immune disorders, as in many cases, only symptomatic relief is possible. It is recommended that preventive measures be integrated into sex education curricula, particularly focusing on painful conditions such as genital herpes, bartholinitis, and noninfectious causes like lichen sclerosus. In cases of genital discharge, precise etiological determination is important, as symptoms may range from individual hygiene to specific infectious agents.

4.1 Background

Vulvitis refers to the inflammation of the vulva and vaginal introitus. The potential causes of vulvar discomfort can be categorized into three groups:

- **Endogenous Factors**: These are internal factors related to the body's own functions or imbalances. A common endogenous factor is estrogen deficiency, which can lead to irritation and inflammation of the vaginal and vulvar tissues. Other endogenous factors include systemic conditions such as diabetes and allergies.
- **Exogenous Factors**: Environmental and external factors like irritants and allergens can trigger skin irritation in the vulvar region. Medications and personal care products with allergens can cause allergic reactions. Poor hygiene can lead

I. Mylonas, *Sexually Transmitted Diseases*,
https://doi.org/10.1007/978-3-031-78204-6_4

to the accumulation of pathogens and irritants, contributing to inflammation and tissue damage. Bacterial, viral, or fungal infections commonly lead to vulvitis.

- **Descending Factors**: Substances or infections from other parts of the body can travel to the vulva, irritating it if they persist or contain infectious agents. Urinary incontinence or fistula leakage can also expose the vulvar area to moisture and irritants, promoting inflammation. Treating the primary source of the problem is often key to effectively treating vulvitis.

Complaints regarding the vulva and vaginal area are exceedingly prevalent, though not all can be attributed to infections. A thorough medical history, along with a meticulous examination, can facilitate the identification and management of many infectious conditions within the vulvovaginal region.

Vulvitis can be differentiated into two main categories:

- **Primary Infections:** Primary infections originate directly in the vulvar area and are not associated with infections elsewhere in the body. These may include:
  - **Yeast Infections:** Caused by an overgrowth of *Candida albicans* fungus, leading to itching, burning, and a thick white discharge.
  - **Bacterial Vaginosis:** Results from an imbalance of normal vaginal bacteria, often causing a fishy odor and gray discharge.
  - **Trichomoniasis:** A sexually transmitted infection caused by a parasite, leading to itching, discharge, and discomfort.
- **Isolated Vulvar Inflammation:** This category refers to inflammation occurring in the vulva without accompanying symptoms in other areas. Causes may include:
  - **Contact Dermatitis:** Irritation from products like scented soaps, detergents, or feminine hygiene products.
  - **Allergic Reactions:** To materials in clothing, spermicides, or other substances that come into contact with the vulva.
  - **Environmental Factors:** Such as prolonged moisture exposure from wet swimsuits or tight clothing.
  - **Skin Conditions:** Eczema or dermatitis localized to the vulvar area.

In some cases, additional symptoms such as painful swelling of the inguinal lymph nodes, dysuria, or dyspareunia may be present. Several diagnostic parameters and options are available for establishing a diagnosis (Table 4.1). The primary objective of any therapeutic intervention is to resolve the underlying condition. However, the effectiveness of therapeutic measures is contingent upon the specific cause or pathogen involved. While infectious conditions are typically easily treatable, immune disorders may present a challenge, often resulting in only partial improvement.

In addition to physical symptoms, *psychological issues* may arise, especially in the context of relationship conflicts, that necessitate resolution. It is advisable to

Table 4.1 Diagnostic approaches for suspected vulvitis or vaginitis

Diagnostic possibilities	Complaints	Comments
Medical history	Acute and short duration of complaints	– Generally indicates infection
		– Injury
		– Intolerance or allergy
	Chronic complaints	– Suggestive of a dermatosis
		– Chronic skin damage
		– Anatomical feature
		– Superinfected skin damage
	Type of complaints	– Itching: Typical of fungal infections
		– Dermatoses (lichen sclerosus, lichen planus)
		– Allergies
		– Skin dryness
		– Parasitic diseases
	Burning complaints	– Common symptom in infections (exception: Candidosis)
		– Lichen planus erosivus
		– Irritant dermatitis
		– Dermatoses
		– Autoimmune diseases
		– Skin damage
Diagnostics in practice	Clinical assessment	– Dermatoses
		– Superinfected skin damage
		– Ulcerating lesions
	Colposcopy	– Vulvitis, vaginitis, cervicitis, urethritis
	Speculum examination	– Vaginitis, cervicitis, urethritis
	Assessment of discharge	– Bacterial vaginosis
	pH value testing	– Bacterial vaginosis
	Microscopy	– Trichomonas, Candida, bacterial vaginosis
	Biopsy	– HPV, malignancy
Diagnostic assistance from a laboratory	Pathogen detection	– Streptococci, staphylococci, intestinal bacteria
	Histology	– Viruses (including human papillomavirus), dermatoses
	Inflammation parameters	– Ascending infection
		– Generalized infection

address the subject of infections and vulvar health with children and adolescents as part of a comprehensive sexuality education program. This should include information on sexually transmitted diseases and sexual hygiene.

Despite the diverse etiologies, the inflammatory response pattern is consistent, characterized by pruritus, burning pain, edema, erythema, and increased genital secretions.

4.2 Common Symptoms

4.2.1 Symptom: Itching

Candidosis (Chap. 36) is recognized as the most prevalent infectious etiology of isolated vulvar pruritus. It is estimated that approximately 20% of women serve as asymptomatic carriers of Candida species within their vaginal flora. The mere detection of Candida species in the absence of clinical symptoms bears no clinical significance outside of pregnancy, as the presence of Candida fungi is also found in normal vaginal secretions. In the differential diagnosis, lichen sclerosus should be considered. Less common causes include parasitic infections such as pediculosis pubis (Chap. 27) and scabies caused by *Sarcoptes scabiei* hominis (Chap. 28), which are primarily classified as noninfectious dermatoses and skin lesions.

Noninfectious dermatoses and skin lesions should also be considered in the differential diagnosis. Lichen sclerosus (Fig. 4.1) is recognized as the most prevalent itchy, inflammatory, and noninfectious dermatosis affecting the vulva. The primary early signs of this condition include persistent itching accompanied by delicate whitish changes of the prepuce, which may be associated with minor constriction of the vaginal canal. Additionally, lichen planus or its chronic variant, lichen planus erosivus, should also be considered in the differential diagnosis.

Vulvar itching may also be attributed to mechanical trauma to the skin. Some women may engage in excessive cleansing practices due to concerns regarding infections and the desire for genital cleanliness. As skin damage increases, it may lead to tearing or the development of persistent scales, resulting in burning discomfort.

Pruritus vulvae can arise from various noninfectious causes that must be addressed in the differential diagnosis (Table 4.2).

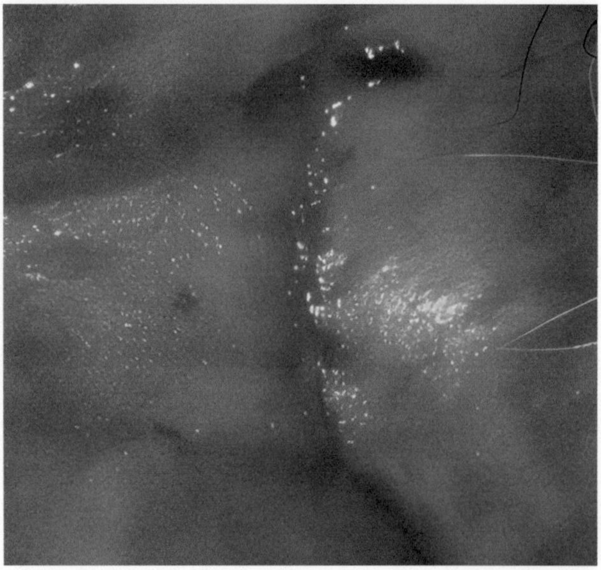

Fig. 4.1 Lichen sclerosus (Mylonas 2016)

Table 4.2 Etiologies of vulvar pruritus

Causes	Frequency	Pathogen
Infectious causes	More common	Candidosis
		Phthiriasis
		Scabies
	Rare	Condylomas (HPV)
		Erythrasma
		Molluscum contagiosum
		Syphilis
Dermatoses		Lichen sclerosus
		Lichen planus
		Lichen simplex
General causes	Frequently	Allergies
		Excessive hygiene
		Injuries
		Scratch marks
	Rare	Depression
		Partner conflict
		Psychogenic
		Sexual disorder

4.2.2 Symptom: Burning and Pain

The two most prevalent etiologies of pain and burning sensations are identified as genital herpes and Bartholin's pseudoabscess (Table 4.3). Genital herpes is recognized as one of the most painful conditions affecting the vulva, attributed to the significant inflammatory response it elicits. Less commonly, Streptococcus A and *Staphylococcus aureus* may also produce analogous symptoms. In patients manifesting symptoms without detectable pathogens, a microbiological swab from the introitus should be performed. However, the presence of intestinal bacteria should not be overstated, as these are typically found in the vulvar region and indicate mere nonpathogenic colonization from the anal area.

Bartholinitis, alternatively termed Bartholin's pseudoabscess, is characterized by localized inflammation of the duct of the apocrine Bartholin's gland, which is approximately 1–2 cm in length. The anatomical positioning of this duct in the vaginal introitus makes it susceptible to contamination from intestinal and vaginal bacteria. Symptoms typically present with an abrupt onset of painful erythema at the posterior commissure, accompanied by an increasingly painful inflammatory swelling of the excretory duct that may enlarge to the size of an egg, leading to protrusion of the labia and constriction of the introitus (Fig. 4.2). The patient may experience significant impairment in ambulation, sitting, and overall functionality. In the acute phase, conservative interventions such as red-light therapy and localized analgesia are recommended, with the consideration of broad-spectrum antibiotics if clinically warranted. Following either spontaneous rupture or surgical incision, relief is

Table 4.3 Causes of vulvar burning sensation and pain

Causes	Frequency	Pathogen
Infectious causes	More common	Abscess
		Acne inversa
		Bartholin's pseudoabscess
		Genital herpes
		Pyoderma fistulans
		Zoster
	Rare	Folliculitis
		Streptococci
		Trichomonads
Dermatoses		M. Adamantiades–Behçet
		Lichen planus erosivus
		Pemphigus
General causes	Frequently	Skin damage
		Injury
	Rare	Irritant dermatitis
		Toxic reaction

achieved through drainage of the inflamed pseudocyst and subsequent suturing of incision margins (marsupialization). Recurrent episodes of bartholinitis often lead to the formation of a Bartholin's retention cyst.

The most common causative organisms of pain and burning sensations are genital herpes and Bartholin's pseudoabscess.

Staphylococcus aureus is a ubiquitous bacterium recognized as the principal pathogen responsible for wound infections, abscess formation, and inflammation of hair follicles or sebaceous glands.

Folliculitis represents an inflammatory condition affecting the hair follicle, typically instigated by *Staphylococcus aureus* (Fig. 4.3). Inflammation involving a hair follicle or sebaceous gland with central necrosis is designated as a furuncle, whereas an extensive and confluent inflammatory process affecting multiple furuncles is termed a carbuncle. Diagnosis is established through clinical findings. Management generally includes the application of local antiseptics or the administration of systemic cephalosporins. Surgical incision is warranted in cases of boils or carbuncles, followed by antiseptic care. Vulvitis attributable to Streptococcus is relatively uncommon. However, in young girls, this pathogen is frequently implicated as the primary cause of vulvitis. If these bacteria are detected in the genital region, even in the absence of clinical symptoms, a course of oral antibiotics, such as penicillin for a duration of 10 days, is warranted (prevention of the severe life-threatening Toxic Shock Syndrome (TSS)). Post-treatment evaluation is critical to ensure the eradication of the pathogen.

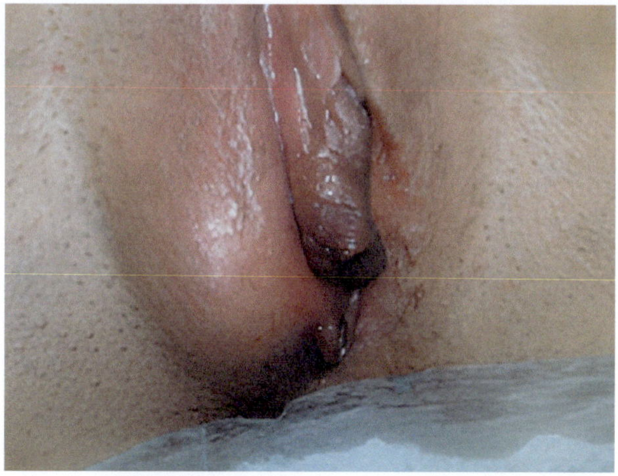

Fig. 4.2 Bartholin's pseudoabscess (Mylonas 2010)

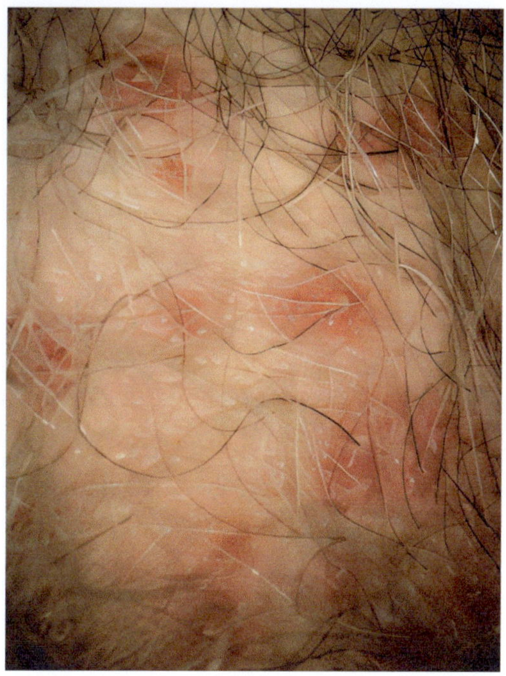

Fig. 4.3 Folliculitis attributed to Staphylococcus aureus (Mylonas and Petersen 2009)

4.2.3 Symptom: Ulcers

Ulcers of the external female genitalia are indicative of chancroid, syphilis, granuloma inguinale, and lymphogranuloma inguinale (Table 6.1), even though these diseases are relatively uncommon in most of the developed countries. Due to the pronounced local and systemic symptoms, differential diagnostic considerations must be made with a detailed medical history, including sexual history, and, if necessary, laboratory tests (Chap. 3).

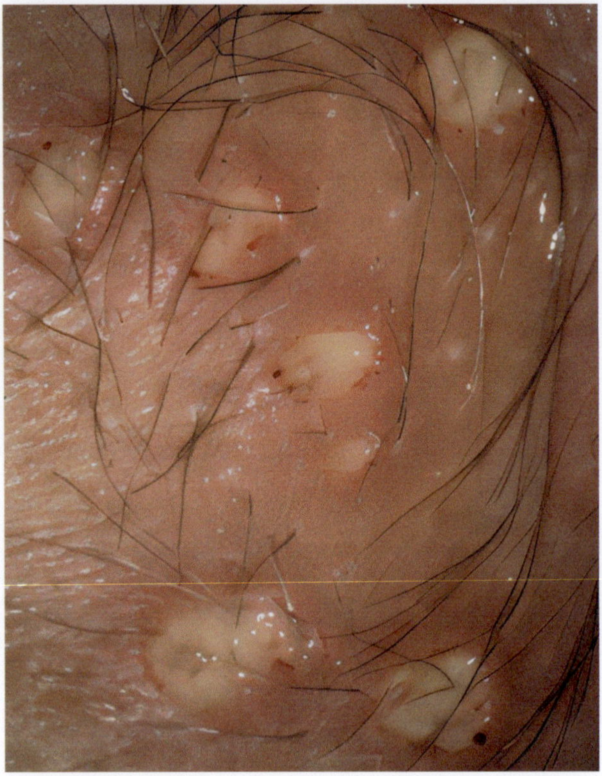

Fig. 4.4 Adamantiades-Behçet disease (Mylonas and Petersen 2009)

Additionally genital herpes (Chap. 20) can manifest as ulcerations, although these efflorescences are more likely to be regarded as erosions. Additionally, basal cell carcinomas, squamous cell carcinomas, Adamantiades–Behçet disease (Fig. 4.4), skin defects caused by scratching in lichen sclerosus, aphthosis, and other chronic inflammatory or scarring processes should be considered in the differential diagnosis.

4.2.4 Symptom: Vulvar Changes Without Symptoms

Vulvar disease can also occur without characteristic symptoms. Patients typically seek medical attention due to concerns about the appearance of their vulva. Occasionally, patients may present with vague complaints during sexual intercourse. In addition to the more common forms of genital warts (Fig. 4.5), it is important to consider the possibility of fibromas and genital malignancies.

Vulvovaginal diseases such as Condylomata acuminata can also occur without characteristic symptoms.

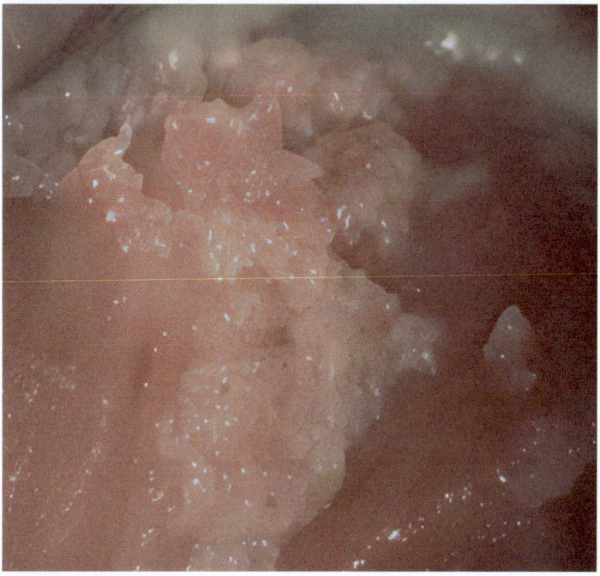

Fig. 4.5 Condylomata acuminata (Mylonas 2016)

4.2.5 Symptom: Vaginal Discharge

Genital discharge constitutes a frequent concern for many women, often perceived primarily as an undesirable odor or a persistent sensation of moisture. Although physiologic vaginal secretions vary across the menstrual cycle and reproductive states, abnormal discharge may represent an underlying pathological process and warrants clinical evaluation (see Figs. 4.6 and 4.7).

Infectious etiologies account for a large proportion of symptomatic vaginitis. The most common infectious causes are vulvovaginal candidiasis (Chap. 36), bacterial vaginosis (Chap. 35), and trichomoniasis (Chap. 23). Other bacterial pathogens—such as *Staphylococcus aureus*, group A streptococci (GAS), and group B streptococci (GBS)—may also produce vaginitis with purulent or abnormal discharge. Noninfectious causes (e.g., foreign bodies, contact dermatitis from topical agents, desquamative inflammatory vaginitis, and atrophic vaginitis) should be considered if microbiological testing is unrevealing.

Because clinical symptomatology is nonspecific, etiological classification of vaginitis requires microbiological or cytological evidence. Laboratory investigations commonly include microscopic examination of wet mounts (with saline and KOH), pH testing, whiff test, Gram stain, culture, antigen detection, or nucleic acid amplification tests (NAATs) as appropriate to the suspected pathogen. Treatment should be guided by the identified organism and, where relevant, by antimicrobial susceptibility results (antibiogram). Empiric therapy may be instituted in selected cases when immediate treatment is indicated and the pretest probability of a specific diagnosis is high, but targeted therapy is preferred whenever possible.

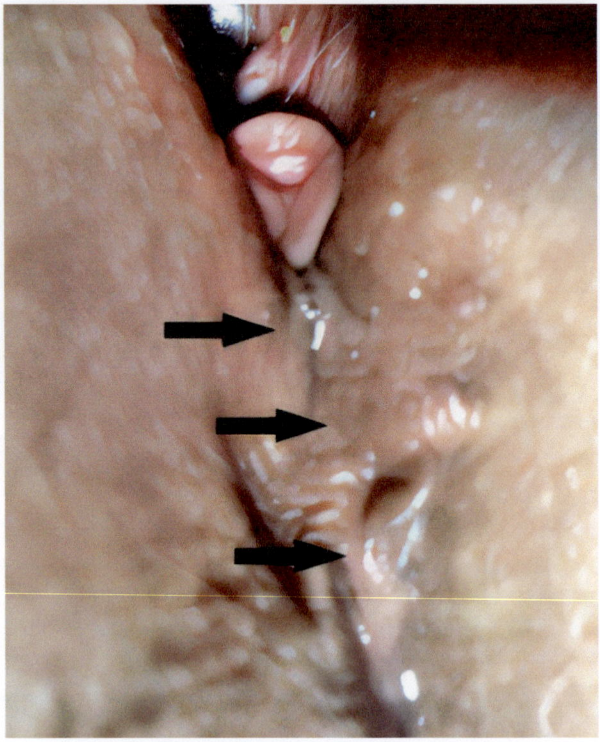

Fig. 4.6 Pronounced genital discharge extending from the vagina to the perianal region under initial examination conditions (Mylonas 2016)

A thorough history and directed symptom review are essential. Clinicians should document the onset, duration, quantity, and temporal pattern of the discharge, and whether it is cyclic or related to sexual activity. Characterization of the discharge—color (white, gray, yellow, green, and bloody), consistency (creamy, curd-like, frothy, thin, and mucoid), and odor (malodorous, fishy, foul, and absent)—is diagnostically informative. Associated symptoms such as vulvar or vaginal pruritus, dysuria, dyspareunia, vulvar burning, pelvic pain, and systemic signs (fever) should be elicited. A focused sexual history—including recent new or multiple partners, condom use, and partner symptoms—must be obtained because of implications for sexually transmitted infections and partner management.

Assessment of personal care practices and exposures is also important. Patients should be asked about menstrual products, intravaginal devices, topical medications, use of vaginal douches, deodorants, perfumed soaps, lubricants, and contraceptive methods (including intrauterine devices). Recent antibiotic use, immunosuppression (including diabetes mellitus and corticosteroid therapy), pregnancy status, and hormone therapy should be recorded because these factors alter vaginal flora and susceptibility to specific infections.

Physical examination should include inspection of the external genitalia, speculum examination of the vagina and cervix, and bimanual palpation when indicated. Findings such as erythema, erosions, visible discharge characteristics, cervical

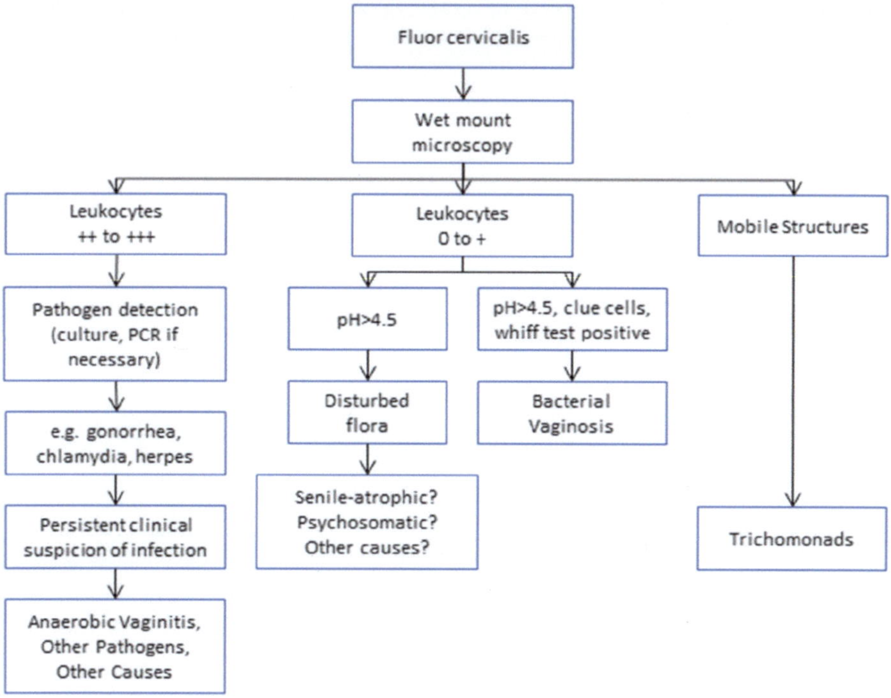

Fig. 4.7 Procedure for managing cervicitis discharge. (Courtesy of I. Mylonas)

exudate, adnexal tenderness, or pelvic masses will direct further diagnostic testing and management.

4.2.6 Symptom: Skin Lesions on the External Genitals

Skin eruptions on the vulva can have various causes and are a common symptom in gynecological practice. These lesions may manifest as redness, vesicles, pustules, or ulcerations and are often indicative of underlying infectious diseases, including sexually transmitted diseases (Table 4.4). Infections such as genital herpes and syphilis typically present with characteristic skin lesions on the vulva. Moreover, bacterial infections like bacterial vaginosis or vulvovaginal candidosis can also result in efflorescence, manifesting as pruritus, burning, and unusual discharge.

Diagnosis and treatment of vulvar and vaginal symptoms and diseases require meticulous clinical examination, often accompanied by specific tests to identify the pathogen. Treatment is contingent upon the specific cause. Potential treatments include antiviral medications, antibiotics, or other targeted therapies. It is essential to consider differential diagnostic considerations when examining skin manifestations (Table 4.4), as diverse diseases can manifest on the vulva.

Table 4.4 Vulvar disorders classified by observed lesions

Efflorescence	Diseases
Blisters	– Chickenpox, contact dermatitis, herpes simplex, herpes zoster
Bullae	– Bullous pemphigoid, impetigo contagiosa, pemphigus vegetans, pemphigus vulgaris
Erythema	– Fixed drug exanthema (acute), intertrigo, psoriasis inversa (synonym: Psoriasis intertriginosa), trichomoniasis, vulvar vestibulitis
Erythema plus lichenification	– Atopic dermatitis, contact dermatitis (chronic), seborrheic dermatitis, tinea cruris
Erythema plus edema	– Bacterial infection, contact dermatitis (acute), erysipelas, fungal infection, gonorrhea, phlegmon
Nodules	– Acrochordon (fibroepithelial polyp), angiofibroma, dermatofibroma, fibroma, fibromyoma, hydradenoma papilliferum, malignant melanoma of the vulva, scabies, syphilis, syringoma
Edema	– Angioedema, Crohn's disease, lymphedema, lymphogranuloma venereum
Papules	– Angiokeratoma, caruncle of the urethra, Fordyce spots (sebaceous hyperplasia), hemangioma, lichen planus, lymphangioma, melanocytic nevus, metastases, molluscum contagiosum, pyogenic granuloma, seborrheic keratosis
Plaques	– Extramammary Paget's disease, leukoplakia, lichen sclerosus, lichen simplex chronicus (squamous cell hyperplasia), plasma cell vulvitis (Zoon's disease), psoriasis
Proliferative papules and/or plaques	– Condylomas (anogenital warts), syphilis, verrucous carcinoma
Ulcerative papules and/or plaques	– Basal cell carcinoma, erosive lichen planus, squamous cell carcinoma
Pustules	– Bacterial infection, fungal infection, hidradenitis suppurativa
Pain in the genital area	– Vulvodynia
Pigmentary changes	– Acanthosis nigricans, benign vulvar melanosis and lentiginosis, erythrasma, functional melanocytic nevus, lentigo simplex, malignant melanoma of the vulva, post-inflammatory hyperpigmentation or hypopigmentation, treponematoses, vitiligo
Ulcers	– Aphthous ulcers, chancroid, genital herpes, granuloma inguinale, lymphogranuloma venereum, M. Adamantiades–Behçet, pyoderma gangraenosum

Key Points

- Vulvitis and vaginitis are inflammatory conditions of the vulva or vagina that commonly present with symptoms like itching, burning, edema, erythema, and increased discharge. The etiology of these conditions can include infections, allergies, inadequate hygiene, or dermatoses.
- Vulvitis is classified as primary infections or isolated inflammation of the vulva, and it can be differentiated from other conditions by medical history and symptoms.
- Painful swelling of the inguinal lymph nodes, dysuria, or dyspareunia may also occur in vulvitis cases.
- Diagnostic parameters, such as clinical examination and tests, can help in making a diagnosis and initiating appropriate treatment.
- Treatment effectiveness depends on the specific cause or pathogen involved, with infections being usually treatable.
- Psychological issues related to relationship conflicts may also arise and require resolution.
- It is recommended to address infections and the vulva in children and adolescents as part of sexuality education, including information on sexually transmitted diseases and sexual hygiene.
- Symptoms of vulvitis, such as itching, can be caused by candidosis, lichen sclerosus, or noninfectious causes like mechanical injuries or excessive washing.
- Burning and pain can be caused by genital herpes, Bartholin's pseudoabscess, or bacterial infections like folliculitis or vulvitis caused by Streptococcus.
- Ulcers on the external genitalia may indicate various conditions like chancroid, syphilis, granuloma inguinale, and lymphogranuloma inguinale.
- Vulvar changes without symptoms can occur, and it is important to consider the possibility of genital warts, fibromas, or genital malignancies.
- Genital discharge can be caused by infections like vulvovaginal fungal infections, bacterial vaginosis, or trichomoniasis.
- Skin lesions on the external genitals can indicate underlying infectious diseases, including STD like genital herpes or syphilis, as well as bacterial infections like bacterial vaginosis or vulvovaginal candidosis.
- Differential diagnosis is necessary for accurate identification of the underlying condition.

Genital Discharge

5

Abstract

Genital discharge is a prevalent symptom that may indicate various gynecological diseases. The etiology of increased discharge can reside in different regions of the genital tract, with infections being the predominant cause. Diagnosis is achieved through a comprehensive medical history and clinical examination to facilitate appropriate treatment. Differentiation is essential among vaginal, cervical, uterine, tubal, and urethral origins of the discharge. The characteristics of the secretions—such as color, consistency, and odor—must also be evaluated. Basic hygiene measures can serve as useful preventive strategies. Additionally, noninfectious etiologies, including hormonal fluctuations or foreign bodies, may also contribute to increased discharge. Precise clarification is substantial to address not only the symptoms but also the underlying conditions.

5.1 Background

An accurate diagnosis is indispensable for effective management of vaginal discharge. This condition can arise from multiple factors, including infections, hormonal changes, and noninfectious causes. Each underlying causative factor necessitates a distinct treatment approach. Administering treatment for vaginal discharge without appropriate diagnosis can result in ineffective or unsuitable management, extended patient discomfort, and potential complications.

- **Targeted Treatment**: Different etiologies of vaginal discharge require specific interventions. Conditions such as bacterial vaginosis, vulvovaginal candidosis, and trichomoniasis are prevalent causes but necessitate distinct antimicrobial or antifungal therapies. By accurately identifying the underlying etiology, healthcare professionals can prescribe the appropriate medication to effectively eradicate the infection and alleviate symptoms.

I. Mylonas, *Sexually Transmitted Diseases*,
https://doi.org/10.1007/978-3-031-78204-6_5

- **Avoiding Unnecessary Treatment**: Accurate diagnosis prevents unnecessary therapy. In certain instances, vaginal discharge may stem from noninfectious origins, such as hormonal alterations or foreign objects. In the absence of a precise diagnosis, patients might receive antibiotics or antifungals that do not address the underlying issue, potentially disrupting the natural balance of the vaginal microbiota. Unwarranted treatment can lead to adverse effects and antibiotic resistance, emphasizing the necessity of identifying the causative agent prior to therapy initiation.
- **Preventing Complications**: Infections leading to vaginal discharge, if left untreated or inadequately managed, can result in complications. For instance, untreated bacterial vaginosis can elevate the risk of preterm labor and postpartum infections. Similarly, untreated sexually transmitted diseases (STD) such as chlamydia or gonorrhea can lead to pelvic inflammatory disease (PID) and subsequent infertility issues. Accurate diagnosis ensures timely detection and appropriate intervention for these infections, thus mitigating the risk of complications.
- **Patient Education and Counseling**: An accurate diagnosis not only facilitates treatment but also empowers healthcare professionals to deliver essential education and counseling to patients. By understanding the etiology of their vaginal discharge, patients can learn about infection prevention, personal hygiene practices, and lifestyle modifications to decrease recurrence risks. Education fosters patient engagement in their care and enhances adherence to prescribed therapies.
- **Identifying Underlying Conditions**: Vaginal discharge may sometimes signify an underlying medical condition, such as hormonal imbalances or malignancies. Accurate diagnosis enables healthcare professionals to identify associated conditions or risk factors, allowing for comprehensive evaluation and management.

5.2 Genital Discharge

Genital discharge is a common presenting symptom that may reflect a spectrum of gynecologic and urologic conditions. Increased mucus production can originate from the lower genital tract—vagina, cervix, and urethra—or from the upper genital tract, including the endometrium and adnexa (fallopian tubes and ovaries); distinguishing the anatomical source is essential because it directs the diagnostic approach and management (Table 5.1).

Infectious processes and microbial colonization are the predominant causes of abnormal discharge, with sexually transmitted organisms among the most important pathogens to consider. Noninfectious causes—such as foreign bodies, atrophic vaginitis, contact dermatitis from topical agents or spermicides, desquamative inflammatory vaginitis, and neoplasia—must also be considered when microbiological testing is unrevealing or clinical features are atypical.

Table 5.1 Characteristics of vaginal discharge

Suspected diagnosis	Consistency	Color	Odor
Bacterial vaginosis	Low viscosity	White-gray	Fishy
Candidosis	Creamy and cheesy	Whitish-yellow	None, musty
Cervical polyps	Medium	Clear (sometimes with a bloody tinge)	None
Chlamydia trachomatis	Medium	Glassy-clear	None
Ectopy	Medium	Clear (sometimes with a bloody tinge)	None
Escherichia coli and other intestinal bacteria	Thin to thick	Greenish	Putrid, sulfurous, slightly musty
Foreign body	Thin to thick	Brownish	Foul-smelling
Gonorrhea	Creamy	Yellowish, purulent	Foul-smelling
Malignoma	Watery	Brown-bloody	Putrid
Parasites	Low viscosity	Yellowish-clear	None, possibly musty
Trichomoniasis	Foamy	Greenish-yellow	Fetid
Tuberculosis	Yellowish	Crumbly	None, possibly foul-smelling

Accurate differential diagnosis requires careful characterization of the discharge (volume, color, consistency, odor, and timing) and a focused clinical examination that includes inspection of the external genitalia, speculum evaluation of the vagina and cervix, and, when indicated, bimanual palpation to assess for uterine or adnexal tenderness or masses. Adjunctive testing—wet-mount microscopy (saline and KOH), pH measurement, whiff test, Gram stain, culture, and nucleic acid amplification tests—should be selected according to the suspected anatomical site and likely pathogens.

Because vaginal and cervical discharges are the most frequent clinical presentations encountered, they are often the initial focus of evaluation; however, clinicians should remain vigilant for signs suggesting upper-tract involvement (e.g., abnormal uterine bleeding, pelvic pain, fever, and cervical motion tenderness) or non-genital sources (e.g., urinary tract infection and proctitis). A systematic, anatomy-based approach ensures appropriate investigation, targeted therapy, and prevention of complications.

Localizations of Genital Discharge:

- Vestibular discharge
- Vaginal discharge
- Cervical discharge
- Uterine discharge
- Tubal discharge
- Urethral discharge

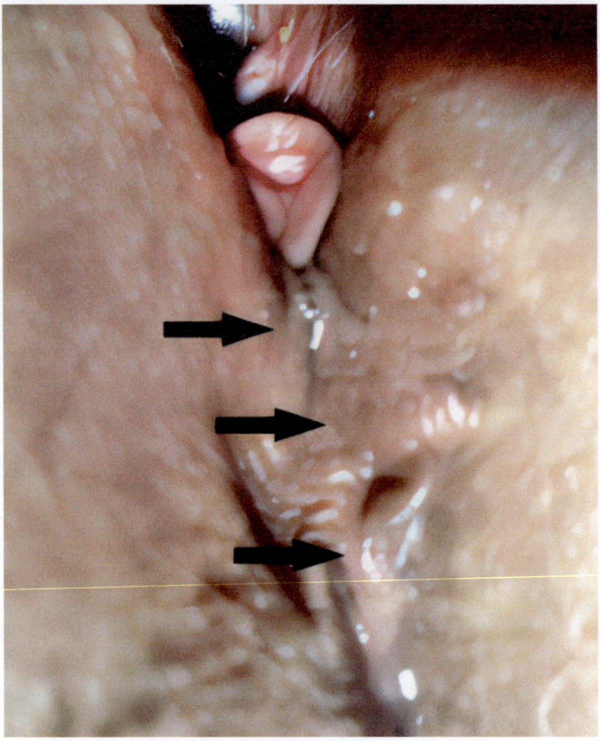

Fig. 5.1 Pronounced genital discharge extending from the vagina to the perianal region under initial examination conditions (Mylonas 2016)

For some women, genital discharge is experienced primarily as an aesthetic concern, most commonly reported as malodour and a persistent sensation of wetness (Fig. 5.1). A focused history should quantify the volume and document the duration and temporal pattern of the discharge (continuous, intermittent, cyclical, or postcoital). Detailed description of color and consistency (e.g., watery, mucoid, frothy, curd-like, and purulent), the presence and character of any odor, and associated symptoms—vulvar or vaginal pruritus, burning, dysuria, dyspareunia, or pelvic pain—must be elicited because these features narrow the differential diagnosis and affect urgency of management. Personal care practices that alter the vulvovaginal environment should be reviewed, including frequency and type of genital cleansing, use of perfumed soaps, cosmetics, intravaginal products or douches, menstrual products, and recent self-treatments. Documentation of recent antibiotics, contraceptive methods, gynecologic procedures, pregnancy status, and sexual exposures is also essential, as these factors modify vaginal flora and influence diagnostic and therapeutic decisions.

5.2.1 Vaginal Discharge

Physiological vaginal secretions maintain a consistent acidic pH between 3.8 and 4.4, are enriched with lactobacilli, contain numerous vaginal epithelial cells, present few to no leukocytes, and are typically odorless. This vaginal environmental system's stability is maintained by lactic acid-producing bacteria (lactobacilli). Disruption to this regulatory mechanism diminishes the physiological protective capacity, facilitating the development of inflammation.

The normal vaginal environment is characterized by:

- pH value < 4.5
- Adequate lactobacilli (assessed via wet mount microscopy)
- Abundant vaginal epithelial cells (assessed via wet mount microscopy)
- Absence of leukocytes (assessed via wet mount microscopy)
- Odorless vaginal discharge
- No subjective complaints
- Lack of inflammation signs

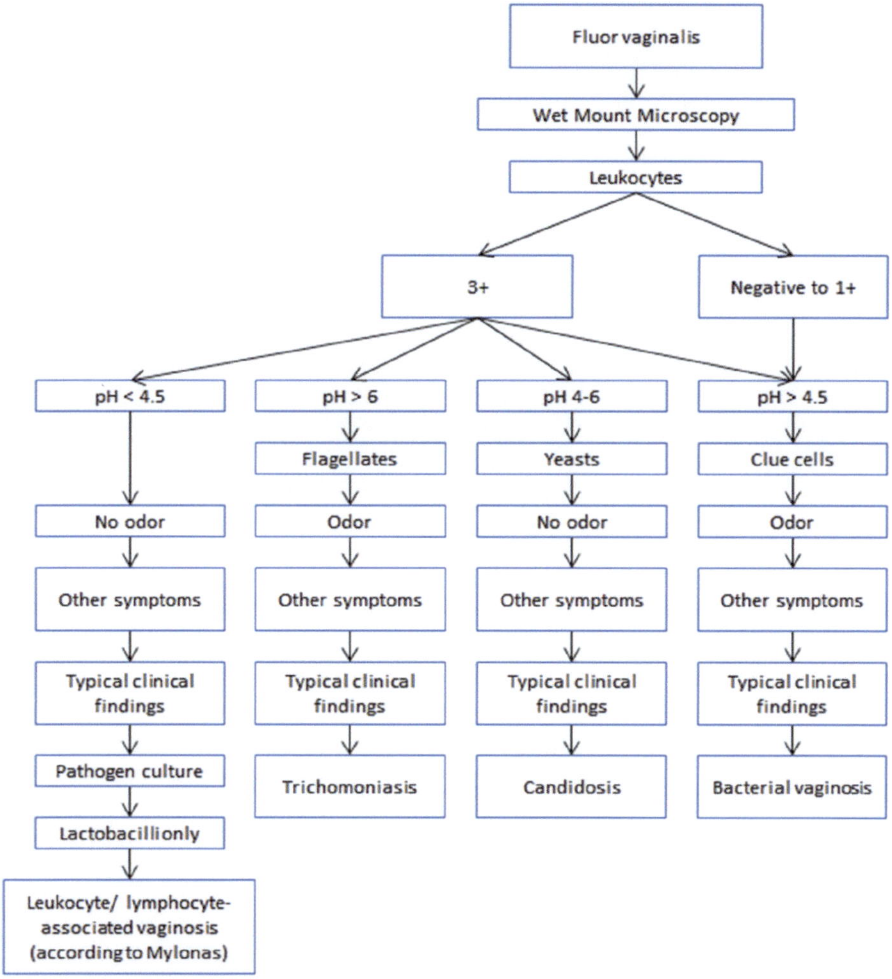

Fig. 5.2 Vaginal discharge treatment algorithm. (Courtesy of I. Mylonas)

Table 5.2 Localization of genital discharge and potential etiologies

Localization	Cause	Comments
Vestibular discharge	Neurovegetative	Increased secretion from vestibular (Bartholin's and Skene's) glands
	Transudation discharge	Mucoid plasma transudate providing lubrication during sexual arousal
Vaginal discharge	Infectious	Includes bacterial vaginosis, candidosis, trichomoniasis, and other bacterial vaginitis
	Estrogen deficiency	Fluor albus (leukorrhea), perimenopausal discharge related to decreased estrogen levels
	Foreign body vaginitis	Common in children; caused by retained tampons, pessaries, or other foreign objects
	Misconduct	Irritation from intimate sprays, douches, or chemical irritants
	Transudation discharge	Occurs during sexual arousal; neurovegetative mechanism
	Desquamation discharge	Increased epithelial cell shedding due to elevated estrogen and progesterone levels (e.g., pregnancy)
	Fluor neonatorum	Physiological discharge in newborns due to withdrawal of maternal placental estrogens; no pathological value
	Psychological causes	Stress-related changes influencing discharge
Cervical discharge	Functional-hormonal	Physiological pre-ovulatory mucus, premenstrual thicker mucus, and cervical hypersecretion
	Infectious	*Chlamydia trachomatis*, *Neisseria gonorrhoeae*, and genital herpes virus infections
	Organic changes	Cervical ectopy, cervical carcinoma, and cervical lacerations
	Psychological causes	Stress-induced alterations
Uterine discharge	Infectious	Pyometra and acute and chronic endometritis
	Organic changes	Endometrial carcinoma, endometrial polyps, and degenerating fibroids
Urethral discharge	Infectious urethritis	Chlamydia and gonorrhea most common; other pathogens (Mycoplasma, Gardnerella, and streptococci) rarely cause significant discharge

Accurate diagnosis of vaginal discharge is essential to ensure appropriate and timely management (Fig. 5.2). Careful assessment of the discharge's appearance and consistency provides useful preliminary diagnostic clues during clinical evaluation (Table 5.2). Clinical patterns should prompt targeted point-of-care testing (pH measurement, whiff/amine test, saline, and KOH microscopy) and appropriate laboratory investigations (Gram stain, culture, and nucleic acid amplification tests) to confirm the suspected etiologic agent and guide therapy.

In relation to the prevalence of infectious vaginitis in the United States, the following statistics have been reported:

- 40–50% have bacterial vaginosis
- 20–25% have vulvovaginal candidosis
- 15–20% have trichomoniasis

Estimates show that 50% of women up to the age of 25 will experience at least one medically diagnosed case of vaginal candidosis. In the United States, two to three million women are diagnosed with trichomoniasis annually, and 20–40% of women attending specialty clinics present with bacterial vaginosis. Noninfectious causes of genital discharge also merit consideration, which include:

- Physiological secretion
- Desquamative inflammatory vaginitis
- Atrophic vaginitis

Additional causes may involve mechanical factors (e.g., foreign bodies) or chemical irritants. Malignant conditions may also contribute to increased discharge, particularly postmenopausal or brownish-bloody discharge, which requires further investigation, potentially through histological examination.

Given the extensive differential diagnosis for vaginal discharge, no symptomatic treatment should be prescribed without a prior diagnosis.

5.2.2 Cervical Discharge

The cervix, composed of a single-layered cylindrical epithelium, is less protected against pathogens compared to the multilayered epithelium of the vulva and vagina. Various factors may induce or modulate cervicitis with associated cervical discharge.

Typical etiologies for cervicitis include:

- Primary infections (e.g., *Chlamydia trachomatis*, *Neisseria gonorrhoeae*, trichomonads, fungi, herpes simplex virus, HPV)
- Cervical pathologies (e.g., erosion, cervical laceration, cervical polyps)
- Ascending vaginal infections (e.g., bacterial vaginosis)
- Psychogenic factors (e.g., libido issues, anorgasmia)

Cervical discharge resulting from an infectious cervicitis is characteristically marked by a significant elevation in leukocyte count, reflecting the intense local immune response within the endocervical canal. Microscopic examination of endocervical secretions typically reveals numerous polymorphonuclear leukocytes, often exceeding 30 cells per high-power field, and may include visible epithelial cell debris and mucus strands. Quantifying leukocytosis in the discharge not only supports the diagnosis of active infection but also helps distinguish infectious cervicitis from noninfectious cervical irritation or physiological mucus variations.

Accurate identification of the causative pathogen is essential for devising an effective treatment plan. Sampling should include separate endocervical swabs for nucleic acid amplification tests (NAATs), culture, and, when indicated, viral PCR assays. Speculum-aided visualization allows direct assessment of mucosal friability, ulcerations, or exudates, while adjunctive tests—such as point-of-care microscopy and pH determination—aid in ruling out concomitant vaginal infections that may contribute to overlapping symptoms.

Epidemiological surveillance data on cervical infections are limited. Clinical studies and surveillance reports consistently identify *Chlamydia trachomatis* as the most prevalent etiologic agent. *Chlamydial cervicitis* often presents subclinically, with minimal overt discharge, yet poses significant risks for ascending infection and subsequent pelvic inflammatory disease. Asymptomatic carriage rates among sexually active women may exceed 5–10%, underscoring the need for routine screening in high-risk populations and pregnant patients.

Herpes simplex virus type II (HSV-2) is another major contributor to cervical inflammation and discharge. Primary HSV-2 cervicitis frequently manifests with copious serosanguinous or clear mucoid exudate, accompanied by ulcerative lesions on the ectocervix. Recurrent HSV-2 episodes tend to produce less discharge but still warrant targeted antiviral therapy to reduce viral shedding and transmission risk.

Human papillomaviruses (HPV), particularly high-risk oncogenic strains, can induce subtle mucosal changes that predispose to increased cervical secretions. While HPV-associated discharge is typically scant and nonpurulent, persistent infections may lead to cervical dysplasia, warranting colposcopic evaluation for abnormal squamocolumnar junction changes and biopsy of suspicious areas.

Protozoan and fungal organisms—including *Trichomonas vaginalis* and Candida species—often coexist with primary cervical pathogens but seldom act as lone causative agents of cervicitis. Trichomonads may be detected in cervical specimens alongside urethral or vaginal involvement, producing a frothy, greenish discharge. Similarly, Candida overgrowth may accompany cervicitis in patients with immunosuppression or biomechanical disruption but is distinguished by its characteristic thick, white "cottage cheese" appearance and pruritic symptoms.

Neisseria gonorrhoeae, while less common in many regions due to widespread screening and treatment programs, remains a classic cause of purulent cervical discharge. Gonococcal exudate is typically yellow to green, profuse, and associated with pronounced cervical erythema and friability. Confirmatory diagnosis relies on NAAT or culture on selective media, and treatment must address potential co-infections with Chlamydia.

Pathogens Associated with Cervicitis:

- Chlamydia trachomatis (serotypes D–K)
- Neisseria gonorrhoeae
- Genital herpes
- Treponema pallidum
- Human papillomaviruses (HPV)
- Other pathogens (e.g., Staphylococcus, Streptococcus, Enterobacteriaceae, anaerobes, and mycoplasmas)

5.2.3 Urethral Discharge

Isolated urethritis is defined as an inflammatory response of the urethral mucosa, which may manifest with or without overt urinary symptoms. Clinically, many patients present with urethral discharge, which varies in appearance from a clear, mucoid exudate to a turbid or purulent fluid. Commonly associated symptoms include dysuria, characterized by a burning sensation during micturition, and urethral pruritus, an itching localized at the urethral meatus. Upon physical examination, expression of discharge from the urethral orifice may be elicited by gentle compression. Microscopic evaluation of urethral swabs typically reveals an elevated number of polymorphonuclear leukocytes, indicating active inflammation.

The predominant causative agent of urethritis is *Neisseria gonorrhoeae*, which induces a marked mucosal inflammatory reaction accompanied by profuse, purulent urethral discharge, mucosal erythema, and edema. When gonococcal infection is excluded—confirmed by negative nucleic acid amplification tests (NAATs) or culture on selective media—the condition is classified as nongonococcal urethritis (NGU). Within NGU cases, *Chlamydia trachomatis* is the most frequently identified pathogen. Infections caused by *C. trachomatis* typically produce a milder, mucopurulent discharge with a less intense inflammatory response compared to gonorrhea. Consequently, systematic screening for chlamydial infection is imperative in all patients presenting with urethritis to ensure appropriate diagnosis and treatment.

A further subset of NGU—referred to as nongonococcal, nonchlamydial urethritis (NGNCU)—includes infections due to other microorganisms, such as *Mycoplasma genitalium*, *Ureaplasma urealyticum*, *Trichomonas vaginalis*, herpes simplex virus (HSV), *Gardnerella vaginalis*, and various streptococcal species. Although these pathogens are less frequently isolated, they can provoke clinically significant urethral inflammation and symptoms. Diagnostic testing employing NAATs for *M. genitalium* and *U. urealyticum* is recommended when clinically indicated. Additionally, empiric therapy targeting *T. vaginalis* or HSV should be considered based on clinical presentation and epidemiological risk.

The clinical classification often includes:

- **Nongonococcal Urethritis (NGU):** Urethritis not caused by *Neisseria gonorrhoeae*.
- **Nongonococcal, Nonchlamydial Urethritis (NGNCU):** Urethritis not caused by *N. gonorrhoeae* or *Chlamydia trachomatis*.

Pathogens warranting consideration during the evaluation of urethral discharge include:

- Herpes simplex virus
- *Mycoplasma genitalium*
- Streptococcal species
- *Trichomonas vaginalis*
- *Ureaplasma urealyticum*

5.3 Conclusions

Accurate diagnosis and targeted treatment of genital discharge are critical in ensuring the well-being of individuals. Genital discharge may signal various gynecological conditions, including infections, hormonal alterations, and noninfectious causes. By accurately identifying the underlying etiology, healthcare professionals can provide focused treatment that mitigates unnecessary interventions and potential complications. Furthermore, precise diagnosis facilitates patient education and counseling, enhancing preventive measures and patient engagement in their care. With proper diagnosis and effective treatment, individuals experiencing genital discharge can achieve symptom resolution, diminish the risk of complications, and improve their overall quality of life.

Key Points

- Genital discharge may arise from infections, hormonal changes, and other factors.
- Various localizations of discharge encompass the vestibule, vagina, cervix, uterus, tubes, and urethra.
- Accurate diagnosis of the underlying cause is essential for effective treatment.
- The characteristics of vaginal discharge, including color, consistency, and odor, provide significant diagnostic insights.
- Infectious origins of vaginal discharge include bacterial vaginosis, vulvovaginal candidosis, and trichomoniasis.
- Noninfectious etiologies, such as physiological secretion, desquamative inflammatory vaginitis, and atrophic vaginitis, carry equal consideration.
- Cervical and urethral discharge each have distinct etiologies and diagnostic implications.
- Accurate diagnosis aids in avoiding unnecessary treatments and mitigating potential complications.
- Patient education and counseling are critical components of managing and preventing genital discharge.
- Recognizing associated underlying conditions related to genital discharge is pivotal for comprehensive patient care.

Ulcerations in the Anogenital Area

6

Abstract

Ulcerations in the anogenital region may arise from various etiology, with sexually transmitted diseases (STD) being a significant contributor. The principal pathogens associated with these genital ulcerations include the herpes simplex virus, Treponema pallidum (syphilis), Haemophilus ducreyi (chancroid), Chlamydia trachomatis (lymphogranuloma venereum), and Klebsiella granulomatis (granuloma inguinale). Although clinical manifestations of these ulcerations may vary, obtaining a comprehensive medical history and conducting a thorough physical examination are imperative for collecting critical information. Accurate diagnosis frequently requires microbiological testing methods, such as serology, polymerase chain reaction (PCR), or biopsy. Treatment is customized to address the specific etiology and identified pathogen; empirical treatment may be considered in certain cases until definitive microbiological results are obtained. Preventive strategies should highlight the consistent use of condoms, vaccination, education on safe sexual practices, and awareness of the risks associated with STDs.

6.1 Background

Ulcerations in the anogenital area frequently present in cases of sexually transmitted diseases (STD). An ulcer is defined as a defect in the skin caused by damage, which typically heals with the formation of scar tissue. Aside from local infections, granulomas and tumors may also undergo ulceration. The ulcerative nature of these diseases facilitates the colonization of additional pathogens, largely due to extensive skin damage. In numerous instances, mixed infections may be present.

Individuals exhibiting anogenital ulcerations are at an increased risk of HIV infection and transmission.

I. Mylonas, *Sexually Transmitted Diseases*,
https://doi.org/10.1007/978-3-031-78204-6_6

6.2 Pathogens

The emergence of anogenital ulcers may be attributed to multiple factors. These painful lesions in the anogenital region can result from infections, dermatological conditions, autoimmune disorders, or trauma (Table 6.1). It is critical to discern the underlying cause to enable an accurate diagnosis and subsequent treatment.

The lesions may be exogenous, vascular, or a consequence of local infections. Nevertheless, most young patients presenting with genital ulcerations have infections caused by sexually transmitted pathogens. Herpes simplex virus types I and II account for up to 80% of cases.

The following pathogens are particularly significant in the context of genital ulcerations:

- ***Herpes Simplex Virus Types I and II***: Causative agents of genital herpes (Chap. 20).
- ***Treponema pallidum***: Etiological agent of primary syphilis (Chap. 16).
- ***Haemophilus ducreyi***: Causative agent of chancroid (Chap. 13).
- ***Chlamydia trachomatis*** Serotypes 1–3: Pathogens responsible for lymphogranuloma venereum (Chap. 17).
- ***Klebsiella granulomatis*** (*Calymmatobacterium granulomatis*): Causative agent of granuloma inguinale (Chap. 19).

It is essential to recognize that anogenital ulcerations may also arise from other infections or conditions. In this context, exclusion of malignant tumors of the vulva is particularly important.

Papillary lesions attributable to sexually transmitted pathogens include:

- Candidosis (Chap. 36).
- Genital warts (Chap. 18).
- Condylomata lata (syphilis) (Chap. 16).
- Pubic lice (Chap. 27).
- Genital herpes (Chap. 20).
- Molluscum contagiosum (Chap. 25).
- Scabies (Chap. 28).

In 25% of patients with genital ulcerations, pathogens remain undetectable despite thorough diagnostic evaluation.

Table 6.1 Causes of ulcerations

	Disease	Skin lesions	Comments
Venereal diseases	Cytomegalovirus (CMV)	Painful, irregular, superficial ulcer often covered with a serous coating	Rare, occurs in isolated cases
	Granuloma inguinale	Painless, nonhardened "flesh-red" ulcer with a clean base; multiple ulcers may be present	May lead to inguinal abscesses
	Human immunodeficiency virus (HIV)	Painful, irregular, superficial ulcer often with a serous coating	Rare, typically seen in isolated cases
	Herpes simplex virus (HSV)	Painful, irregular superficial ulcers on an erythematous base; lesions may crust over	Both HSV-1 and HSV-2 can cause these lesions
	Lymphogranuloma venereum	Primary lesion is often unnoticed; may appear as a small, painless papule or ulcer	Usually accompanied by painful inguinal lymphadenopathy
	Primary syphilis	Single, painless ulcer with hardened edges and a clean base	Classic manifestation of a sexually transmitted infection
	Secondary syphilis	Multiple painless, superficial ulcers	Classic manifestation of a sexually transmitted infection
	Chancroid	Painful, irregular soft ulcer with a necrotic base; may present as multiple ulcers	Often accompanied by inguinal blisters
Nonvenereal diseases	Aphthous efflorescence	Painful, irregular ulcers with erythematous borders and a white fibrin coating	Frequently associated with oral ulcers
	Erosive lichen planus	Nonspecific superficial ulcerations	Often linked to oral lesions
	Erythema multiforme	Superficial erosions	May occur alongside stomatitis or bullous eruptions on the palms and soles
	Fixed drug eruptions	Well-defined, dark red superficial erosions	Typically associated with a history of recent medication use
	M. Adamantiades–Behçet	Painful, flat, irregular ulcers with erythematous borders and a white fibrin coating	Associated with oral ulcers, uveitis, arthritis, and vasculitis

(continued)

Table 6.1 (continued)

	Disease	Skin lesions	Comments
	Crohn's disease	Ulcerative perineal granulomas; may lead to scarring or fistula formation	Associated with inflammatory bowel disease; anal fissures may also be present
	Squamous cell carcinoma	Irregular, brittle ulcerations	More common in elderly patients with indolent, nonhealing ulcers
	Reiter syndrome	Painless, serpiginous superficial erosions with raised, erythematous edges	Typically associated with urethritis, arthritis, or conjunctivitis
	Trauma	Variable morphology	Related to a history of trauma (e.g., episiotomy)

6.3 Risk Factors

There are no risk factors uniquely associated with sexually transmitted infections (STIs) that cause ulcerations in the anogenital region; rather, these ulcerative conditions share the general risk factors common to STIs (refer to Sect. 2.5 for a comprehensive overview). These include behaviors and circumstances such as unprotected sexual intercourse, multiple sexual partners, previous history of STIs, inconsistent condom use, and certain demographic or socioeconomic factors. Despite the absence of condition-specific risk factors, it remains essential to thoroughly evaluate patients presenting with anogenital ulcerations for these established general STI risk factors. A detailed sexual history and risk assessment facilitate accurate diagnosis, appropriate testing, and targeted counseling aimed at both treatment and prevention of further transmission.

Risk Factors for STD to be Investigated:

- Persons with anogenital ulcers.
- New partners.
- Partners who have traveled to endemic areas.
- HIV-infected sexual partners.
- Partners of unknown status.
- Travel abroad to endemic areas (including sexual partners).
- History of genital lesions.
- Previous instances of sexually transmitted diseases.
- Substance abuse (including within sexual partnerships).
- History of homosexuality in male partners (MSM, men who have sex with men).

6.4 Clinical Manifestation

Ulcerative lesions may occur not only in the genital region (Fig. 6.1) but also in the anal area, especially in response to changes in sexual practices (Fig. 6.2). Thus, a comprehensive examination of the entire anogenital area is warranted. Each patient presenting with a genital ulcer should undergo an extensive medical history review, including a sexual history. All relevant risk factors (Sect. 2.5) should be assessed.

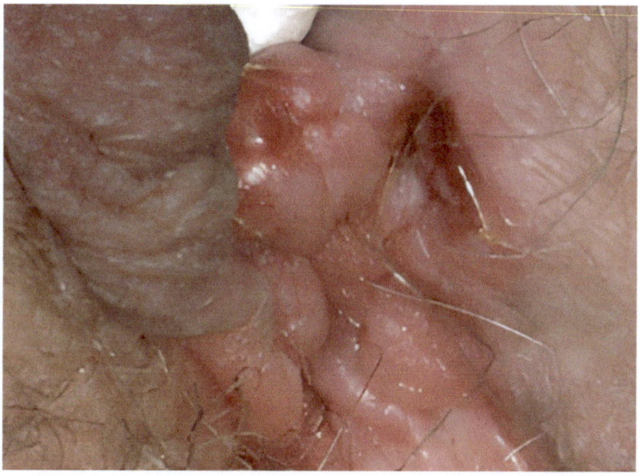

Fig. 6.1 Small genital ulcer (Mylonas 2016)

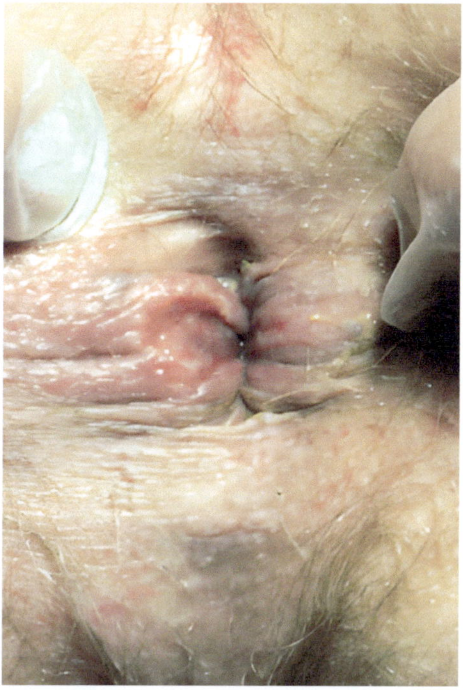

Fig. 6.2 Perianal primary manifestation of chancroid (Caspary et al. 2006)

Papillary changes often represent the initial manifestations but may no longer be visible in the majority of ulcer disease cases (Fig. 6.3). The temporal relationship between efflorescences and symptoms is critical. Chronic changes or ulcerations are more indicative of HPV infection or malignancy, whereas acute symptoms, particularly linked to sexual intercourse, suggest a sexually transmitted infection (Fig. 6.4).

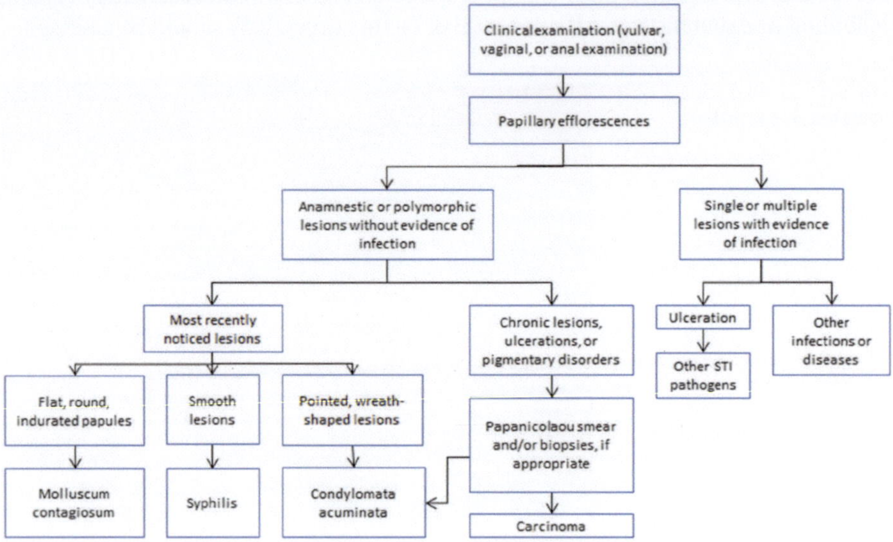

Fig. 6.3 Procedure for assessing papular lesions (Courtesy of I. Mylonas)

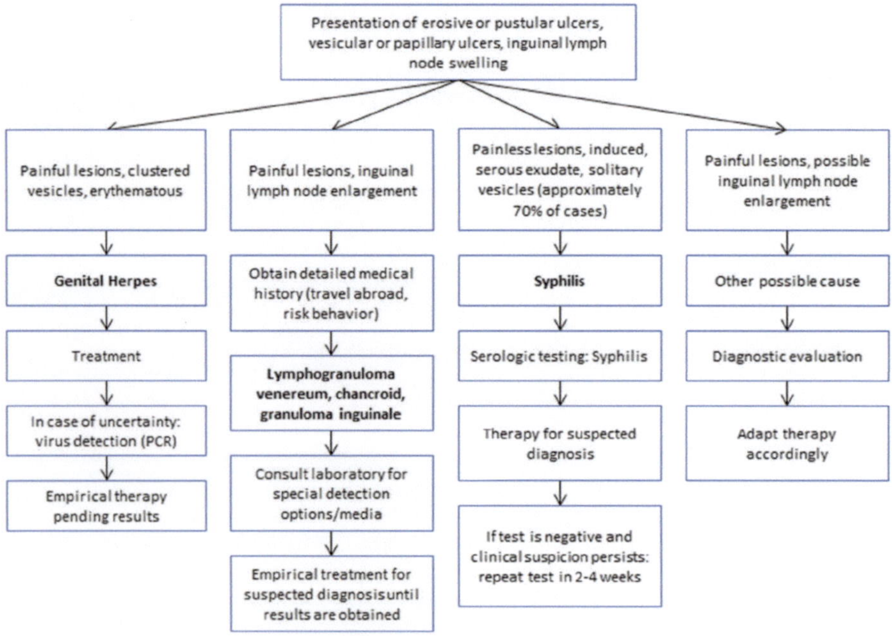

Fig. 6.4 Ulcerations in the anogenital region (Courtesy of I. Mylonas)

Clinical Examination of Ulcerative Lesions

During the clinical examination, ulcers typically present with distinctive visual features and are often encircled by inflamed tissue characterized by erythema, edema, and tenderness. Key aspects to assess include ulcer morphology, skin texture, and the patient's pain profile, all of which yield essential diagnostic insights. Detailed inspection of the ulcer's margins (whether undermined, well-defined, or rolled), the nature of the base (granulating, sloughy, or necrotic), and the quality of any exudate (serous or purulent) plays a pivotal role in distinguishing between different ulcer etiologies.

Serous exudate—clear, watery fluid lacking cellular debris—typically indicates a noninfectious or early inflammatory process, whereas purulent discharge—opaque fluid rich in neutrophils and bacteria—strongly suggests a bacterial infection. Moreover, the surrounding perilesional skin may exhibit warmth, induration, or fluctuance, further supporting an infectious cause.

Correlating these clinical observations with a thorough patient history (including onset, systemic symptoms, comorbidities, and recent trauma) and targeted laboratory or imaging studies (e.g., microbiological cultures, biopsy, and Doppler ultrasound) refine the differential diagnosis. Collectively, these findings underscore the importance of a systematic approach to ulcer assessment, ensuring prompt identification of infectious agents and facilitating appropriate therapeutic interventions (Table 6.2).

Table 6.2 Characteristics of ulcers

Characteristic	Syphilis	Granuloma inguinale	Herpes Simplex Virus (HSV)	Lymphogranuloma venereum (LGV)	Chancroid
Incubation period	9–90 days	8–80 days	2–7 days	7–21 days	1–14 days
Primary lesion	Papule	Papule	Vesicles	Papule, pustule, or vesicle	Papule or pustule
Quantity	Usually solitary	Variable	Several	Usually solitary	Several
Size (mm)	5–15	Variable	1–10	2–10	2–20
Margins	Well defined, raised, round or oval	Variable, increased, irregular	Erythematous	Raised, round or oval	Frayed, irregular
Base	Red, smooth, nonpurulent	Red, rough	Red, smooth, serous liquid	Variable	Purulent exudate
Induration	++	++	–	–	–
Pain	–	+	++	±	++

– = Absent
± = Variable/Moderate
+ = Sometimes/Strongly
++ = Pronounced/Very Strong

Key characteristics of ulcers include:

- Ulcer base (granular, purulent, bloody).
- Edge of the ulcer (raised, undermined, at skin level).
- Consistency of tissue surrounding the ulcer (soft, coarse, hard).
- Condition of skin around the ulcer (unresponsive, inflamed, reddened, weeping, raised, infiltrated).
- Pain associated with the ulcer.

6.5 Diagnosis

Diagnostic Approach to Anogenital Ulcerations

A definitive diagnosis of anogenital ulcerations cannot typically be achieved by medical history and physical examination alone, as clinical features often suggest but do not conclusively identify the causative pathogen. Consequently, microbiological and histopathological investigations are indispensable for accurate etiological determination and guiding effective management.

All patients presenting with genital ulcers should undergo comprehensive serological screening for syphilis, incorporating both non-treponemal tests (e.g., rapid plasma reagin [RPR] and venereal disease research laboratory [VDRL]) and treponemal-specific assays to optimize diagnostic sensitivity and specificity. When herpes simplex virus (HSV) infection is suspected—based on clinical signs such as vesicular prodrome, recurrent ulcerations, or significant pain—polymerase chain reaction (PCR) testing of lesion swabs is the preferred diagnostic tool to confirm HSV type and quantify viral load.

For other suspected infectious agents, close collaboration with the microbiology laboratory is essential to select appropriate culture media and molecular diagnostic assays. For instance, if chancroid (*Haemophilus ducreyi*) or lymphogranuloma venereum (LGV; *Chlamydia trachomatis* serovars L1–L3) are considered, specialized culture techniques and targeted nucleic acid amplification tests (NAATs) must be employed. Additionally, in patients with relevant epidemiological risk factors or travel history, investigation for granuloma inguinale caused by *Klebsiella granulomatis*—utilizing special staining methods and PCR—is warranted.

In cases where lesions persist, display atypical features, or fail to respond to standard antimicrobial therapy, a punch or excisional skin biopsy with subsequent histopathological examination is critical. Tissue analysis aids in excluding noninfectious etiologies, such as malignancies (e.g., squamous cell carcinoma), inflammatory dermatoses (e.g., fixed drug eruption, lichen planus), or vasculitis, thereby refining the differential diagnosis and preventing inappropriate treatment.

In summary, an effective diagnostic workup for anogenital ulcers should integrate:

1. Syphilis serology using both non-treponemal and treponemal tests
2. HSV PCR testing when clinically indicated
3. NAATs for *Chlamydia trachomatis* and *Neisseria gonorrhoeae* in patients with relevant risk factors
4. Specialized culture or molecular assays for less common pathogens, such as *H. ducreyi* and *K. granulomatis*, coordinated with the microbiology laboratory
5. Histopathological evaluation through skin biopsy for chronic, atypical, or treatment-resistant lesions suspected; consultation with the laboratory to determine necessary culture media and procedures is advisable.

Concurrent HIV infections may change the typical appearance of genital ulcerations, leading to variations in management depending on the patient's known HIV status.

6.6 Treatment

6.6.1 Drug Therapy

The pharmacotherapeutic approach is determined by the established etiology and the principal pathogen. Management is to be pathogen-directed whenever possible; empiric therapy is to be instituted when prompt treatment is required and is to be refined once laboratory results are obtained.

Given the epidemiological context, empirical therapy for genital herpes should be considered in most cases of genital ulcers, especially where symptoms and efflorescences are characteristic.

Empiric antimicrobial therapy for suspected *Treponema pallidum* (syphilis), *Chlamydia trachomatis* L1–L3 (lymphogranuloma venereum, LGV), *Klebsiella granulomatis* (granuloma inguinale and donovanosis), and *Haemophilus ducreyi* (chancroid) should be determined after assessment of epidemiologic, clinical, and social factors. The decision to initiate empiric treatment is to be individualized and documented; the following considerations are to be applied.

Indications Favoring Empiric Therapy

- **Epidemiologic Exposure:** Recent travel to or residence in regions with endemic disease prevalence, or sexual contact with persons from high-prevalence areas, increases the pretest probability and supports empiric treatment.

- **Clinical Features:** Characteristic ulcer morphology, regional lymphadenopathy (e.g., tender inguinal adenopathy in LGV), or progressive ulcerative disease without response to standard local care should prompt consideration of empiric therapy.
- **High Clinical Suspicion with Pending or Unavailable Diagnostics:** When laboratory testing is delayed, inaccessible, or unreliable, empiric therapy may be warranted to reduce morbidity and transmissibility.
- **Limited Capacity for Follow-Up:** Empiric treatment is to be strongly considered for patients with anticipated poor follow-up (homelessness, unstable housing, substance use disorder, inability to be contacted, or likely nonadherence) to ensure prompt management and public-health control.
- **Coexisting Sexually Transmitted Diseases:** Presence of other STDs or high-risk sexual behavior increases likelihood of coinfection and may justify broader empiric coverage.

Possible Approach to Empiric Therapy

- **Obtain specimens for appropriate diagnostic** testing (NAAT/PCR for HSV and *C. trachomatis* when indicated, serology and dark-field microscopy for syphilis, culture or PCR for *H. ducreyi*, and biopsy for donovanosis if available) prior to administration of antimicrobials whenever feasible.
- **Select empiric agents** guided by local epidemiology and resistance patterns (institutional antibiogram) and standard (guideline) recommendations.
- **Arrange Expedited Follow-Up and Partner Notification:** Patients receiving empiric therapy must be scheduled for timely reassessment (typically within 48–72 h for severe or progressive disease) and instructed about partner notification and testing according to local public-health protocols.
- **Reassess and Modify Therapy:** Empiric therapy is to be reviewed and adjusted when diagnostic results are available, clinical response is documented, or additional information regarding exposures is obtained.

Requirements for empirical syphilis treatment:

- Detection of pathogens through dark-field microscopy.
- Positive results from direct or indirect immunofluorescence antibody tests or PCR.

Persistent high suspicion of syphilis infection or historical suspicion of contact with syphilis-infected partners, despite:

- Negative dark-field microscopy.
- Negative HSV antibody test.
- Negative cultures for Haemophilus ducreyi.
- Insufficient follow-up assurance (e.g., noncompliance).

6.6.2 Further Measurements

If strong suspicion of syphilis infection persists despite negative results from dark-field microscopy, HSV tests, and cultures for *Haemophilus ducreyi*, further measures should include an HIV test. Patients with syphilis, lymphogranuloma venereum, or chancroid are at an elevated risk for coinfection with HIV. The timing of the HIV antibody test should be considered, given that genital ulcerations increase the risk of HIV transmission. If necessary, an additional HIV test for patients with existing anogenital ulcerations can be conducted after 12 weeks.

6.7 Differential Diagnosis

The etiology of anogenital ulcerations is diverse (Table 6.1). Differential diagnosis should include sexually transmitted diseases such as genital herpes and syphilis, inflammatory conditions like Crohn's disease or ulcerative colitis, fungal infections like candidosis, and traumatic injuries resulting from friction or mechanical harm. Less common causes may involve tumors or autoimmune disorders.

6.8 Prevention

For patients lacking immunity to hepatitis B virus, vaccination should be recommended. Discussion regarding the potential for HPV vaccination is also advised.

To prevent subsequent infections, it is critical to inform the patient's sexual partner of their risks.

Additionally, patients should receive education on the risks associated with unprotected sexual intercourse and the importance of safe sexual practices as part of comprehensive sexual health education.

Key Points

- Ulcerations in the anogenital area may stem from various causes, including infections from sexually transmitted pathogens.
- Genital ulcerations may be associated with several pathogens, including herpes simplex virus, *Treponema pallidum* (syphilis), *Haemophilus ducreyi* (chancroid), *Chlamydia trachomatis* (lymphogranuloma venereum), and *Klebsiella granulomatis* (granuloma inguinale), among others.

(continued)

- It is advisable to inquire about risk factors for sexually transmitted diseases when evaluating affected patients, as such factors can aid in diagnosis.
- Clinical presentation of genital ulcerations may vary; however, a comprehensive history and examination can yield valuable insights.
- Accurate diagnosis often necessitates the use of microbiological tests, including serology, PCR, or biopsy.
- The therapeutic approach is contingent upon the identified etiology and corresponding pathogen; in some instances, empirically derived therapeutic strategies may be appropriate.
- Preventive measures include the use of condoms, vaccination against hepatitis B and HPV, and education on safe sexual practices and the risks associated with sexually transmitted infections.

Cervicitis

7

Abstract

Cervicitis is defined as inflammation of the cervix, induced by various pathogens, including *Chlamydia trachomatis*, *Neisseria gonorrhoeae*, trichomonads, fungi, herpes viruses, and human papillomavirus (HPV). Symptoms may present as discharge, bleeding, and pelvic pain: However, in some cases, the condition remains asymptomatic, which facilitates its transmission. Gynecological examinations and microbiological tests are utilized to identify the pathogens responsible for cervicitis. Potential complications encompass ascending infections, including salpingitis and pelvic inflammatory disease (PID), which may result in infertility. Additionally, the pathogens can be transmitted during pregnancy and birth, causing severe infections in newborns. Treatment is depending on the isolated microorganism. Additionally, it is recommended that patients receive education, that their partners undergo treatment, and that the use of condoms be encouraged.

7.1 Background

The cervix, characterized by a single-layered cylindrical epithelium, exhibits less defense against pathogenic microorganisms compared to the multilayered vulvar and vaginal epithelium. Several factors can contribute to the onset or exacerbation of cervicitis, which include:

- Primary infections (e.g., *Chlamydia trachomatis*, *Neisseria gonorrhoeae*, trichomonads, fungi, herpes viruses, HPV).
- Anatomical abnormalities of the cervix (e.g., erosion, cervical laceration, cervical polyps).
- Ascending vaginal infections (e.g., bacterial vaginosis).
- Psychogenic factors (e.g., frustration of libido, anorgasmia).

I. Mylonas, *Sexually Transmitted Diseases*,
https://doi.org/10.1007/978-3-031-78204-6_7

7.2 Pathogens

The predominant pathogens associated with cervicitis are *Chlamydia trachomatis* and *Neisseria gonorrhoeae*. While current epidemiological data is lacking, it is presumed that the majority of cervicitis cases are attributed to *Chlamydia trachomatis*, herpes simplex virus (HSV) type II, and papillomaviruses. It is important to note that trichomonads and fungi can also contribute to cervicitis; however, instances of cervicitis solely caused by these pathogens have primarily been documented through case studies (Table 7.1).

Table 7.1 Common pathogens associated with cervicitis

Pathogen	Clinical presentation	Comments	See chapter
Chlamydia trachomatis (serotypes D–K)	– Aqueous-clear discharge – Possibly purulent or bloody-tinged discharge – No significant complaints (approx. 90%) – Rarely dysuria – Contact bleeding	– Most common form of acute cervicitis – Transmission through sexual intercourse	Chapter 17
Neisseria gonorrhoeae	– Cervical discharge (80–90%) – Purulent, painful urethritis	– Often associated with other sexually transmitted infections	Chapter 14
Genital herpes	– Erosions and ulcerations – Possible discharge – Superinfection	– Isolated cervicitis due to HSV is expected mainly in recurrent genital herpes – Often associated with vulvitis/vaginitis	Chapter 20
Syphilis	– Typical primary chancre – Single, painless papule – Transition to painless ulcer	– Occasionally affects the portio – Absence of inguinal lymph node swelling – Discovery of primary infection is often coincidental	Chapter 16
HPV	– Condylomata acuminata – No symptoms	– Discovery of primary infection is often coincidental – Frequent coinfection of the vulva and vagina	Chapter 18
Other bacteria	– Cervical discharge – Often no further symptoms	– Possible pathogens: Staphylococci, streptococci, Enterobacteriaceae, anaerobes, mycoplasma – Isolated cervicitis caused by these bacteria is rare – Frequent coinfection of the vagina or endometritis	

7.3 Clinical Manifestation

Acute cervicitis presents a significant diagnostic challenge, as it may be clinically indistinguishable from other disorders of the female genital tract. The condition frequently occurs without symptoms, with up to 80% of patients remaining asymptomatic. This asymptomatic presentation is clinically significant because it facilitates ongoing pathogen transmission and delays appropriate treatment initiation.

The nonspecific nature of cervicitis symptoms when present—including abnormal vaginal discharge, intermenstrual bleeding, dyspareunia, and dysuria—overlaps considerably with other gynecological conditions, such as vaginitis, bacterial vaginosis, and pelvic inflammatory disease. This symptom overlap complicates differential diagnosis and may lead to misdiagnosis or delayed recognition of the condition.

Subclinical cervicitis poses particular public health concerns because infected individuals remain unaware of their condition while potentially transmitting sexually transmitted infections to partners. The inflammatory process disrupts the cervical mucosal barrier, increasing both HIV acquisition risk and viral shedding, thereby enhancing transmission potential. Additionally, untreated cervicitis may ascend to involve the upper genital tract, resulting in serious complications, including pelvic inflammatory disease, chronic pelvic pain, infertility, and ectopic pregnancy. The diagnostic complexity is further compounded by the fact that up to 83% of cervicitis cases remain of unknown etiology despite thorough microbiological investigation. Even when common sexually transmitted pathogens such as *Chlamydia trachomatis* and *Neisseria gonorrhoeae* are identified, they account for only 25% of cases. This high proportion of cases with unidentified etiology underscores the need for empirical treatment approaches in high-risk populations.

Given these diagnostic challenges and the potential for serious sequelae, clinical suspicion should remain high for cervicitis in sexually active women presenting with genital symptoms, and screening protocols should be implemented for high-risk populations to reduce adverse outcomes.

Symptoms that may indicate cervicitis include:

- Hyperemia and fragility of the cervical epithelium (leading to easy bleeding).
- Mucopurulent cervicitis (e.g., due to Chlamydia, Neisseria gonorrhoeae) presenting with yellowish, mucopurulent, foul-smelling discharge.
- Vesicular lesions, erosions, and bleeding (e.g., associated with genital herpes).
- General symptoms are often absent.

7.4 Diagnosis

Cervicitis diagnosis is established through clinical examination, microbiological identification of pathogens, and supplementary diagnostic tests as necessary. This comprehensive approach is essential to accurately ascertain the cause of the inflammation.

- **Clinical Examination**: During gynecological examination, the cervix may be coated with yellowish, thick mucus. Palpation may elicit pain, and contact bleeding may occur due to the vulnerability of the cervical epithelium during the examination. However, clinical examination alone is frequently inadequate for determining the specific cause of cervicitis.
- **Wet Mount Microscopy/Phase-Contrast Microscopy**: Cervical discharge (See Sect. 5.2.2) in cases of cervicitis typically contains numerous leukocytes, usually exceeding 25 leukocytes per field at 400× magnification, without the presence of visible pathogens in the native preparation. Microscopy of the native preparation alone is often insufficient for identifying the specific cause of cervicitis.
- **Microbiological Examination**: Cervical swabs are collected to identify potential infectious agents such as *Chlamydia*, gonococci, herpes viruses, or, in uncertain cases, *Trichomonas*. Advanced methodologies, including PCR testing, enhance the accuracy of pathogen identification.
- **Colposcopy**: This procedure permits a more detailed assessment of cervical changes and abnormalities.
- **Additional Tests**: Depending on the suspected diagnosis, further examinations such as HPV DNA testing or imaging procedures may be warranted.

Consequently, the diagnosis of cervicitis is derived from a combination of clinical examination, microbiological pathogen identification, and additional diagnostic investigations as required. This thorough approach is vital for accurately identifying the precise cause of inflammation.

Serological detection of infectious diseases is ineffective for diagnosis of a cervicitis.

7.5 Complications

Upper Genital Tract Complications

- **Pelvic Inflammatory Disease (PID)** constitutes the most severe complication of cervicitis, occurring when infectious agents ascend from the cervix to involve the endometrium, fallopian tubes (salpingitis), ovaries, and adjacent pelvic structures. The incidence of PID varies between 20% and 80%, influenced by factors, such as diagnostic delay, coinfections, and host immune response. Evidence indicates that delayed treatment of *Chlamydia trachomatis* cervicitis increases the risk of PID and subsequent infertility by approximately threefold.

- **Infertility** affects nearly 20% of women who develop PID. This results from persistent inflammation and fibrosis causing tubal occlusion and disruption of normal tubal function, impairing ovum transport and fertilization. Importantly, asymptomatic or subclinical infections can still provoke silent tubal damage, leading to infertility.
- **Ectopic Pregnancy** risk escalates significantly following PID secondary to cervicitis. Salpingitis increases the risk of ectopic gestation by approximately tenfold compared to the general population. Approximately 7–10% of pregnancies following salpingitis are ectopic. Moreover, nearly 40% of women with a history of one ectopic pregnancy fail to conceive intrauterine pregnancies subsequently.
- **Chronic Pelvic Pain** develops in about 40% of women after PID episodes. This chronic discomfort is attributed to adhesions, ongoing inflammation, and structural distortion of pelvic organs. Chronic cervicitis contributes to recurrent PID, with recurrence rates reaching 82% in untreated cases compared to 24% in patients treated with cervical electrocauterization.

Pregnancy and Neonatal Complications

- **Preterm Birth** is strongly associated with cervical infections. The prevalence of chlamydial cervicitis in women presenting with preterm labor is significantly elevated at 22.9%, compared to 5.7% in women delivering at term. Cervical inflammation compromises epithelial integrity, facilitating ascending infection and triggering premature uterine contractions.
- **Premature Rupture of Membranes (PROM)** occurs more frequently in women with persistent cervicitis. Bacterial colonization, notably with *Ureaplasma urealyticum* (34.5%) and *Enterococcus* spp. (27.6%), correlates with increased PROM and preterm birth rates. Antimicrobial therapy effectively reduces these adverse outcomes, confirming the infectious etiology.
- **Vertical Transmission** of pathogens from mother to neonate occurs in approximately 53.9% of colonized mothers during delivery. The predominant transmitted organisms include *Escherichia coli* (16.4%), *Candida* spp. (6.3%), and *Klebsiella* spp. (3.6%). Prolonged labor exceeding 12 h increases transmission risk by 2.23-fold, whereas low birth weight (<2500 g) enhances this risk by 5.38-fold.
- **Neonatal Infections** primarily present as conjunctivitis but may progress to severe conditions, such as pneumonia, meningitis, sepsis, septic arthritis, and endocarditis. *Chlamydial pneumonia* is characterized by staccato cough, tachypnea, and bilateral pulmonary infiltrates in infants aged 1–3 months, necessitating a 14-day antibiotic regimen.

HIV Transmission and Susceptibility

- **Increased HIV Susceptibility and Transmission** is observed in women with cervicitis through multiple mechanisms: disruption of the cervical mucus barrier, recruitment of HIV target cells (e.g., CD4+ T lymphocytes), and elevated local proinflammatory cytokines. A direct correlation exists between the presence of cervicitis and HIV RNA detection in cervical secretions.
- **HIV-Positive Women** with cervicitis who utilize hormonal contraceptives demonstrate a threefold increased incidence of cervical chlamydial infection and a 1.6-fold increased incidence of nonspecific cervicitis. These effects may be mediated by enhanced viral replication within inflamed tissues, epithelial barrier compromise, and increased shedding of infected cells.
- **Immune Activation Post-Sexual Exposure** induces rapid increases in genital tract inflammatory markers and expands the population of HIV target cells (notably Th17 and activated T cells) within 72 h after unprotected intercourse, thereby heightening vulnerability to HIV acquisition.

Long-Term Reproductive Health Impact

- **Tubo-ovarian Abscesses (TOA)** develop in approximately 15% of women with untreated or inadequately treated salpingitis. TOAs may rupture, precipitating acute abdomen, peritonitis, and septic shock requiring emergent intervention.
- **Hydrosalpinx**, characterized by fimbrial obstruction and accumulation of serous fluid within the fallopian tube, frequently remains asymptomatic but may cause pelvic pressure, chronic pain, dyspareunia, and contribute to infertility due to impaired tubal function.
- **Fitz-Hugh-Curtis Syndrome**, or perihepatitis, arises from the extension of pelvic infection to the hepatic capsule, commonly associated with gonococcal or chlamydial salpingitis. It manifests as sharp right upper quadrant pain aggravated by respiration or movement.

Cervicitis caused by sexually transmitted pathogens poses significant risks for acute complications, such as PID and infertility, as well as long-term reproductive morbidity, including ectopic pregnancy, chronic pelvic pain, and tubo-ovarian abscess formation. Pregnancy complications such as preterm birth, PROM, vertical transmission of pathogens, and neonatal infections are also closely linked to cervical infections.

7.6 Treatment

The therapeutic approach is contingent upon the specific pathogen implicated.

7.7 Prevention

- **Sexuality Education**: Comprehensive education concerning sexuality, sexually transmitted diseases (STD), and sexual hygiene is crucial for children and adolescents. This education should be age-appropriate and encompass the physical, emotional, and social dimensions of sexual health.
- **Partner Treatment**: It is advisable to treat both the patient and their sexual partner(s) for infections such as *Chlamydia* and *Neisseria gonorrhoeae* to mitigate the risk of reinfection. This strategy assists in breaking the transmission cycle and ensuring effective management of the infection.
- **Condom Use**: Regular and correct use of condoms provides significant protection against various STDs, including *Chlamydia* and *Neisseria gonorrhoeae*. Consistent utilization of condoms is an essential component of STD prevention strategies.

Key Points

- Cervicitis is induced by various pathogens, including *Chlamydia* and *Neisseria gonorrhoeae*.
- Contributing factors to the development of cervicitis include infections, cervical diseases, and psychogenic causes.
- Clinical manifestations can be challenging to differentiate; some cases may be asymptomatic.
- Symptoms indicative of cervicitis may encompass hyperemia, mucopurulent discharge, bleeding, and occasionally general symptoms.
- Diagnosis typically involves gynecological examination and pathogen detection.
- Potential complications include ascending infections leading to infertility and risks during pregnancy affecting newborns.
- Treatment strategies are pathogen-specific. Preventive measures include education and condom use.

Pelvic Inflammatory Disease (PID) 8

Abstract

Pelvic inflammatory disease (PID) is defined as an inflammation of the fallopian tubes and ovaries. In the majority of instances, this condition is initiated by bacteria originating from the lower genital tract, which gain access to the abdominal cavity, subsequently infecting the uterus, fallopian tubes, and ovaries. The most prevalent pathogens identified are *Chlamydia trachomatis* and *Neisseria gonorrhoeae*, although other microorganisms from the vaginal flora may also contribute to the infection. The diagnosis of PID poses challenges due to the variability and non-specific nature of the symptoms. Diagnostic procedures typically include physical examination, laboratory tests, imaging, and laparoscopy. Treatment usually consists of antibiotic therapy, while severe cases may necessitate surgical intervention. Preventative strategies focus on promoting sexual hygiene, facilitating early detection of lower genital tract infections, and encouraging consistent condom use. Complications arising from PID can include infertility, ectopic pregnancy, and chronic pelvic or upper abdominal pain.

8.1 Background

Pelvic Inflammatory Disease (PID) is defined as an inflammatory condition affecting the internal female reproductive organs. This disease typically occurs when bacteria from the lower genital tract ascend into the abdominal cavity, causing infections in the uterus, fallopian tubes, and ovaries. However, the infection can also descend or result from surgical interventions.

I. Mylonas, *Sexually Transmitted Diseases*,
https://doi.org/10.1007/978-3-031-78204-6_8

8.2 Pathogen and Pathogenesis

A variety of pathogens can contribute to the clinical presentation of PID. In addition to the primary pathogens, *Chlamydia trachomatis* and *Neisseria gonorrhoeae*—though not the most common—can also be identified within the vaginal flora. Pathogens causally linked to PID include anaerobes, *Gardnerella vaginalis*, *Haemophilus influenzae*, *Enterobacteriaceae*, and *Streptococcus agalactiae* (Table 8.1). Furthermore, *cytomegaloviruses*, mycoplasmas, and *Ureaplasma urealyticum* are discussed as potential etiological agents. However, mixed cultures frequently complicate the identification of the primary pathogen. *Actinomyces* has been recognized as a cause of PID in select cases, particularly in association with the use of an intrauterine device (IUD). *Peptostreptococci*, *Bacteroides*, and other obligate anaerobes are often encountered in older patients with PID.

Identification of *Chlamydia trachomatis* and/or *Neisseria gonorrhoeae* occurs in approximately one-third of cases, notably in the United States.

Anaerobic gram-negative bacteria and mycoplasmas (e.g., *Mycoplasma hominis* and *Ureaplasma urealyticum*) are, in many instances, observed in women with bacterial vaginosis and have been isolated from the upper genital tract in instances of endometritis and salpingitis.

Bacterial vaginosis has been associated with both acute and subclinical PID in the absence of existing gonococcal or chlamydial infections.

Table 8.1 Potential pathogens responsible for pelvic inflammatory disease (PID)

Pathogen category	Pathogen	Frequency/comments
Sexually transmitted pathogens	*Neisseria gonorrhoeae*	10–15% of gonorrhea infections progress to PID
	Chlamydia trachomatis	10–20% of chlamydial infections lead to PID
	Mycoplasma genitalium	Found in 4–22% of PID cases; up to 60% in post-abortal PID
	Herpes simplex virus (HSV)	Rarely a primary cause
Anaerobic pathogens	*Peptostreptococcus* spp.	7–8% when detected alone; part of polymicrobial anaerobic flora
	Bacteroides spp., *Prevotella* spp.	Common anaerobic flora; anaerobes account for 25–50% of infections
	Peptococcus spp.	Part of anaerobic flora; estimated 5–10%
	Actinomyces spp.	<1%; mostly associated with intrauterine device (IUD) use

(continued)

Table 8.1 (continued)

Pathogen category	Pathogen	Frequency/comments
Aerobic pathogens	*Streptococcus* spp. (incl. Group B)	20–46%, varies by diagnostic method and population
	Staphylococcus spp.	16–32%, includes coagulase-negative staphylococci and *S. aureus*
	Escherichia coli and *Enterobacteriaceae*	17–19%
	Haemophilus influenzae	Rare; usually respiratory co-infection
Suspected or unclear association	*Gardnerella vaginalis*	Linked to bacterial vaginosis; direct role in PID unclear
	Trichomonas vaginalis	Rarely sole pathogen; may increase infection risk
	Mycoplasma hominis	0.7–11%, varies regionally and by detection method
	Ureaplasma urealyticum	20–30% in some populations; pathogenic role debated
	Ureaplasma parvum	Often coexists with *U. urealyticum*; clinical relevance uncertain
	Cytomegalovirus (CMV)	Rare; generally not a primary cause

Additional notes:

- Polymicrobial infections involving both aerobic and anaerobic bacteria are common in adnexitis
- Frequencies depend on population studied and diagnostic method (culture vs. PCR) and are approximate
- IUD use is associated with increased *Actinomyces* spp. prevalence

Women with PID typically present with a range of non-specific symptoms, complicating both diagnosis and treatment. For instance, women with subacute PID may exhibit few or no lower abdominal symptoms, despite having underlying conditions such as endometritis or salpingitis. An increased risk of subclinical PID, six-fold, corresponds to *Chlamydia trachomatis* infections, while a fourfold increased risk correlates with infections caused by *Neisseria gonorrhoeae*.

Recent reports have associated *Mycoplasma genitalium* (Chap. 21), a pathogen noted for its increasing frequency in non-gonococcal urethritis (Sect. 14.4.1.3) and cervicitis (Chap. 7), with the etiology of PID.

The predominant mechanism of PID development is via ascending infections from the lower genital tract to the uterus, fallopian tubes, and ovaries. Nevertheless, pathogens can also infiltrate the internal organs through alternative routes.

8.2.1 Common Routes of Infection in Gynecology

- **Ascending Infection:** The most common route, where microorganisms ascend through the cervix, infecting the uterine mucosa, often without overt clinical symptoms. Progression allows pathogens to traverse the fallopian tubes toward the ovaries, potentially resulting in unilateral disease with varying severity, culminating in pelvic peritonitis.

- **Descending Infection:** Occurs when pathogens enter the uterine mucosa via the vagina, frequently due to sexually transmitted infections. Additionally, infections may arise from conditions such as appendicitis, peritonitis, or inflammatory bowel disease.
- **Postoperative Infection:** Defined as infections occurring post-surgical procedures. Although rare after gynecological interventions, preexisting vaginal infections elevate the risk of postoperative intra-abdominal infections, warranting preoperative evaluations, including phase contrast microscopy.
- **Hematogenous Infection:** Involves pathogens spreading through the bloodstream, as observed in conditions like tuberculosis, which can disseminate infectious agents to the internal female genital tract.

The onset of PID may be influenced by several predisposing factors, including:

- Menstruation.
- Intrauterine device (IUD) use.
- Dilation and Curettage (D&C).
- Birth or bed confinement.
- Diagnostic procedures (e.g., hysteroscopy, hysterosalpingography).
- Promiscuity.
- Premature sexual intercourse.

Cervical infection caused by microorganisms damages the endocervical canal, facilitating the ascent of pathogens. Notably, *Neisseria gonorrhoeae*, *Chlamydia trachomatis*, *Mycoplasma hominis*, *Mycoplasma genitalium*, and other bacterial entities can adhere to spermatozoa, enhancing their potential to ascend through the genital tract. The loss of the cervical mucus during menstruation, together with the act of menstruation itself, elevates the risk of microbial ascension from the vagina and cervix into the upper genital tract. Furthermore, younger women exhibit a larger cervical ectopia due to elevated hormone levels at menarche, providing an increased adhesion surface for bacterial pathogens.

The subsequent ascension results in tubal inflammation characterized by edematous tissue swelling and leukocytic infiltration of the stroma. Additional complications can include:

- Fibrinous adhesions inducing alterations in the fallopian tubes, such as lumen displacement, fimbrial adhesion, uterine tubal ostium displacement, and perisalpingitis.
- Accumulation of exudate leading to fallopian tube distension, resulting in hydro-, pyo-, or hematosalpinx.

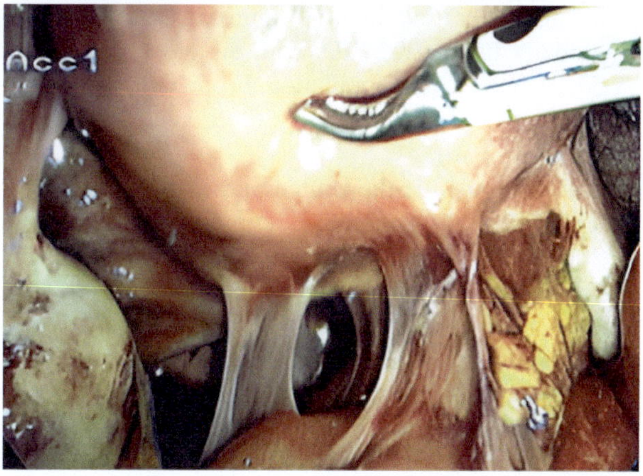

Fig. 8.1 Significant adhesions on the posterior uterine wall in acute pelvic inflammatory disease (PID) (Mylonas 2016)

- In the absence of adhesions, infectious exudate may lead to pelvic peritonitis.
- A significant volume of pus within the pouch of Douglas may culminate in a Douglas abscess.
- Ovarian involvement can occur, manifesting as perioophoritis or tubo-ovarian abscess, and potentially leading to perihepatitis (*Fitz-Hugh–Curtis syndrome*) (Fig. 17.2).
- Inflammation may involve the greater omentum or intestine, referred sometimes as inflammatory adnexal tumor (pseudotumor). After the acute inflammation resolves, connective tissue remodeling takes place during the healing phase. This process may lead to the formation of rigid and immobile tubes, accompanied by varying degrees of surrounding salpingeal adhesions (Fig. 8.1).

8.3 Epidemiology

The estimated prevalence of PID in women is approximately ten per 1000 individuals. To date, only a limited number of studies have sought to delineate the prevalence and incidence of PID. Projections for the United States suggest that approximately one million women receive treatment for PID annually. The incidence of PID is notably higher in developing nations compared to the Western world; for example, a remote community in the Northern Territory of Australia reported a 32% incidence of PID among indigenous women. In Europe, estimates indicate that about 1% of women are affected by PID. The average age of onset ranges from 15 to 39 years, with 70% of patients being younger than 25 years. Nulliparous women experience PID at approximately double the rate of women with a history of at least one full-term pregnancy.

- **Global Overview:** Pelvic Inflammatory Disease (PID) remains a significant global health concern, affecting millions of women of reproductive age worldwide. The epidemiology of PID varies across different regions and has shown changes over time. In 2019, approximately 1.05 million women aged 15-49 years globally had active PID, with an age-standardized prevalence rate (ASPR) of 53.19 per 100,000 population. From 1990 to 2019, while the absolute number of PID cases increased by 36.66%, the ASPR exhibited a slight decline (EAPC: -0.50).

- **United States:** In the United States, the prevalence of self-reported lifetime PID among sexually experienced reproductiveaged women was estimated at 4.4% in 2013-2014, equating to approximately 2.5 million women aged 18-44 years. The Centers for Disease Control and Prevention (CDC) estimates that over 1 million women experience an episode of PID annually, resulting in about 2.5 million office visits and 125,000-150,000 hospitalizations.
- **Europe:** In Western Europe, the ASPR of PID was relatively low at 27.45 per 100,000 population in 2019. Nevertheless, Western Europe was the only region with significantly increasing PID trends. Conversely, Eastern Europe experienced declining PID trends but increasing ectopic pregnancy trends.
- **Asia:** Southeast Asia reported the lowest ASPR of PID at 17.77 per 100,000 population in 2019, whereas East Asia had a slightly higher rate of 34.20 per 100,000.
- **Africa:** Western Sub-Saharan Africa had the highest ASPR of PID globally at 116.02 per 100,000 population in 2019, followed by Central Sub-Saharan Africa at 83.49 per 100,000. These regions bear a disproportionately high burden of PID compared to other parts of the world.
- **Latin America:** Although specific data for Latin America was not provided, Southern Latin America was noted for having one of the highest age-standardized incidence rates of ectopic pregnancy, often a complication of PID.

8.4 Clinical Manifestation

8.4.1 Gynecology

The clinical presentation of **acute pelvic inflammatory disease (PID)** varies widely, ranging from mild, often unnoticed subclinical forms to severe, life-threatening inflammatory conditions. This variability poses a diagnostic challenge, as up to 75% of women with tubal occlusion have never experienced PID symptoms severe enough to prompt antibiotic treatment. PID encompasses distinct clinical categories with differing presentations and severity.

Classification of PID

- **Acute PID (≤30 days duration)** usually presents with severe, bilateral lower abdominal pain, frequently accompanied by fever above 38.3 °C (101 °F). The pain typically develops within 10 days and may be associated with nausea, vomiting, and peritoneal irritation signs. Gonococcal PID often has a rapid onset with higher fevers and prominent cervical discharge, whereas chlamydial PID tends to have a longer duration but milder pain and elevated inflammatory markers (Table 8.2).

Table 8.2 Clinical symptoms of acute pelvic inflammatory disease

Symptoms	Comments
Pain	– A sudden and acute onset of severe lower abdominal pain may be noted
	– Abdominal pain can present as either unilateral or bilateral
Temperature	– The presence of fever or subfebrile temperatures should be documented
General condition	– Nausea has been reported by the patient
	– Abdominal distension (meteorism) may be observed
	– Alternating episodes of constipation and diarrhea are experienced
Gynecological findings	– A foul-smelling, yellowish-green vaginal discharge has been observed
	– Postmenstrual spotting has been reported by the patient
	– Dyspareunia (pain during sexual intercourse) may occur
	– Tenderness upon palpation of the adnexa is noted, possibly accompanied by palpable, doughy adnexal masses
	– Tension within the lower abdomen may be present; caution is advised for potential pelvic peritonitis
	– Cervical motion tenderness (sliding cervical pain) is observed
	– A palpable mass in the small pelvis may indicate the presence of abscesses, such as pyosalpinx, tubo-ovarian abscess, or Douglas abscess
Ultrasound	– Free fluid may be detected in the pouch of Douglas
	– Imaging may reveal thickened fallopian tubes (sactosalpinx) and enlarged or indistinct ovaries
	– Sonography, in conjunction with findings from the bimanual pelvic examination, serves as an essential follow-up diagnostic tool
Wet mount microscopy	– Laboratory findings may indicate bacterial vaginosis, along with the presence of leukocytes, erythrocytes, cocci, and reduced counts of Döderlein bacilli
	– Microbiological cervical smear testing is beneficial in selected cases and should be conducted prior to the initiation of antibiotic therapy
Laboratory	– Laboratory assessments may reveal elevated white blood cell count (WBC) and increased C-reactive protein (CRP) levels
	– Beta-human chorionic gonadotropin (beta-hCG) levels should be negative
	– Urine sediment analysis is expected to be negative
	– An assessment of the coagulation profile (prothrombin time, partial thromboplastin time) should be performed
Laparoscopy	– Hyperemia of the internal genitalia may be noted
	– The presence of inflammatory exudates is a consideration
	– Possible conditions include pyo-, hydro-, or sactosalpinx
	– Exudative fluid accumulation may be detected in the abdominal cavity
	– Intraoperative swabs obtained from the fallopian tubes possess diagnostic value
	– Swabs collected from the pouch of Douglas are considered to have less clinical significance

- **Subacute PID** is characterized by persistent lower abdominal pain, low-grade fever, and well-defined palpable adnexal tenderness. Physical examination reveals cervical motion tenderness (the classic "chandelier sign"), uterine tenderness, and adnexal tenderness, which are the minimal clinical criteria for PID diagnosis. Additional findings may include mucopurulent cervical discharge, cervical friability, and abundant white blood cells on saline microscopy of vaginal fluid (Table 8.3).
- **Chronic PID (>30 days duration)** manifests with ongoing adnexal tenderness without fever, though intermittent exacerbations with acute symptoms may occur. Long-term consequences include chronic pelvic pain, affecting approximately 12% after one PID episode, 30% after two episodes, and over 60% after three or more episodes (Table 8.4).

Clinical Manifestations

- **Lower abdominal pain** is the most common symptom, occurring in about 95% of PID patients. Pain is typically bilateral but may be unilateral despite bilateral involvement. It can radiate to the upper abdomen and is often accompanied by nausea and vomiting when severe.
- **Abnormal vaginal discharge** occurs in approximately 75% of patients with gonococcal or chlamydial PID, usually presenting as mucopurulent, yellow-green discharge from the endocervical canal. This discharge differs distinctly from normal physiological secretions in color, consistency, and odor.
- **Menstrual irregularities**—including intermenstrual bleeding or menorrhagia—occur in around 40% of patients, primarily due to coexisting endometritis. Dysmenorrhea frequently worsens due to pelvic inflammation and scarring.
- **Dyspareunia**, especially deep pelvic pain during intercourse, is common due to pelvic inflammation and increased sensitivity; this symptom may persist long term as a result of adhesion formation.

Table 8.3 Clinical symptoms of subacute pelvic inflammatory disease

Symptoms	Comments
Pain	– Lower abdominal pain with tenderness in the adnexal area
Temperature	– Subfebrile to normal temperatures
Gynecological findings	– Relatively well-defined palpable findings in the adnexal area
	– Sometimes sliding cervical pain
	– Dysmenorrhea
	– Dyspareunia
Laboratory	– Often shows inconspicuous results
	– Sometimes presents with low leukocytosis
	– Occasionally borderline C-reactive protein (CRP)
Ultrasound	– Sometimes reveals thickened tubes
	– Occasionally shows uterine loosening
Laparoscopy	– Minor hyperemia of the internal genitals
	– Sometimes presents inflammatory deposits
	– Intraoperative swabs from the salpinges may be warranted

Table 8.4 Clinical symptoms of chronic pelvic inflammatory disease

Symptoms	Comments
Pain	– Pressure sensitivity is often localized to the adnexal region
	– Continuous lower abdominal pain may be reported
	– Low back pain can occur, potentially due to adhesions
Ultrasound	– Thickened, stationary fallopian tubes may occasionally be observed
	– Results are often inconclusive
Laboratory	– Findings may frequently be inconspicuous
	– Low leukocytosis may sometimes be indicated
	– Borderline levels of C-reactive protein (CRP) may be noted occasionally
Temperature	– Elevation is typically not present
Gynecological findings	– Recurrent vaginal discharge has been reported
	– Dysmenorrhea is frequently experienced
	– The presence of retroflexio uteri fixata (fixed retroverted uterus) may be noted
	– Dyspareunia is a common symptom
Wet mount microscopy	– Characteristic features may intermittently present
	– Elevated leukocyte counts may be detected
	– The presence of erythrocytes and cocci has been observed
	– A decrease in Döderlein bacteria is often evident
Laparoscopy	– Minor hyperemia of the internal genitals may be noted
	– Inflammatory deposits may sometimes be revealed
	– Intraoperative swabs of the salpinges may be collected, although findings are often insignificant
	– Pressure sensitivity is often localized to the adnexal region

- **Urinary symptoms** such as dysuria and increased frequency occur in approximately 15% of women with PID. These symptoms are caused by bladder irritation secondary to adjacent pelvic inflammation.
- **Fever** is present in about 40% of cases, predominantly in those with severe disease. When present, fever generally exceeds 38.3 °C and may be accompanied by chills and systemic signs of toxicity.

Specific Clinical Signs

- **Cervical motion tenderness** detected during bimanual examination is a hallmark sign of PID indicative of pelvic peritoneum inflammation.
- **Palpable adnexal masses** suggest tubo-ovarian abscess (TOA), which occurs in about 10–15% of hospitalized PID patients.
- **Retroflexed fixed uterus (retroflexio uteri fixata)** may develop due to chronic PID-related adhesions and scarring, contributing to chronic pelvic pain and dyspareunia.

Severe Complications and Life-Threatening Presentations

- **Tubo-ovarian abscess** is a serious complication presenting with sudden severe pelvic pain, high fever, tachycardia, and abdominal distension. Physical examination reveals generalized abdominal guarding and rebound tenderness, often limiting detailed pelvic examination.

- **Ruptured tubo-ovarian abscess** constitutes a medical emergency characterized by diffuse peritonitis, septic shock, and potential mortality. Symptoms include severe abdominal pain, high fever (up to 39.5 °C), vomiting, and peritoneal irritation signs.
- **Fitz-Hugh-Curtis syndrome (perihepatitis)** may develop as an extension of salpingitis, causing pleuritic right upper quadrant pain radiating to the right shoulder due to inflammation of the liver capsule.

Diagnostic Challenges

The broad variability in clinical features makes diagnosing PID difficult. Many patients have minimal or no symptoms, while others present with acute severe illness. The absence of fever and normal white blood cell counts do not rule out PID. Subclinical PID can remain asymptomatic yet still cause serious reproductive complications such as infertility, ectopic pregnancy, and chronic pelvic pain. Therefore, a high index of suspicion is necessary in sexually active women presenting with lower abdominal pain, abnormal vaginal discharge, or menstrual irregularities—especially in high-risk populations. Prompt empirical treatment is essential once minimum clinical criteria are met to prevent long-term reproductive damage and life-threatening sequelae.

The diversity in symptom type and severity contributes to misdiagnoses in approximately 40–50% of cases.

8.4.2 Pregnancy

PID during pregnancy is a very rare event; prevalence is estimated at <0.1% of all pregnancies. Physiological changes of gestation, particularly formation of the cervical mucus plug from approximately 12 weeks' gestation, create a natural barrier to ascending bacterial infection.

Epidemiology and Risk Factors

- In systematic reviews, only 49 documented cases of pelvic inflammatory disease (PID) during pregnancy were identified since 1971.
- Mean gestational age at diagnosis was 19.0 ± 10.3 weeks; mean maternal age was 25 ± 6.3 years.
- The following specific risk factors for pregnancy-associated PID have been described:
  - Maternal pelvic anatomic abnormalities (structural predisposition)
  - History of sexually transmitted infection prior to conception
  - Recent pelvic surgery or invasive pelvic procedures
  - In vitro fertilization (IVF) or oocyte retrieval, which have been associated with increased infection risk

Clinical Presentation and Complications

- Severe maternal complications were frequently reported: 62.8% of patients required exploratory laparotomy; 32.6% underwent unilateral salpingo-oophorectomy; 25.6% underwent appendectomy.
- Sepsis occurred in approximately 7% of cases and was associated with three neonatal deaths.
- Fetal and neonatal outcomes were affected: of 49 documented pregnancies, 26 (60.5%) resulted in live births with a mean gestational age of 33.8 ± 5.1 weeks; 17 cases (39.5%) resulted in nonviable pregnancy outcomes (spontaneous abortion and intrauterine fetal demise).

Pregnancy-Associated Risks

- PID in early pregnancy (<12 weeks) has been associated with an increased risk of chorioamnionitis and spontaneous abortion.
- In a Taiwanese cohort study of >30,000 women with PID, preterm birth occurred in 1.84% versus 1.63% in controls. The adjusted hazard ratio (aHR) for preterm birth was 1.864 ($p < 0.001$).
- The systemic inflammatory response during PID may lead to placental insufficiency, intrauterine growth restriction (IUGR), and premature rupture of membranes.
- Vertical transmission of bacterial pathogens is considered rare; however, maternal sepsis can cause fetal distress and neonatal death.

8.5 Diagnosis

The diagnosis of Pelvic Inflammatory Disease (PID) presents significant challenges and is determined by a thorough medical history, clinical examination, imaging procedures—including invasive diagnostics—and the collection of clinical-chemical and microbiological data. The diagnostic assessment includes a range of examination methods broadly categorized into five main categories:

- **Physical Examination:**
  - **Palpation and Inspection:** The examination may reveal pressure pain in the adnexa and potential defensive rigidity in the lower abdomen. Cervical sliding pain and the presence of masses in the small pelvis, such as abscesses (e.g., pyosalpinx, tubo-ovarian abscess, Douglas abscess), may also be observed.
- **Laboratory Tests:** Various laboratory tests are employed to assess the inflammatory status of the patient, including:
  - **Blood Count:** Evaluates the presence of infection or inflammation.
  - **Erythrocyte Sedimentation Rate (ESR):** This test is utilized to detect inflammation within the body.
  - **C-Reactive Protein (CRP):** Serves as an indicator of acute inflammation.
  - **β-hCG:** Rules out pregnancy-related concerns.

  - **Urine Sediment:** Identifies urinary tract involvement.
  - **Coagulation Status (Quick Value, Prothrombin Time—PTT):** Assesses coagulation function.
- **Ultrasound:** This imaging modality assists in identifying:
  - **Free Fluid:** Presence within the Douglas space.
  - **Thickened Fallopian Tubes:** Suggestive of inflammation or infection.
  - **Enlarged or Blurred Ovaries:** Indicative of ovarian involvement. These findings, coupled with bimanual palpation results, serve as an effective follow-up tool.
- **Wet Mount Microscopy/Native Preparation:** Microscopic analysis of native preparations may reveal:
  - **Bacterial Vaginosis:** Indicated by the presence of clue cells.
  - **Leukocytes and Erythrocytes:** Reflective of inflammation and infection.
  - **Cocci:** Suggestive of a bacterial infection.
  - **Lack of Lactobacilli:** Indicates disturbed vaginal flora. In select instances, a microbiological cervical smear may be beneficial, particularly prior to the initiation of antibiotics.
- **Laparoscopy:** This minimally invasive surgical technique can identify a spectrum of pathological findings, including:
  - **Massive Hyperemia:** Of the internal genital structures.
  - **Inflammatory Deposits:** Present on pelvic structures.
  - **Pyometra:** Infection of the uterine cavity.
  - **Hydroperitoneum:** Fluid accumulation in the abdominal cavity.
  - **Sactosalpinx:** Presence of fluid-filled fallopian tubes.
  - **Exudate:** Observed in the abdominal cavity. Intraoperative smears from the fallopian tubes can yield valuable diagnostic information; however, smears obtained from the Douglas space are generally less informative.

Diagnosis of subacute or chronic PID is conducted similarly to that of acute PID.

It is not necessary for all criteria to be met for a diagnosis to be established. Although lower abdominal discomfort is the most common symptom, some women may present with only mild or even absent symptoms despite underlying evidence of infection and inflammation of the uterine lining.

8.5.1 Clinical Examination

- **Palpation Findings:** During examination, the following findings may be identified:
  - **Unilateral or Bilateral Pressure Pain:** May be accompanied by palpable, doughy adnexal masses.

  - **Pain on Palpation:** Pain may be elicited during examination.
  - **Tumors in the Small Pelvis with Abscessation:** This includes conditions such as pyosalpinx, tubo-ovarian abscess, or Douglas abscess.
- **Sensitivity of Palpation Findings:**
  - **Cervical Sliding Pain:** Approximately 92% sensitivity when compared to histologically confirmed endometritis.
  - **Painful Adnexal Swelling:** Observed in 94% of patients.
  - **Uterine Tension:** Present in 96% of patients.
  - **Combination of Criteria:** Utilizing all three criteria (cervical sliding pain, painful adnexal swelling, and uterine tension) results in a sensitivity reduction to 83%.
- **Phase-Contrast Microscopy of the Native Preparation:** Evaluation of a native preparation obtained from the vagina or cervical canal may show:
  - **Leukocytes:** Indicative of inflammation.
  - **Erythrocytes:** Presence of blood cells.
  - **Cocci:** Suggestive of bacterial infection.
  - **Lactobacilli:** Limited in number, suggesting disrupted vaginal flora.
  - **Trichomonads:** Indicating possible trichomoniasis.
- **Microbiological Diagnosis:** To ascertain the presence of specific microorganisms, a microbiological cervical smear should be performed. This includes:
  - **Culture and Resistance Testing:** Particularly for *Chlamydia trachomatis* and *Neisseria gonorrhoeae*, where relevant prevalence exists.
  - **Timing of Swab Collection:** It is advisable to collect the swab before antibiotic administration to ensure accurate culture and sensitivity results.

8.5.2 Radiological Procedures

Ultrasound:

- **Findings:** Sonography typically reveals the presence of free fluid within the Douglas space, thickened fallopian tubes (sactosalpinx), and enlarged or blurred ovaries (Fig. 8.2).
- **Monitoring:** Combined with bimanual palpation performed at regular intervals, ultrasound facilitates effective monitoring of disease progression.
- **Transvaginal Ultrasound:** This minimally invasive procedure enhances diagnostic capabilities for evaluating PID; however, its sensitivity ranges from 32–81%, which is lower than that of laparoscopy.

Magnetic Resonance Imaging (MRI):

- **Potential Utility:** MRI may represent a useful alternative diagnostic tool for PID.
- **Limitations:** Current data supporting its use are limited; moreover, MRI is cost-prohibitive and impractical for routine clinical application.

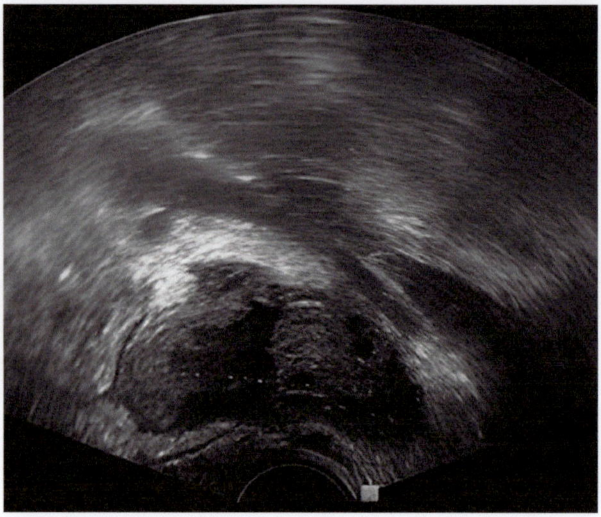

Fig. 8.2 Sonographic image indicating a tubo-ovarian abscess (Mylonas 2016)

8.5.3 Laboratory Diagnostics

Laboratory Tests: These should be implemented to gather comprehensive diagnostic information, including:

- **Complete Blood Count with Differential:** Evaluates overall health and identifies various disorders, including infections and inflammation.
- **Erythrocyte Sedimentation Rate (ESR):** Useful for assessing inflammatory processes, where feasible.
- **C-Reactive Protein (CRP) Value:** An elevated level indicates acute inflammation.
- **β-hCG:** Used to rule out pregnancy-related complications.
- **Urine Sediment:** To exclude urinary tract infections.
- **Coagulation Status:** Includes Quick value (Prothrombin Time, PT), Partial Thromboplastin Time (PTT), and platelet count to evaluate clotting ability.

The World Health Organization (WHO) advocates for a symptom-oriented approach to the diagnosis and management of PID. In the presence of symptoms such as lower abdominal pain or tenderness on palpation, immediate treatment initiation is recommended to prevent complications and improve outcomes, without waiting for laboratory test results.

8.5.4 Surgical Measures

At present, pelvic inflammatory disease (PID) can be confirmed through diagnostic laparoscopy or histopathological examination of biopsies obtained from the endometrium or fallopian tubes. However, neither method demonstrates high accuracy. The diagnostic accuracy of laparoscopy is estimated to range from 25% to 50% when compared to minibiopsy of tubal tissue. Histologically confirmed endometritis shows a sensitivity of 70–89% and a specificity of 67–92% when correlated with laparoscopically diagnosed salpingitis.

Confirmation of PID:

- **Diagnostic Laparoscopy:** Provides visual confirmation of the disease, albeit with a diagnostic accuracy of 25–50% compared to tubal tissue (mini) biopsies.
- **Histopathological Examination:** Biopsies from the endometrium or salpinges have demonstrated a sensitivity of 70–89% and specificity of 67–92% in confirming histologically diagnosed endometritis compared to laparoscopically diagnosed salpingitis.

Challenges in Current Diagnostic Methods:

- **Variability in Accuracy:** Both laparoscopy and histopathology have limitations concerning their sensitivity and accuracy.
- **Invasiveness:** Laparoscopy is an invasive procedure and is not routinely employed due to associated surgical risks and costs.

Laparoscopy in PID Diagnosis:

- **Advantages:**
  - **Reliable Diagnosis:** Allows for detailed assessment of disease extent.
  - **Differential Diagnosis:** Assists in ruling out other conditions, including appendicitis and inflammatory bowel disease.
  - **Pathogen Detection:** Enhances the identification of infectious agents.
  - **Therapeutic Options:** Facilitates immediate therapeutic interventions, including surgical procedures and lavage.
- **Disadvantages:**
  - **Hospitalization:** Requires inpatient care.
  - **High Costs:** Involves substantial expenses associated with surgical and hospital resources.
  - **Surgical Risks:** Carries inherent risks due to its invasive nature.

Utility of Laparoscopy: Laparoscopy is advantageous for diagnosing acute PID and is also valuable for recognizing chronic and past conditions. Findings during laparoscopy may encompass:

- **Massive Enlargement:** Notable enlargement of internal genital structures.
- **Inflammatory Deposits:** Presence of inflamed tissues.
- **Tubal Pathologies:** Including pyosalpinx, hydrosalpinx, or sactosalpinx.
- **Exudate:** Fluid accumulation within the abdominal cavity.

Intraoperative Swabs:

- **Salpingitis Swabs:** Should be dispatched to the laboratory in appropriate transport media to identify oxygen-sensitive obligate anaerobes.
- **Douglas Space Smears:** Generally considered less informative and not routinely recommended.

Obtaining smears from the Douglas pouch is of limited diagnostic value.

8.5.5 Pregnancy

In a Scandinavian study involving 2501 women with clinically suspected PID, sterility was observed in 16% of women with laparoscopically confirmed salpingitis, compared to 2.7% in the control group. Tubal infertility, accounting for approximately one-quarter of all infertility cases, was noted in 10.8% of subjects.

Sterility can result from tubal occlusion, with associations noted to antibodies against *Chlamydia trachomatis* or gonococci in various retrospective case-control studies. The likelihood of developing infertility increases approximately twofold with each subsequent episode of PID, reaching roughly 40% after three or more episodes. Infertility rates are markedly elevated in populations with a high prevalence of PID coupled with limited access to medical care. Chronic lower abdominal pain post-episode is noted in approximately 20–30% of women, significantly impacting both physical and mental health.

PID during pregnancy is rare, particularly after the first trimester. Pregnant patients presenting with PID should be hospitalized for further evaluation and parental therapy due to increased morbidity risks for both mother and fetus.

8.6 Treatment

8.6.1 General Consideration

Any patient presenting with acute PID should be admitted to the hospital, and treatment should commence immediately.

It is advisable to initiate therapy prior to any further diagnostic evaluations, as delays are associated with an elevated risk of sterility and chronic lower abdominal issues.

- **Outpatient Treatment:** Mild cases of PID, characterized by the absence of palpable tumors or significant ultrasound findings and excluding appendicitis, may be managed on an outpatient basis.
- **General Measures:**
  - **Bed Rest:** Patients are advised to minimize activity.
  - **Ice Packs:** Application of ice packs to the affected area can help reduce inflammation.
  - **Pain Management:** Analgesics and spasmolytics should be administered for relief.
  - **Diabetes Monitoring:** For diabetic patients, continuous monitoring and management of their condition is essential.
- **Resorption-Promoting Measures:** Following the acute phase, various physical measures may assist in promoting resorption and mitigating inflammation, though clinical efficacy may be uncertain:
  - **Cold Application:** Cold compresses.
  - **Priesnitz Compresses and Wraps:** Traditional methods aimed at reducing inflammation.
  - **Ascending Sitz Baths:** Improve circulation and alleviate discomfort.
  - **Short Wave Treatment:** Employs electromagnetic fields for therapeutic benefit.
  - **Mud Packs:** Utilized for their anti-inflammatory properties.
- **Pharmacological Interventions:**
  - **Antibiotic Therapy:** Should be informed by an antibiogram when available. Broadspectrum antibiotics are recommended for initial empirical treatment. Key considerations include:
    - **Broad-Spectrum Coverage:** Selecting antibiotics that are effective against major aerobic and anaerobic bacteria.
    - **Combination Therapy:** Caution is advised against combining bactericidal and bacteriostatic antibiotics due to potential pharmacological interference, reduced effectiveness, and increased risk of resistance.
    - **Triple Antibiotic Therapy:** Despite its theoretical advantage of broader coverage, practical challenges such as adverse effects and drug interactions exist, along with limited supporting clinical evidence.
  - **Recommended Regimen:** A combination of a fluoroquinolone with metronidazole is favored by many experts for its superior efficacy compared to traditional cephalosporin-based therapies.
- **Therapy Adjustment:**
  - Modifications should be made based on antibiogram results.
  - **Chronic PID:** Extended therapy duration up to 3 weeks is recommended for chronic cases.
- **Surgical Interventions:** If medical therapy is ineffective, surgical options should be considered:
  - **Laparoscopy/Laparotomy:** Indicated for persistent fever, unresolved adnexal masses, or deterioration in the patient's overall condition.

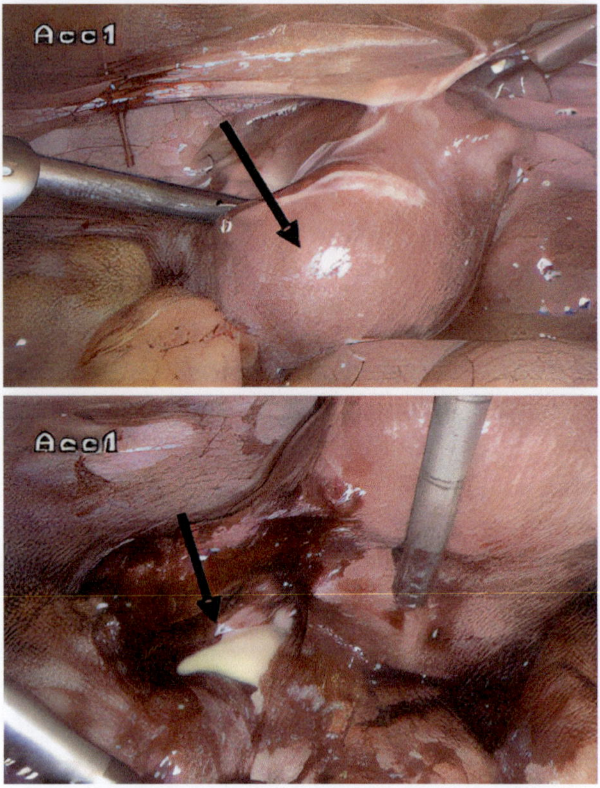

Fig. 8.3 Tubo-ovarian abscess in the left adnexa. Abundant purulent material is discharged upon incision of the abscess (Mylonas and Friese 2009)

- **Abscess Management:** In cases involving Douglas, ovarian, or tubo-ovarian abscesses (Fig. 8.3), inpatient treatment is critical.
- **Personalized Approach:** Surgical treatment should be individualized according to the patient's age, reproductive goals, and overall health status.

From an infectious disease management perspective, it is advisable to remove any intrauterine device (IUD) that has been inserted.

8.6.2 Antimicrobial Therapy

8.6.2.1 Outpatient Therapy

8.6.2.1.1 General Consideration

- In certain cases, pelvic inflammatory disease (PID) can be managed on an outpatient basis, provided specific criteria are met (Table 21).

- **Requirements for Outpatient Therapy:**
  - **Mild PID:** Symptoms are not severe.
  - **Absence of Palpable Tumor:** No tumors are detected upon examination.
  - **Absence of Ultrasound Findings:** No significant abnormalities are observed in ultrasound imaging.
  - **Exclusion of Appendicitis:** Appendicitis must be ruled out as a differential diagnosis.
- **Follow-Up:**
  - **Re-examination:** Patients treated on an outpatient basis should be reexamined and assessed 2–3 days after initiating therapy.
  - **Hospital Admission Criteria:** If no clinical improvement is noted, the patient should be admitted to the hospital, and parenteral therapy should be initiated.
- **Considerations for Specific Patient Populations:** Short-term and monotherapies may be particularly beneficial for:
  - **Low Compliance:** Patients who may struggle with adhering to complex treatment regimens.
  - **Limited Access to Medical Care:** Individuals who have difficulty accessing healthcare services.
  - **Low Socioeconomic Status:** Women from disadvantaged backgrounds are at an elevated risk of sexually transmitted diseases (STD) and subsequent PID. These individuals often report a higher number of sexual partners, more frequent partner changes, and greater cervical ectopia, all of which contribute to their increased biological susceptibility to infections.

8.6.2.1.2 Global Outpatient Treatment Options for Pelvic Inflammatory Disease

- **Ofloxacin and Metronidazole**
  - **Dosage and Duration:** Ofloxacin 400 mg orally twice daily, plus metronidazole 500 mg orally twice daily for 14 days.
  - **Note:** Ofloxacin, a racemate exhibiting reduced efficacy, should be substituted with levofloxacin, a more potent alternative, when available.
- **Amoxicillin/Clavulanic Acid and Metronidazole**
  - **Dosage and Duration:** Amoxicillin/clavulanic acid 875/125 mg orally twice daily, plus metronidazole 500 mg orally three times daily for 10–14 days.
  - **Note:** Not recommended in some countries due to limited efficacy against some bacteria and the potential for resistance.
- **Ciprofloxacin and Metronidazole**
  - **Dosage and Duration:** Ciprofloxacin 500 mg orally twice daily, plus metronidazole 500 mg orally twice daily for 14 days.
  - **Note:** Avoid this regimen if *Chlamydia trachomatis* is suspected.
- **Ceftriaxone, Doxycycline, and Metronidazole**
  - **Dosage and Duration:** Ceftriaxone 500 mg intramuscularly or intravenously as a single dose, plus doxycycline 100 mg orally twice daily, plus metronidazole 500 mg orally twice daily for 14 days.
  - **Note:** A recommended option for broad-spectrum coverage, including anaerobes.

- **Levofloxacin and Metronidazole**
  - **Dosage and Duration:** Levofloxacin 500 mg orally once daily, plus metronidazole 500 mg orally twice daily for 14 days.
  - **Note:** A recommended option for broad-spectrum coverage, including anaerobes.
- **Moxifloxacin and Metronidazole**
  - **Dosage and Duration:** Moxifloxacin 400 mg orally once daily, plus metronidazole 500 mg orally twice daily for 14 days.
  - **Note:** While effective for broad-spectrum coverage, this regimen may be theoretically less optimal to other combinations.
- **Amoxicillin/Clavulanic Acid, Doxycycline, and Metronidazole**
  - **Dosage and Duration:** Amoxicillin/clavulanic acid 875/125 mg orally twice daily, plus doxycycline 100 mg orally twice daily, plus metronidazole 500 mg orally twice daily for 14 days.
  - **Note:** Not recommended in some countries due to limited coverage against key pathogens and increased resistance risks.

Empirical therapy without metronidazole is strongly discouraged due to the high prevalence of anaerobic bacteria in pelvic inflammatory disease (PID) cases, as regimens incorporating metronidazole are essential to ensure adequate anaerobic coverage. The combination of bacteriostatic agents, such as doxycycline, with bactericidal agents, such as ceftriaxone, may reduce the effectiveness of the bactericidal drugs and should be carefully evaluated to avoid compromising treatment efficacy. Additionally, the implementation of triple antibiotic therapy can be challenging in some regions due to limited availability of medications or constraints in healthcare infrastructure, and concerns about antibiotic resistance further complicate its use in such settings.

8.6.2.2 Inpatient Therapy

8.6.2.2.1 General Consideration

- **Criteria for Inpatient Treatment:** Inpatient treatment should be considered if any of the following criteria are met:
  - **Potential Appendicitis:** Appendicitis cannot be excluded.
  - **Systemic Symptoms:** Presence of fever, nausea, or vomiting.
  - **Peritonitis:** Signs of inflammation or infection within the peritoneal cavity.
  - **Adnexal Findings:** Particularly the presence of a tubo-ovarian abscess (Fig. 8.3).
  - **Specific Patient Groups:** Adolescents or pregnant women.
  - **Non-Response to Oral Therapy:** No improvement reported after a maximum of 48 h of oral therapy.
  - **Transition from Parenteral to Oral Therapy:**
    - A 48-h period should elapse between the initiation of antibiotic therapy and the commencement of oral therapy.
    - It is anticipated that lower abdominal discomfort and other symptoms of acute PID will resolve within 48–72 h of starting antibiotic therapy.

- **Further Diagnostic Procedures:**
  - **Lack of Symptom Improvement:** If no improvement is observed within 48–72 h, additional diagnostic assessments should be conducted.
  - **Consideration of Laparoscopy:** Laparoscopy may be used as a diagnostic tool to further investigate persistent symptoms.

8.6.2.2.2 Global Inpatient Treatment Options for Pelvic Inflammatory Disease

- **Ciprofloxacin and Metronidazole**
  - **Dosage and Duration:** Ciprofloxacin 400 mg intravenously twice daily, plus metronidazole 500 mg three times daily, intravenously or orally, for 10–14 days.
  - **Note:** Use only when infection with *Chlamydia trachomatis* is not suspected.
- **Levofloxacin and Metronidazole**
  - **Dosage and Duration:** Levofloxacin 500 mg intravenously twice daily, plus metronidazole 500 mg three times daily, intravenously or orally, for 10–14 days.
  - **Note**: Provides broad-spectrum coverage, including anaerobic bacteria.
- **Moxifloxacin and Metronidazole**
  - **Dosage and Duration:** Moxifloxacin 400 mg intravenously once daily, plus metronidazole 500 mg three times daily, intravenously, for 10–14 days.
  - **Note:** Effective for anaerobic coverage but may not be as comprehensive as other regimens.
- **Amoxicillin/Clavulanic Acid and Metronidazole**
  - **Dosage and Duration:** Amoxicillin/clavulanic acid 2.2 g intravenously three times daily, plus metronidazole 500 mg three times daily, intravenously, for 10–14 days.
  - **Note:** Suitable for broad-spectrum coverage but may not cover all specific pathogens. Not recommended in some countries due to limited efficacy against some bacteria and the potential for resistance.
- **Ampicillin/Sulbactam and Metronidazole**
  - **Dosage and Duration:** Ampicillin/sulbactam 3 g intravenously four times daily, plus doxycycline 100 mg twice daily, orally or intravenously, for 10–14 days.
  - **Note:** Effective against a broad range of pathogens, including anaerobic bacteria. Not recommended in some countries due to limited efficacy against some bacteria and the potential for resistance.
- **Clindamycin and Gentamicin**
  - **Dosage and Duration:** Clindamycin 900 mg intravenously three times daily, plus gentamicin (initial dose of 2 mg/kg intravenously or intramuscularly, followed by 1.5 mg/kg three times daily), intravenously, for 10–14 days.
  - **Note:** Useful for severe infections. However, the combination may be pharmacologically suboptimal due to bacteriostatic/bactericidal interactions. Not recommended in some countries due to limited efficacy against some bacteria and the potential for resistance.

- **Piperacillin/Tazobactam and Doxycycline**
  - **Dosage and Duration:** Piperacillin/tazobactam 4.5 g intravenously three times daily, plus doxycycline 100 mg orally twice daily, for 7–14 days.
  - **Note:** Provides broad coverage but is often reserved for severe or complicated cases. However, the combination may be pharmacologically suboptimal due to bacteriostatic/bactericidal interactions. Sometimes metronidazole 500 mg three times daily, intravenously, for 10–14 days is being added together or instead of doxycycline.

Empirical regimens without metronidazole are not recommended for pelvic inflammatory disease (PID) due to the high prevalence of anaerobic bacteria, as anaerobic coverage is essential to prevent severe complications. A three-times-daily regimen of metronidazole (500 mg per dose) is generally preferred, with international guidelines recommending a total daily dose of 1000–1500 mg (administered as 500 mg two to three times daily). Some guidelines suggest a reduced dose of 400 mg two to three times daily, representing a reduction of 20–45%. Ciprofloxacin should be used only in cases where *Chlamydia trachomatis* infection is not suspected. The combination of bacteriostatic agents, such as tetracyclines, macrolides, or clindamycin, with bactericidal agents, such as beta-lactams, fluoroquinolones, or aminoglycosides, can decrease the efficacy of bactericidal agents due to pharmacological incompatibility. Furthermore, triple antibiotic therapy (e.g., ceftriaxone intramuscularly combined with doxycycline and potentially metronidazole) may be impractical in certain regions because of healthcare infrastructure limitations, including medication availability and intramuscular administration capabilities. Concerns regarding antibiotic resistance further complicate the use of such regimens on a global scale.

8.6.3 Care Situation

Many women rely on emergency departments and (specialist) outpatient clinics for the diagnosis and treatment of their conditions. Therefore, the need for rapid diagnosis and timely treatment, along with a significantly lower decision threshold, is crucial, as the likelihood of follow-up care is often low.

The risk of long-term sequelae (e.g., infertility and chronic pelvic pain) increases if treatment is delayed. Thus, it is paramount that women receive prompt care when they first present to the healthcare system.

Notably, 20% of patients presenting to the emergency department with lower abdominal pain were not treated or received treatment that deviated from recommendations. A retrospective analysis of 121 cases of PID in 2004 demonstrated poor adherence to treatment guidelines:

- Detailed History: 14%.
- Physical Examination: 22%.
- Comprehensive Diagnostic Tests: 71%.
- Prescription of Antibiotics: 32%.
- Instructions for Safer Sex: 15%.

Overall, these findings suggest that physicians often prescribe antibiotics for shorter durations to achieve better compliance or to align with financial constraints, resulting in suboptimal diagnosis and treatment in both outpatient and inpatient settings.

HIV-positive patients with PID typically experience a more severe course compared to their uninfected counterparts, exhibiting a higher risk of developing tubo-ovarian abscesses and increased rates of laparoscopic or surgical interventions, including extirpation and hysterectomy. Close monitoring of these patients is essential.

8.7 Differential Diagnosis

A variety of gynecological and non-gynecological conditions must be considered in the differential diagnosis of acute abdominal pain. Gynecological causes may include:

- Pelvic Inflammatory Disease (PID).
- Salpingitis.
- Endometriosis.
- Myoma necrosis.
- Ovarian cyst rupture.
- Pedicle torsion.

Additionally, pregnancy-related factors such as miscarriage, ectopic pregnancy, premature placental abruption, and preterm labor can also result in abdominal pain. Non-gynecological causes include:

- Appendicitis.
- Diverticulitis.
- Urinary tract infection.
- Ileus.
- Ureteral stones.

Minor triggers such as menstruation, constipation, and a full bladder may also lead to abdominal pain. The most critical and prevalent differential diagnoses include appendicitis, diverticulitis, and ectopic pregnancy (Table 8.5).

Table 8.5 Important differential diagnoses of pelvic inflammatory disease (PID)

Criteria	PID	Appendicitis	Ectopic pregnancy	Diverticulitis
General				
Age (15–25 years)	+++	+/–	++	–
Pregnancy	–	–	+++	–
Symptoms				
Defense tension	++	+++	++	+
Pulling on both sides	+++	–	–	–
Standing on one side	–	+++	+++	–
Fever (over 38 °C)	++	+++	–	++
Vaginal discharge	+++	–	+	–
Cramp-like	+	++	++	++
Pain upon release	–	+++	–	+
McBurney point	–	+++	–	–
Urinary problems	+	+	+	–
Kidney palpation	–	–	–	–
Sliding cervical pain	+++	–	++	–
Bowel irregularities	+	+++	+	++
Nausea and vomiting	+	+++	+	+
Lower abdominal pain	+	++	+	++
Laboratory				
Elevated CRP	+++	+++	–	++
Leukocytosis	+++	+++	–	++
Sonography				
Adnexal mass	+++	–	++	–
Visualized tube	–	–	+++	–
Extrauterine sac	–	–	+++	–
Free fluid	+++	+	+++	–
Dilated renal pelvis	–	–	–	–
Empty uterine cavity	–	–	+++	–
Blurred ovaries	++	–	–	–
Thickened bowel wall	–	–	–	+++
Complications	Concomitant appendicitis	Accompanies PID	–	–
	Pelveoperitonitis	Perforation	Tubal rupture	Pelveoperitonitis
	Ectopic Pregnancy	Ectopic Pregnancy	Sepsis	Abscess formation

– = never/very rarely; + = rarely; ++ = frequently; +++ = very frequently

8.8 Prevention

Given the diagnostic challenges associated with PID, implementing prophylactic measures is essential. Preventing pelvic inflammatory disease begins with providing adequate sexual hygiene education for children and adolescents. Early detection of infections in the lower genital tract is similarly crucial. The insertion of an intrauterine device (IUD) for contraceptive purposes is not recommended for nulliparous women and individuals with diabetes.

Additionally, early detection of sexually transmitted diseases (STD) and the provision of counseling and prevention strategies can contribute to reducing PID incidence.

The most effective method for preventing PID is to promote the primary prevention of sexually transmitted diseases. Research has demonstrated the impact of consistent condom use on the prevention of infections with *Neisseria gonorrhoeae* and *Chlamydia trachomatis*. Among 684 sexually active women, consistent condom use was associated with a 30–60% reduction in recurrent PID. Consequently, the limited data available suggest that barrier contraception, particularly condoms, may offer .protection against PID.

Key Points

- PID represents inflammation of the internal female reproductive organs, notably the fallopian tubes and ovaries. It is typically the consequence of an ascending infection but can also arise via descending routes or postoperatively.
- Identified risk factors for PID include menstruation, intrauterine devices (IUDs), diagnostic procedures, promiscuity, and early sexual activity.
- Clinical manifestations of PID can vary widely, but the most common symptoms are abdominal pain, fever, nausea, and vaginal discharge.
- The clinical picture of PID can range from mild cases with few symptoms to severe, life-threatening forms of inflammation.
- PID may present in three distinct forms: acute, subacute, and chronic.
- Typical symptoms of acute PID include severe lower abdominal pain and fever.
- Subacute PID is characterized by pain, tenderness in the lower abdomen, and palpable findings in the adnexal area.
- Chronic PID may present with tenderness in the adnexa without an increase in temperature.
- Diagnosing PID is challenging, necessitating a comprehensive medical history, thorough clinical examination, imaging techniques, and laboratory tests.

(continued)

- Clinical examination findings may include adnexal tenderness, cervical tenderness, and tumor formation in the pelvis.
- Laboratory tests can indicate inflammatory parameters and other relevant metrics. Ultrasound examinations often reveal free fluid within the Douglas space, as well as thickened fallopian tubes and enlarged ovaries.
- Laparoscopic evaluation can facilitate establishing a reliable diagnosis, excluding differential diagnoses, and enhancing pathogen detection.
- PID during pregnancy can lead to various complications, necessitating the implementation of specific diagnostic and therapeutic procedures.
- Women with a history of PID are at increased risk of infertility, chronic lower abdominal pain, and ectopic pregnancies.
- It is recommended that therapy be initiated before conducting additional diagnostic procedures to avoid delays.
- In the case of mild PID without complications, outpatient treatment may be considered a viable option.
- General measures such as bed rest, application of ice packs, and administration of analgesics may be beneficial. Antibiotic therapy should be provided for an appropriate duration.
- If pharmacological intervention proves ineffective, surgical options, such as laparoscopy or laparotomy, may be required.
- Differential diagnoses, including appendicitis, diverticulitis, and ectopic pregnancy, should be kept in mind when treating PID.
- Preventive strategies for reducing PID incidence include sexual hygiene education, early detection of lower genital tract infections, and promotion of condom use.

Urethritis

9

Abstract

Urethritis is characterized by inflammation of the urethra, typically presenting symptoms such as dysuria and urethral discharge. The primary pathogens associated with urethritis include *Neisseria gonorrhoeae* and *Chlamydia trachomatis*. When these pathogens are excluded, the condition may be classified as nongonococcal urethritis (NGU) or nongonococcal nonchlamydial urethritis (NGNCU). Other potential causative agents include mycoplasma and herpes simplex virus. Diagnosis is based on the analysis of urethral discharge, urine, and smears, with the identification of granulocytes in the smear serving as an indicator of urethritis. Immediate initiation of antibiotic therapy is recommended. If symptoms persist, reevaluation is warranted, as recurrent or persistent urethritis may suggest the involvement of other pathogens or resistant organisms. When symptoms are present without isolation of a pathogen, often accompanied by burning and itching, specialized clinical examinations should be conducted, and individualized treatment should be implemented.

9.1 Acute Urethritis

9.1.1 Background

Urethritis can be categorized into infectious and non-infectious forms. Infectious urethritis can be further divided into bacterial, viral, and trichomoniasis. Non-infectious urethritis includes irritative urethritis, allergic urethritis, and trauma-related conditions. Isolated urethritis is more commonly observed in males, while females frequently present with concurrent cystitis. Dysuria without evidence of bacteria in midstream urine is categorized as acute urethral syndrome; inflammation of Skene's glands may also be present.

I. Mylonas, *Sexually Transmitted Diseases*,
https://doi.org/10.1007/978-3-031-78204-6_9

9.1.2 Pathogen

The primary pathogen implicated in urethritis is *Neisseria gonorrhoeae*. If urethritis is unrelated to this pathogen, it is classified as nongonococcal urethritis (NGU). *Chlamydia trachomatis* may also be identified as a causative factor. If neither *Neisseria gonorrhoeae* nor *Chlamydia trachomatis* is involved, the condition is often referred to as nongonococcal nonchlamydial urethritis (NGNCU).

The significant pathogens associated with acute urethritis include:

- **Major Pathogens:**
  - ***Chlamydia trachomatis.***
  - ***Neisseria gonorrhoeae.***
- **Other Pathogens:**
  - ***Trichomonas vaginalis.***
  - **Herpes simplex virus.**
  - ***Mycoplasma genitalium.***
  - ***Ureaplasma urealyticum.***
- **Very Rare Pathogens:**
  - ***Candida albicans.***
  - **Adenoviruses.**

9.1.3 Clinical Manifestation

Isolated urethritis is characterized by urethral inflammation that manifests as dysuria, urethral discharge, and meatal irritation. Discharge may range from mucopurulent to frankly purulent in appearance (see Fig. 9.1). In gonococcal urethritis, symptoms typically emerge 2–6 days after exposure, whereas nongonococcal urethritis—most often due to *Chlamydia trachomatis*, *Mycoplasma genitalium*, or *Ureaplasma urealyticum*—presents after an incubation period of approximately 2–3 weeks. Up to 25% of cases remain asymptomatic, underscoring the importance of screening in at-risk populations.

Key clinical features include:

- Dysuria: burning or pain on urination
- Urethral Discharge: mucopurulent or purulent, often most noticeable on morning awakening
- Distal Urethral or Meatal Irritation: pruritus, erythema, or tenderness

In women, urethritis may occur without concurrent cervicitis; therefore, obtain first-void urine for NAATs and collect endocervical or vaginal swabs for Gram stain, culture, and amplification assays. Prompt specimen collection and targeted testing facilitate accurate diagnosis, enable detection of coinfections, and guide appropriate antimicrobial therapy.

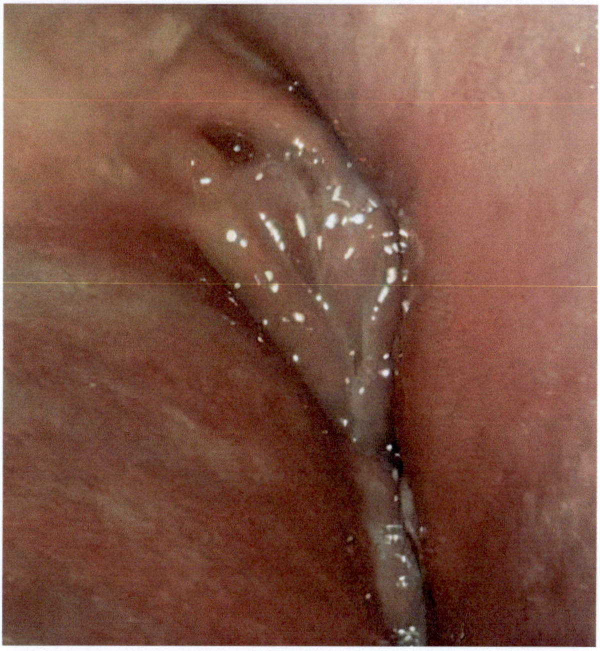

Fig. 9.1 Severe purulent urethritis caused by gonococci (Mylonas 2016)

Dysuria and pollakiuria may also indicate urethritis but are often misinterpreted as cystitis.

9.1.4 Diagnosis

Presence of urethral discharge should be utilized for microbiological examination. Additionally, endourethral swabs may be collected (Fig. 9.2).

The detection of granulocytes in the smear is indicative of urethritis.

Clinical evaluation of suspected urethritis requires targeted specimen collection to optimize pathogen detection.

Initially, assess for visible urethral discharge, which should be promptly collected for Gram staining, microscopy, and culture. If discharge is minimal or absent, obtain endourethral swabs using a flexible, small-bore swab inserted 2–4 cm into the urethra and gently rotated (see Fig. 9.2).

A noninvasive alternative is first-void urine (FVU) collection, suitable for nucleic acid amplification tests (NAATs) and quantitative microscopy. Patients should be instructed to provide the initial 10–20 mL of their first morning urine stream, as this

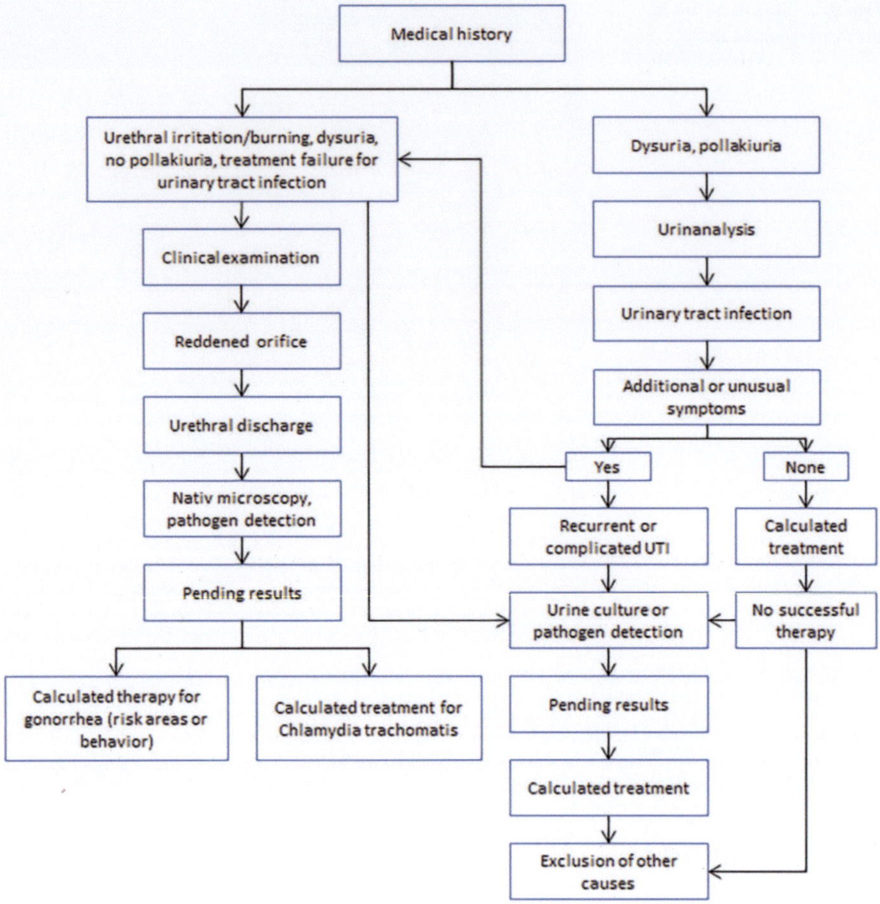

Fig. 9.2 Diagnostic procedure for suspected urethritis. (Courtesy of I. Mylonas)

contains the highest concentration of urethral epithelial cells, leukocytes, and pathogens. If morning collection is not feasible, advise a minimum of 2–4 h of urinary abstinence before sample collection to enhance specimen quality.

For a more detailed assessment of infection site, a three-stream urine collection may be performed approximately 2 h after the last void. However, collection of the final void is not always feasible in clinical settings and may be omitted when impractical.

1. First Portion (Initial 10–20 mL): Reflects urethral flora and leukocyte count, aiding in diagnosing urethritis.
2. Midstream Portion: Minimizes urethral contamination and is useful for detecting bladder infection.
3. Final Portion: May capture organisms ascending into the bladder or kidneys, assisting in evaluation for cystitis or pyelonephritis.

Microscopic examination of each fraction for white blood cell counts and bacterial casts helps differentiate lower from upper urinary tract involvement.

Specimens should be processed immediately when possible. If transport exceeds 2 h, samples must be refrigerated at 2–8 °C to preserve integrity.

Differential diagnoses for urethritis may include:

- Fever and chills.
- Hematuria.
- Pollakiuria.
- Nocturia.
- Urgency symptoms.
- Lymphadenopathy.

In females, a burning sensation during urination frequently suggests a urinary tract infection (UTI), and symptoms such as pollakiuria and dysuria may similarly indicate such an infection.

9.1.5 Therapy

9.1.5.1 Antimicrobial Therapy

Empirical therapy for a urethritis should primarily focus on *Chlamydia trachomatis*. In cases of high clinical suspicion or prevalent gonorrhea, the most appropriate treatment should be implemented (Sect. 14.6). This principle extends to infections caused by *Trichomonas vaginalis*, warranting empirical treatment in high-prevalence areas.

Antibiotic therapy should commence promptly upon diagnosis of urethritis, even prior to microbiological smear test results.

Tetracyclines and macrolides are effective against *Chlamydia trachomatis*, although instances of treatment-refractory infections have been documented. Azithromycin has emerged as the preferred therapy, particularly in Anglo-American regions. Other macrolides (e.g., erythromycin) or fluoroquinolones (e.g., levofloxacin) may also be employed (Table 9.1). These treatments have demonstrated efficacy against *Chlamydia trachomatis* and associated urinary tract pathogens; however, tetracyclines and increasingly azithromycin are ineffective against *Mycoplasma genitalium*.

Symptoms may persist for up to seven days following the cessation of therapy.

Table 9.1 Treatment options for acute urethritis with limited efficacy against *Mycoplasma genitalium*

Indication	Medication	Dosage	Duration
Treatment	Azithromycin	Day 1: 500 mg orally once Days 2–5: 250 mg orally once	5 days
	Doxycycline	100 mg orally twice daily	7 days
First alternative	Moxifloxacin	400 mg orally once daily	7–10 days
Second alternative	Erythromycin	500 mg orally four times daily	7–10 days
	Erythromycin ethylsuccinate	800 mg orally four times daily	7–10 days
	Roxithromycin	150 mg orally twice daily	7–10 days
	Levofloxacin	500 mg orally once daily	7 days

9.1.5.2 Further Measures

Subsequent behavioral measures should be thoroughly discussed with the patient. In most instances, follow-up examinations to confirm treatment success are unnecessary. Patients should be informed that symptoms *may continue for up to 1 week* after treatment completion. If symptoms return within 30 to 90 days after treatment, reevaluation is necessary, as this may indicate recurrent or persistent urethritis.

9.1.5.3 Treatment of the Partner

It is recommended to notify sexual partners who were active within 60 to 90 days prior to the onset of symptoms. If no sexual partners are identified during this period, the most recent partner should be informed. Testing and treatment of sexual partners are recommended; treatment should be empirical, irrespective of clinical findings or pending laboratory results.

9.1.5.4 Measures Following Treatment Completion

- Unprotected sexual intercourse should be avoided for up to 7 days post-initiation of therapy.
- Usage of condoms during sexual intercourse is highly recommended.
- Follow-up examinations after successful treatment are not advised. If deemed necessary, a follow-up should occur at the earliest opportunity, ideally within 3 weeks post-treatment, to mitigate the risk of false-positive results, particularly with molecular biological diagnostic methods.
- Persistent or recurrent symptoms within a week after treatment completion warrant reexamination and assessment.
- The presence of symptoms alone, without supportive laboratory findings or clinically significant results, does not justify the initiation of a new treatment regimen.
- In the event of urethritis diagnosis, immediate antibiotic therapy should be commenced, even in the absence of microbiological confirmation.

9.2 Recurrent or Persistent Urethritis

9.2.1 Background

Recurrent or persistent urethritis poses significant diagnostic and therapeutic challenges. This condition is defined as symptomatic urethritis occurring 30–90 days following treatment for acute non-gonococcal urethritis in approximately 10–20% of cases. In such cases, the presence of resistant microorganisms should be considered. Additionally, reinfection from a new or inadequately treated partner, along with issues related to poor adherence to antibiotic therapy (for instance, due to gastrointestinal side effects), must also be taken into account.
Key aspects to consider in recurrent or persistent urethritis include:

- Possible infections with other, non-sexually transmitted pathogens.
- The presence of resistant microorganisms.
- Incomplete or inappropriate medication administration.
- Reinfection by a new or untreated partner.
- Other potential causes such as urinary tract infections, neoplasms, or urethral strictures.

9.2.2 Pathogen

The etiology of recurrent or persistent urethritis appears to be multifactorial. *Mycoplasma genitalium* has been identified as a potential causative agent in 20–40% of cases. Similarly, *Ureaplasma urealyticum* has been associated with chronic NGU, although the precise correlation remains undefined.

9.2.3 Clinical Manifestation

Symptoms are consistent with those observed in acute urethritis.

9.2.4 Diagnosis

Diagnosis corresponds with that of acute urethritis. However, the following considerations should be addressed:

- Confirmation of urethritis should be established both clinically and through laboratory assessments.
- Urethral swabs should be tested for the presence of *Trichomonas vaginalis*. If ulcerative lesions are prominent, testing for herpes simplex should also be conducted.
- Examination of urethral swabs or urine for *Ureaplasma urealyticum* and *Mycoplasma genitalium* is recommended.

9.2.5 Therapy

9.2.5.1 Antimicrobial Therapy

- **Current Treatment Protocols**: Current guidelines throughout the world do not sufficiently address *Mycoplasma genitalium*. Given the rising prevalence of antibiotic resistance, especially noted with single doses of azithromycin, treatment courses longer than 5 days are now frequently advocated (Table 9.2).
- **Management of Recurrent Nongonococcal Urethritis (NGU)**: Retreatment protocols must include coverage for both *Mycoplasma genitalium* and *Trichomonas vaginalis*, particularly in areas with a high prevalence of these pathogens.
- **Macrolide Utilization**: Should macrolides have been utilized in the initial treatment regimen, an alternative antibiotic class should be chosen for follow-up therapy to prevent the emergence of resistance.
- **Urological Examination**: A urological examination is essential for differentiating urethritis from other urological conditions such as urinary tract infections, neoplasms, or urethral strictures.
- **Symptom Resolution**:
  – **Spontaneous Resolution**: Symptoms may resolve spontaneously, though this process can extend over several months.
  – **Symptomatic Therapy**: During this period, symptomatic treatments with analgesics and nonsteroidal anti-inflammatory drugs (NSAIDs) may provide relief.

9.2.5.2 Further Measures

Further behavioral discussions with the patient are recommended. In addition to previously mentioned measures (Sect. 2.8, page 25), consider:

- Treatment of sexual partners for infections with *Trichomonas*, *Chlamydia trachomatis*, and *Mycoplasma*.
- Exclusion of diabetes mellitus and immunodeficiency diseases (e.g., HIV) as potential underlying causes in recurrent or persistent urethritis.

Table 9.2 Treatment options for recurrent or persistent urethritis with limited efficacy against *Mycoplasma genitalium*

Indication	Medication and dosage	Duration
Treatment	Azithromycin 1.5 g orally as a single dose plus metronidazole 500 mg orally twice daily	5 days
	Erythromycin 500 mg orally four times daily for 21 days plus Metronidazole 500 mg orally twice daily	5 days
First alternative	Moxifloxacin 400 mg orally once daily for 7–10 days plus Metronidazole 500 mg orally twice daily	5 days
Second alternative	Clarithromycin 500 mg orally twice daily for 21 days plus Metronidazole 500 mg orally three times daily	5 days
	Roxithromycin 300 mg orally once daily for 21 days plus Metronidazole 500 mg orally three times daily	5 days

- The administration of a single dose of azithromycin is no longer considered advisable.
- While effective against *Chlamydia trachomatis* and other pathogens, neither tetracyclines nor azithromycin are effective against *Mycoplasma genitalium*.

Symptoms may persist for up to 7 days post-therapy cessation.

9.2.5.3 Treatment of the Partner

Sexual partners who were active within 60 to 90 days prior to the onset of symptoms should be informed. If no sexual partners are identified within this time frame, the most recent partner should be notified. Testing and treatment of partners are advised; treatment should be empirical, regardless of clinical findings or laboratory results.

Subsequent behavioral measures should be clearly communicated to the patient. In most cases, follow-up examinations to confirm treatment success are not necessary. The patient should be informed that symptoms may persist for up to one week following the completion of treatment. If symptoms recur within 30 to 90 days post-treatment, reassessment is necessary, as this may indicate recurrent or persistent urethritis.

9.2.5.4 Measures Following Treatment Completion

- Unprotected sexual intercourse should be avoided for up to 7 days post-initiation of therapy.
- Strong emphasis should be placed on the use of condoms during sexual intercourse.
- Follow-up examinations post successful treatment are not advised. If necessary, follow-up assessments should be performed at the earliest convenience, ideally within 3 weeks of treatment completion. Increased risk of false-positive results is associated with examinations conducted too soon, particularly with molecular biological diagnostic procedures.
- Should symptoms persist or recur within a week of treatment completion, reexamination and assessment are recommended.
- Mere presence of symptoms without laboratory or clinically significant findings does not justify the initiation of a new therapeutic regimen.
- Upon diagnosis of urethritis, immediate antibiotic therapy should be initiated, even in the absence of microbiological test results.

9.3 Complaints Without Pathogen Isolation

- **Presenting Symptoms**: Patients frequently present with urethritis symptoms, including mild itching and burning during urination. In many instances, cultures yield negative results. Standard antibiotic treatment for suspected cystitis (e.g.,

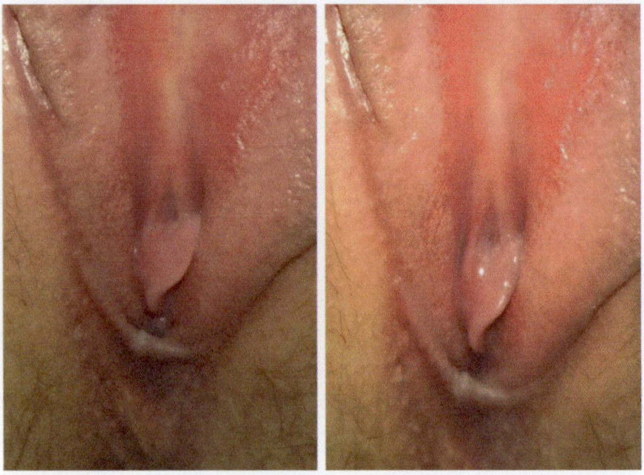

Fig. 9.3 Maneuver for suspected urethritis without confirmed pathogen. Fluid formation at the urethra is observable on the right before the patient contracts the pelvic floor muscle on the left (Mylonas 2024). (Courtesy of I. Mylonas)

fosfomycin, cotrimoxazole, amoxicillin, or ciprofloxacin) often fails to alleviate symptoms. Urological examinations, including cystoscopy, usually do not reveal a cause.

- **Clinical Examination**:
  - **Observations**: Physical examination commonly shows no significant findings, such as increased urine secretion or marked erythema at the meatus. Vulvovaginitis and cervicitis typically remain undetectable.
  - **Procedure (According to Mylonas)**:
    - **Preparation**: Ensure the introitus area is not disinfected, and avoid vaginal ultrasound examination. The patient should ideally have an empty bladder, although the procedure can be performed with a full bladder. Prepare a cotton swab or eyelet and a microscope slide.
    - **Specimen Collection**: Insert the lower blade of a split speculum into the posterior fornix. Instruct the patient to contract their pelvic floor muscles three times to simulate urination. Collect any observed fluid (Fig. 9.3) from the meatus with i.e. a cotton swab, and transfer it to a microscope slide containing physiological saline.
    - **Wet Mount Microscopy**: Examine the slide under phase contrast microscopy. Presence of leukocytes denotes an inflammatory response. In their absence, urethritis is unlikely.
- **Further Examination Findings**:
  - **Genital Discharge**: Due to pelvic muscle tension and speculum positioning, genital fluid may accumulate below the cervix. Conduct a microscopic evaluation of the vaginal secretion. If copious yellow or green discharge is noted, perform a microbiological examination, as it may have contacted the urethra.

Table 9.3 Treatment strategies for urethritis-like symptoms without pathogen isolation following positive leukocyte detection in phase-contrast microscopy (according to Mylonas)

Indication	Medication	Dosage	Duration
Standard	Azithromycin	Day 1: 500 mg orally once, followed by 250 mg orally (days 2–5)	5 days
Alternative	Moxifloxacin	400 mg orally once daily plus	14 days
	Octenidine dihydrochloride	Vaginal therapeutic once daily or	7 days
	Dequalinium chloride	Once daily for 6 days	
In complicated cases (according to Mylonas)[a]	Doxycycline	100 mg orally twice daily followed by	7 days
	Pristinamycin[a]	1000 mg orally four times daily	10 days

[a]The options provided are intended for cases where pathogen isolation is not feasible, yet positive leukocyte detection is observed through wet mount microscopy following clinical evaluation. In complicated cases, alternative medications, such as doxycycline or pristinamycin, may be considered. It is essential to consider individual patient factors and specific diagnostic findings when determining the most appropriate treatment strategy

- **Treatment Recommendations** (Table 9.3):
  - **Azithromycin for Urethritis**: If leukocytes are identified in the meatus smear:
    - **Dosage**: Azithromycin 500 mg on day 1, followed by 250 mg daily for days 2–5.
    - **Symptomatic Improvement**: Most patients experience significant relief, though some may suffer persistent or recurrent symptoms.
  - **Alternative Medications**:
    - **Moxifloxacin**: 400 mg daily for 14 days, potentially combined with vaginal therapeutic agents such as octenidine dihydrochloride for 7 days or dequalinium chloride for 6 days.
    - **Doxycycline and Pristinamycin**: Doxycycline 100 mg twice daily for 7 days, followed by pristinamycin 1000 mg four times daily for 10 days. It should be noted that pristinamycin is unavailable in many countries but can be obtained through international pharmacies.
- **Microbiological Findings**:
  - **Pathogen-Specific Treatment**: Treatment should be guided by antibiogram results.
  - **Bacterial Vaginosis**:
    - **Local Treatment**: Metronidazole vaginal cream for 7 days.
    - **Systemic Treatment**: Azithromycin.
    - **Partner Treatment**: Partners should receive similar treatment if leukocytes are found in phase-contrast microscopy, including azithromycin therapy.
- **Conclusions**: Most patients will experience symptom resolution with appropriate treatment; however, approximately 20% may encounter recurrent symptoms within 1 year, necessitating continued monitoring and potentially repeated or adjusted therapeutic interventions.

Key Points

- Urethritis, defined as inflammation of the urethra, presents with a range of symptoms, including dysuria (painful urination) and urethral discharge.
- Isolated urethritis primarily affects men, although women frequently present with both urethritis and cystitis.
- **Acute urethritis** is characterized by sudden inflammation of the urethra.
  - **Acute urethral syndrome** is linked to dysuria and inflammation of the urethral glands.
  - The most common causative agent is *Neisseria gonorrhoeae*, while nongonococcal urethritis (NGU) is attributed to other pathogens, such as *Chlamydia trachomatis*.
  - Symptoms commonly include urethral discharge, dysuria, and urethral itching.
  - Diagnosis is established through the detection of segmented granulocytes in smears.
  - Urine samples can also be utilized for diagnostic purposes.
  - Empirical therapy should target *Chlamydia trachomatis*, and antibiotic treatment must commence immediately upon diagnosis of urethritis, even if microbiological results are pending.
  - It is essential to inform and, if necessary, treat sexual partners.
  - Patients should be advised to avoid unprotected sexual intercourse and to use condoms.
  - Follow-up examinations are generally unnecessary after treatment completion.
  - Reevaluation is warranted if symptoms persist or recur.
- **Recurrent or Persistent Urethritis.**
  - Recurrent or persistent urethritis may develop approximately 30–90 days after completing treatment for acute urethritis.
  - Potential causes include resistant microorganisms, inadequate medication adherence, reinfection by a new or untreated partner, and infections with other pathogens or urological conditions.
  - *Mycoplasma genitalium* is a notable common cause.
  - Diagnosis relies on clinical evaluations and laboratory tests, including the detection of *Ureaplasma urealyticum* and *Mycoplasma genitalium*.
  - Standard treatment protocols may not effectively address *Mycoplasma genitalium*, necessitating prolonged therapy or alternative antibiotics in such cases.
  - It is recommended that the sexual partners of the affected individuals be informed, tested, and treated.
  - Additional behavioral measures may be indicated, including condom use and assessment for diabetes or other immunodeficiency conditions.

(continued)

- In instances where pathogen isolation is lacking, specialized diagnostic examinations utilizing phase contrast microscopy may facilitate diagnosis.
- The treatment plan may encompass a variety of antibiotics, contingent on diagnostic findings.
- Symptoms may persist for up to 1 week following treatment completion.
- Post-therapy, behavioral measures should be discussed comprehensively with the patient.
- Follow-up examinations are typically unnecessary.

Pharyngitis 10

Abstract

Pharyngitis, characterized as a prevalent throat infection, is frequently caused by viruses, notably rhinoviruses, though bacterial etiologies such as Streptococcus spp. are also implicated, albeit less commonly. Laryngitis may accompany pharyngitis in some instances. Symptoms include sore throat, erythema, edema, and dysphagia, with a slight fever potentially present. Accurate diagnosis can be challenging due to the variability of symptoms. Standard diagnostic protocols involve throat swabs for bacterial pathogen detection, while serological tests play a crucial role in identifying viral causes. The treatment of choice is typically symptomatic; however, in instances of pharyngitis linked to sexually transmitted diseases (STD), targeted therapies are essential. Regular handwashing is emphasized as an effective preventative measure. If sexually transmitted diseases are suspected, appropriate testing and extended treatment are imperative.

10.1 Background

Pharyngitis refers to the inflammation of the pharynx or tonsils, with potential causes including bacterial, viral, or fungal pathogens. It is generally the most prevalent symptom of illness, especially during the cold months. Approximately 20% of pharyngitis cases may also involve laryngitis, defined as inflammation of the larynx. Secondary infections with Group A Streptococcus or *Haemophilus influenzae* may frequently occur. It is essential to recognize that pharyngitis can be symptomatic of several sexually transmitted infections. Nevertheless, other factors—such as viral infections, bacterial infections, allergies, and environmental irritants—can also precipitate pharyngitis. Therefore, the presence of pharyngitis alone is *insufficient* to indicate a sexually transmitted infection.

I. Mylonas, *Sexually Transmitted Diseases*,
https://doi.org/10.1007/978-3-031-78204-6_10

For suspected sexually transmitted diseases, obtaining a precise diagnosis is critical. In particular, if pharyngitis symptoms manifest alongside suspicion of an STD, comprehensive further testing should be conducted to ensure accurate diagnosis and treatment.

10.2 Pathogen

Various pathogens are implicated in the etiology of pharyngitis. Viral pharyngitis is often associated with upper respiratory infections, most commonly caused by rhinoviruses and coronaviruses, with additional contributions from parainfluenza, respiratory syncytial virus, influenza, and adenoviruses (Table 10.1). Specific presentations may also be linked to other viruses, including adenoviruses, coxsackieviruses, human herpesvirus 6, or cytomegalovirus (CMV). Selected sexually transmitted diseases can manifest with pharyngitis; specifically, cases of gonorrhea, chlamydial infections, or syphilis may present pharyngitis as a prominent symptom.

10.3 Epidemiology

Pharyngitis is a prevalent condition frequently associated with upper respiratory tract infections. Viruses, including rhinovirus, coronavirus, adenovirus, and parainfluenza virus, constitute the primary causative agents of pharyngitis. Bacterial pharyngitis is predominantly due to β-hemolytic group A streptococci, accounting for an estimated 15–30% of cases in children. Fungal pharyngitis primarily affects immunocompromised individuals. In summary, pharyngitis largely represents a viral illness, though bacterial causes also exist. Data regarding sexually transmitted pathogens related to pharyngitis remain limited.

Table 10.1 Pathogens associated with pharyngitis

Viral pathogens (very common)	Bacterial pathogens (less common)	Fungal infection (very rare)	Special cases
– Adenoviruses	– Anaerobic mixed infections	– Candida and others	– Diphtheria
– CMV	– *Bordetella pertussis*		– *Coxiella burnetii*
– Coronaviruses	– Chlamydia		– Gonococci
– Coxsackie virus	– Mycoplasma		– Mycobacteria
– EBV	– *Neisseria meningitidis*		– Treponemas
– Echoviruses	– Streptococci		– Tetanus
– Enteroviruses			
– HSV			
– Influenza viruses			
– Parainfluenza virus			
– Rhinoviruses			
– RSV			

10.4 Clinical Manifestation

Clinically, pharyngitis is characterized by diffuse erythema of the oropharyngeal mucosa, often accompanied by edema and prominent lymphoid follicles. Patients may present with a range of symptoms, including stridor, dysphagia, cough, and general throat irritation. Common complaints also include odynophagia (painful swallowing), a sensation of scratching or burning in the throat, and dryness. In some cases, a low-grade fever may be present, particularly in acute infections.

Chronic pharyngitis is frequently associated with persistent symptoms, such as ongoing swallowing difficulties, a chronic cough, and a frequent urge to clear the throat. These symptoms can significantly impact quality of life and may require comprehensive evaluation.

Although certain clinical features may suggest specific etiological agents, definitive diagnosis of pharyngitis can be challenging due to the wide variety of possible pathogens—including viral, bacterial, fungal, and sexually transmitted organisms—and the overlapping clinical presentations they produce. Diagnostic accuracy often requires targeted laboratory investigations, such as throat cultures, nucleic acid amplification tests (NAATs), or serologic assays.

Sexually transmitted pharyngitis, caused primarily by *Neisseria gonorrhoeae*, *Chlamydia trachomatis*, and less commonly *Treponema pallidum*, frequently presents with clinical signs indistinguishable from those caused by other pathogens. Because of this overlap, establishing a causal relationship requires a thorough and sensitive approach, including detailed sexual history taking and, when indicated, additional genital or extragenital examinations and testing. Recognizing the possibility of sexually transmitted infections in patients with pharyngitis is critical for appropriate diagnosis, treatment, partner notification, and prevention of further transmission.

Certain sexually transmitted infections, such as gonorrhea, chlamydial infections, or syphilis, may also result in pharyngitis following orogenital exposure.

10.5 Diagnosis

In bacterial infections, laboratory indicators such as elevated C-reactive protein (CRP) levels or leukocytosis may suggest infection. A variety of diagnostic procedures are utilized to ascertain the specific etiology. When bacterial infection is suspected, throat swabs are warranted. In cases where a viral (or some bacterial) etiology is suspected, serological assays may be employed to identify antibodies to specific pathogens, including adenoviruses, coxsackieviruses, echoviruses, influenza A/B, and chlamydia.

If conditions such as Plummer–Vinson syndrome or Sjögren's syndrome are suspected, further diagnostic evaluation may be indicated, including assessments for SS-A and SS-B antibodies and expedited mononucleosis tests if indicated.

When sexually transmitted diseases are suspected, additional clinical evaluations and pathogen detection procedures must be conducted. Typically, suspicion arises from the medical history indicating exposure, potentially supplemented by observed anogenital findings.

10.6 Treatment

Management of uncomplicated pharyngitis is primarily symptomatic. To alleviate discomfort, over-the-counter throat lozenges, preferably sugar-free, are recommended to soothe the inflammatory sensation. It is advisable to avoid nicotine and alcohol during illness, as these substances may adversely impact recovery. For mild fever, cold compresses applied to the calves may provide symptomatic relief. In cases of severe pain, analgesics such as paracetamol or ibuprofen may be administered.

In addition to pharmacological interventions, adherence to general hygiene practices is crucial for curbing infection transmission and aiding the healing process.

If specific etiologies of pharyngitis are suspected, targeted treatment should be tailored according to the implicated cause.

10.7 Differential Diagnosis

Differential diagnosis of pharyngitis involves distinguishing between various causes of throat inflammation, which can be viral, bacterial, or non-infectious (Table 10.2). Non-infectious causes may include allergies, gastroesophageal reflux disease (GERD), and irritants like smoking. Correct diagnosis is crucial for appropriate management, as bacterial infections may require antibiotics, while viral infections are typically self-limiting.

When evaluating dysphagia as a symptom of pharyngitis, various potential causes should be considered. These include diverse pathogens such as bacteria or viruses (Table 10.2). Additionally, certain pharmacological agents, notably anticholinergics, as well as nasal drops or arsenic exposure, may contribute to swallowing difficulties. Systemic conditions such as diabetes mellitus or Plummer-Vinson syndrome should also be evaluated as potential dysphagia triggers. Furthermore, neurological conditions (e.g., glossopharyngeal nerve paresis) and autoimmune disorders (e.g., pemphigus, scleroderma) are relevant considerations. Chronic inflammatory conditions, including pharyngitis chronica hyperplastica or

Table 10.2 Differential diagnostic features of pharyngitis

Pathogen	Redness	Ulcers	Fever	LN	Further Symptoms
Adenoviruses	++	–	+	–	Exudate
Anaerobic mixed infections	++	++	+	+	–
Bordetella pertussis	+	–	+++	–	Exudate
Candida	++	–	–	–	White coating
Chlamydia	+	–	+	–	Purulent exudate
CMV	+	+	+	–	–
Coronaviruses	++	–	–	–	–
Coxiella burnetii (*)	–	–	++	–	–
Coxsackie virus	++	–	+++	–	Bubbles
Diphtheria	++	++	+++	–	Pseudomembranous coatings
EBV	++	++	++	+++	Gray wipeable coating
Echoviruses	+	–	+	–	–
Enteroviruses	+	–	+	–	–
Gonococci	+	–	+	–	Purulent exudate
HSV	++	++	–	+	Blisters, ulcers
Influenza viruses	+	–	+++	–	–
Mycobacteria (*)	+	++	++	–	–
Mycoplasma	+	–	+	–	Purulent exudate
Neisseria meningitidis (*)	++	+	+++	++	Purulent exudate
Parainfluenza virus	+	–	++	–	–
Rhinoviruses	++	–	–	–	Exudate
RSV	+	–	++	–	Exudate
Streptococci	+++	+	+++	++	Thick purulent exudate
Treponemas	+	++	+	–	–

*Only isolated reports

– = no symptoms; + = mild symptoms; ++ = moderate symptoms; +++ = severe symptoms; LN = lymphnodes

Note: Symptoms can vary among patients, and not all symptoms may be present

pharyngitis lateralis, along with dry mucous membranes (pharyngitis sicca), should also be assessed. Other potential causes of dysphagia include Sjögren's syndrome and uremia.

10.8 Prevention

To reduce the risk of pharyngitis, it is essential to address individual risk factors, such as malnutrition and the use of irritants like tobacco and alcohol. Hand hygiene, particularly handwashing with soap, is a straightforward yet effective method for preventing infections such as pharyngitis.

In cases where sexually transmitted diseases are suspected, consideration of pharyngitis is advisable. Treatment duration may be extended in the event of pharyngeal involvement, as observed in cases of gonorrhea.

Key Points

- Pharyngitis constitutes inflammation of the throat or tonsils and may arise from various etiological factors, including bacterial, viral, or fungal pathogens.
- Approximately 20% of pharyngitis cases are accompanied by laryngitis.
- Pharyngitis may coexist with sexually transmitted infections; however, it is not solely attributable to such illnesses.
- Determining the precise etiology can be achieved through throat swabs, serological testing, and additional diagnostic procedures.
- Treatment is predominantly symptomatic and may encompass the use of analgesics, throat lozenges, and compresses.
- For specific etiologies, including select bacterial infections, targeted antibiotic therapy may be indicated.
- A thorough differential diagnosis for dysphagia should encompass a range of potential causes, including infections, pharmacological effects, and systemic diseases.
- Preventative strategies to avert pharyngitis include a balanced diet, avoidance of harmful substances, and regular handwashing.
- In cases of suspected sexually transmitted disease, prompt diagnosis and, if necessary, extended treatment are crucial.

Proctitis

11

Abstract

Proctitis is defined as inflammation of the rectum, which may result from infections, including sexually transmitted diseases (STD), particularly those contracted during anal intercourse, or as a concomitant symptom of other gastrointestinal disorders. The etiology of proctitis is multifactorial, involving various pathogens, such as bacteria, viruses, and parasites, notably *Entamoeba histolytica*. Symptoms typically include painful and bloody defecation, inguinal lymphadenopathy, and discomfort in the perianal region. Diagnostic sigmoidoscopy may reveal ulcerations, edema, and fissures. Diagnosis is confirmed through the examination of samples collected via smears, biopsies, and serological tests, with polymerase chain reaction (PCR) being the preferred method for pathogen identification, including *Chlamydia trachomatis* and Herpes simplex. Treatment protocols are pathogen-specific, and preventive counseling is crucial.

11.1 Background

The term "proctitis" is used to describe the isolated inflammatory disease of the rectum. The etiology of proctitis encompasses a wide spectrum of potential causative factors, including infections caused by bacteria, viruses, or fungi. Additionally, inflammatory bowel diseases (IBD), such as Crohn's disease or ulcerative colitis, have been identified as significant contributing factors. Furthermore, the effects of radiation therapy administered to the pelvic region have been observed to result in proctitis. Sexually transmitted diseases (STDs), such as gonorrhea or syphilis, and irritation or injury to the rectum, are additional etiological factors that should be considered.

I. Mylonas, *Sexually Transmitted Diseases*,
https://doi.org/10.1007/978-3-031-78204-6_11

11.2 Pathogen

Bacteria and viruses have been identified as potential triggers for proctitis, with parasites also playing a distinguished role. Direct infections during anal intercourse are common among STDs. However, pathogens such as *Entamoeba histolytica* and *Giardia intestinalis* may also be implicated.

Besides direct infection, various inflammatory conditions can lead to rectal involvement.

11.3 Epidemiology

Sexually transmitted diseases (STD) are a major cause of proctitis, particularly among men who have sex with men (MSM). The most frequently implicated pathogens include *Chlamydia trachomatis*, *Neisseria gonorrhoeae*, herpes simplex virus (HSV), and *Treponema pallidum* (syphilis). Data on female patients with STD-related proctitis remain scarce.

Pathogen Distribution: A retrospective analysis of clinical proctitis cases in MSM revealed the following distribution of causative agents:

Gonorrhea: 30%
Chlamydia: 19%
Herpes simplex virus (HSV): 16%
Syphilis: 2%

Recently, Mpox (formerly referred to as monkeypox) has been identified as a potential cause of sexually acquired proctitis, further expanding the list of relevant pathogens in this context.

Risk Factors: The primary risk factor for STI-related proctitis is receptive anal intercourse. Additional contributing factors that increase vulnerability to infection include:

HIV positivity
High-risk sexual behaviors
Use of shared sex toys

Global Epidemiology and Trends: The worldwide epidemiology of infectious proctitis exhibits significant variation across regions. Key observations include:

Undocumented Prevalence: The specific prevalence of individual pathogens remains underreported due to limited data.

Determinants of Infection: Rates of infection are influenced by sexual practices, condom usage, and the number of sexual partners.

Recent Trends

Decline in Case Numbers: A noticeable decline in infectious proctitis rates has been observed in recent years, likely driven by public awareness campaigns linking sexual behaviors, particularly HIV transmission, to infection risks.

Resurgence in Cases: Despite earlier declines, a resurgence in infectious proctitis has been documented globally.

This trend has been particularly evident in the United States and Europe, where cases of STIs leading to proctitis have risen.

Future Outlook: An overall global increase in proctitis cases is anticipated, driven by evolving sexual behaviors and gaps in preventive measures.

11.4 Clinical Manifestation

Ulcerative efflorescence of the perianal skin often indicates an infection with a sexually transmitted pathogen.

Due to the high incidence of secondary infections, rectal lesions are frequently associated with significant pain.

Inguinal lymphadenopathy is a common clinical finding, and patients often report painful, occasionally bloody, defecation. Granulomatous changes may lead to strictures, perianal abscesses, and, in the absence of treatment, fistula formation. Proctitis caused by *Chlamydia trachomatis* may present asymptomatically.

During a sigmoidoscopy, erythematous changes and purulent exudate may be evident. Complications can include ulcerations, edema, and fissures.

Infections associated with the herpes simplex virus (HSV) may present as asymptomatic infections or cause severe perianal pain; symptoms may also include constipation and fever. Characteristic vesicular lesions may develop on the skin, while ulcers can manifest within the anal canal. Rarely, cytomegalovirus (CMV) has been implicated in proctocolitis, resulting in painful perianal ulcerations and fissures, particularly in immunocompromised patients, such as those with HIV.

11.5 Diagnosis

Rapid pathogen detection is crucial when proctitis is suspected. The diagnostic approach typically involves:

Sigmoidoscopy: This procedure allows for the collection of smears and biopsies for analysis. It enables direct visualization of the rectal lining and collection of samples for further testing.

Serological Testing:

Treponema pallidum (Syphilis): Serological tests are the standard for laboratory diagnosis, though they may be insensitive in early primary syphilis.

Serological testing for herpetic infections or CMV may have limited utility in the context of proctitis.

Nucleic Acid Amplification Techniques: Polymerase chain reaction (PCR) is the preferred method for direct detection of:

Chlamydia trachomatis

Cytomegalovirus (CMV)

Herpes simplex virus (HSV)

Additional Tests (Blood tests): Can show signs of infections or other conditions causing proctitis.

Stool Tests: May reveal signs of infections.

Rectal Cultures: Can identify bacterial infections.

11.6 Treatment

The treatment approach is guided by the specific pathogen involved.

Treatment is pathogen-specific and may include:

Antibiotics: For bacterial infections like Chlamydia or gonorrhea, antibiotics are the primary treatment. The choice of antibiotic depends on the specific pathogen identified.

Antiviral Medications: For viral causes, such as HSV or CMV.

Antiparasitic Medications

Patient Education: Patients must be comprehensively informed about:

Risks of contracting sexually transmitted pathogens through unprotected sexual intercourse.

Importance of safer sex practices, including consistent condom use.

Follow-Up: Regular follow-up is essential to ensure treatment effectiveness and prevent recurrence or transmission.

11.7 Differential Diagnosis

A thorough differential diagnosis of proctitis must consider a range of conditions that may present similarly, exhibiting symptoms such as pain, bleeding, and rectal mucus. The following conditions should be evaluated:

- **Hemorrhoids:**
  - **Symptoms:** Pain, blood in the stool, and rectal mucus related to inflamed hemorrhoids.

  - **Rationale:** Hemorrhoids can simulate the symptomatic picture of proctitis and warrant detailed investigation.
- **Anal Fissures:**
  - **Symptoms:** Tears in the anal canal causing pain and bleeding during bowel movements.
  - **Rationale:** These symptoms can be mistakenly attributed to proctitis, necessitating careful examination.
- **Infectious Intestinal Diseases:**
  - **Examples:** Bacterial or viral intestinal infections.
  - **Symptoms:** Diarrhea, abdominal pain, and rectal bleeding may resemble proctitis.
- **Inflammatory Bowel Diseases (IBD):**
  - **Types:**
    Crohn's Disease: Inflammation throughout the gastrointestinal tract, potentially affecting the rectum.
    Ulcerative Colitis: Primarily affects the colon and rectum, leading to ulceration.
  - **Symptoms:** Rectal inflammation, pain, and bleeding, often confused with proctitis.
- **Rectal Ulcers or Polyps:**
  - **Symptoms:** Bleeding and pain localized to the rectum.
  - **Rationale:** These conditions must be distinguished from proctitis through endoscopic evaluation.
- **Sexually Transmitted Diseases (STD):**
  - **Examples:** Gonorrhea, syphilis.
  - **Symptoms:** Rectal inflammation and discharge analogous to proctitis.
  - **Important Note:** Pharyngeal involvement should be considered, particularly in cases of gonorrhea, which may necessitate extended treatment.
- **Irritable Bowel Syndrome (IBS):**
  - **Symptoms:** Abdominal discomfort, altered bowel habits, and flatulence.
  - **Rationale:** IBS can mimic proctitis symptoms; a detailed history and functional assessments are important.
- **Anal Fistulas or Abscesses:**
  - **Symptoms:** Pain, swelling, and inflammation in the anal region.
  - **Rationale:** Similar presentations require differentiation through clinical examination and imaging studies.
- **Chronic Constipation:**
  - **Symptoms:** Prolonged constipation leading to irritation and inflammation of the rectal mucosa.
  - **Rationale:** This condition may mimic proctitis and necessitates appropriate management.
- **Malignancies:**
  - **Symptoms:** Tumors present in the rectum manifesting as pain and bleeding.
  - **Rationale:** Although infrequent, malignancies must be ruled out via imaging and biopsy.

- **Proctalgia Fugax:**
  - **Description:** Sudden, severe rectal pain occurring without identifiable cause.
  - **Rationale:** It is a diagnosis considered subsequent after ruling out other conditions.

11.8 Prevention

Prophylactic measures for proctitis should focus on preventing rectal inflammation:

- Individuals are advised to minimize rectal injury by adopting gentle practices related to bowel movements and the use of mild cleansing agents.
- Safe sex practices are critical to mitigate risks associated with sexually transmitted infections.
- Long-term use of laxatives should be avoided, and a diet rich in fiber is recommended to maintain healthy intestinal flora and stool regulation.
- Limiting alcohol and nicotine consumption is advisable, as these substances can irritate the gastrointestinal tract.
- Adequate hydration is essential to promote optimal bowel function.
- For individuals with preexisting inflammatory bowel diseases such as Crohn's disease or ulcerative colitis, regular medical evaluations and adherence to treatment plans are crucial to reduce the risk of proctitis.
- The long-term use of certain medications, including antibiotics that may alter the intestinal environment, should also be avoided.

Key Points

- Proctitis can arise from a variety of factors, including infections, inflammatory bowel diseases, radiotherapy, sexually transmitted diseases, and irritation or injury to the rectum.
- Various pathogens, such as bacteria, viruses, and parasites, can cause proctitis, including STDs like gonorrhea and syphilis.
- Symptoms commonly include ulcerative efflorescence of the perianal skin, painful defecation, inguinal lymphadenopathy, erythematous changes, and lesions in the rectum.
- Diagnostic modalities consist of smears, biopsies, and serological tests.
- Treatment is individualized based on the underlying cause and typically incorporates educational components about safer sex practices and prevention strategies to avert further infections.

Lymphadenopathy or Lymphadenitis 12

Abstract

Lymphadenopathy is characterized as an altered state of lymph nodes, marked by changes in size and consistency. It can present as either localized or generalized. Lymphadenitis, on the other hand, is defined as inflammation of the lymph nodes, characterized by painful swelling and the potential formation of a fistula. Acute lymphadenitis is frequently attributed to infectious etiologies, whereas chronic variants are often linked to hyperplasia and typically present as painless. Localized lymphadenopathy is generally associated with a primary lesion, whereas generalized lymphadenopathy may arise from multiple causes, including infections and hypersensitivity reactions. Inguinal lymphadenopathy is commonly associated with sexually transmitted infections. Diagnosis typically necessitates the employment of imaging techniques, with treatment strategies varying based on the underlying cause.

12.1 Background

Lymphadenopathy is identified as a modification in the size and/or consistency of a lymph node or a collection of lymph nodes (regional lymphadenopathy). This condition can also manifest in a generalized form, affecting multiple sites and groups of lymph nodes.

Lymphadenitis is characterized as an inflammatory response in lymph nodes. During the acute inflammatory phase, swelling and hyperplasia of the cells along the sinus wall, leukocyte infiltration, and edema occur. This results in an expansion of the lymph node capsule, which causes localized pain. In some cases, the lymph node may rupture through the skin, leading to a draining fistula.

Lymphadenitis can be classified into acute and chronic forms. Acute lymphadenitis is chiefly caused by infectious agents. Chronic lymphadenitis is often associated with lymph node proliferation and may present as either follicular hyperplasia

I. Mylonas, *Sexually Transmitted Diseases*,
https://doi.org/10.1007/978-3-031-78204-6_12

or paracortical lymphoid hyperplasia, depending on the underlying cause of inflammation; such lymph nodes are often painless.

Further frequently used alternative subdivisions include:

- Inflammatory lymphadenopathy.
- Lymphadenopathy associated with lymphoproliferative diseases.
- Infiltrative lymphadenopathy secondary to malignant diseases.
- Reactive lymphadenopathy, which may have infectious or noninfectious origins.

12.2 Localized Lymphadenopathy

Localized lymphadenopathy is characterized by the involvement of no more than two adjacent groups of lymph nodes. This condition may be acute or chronic and is typically related to a primary lesion (Table 12.1).

The lymph nodes in the head and neck region are categorized into various anatomical and clinical areas. Adenopathies in this region may correlate with primary foci of infection or acute viral diseases. The lymphatic nodes of the axilla drain regions including the arm, portions of the chest wall, back, and breasts. Inguinal lymphadenopathy is frequently observed and may arise from injuries or antecedent infections in the lower extremities. The abdominal and retroperitoneal lymph nodes facilitate drainage from the abdominal, retroperitoneal, and pelvic organs. Accurate identification and characterization of these lymph nodes usually necessitate advanced imaging techniques, including:

Table 12.1 Localization of enlarged lymph nodes and associated conditions

Localization	Associated disease or condition
Occipital	Scalp infections, insect bites, head lice, allergy to hair shampoo
Postauricular	Rubella, infected pierced ears, external otitis, HIV infection
Preauricular	Eye and conjunctival infection, tularemia
Posterior cervical	Toxoplasmosis
Submental	Tooth and oral cavity infections
Cervical and submandibular	Infections of the oral cavity, infectious mononucleosis, cytomegalovirus, HIV, tuberculosis
Supraclavicular	Neoplasia
Mediastinal	Sarcoidosis, tuberculosis, histoplasmosis, blastomycosis, anthrax, neoplasia (lymphoma, metastases)
Axillary	Cat scratch disease, purulent infections of the arm, neoplasia
Epitrochlear	Viral diseases, cat scratch disease, tularemia, hand infections, secondary syphilis
Abdominal/retroperitoneal	Tuberculosis, yersiniosis, neoplasia
Pelvis	Sexually transmitted infections, neoplasia
Inguinal	Genital herpes, syphilis, lymphogranuloma venereum, granuloma inguinale, filariasis, scabies mite infestation, neoplasia

- **Ultrasound (US):** A noninvasive imaging modality that uses high-frequency sound waves to visualize lymph nodes. It is particularly useful for identifying the characteristics of superficial lymph nodes, assessing their size, shape, and vascularity, and aiding in differentiating between benign and malignant processes.
- **Computed Tomography (CT):** This imaging technique provides detailed images of the body's internal structures. CT scans are often employed to evaluate enlarged lymph nodes in the thorax, abdomen, and pelvis, allowing for assessment of lymph node size, number, and any associated masses or infiltrative diseases.
- **Magnetic Resonance Imaging (MRI):** MRI is utilized for its superior soft tissue contrast, particularly in complex anatomical regions. It may be employed to evaluate lymphadenopathy in the head, neck, or pelvic areas, allowing for detailed visualization of lymph node morphology and surrounding structures.
- **Positron Emission Tomography (PET):** Often combined with CT (PET/CT), this imaging technique aids in identifying metabolically active lymph nodes that may suggest malignancy. It is especially valuable in evaluating lymphadenopathy related to lymphoproliferative disorders.
- **Fine Needle Aspiration Cytology (FNAC):** While not an imaging technique, FNAC is often guided by ultrasound or CT. This procedure involves the aspiration of cells from a lymph node for cytological examination, providing rapid diagnostic information regarding the nature of lymphadenopathy.

12.3 Generalized Lymphadenopathy

Generalized lymphadenopathy may result from various conditions, including infectious diseases such as dengue fever, filariasis, leishmaniasis, histoplasmosis, tuberculosis, brucellosis, toxoplasmosis, and leptospirosis. Viral infections, including rubella, measles, chickenpox, hepatitis A and B, Epstein-Barr virus (EBV), cytomegalovirus (CMV), and HIV, can also lead to this condition. Bacterial infections, such as brucellosis and leptospirosis, as well as noninfectious causes, such as hypersensitivity reactions induced by medications, may also contribute to generalized lymphadenopathy.

- **Acute generalized infectious lymphadenopathy** (Table 12.2) is commonly attributable to viral agents, particularly in pediatric populations.
- **Acute generalized noninfectious lymphadenopathy** (Table 12.3) is mostly linked to hypersensitivity reactions to medications. Resolution is typically observed upon discontinuation of the offending agent.
- **Chronic generalized infectious lymphadenopathy** (Table 12.2) is less frequently caused by viral agents, with HIV as a notable exception. Possible etiological factors include bacterial and fungal infections such as tuberculosis, syphilis, histoplasmosis, and cryptococcosis.

Table 12.2 Differential diagnosis of infectious lymphadenopathy

Etiology	Local	Generalized	Regional
Bacteria (acute)	Anthrax	+	
	Cat scratch disease	+	+
	Chlamydia trachomatis		
	Diphtheria	+	
	Haemophilus ducreyi	+	
	Klebsiella granulomatis	+	
	LGV	+	
	Malleus	+	
	Melioidosis		+
	Plague	+	
	Rat bite fever	+	+
	Rickettsia		
	Scarlet fever	+	+
	Staphylococci	+	
	Streptococci	+	
	Syphilis	+	+
	Tuberculosis	+	+
	Tularemia	+	
	Typhus fever		+
Viruses	Adenovirus	+	
	CMV		+
	Dengue fever		+
	EBV		+
	Herpes simplex	+	+
	HIV/AIDS		+
	Lassa fever		+
	Measles		+
	Rubella	+	+
	Viral hepatitis	+	
	West Nile fever		+
	Zika virus	+	
Mycoses	Coccidioidomycosis	+	
	Cryptococcosis	+	+
	Histoplasmosis		+
	Paracoccidioidomycosis	+	
Protozoa	African trypanosomiasis	+	+
	Chagas disease		+
	Kala-azar		+
	Leishmaniasis	+	
	Toxoplasmosis	+	
Helminths	Filariasis		+
	Loa loa	+	
	Onchocerciasis	+	

- In **chronic generalized noninfectious lymphadenopathy** (Table 12.3), neoplastic origins are often implicated, with underlying conditions potentially including lymphoreticular neoplasms such as Hodgkin's disease, non-Hodgkin's lymphomas, and chronic lymphocytic leukemia.

Table 12.3 Differential diagnosis of noninfectious lymphadenopathy

	Etiology	Regional	Generalized
Noninfectious lymphadenopathy	Drug hypersensitivity		+
	Connective tissue disorders		+
	Castleman's disease	+	
	Kawasaki disease	+	
	Kikuchi disease	+	
	Rosai-Dorfman disease	+	
	Sarcoidosis		+
	Silicone breast implant	+	
Malignancy	Leukemia		+
	Metastatic carcinoma	+	+
Nonmalignant (infiltrative)	Lipid storage disease		+
	Amyloidosis		+
Primary lymphoproliferative	Angioimmunoblastic lymphadenopathy		+
	Lymphoma		+
	Malignant histiocytosis		+
Pharmaceuticals	Examples: Allopurinol, atenolol, captopril, carbamazepine, cephalosporins, hydralazine, penicillin, phenytoin, pyrimethamine, sulfonamides		+

12.4 Inguinal Lymphadenopathy

Inguinal lymphadenopathy is prevalent, with the most common causes being sexually transmitted diseases and metastatic genital tumors. Parasitic etiologies are also significant, particularly in developing nations.

- **Sexually transmitted diseases:**
  - **Chancroid (*Haemophilus ducreyi*):** Characterized by a painful, nonindurated ulcer that may develop within 1 day to several weeks following inoculation, accompanied by swelling and pain in the inguinal lymph nodes.
  - **Lymphogranuloma Venereum (*Chlamydia trachomatis* serovars L1, L2, L3):** Initially presents with vesicular lesions after 1–2 weeks, often asymptomatic. Inguinal lymphadenopathy appears 1–6 weeks post-cessation of vesicles, typically manifesting as painful lymph node enlargement, with bilateral involvement in 30–40% of cases.
  - **Syphilis:** Moderately enlarged, nonpurulent, and painless lymph nodes may indicate a primary syphilis. Chancroid ulcers typically appear 14-30 days after inoculation and present as nonexudative lesions. Generalized lymphadenopathy in secondary syphilis is characterized by a characteristic pattern of enlargement of the epitrochlear lymph nodes.
  - **Genital herpes** is marked by classic vesicular lesions along with inguinal lymphadenopathy.

  - **Granuloma Inguinale (Donovanosis):** Caused by Klebsiella (Calymmatobacterium) granulomatis, presenting as a painless ulcer with a slightly bleeding, red surface. This condition is also referred to as pseudobubo.
- **Parasitic lymphadenopathy:**
  - **African Trypanosomiasis (Sleeping Sickness):** Clinical manifestations include lymphadenopathy, with affected nodes being nonpainful and a large, mobile lymph node (Winterbottom sign).
  - **American Trypanosomiasis (Chagas Disease):** Lymphadenopathy occurs in approximately two-thirds of acute cases, often accompanied by hepatosplenomegaly and local edema.
  - **Filariasis:** Symptoms include fever and inguinal or axillary lymphadenopathy, along with lymphatic reactions.
  - **Leishmaniasis:** Lymphadenopathy often precedes skin lesions, particularly prevalent in South America, with *Leishmania major* infections common in equatorial Africa.
  - **Onchocerciasis (River Blindness):** Moderate lymphadenopathy is frequently seen in the groin area.
  - **Toxoplasmosis:** Lymphadenopathy is a common feature of primary Toxoplasma infections, predominantly affecting the neck, axillae, and groin. The lymph nodes tend to be discrete, variable in consistency, and rarely purulent or ulcerated.
  - ***Wuchereria bancrofti* Infection:** Characterized by extensive lymphadenopathy, eosinophilia, hydrocele, and elephantiasis.

12.5 Assessment and Treatment

12.5.1 Head and Neck Lymphadenopathy

The oropharyngeal cavity (including dental structures) is the most common cause of lymph node swelling in the head and neck, followed closely by the nasal cavity and skin conditions. In younger patients, distinguishing enlarged lymph nodes from conditions such as epidermal cysts, thyroglossal cysts, or branchiogenic cysts is essential. Symmetrical enlargements are typically benign and viral in origin, whereas unilateral enlargements require a comprehensive differential diagnosis, including consideration of viral infectious diseases. Common causes of unilateral enlargement are bacterial agents, cat scratch disease, toxoplasmosis, and neoplasia. If asymmetrical cervical lymph node enlargement persists over an extended period and serological tests yield negative results, a fine needle biopsy is usually indicated. Rarely, cervical lymphadenopathies may arise from Kimura's disease (eosinophilic hyperplastic lymphogranulomatosis) and Gianotti-Crosti syndrome (associated with hepatitis B in children).

12.5.2 Axillary Lymphadenopathy

Unilateral axillary lymphadenopathy may be spurred by local infectious processes affecting the arm and hand, hidradenitis suppurativa, cat scratch disease, HIV infection, toxoplasmosis, tularemia, streptococcal and staphylococcal lymphadenitis, sleeping sickness, and African trypanosomiasis. Post-vaccination lymphadenopathy has been consistently observed following smallpox vaccinations and, on occasion, following anthrax vaccinations—similarly noted with measles vaccinations. The Bacille-Calmette-Guérin (BCG) vaccination may also lead to localized lymph node enlargement.

Asymptomatic unilateral axillary lymph node enlargement typically suggests a neoplastic origin, while bilateral enlargement can stem from a variety of diseases, including viral, bacterial or protozoal infections as well as neoplasia, allergic reactions, and noninfectious inflammatory processes.

12.5.3 Thoracic Lymphadenopathy

The most prevalent causes of thoracic lymphadenopathy include tumors, tuberculosis, sarcoidosis, endemic fungal infections, and anthrax. In children, mediastinal lymph node enlargement commonly occurs in primary tuberculosis and may present as unilateral or bilateral, with or without visible pulmonary signs on X-ray. In adults, unilateral enlargement of mediastinal and hilar lymph nodes in the absence of symptoms often signifies tumor-related origins. Exceptions include individuals infected with the human immunodeficiency virus (HIV) and those residing in areas endemic to tuberculosis or fungal infections (e.g., cryptococcosis, histoplasmosis, and coccidioidomycosis). Sarcoidosis frequently leads to bilateral hilar lymphadenopathy in asymptomatic young adults.

12.5.4 Sexually Transmitted Diseases and Abdominal Lymphadenopathy

Abdominal lymphadenopathy is most frequently associated with neoplastic conditions, including lymphomas, metastatic carcinomas, and other malignancies. Infectious causes, though less common, also contribute to abdominal lymph node enlargement. Among infectious etiologies, mesenteric and intestinal tuberculosis are notable, particularly in endemic regions, presenting with caseating granulomatous lymphadenitis. Other bacterial infections such as *Yersinia enterocolitica* can cause mesenteric lymphadenitis resembling appendicitis, especially in children and young adults. Rare infections like Whipple's disease, caused by *Tropheryma whipplei*, may involve mesenteric nodes alongside systemic manifestations. Intestinal anthrax, although exceedingly rare, can also produce localized lymphadenopathy.

Additionally, mesenteric lymphadenopathy is a recognized feature of inflammatory bowel diseases (IBD), particularly Crohn's disease. In this context, lymph node enlargement reflects the chronic inflammatory process affecting the intestinal wall and regional lymphatic structures.

While STDs primarily cause lymphadenopathy in inguinal and pelvic regions, certain systemic infections such as HIV may lead to generalized lymphadenopathy, including intra-abdominal nodes. Furthermore, secondary infections or neoplastic complications related to STDs may occasionally manifest with abdominal lymph node involvement.

Comprehensive evaluation of abdominal lymphadenopathy necessitates integration of clinical history, imaging studies (such as ultrasound, CT, or MRI), microbiological investigations, and sometimes histopathological examination through biopsy to establish an accurate diagnosis and guide appropriate treatment.

12.5.5 Pelvic Lymphadenopathy

Enlargement of pelvic lymph nodes may present with a variety of symptoms, which largely depend on the underlying etiology. Common clinical features include:

- Pain or discomfort localized to the pelvic region
- A sensation of pressure or fullness in the lower abdomen
- Swelling, firmness, or palpable masses in the groin or pelvic area
- Generalized malaise or nonspecific systemic symptoms such as fever or fatigue

Pelvic lymphadenopathy can arise from numerous causes. Asymptomatic unilateral lymph node enlargement often suggests a neoplastic process, whereas bilateral enlargement is more likely associated with a broad spectrum of conditions, including viral, bacterial, or protozoal infections; malignancies; allergic reactions; and noninfectious inflammatory diseases.

Sexually transmitted diseases, particularly *Neisseria gonorrhoeae* and *Chlamydia trachomatis*, are common infectious causes and may lead to reactive lymphadenopathy in the pelvic and inguinal regions. Inflammatory bowel diseases (IBD), such as Crohn's disease and ulcerative colitis, can cause mesenteric and pelvic lymph node enlargement due to chronic inflammation.

Advanced gynecologic malignancies—including cervical, ovarian, and endometrial cancers—frequently involve regional lymph nodes and may present clinically with pelvic lymphadenopathy. Autoimmune disorders such as systemic lupus erythematosus and rheumatoid arthritis can also cause lymph node enlargement secondary to systemic inflammation.

Assessment and Management

Evaluation of pelvic lymphadenopathy requires a thorough clinical history, physical examination, and appropriate diagnostic investigations. Imaging modalities such as pelvic ultrasound, computed tomography (CT), or magnetic resonance imaging (MRI) are essential to assess the size, number, and characteristics of lymph nodes. Laboratory testing should include screening for infectious agents, autoimmune markers, and tumor markers where indicated. Biopsy or fine-needle aspiration may be necessary for definitive diagnosis.

Treatment is directed at the underlying cause: antimicrobial therapy for infections; immunosuppressive agents for autoimmune diseases; and oncologic management, including surgery, chemotherapy, or radiotherapy for malignancies. Symptomatic relief may involve analgesics and supportive care. Multidisciplinary collaboration among gynecologists, infectious disease specialists, oncologists, and rheumatologists is often required for optimal patient outcomes.

12.5.6 Inguinal Lymphadenopathy

Enlargement of inguinal lymph nodes is a common clinical finding associated with a variety of sexually transmitted infections (STIs). Among the most frequent infectious causes are syphilis, chancroid, lymphogranuloma venereum (LGV), granuloma inguinale (donovanosis), genital herpes, pubic lice (phthiriasis pubis), and human immunodeficiency virus (HIV) infection. These conditions often provoke localized lymphadenitis due to the proximity of lymphatic drainage from the genital and perineal regions.

In women, additional sources of inflammation contributing to inguinal lymphadenopathy include infections of the Bartholin and Skene glands located in the labia, which may lead to abscess formation and secondary lymph node involvement. Beyond sexually transmitted pathogens, other infectious etiologies such as *Bartonella henselae* (cat scratch disease), purulent bacterial infections of the lower extremities, and *Toxoplasma gondii* infection should be considered.

The differential diagnosis must also account for parasitic and zoonotic diseases, especially in endemic regions or in patients with relevant travel history. Filariasis caused by *Wuchereria bancrofti* and related filarial species can lead to chronic lymphadenopathy and lymphedema. Onchocerciasis (river blindness) may present with regional lymph node enlargement in affected areas. Additionally, human plague (*Yersinia pestis* infection) can cause painful, swollen inguinal lymph nodes (buboes) in endemic zones.

Given this broad range of potential causes, a thorough clinical evaluation—including detailed sexual, travel, and exposure histories—is essential. Diagnostic workup may involve serologic testing, microbiological cultures, molecular assays, imaging studies, and, when indicated, lymph node biopsy to establish an accurate diagnosis and guide appropriate treatment.

Key Points

- Lymphadenopathy describes changes in lymph node size and consistency, which can be either localized (in up to two adjacent regions) or generalized (affecting multiple regions).
- Lymphadenitis refers to inflammation of the lymph nodes, which is typically painful in acute infections, whereas chronic forms are often painless and characterized by cellular proliferation.
- Localized lymphadenopathy usually arises as a response to a primary lesion, such as infections in the head and neck area, arm, chest, lower abdomen, or lower extremities.
- Generalized lymphadenopathy has diverse causes, including viral infections (e.g., Epstein-Barr virus and HIV), bacterial infections (e.g., tuberculosis and syphilis), parasitic diseases, drug-induced hypersensitivity reactions, and lymphoproliferative or neoplastic disorders.
- Inguinal lymphadenopathy commonly occurs in sexually transmitted infections, such as syphilis, lymphogranuloma venereum (LGV), genital herpes, as well as parasitic infections like trypanosomiasis and filariasis.
- Diagnostic imaging techniques such as computed tomography (CT) and magnetic resonance imaging (MRI) are often necessary, especially to evaluate abdominal and retroperitoneal lymph node abnormalities.
- Abdominal lymphadenopathy is predominantly of neoplastic origin, while infectious causes are comparatively rare.
- Pelvic lymph node enlargement is frequently associated with sexually transmitted infections, inflammatory diseases, or malignant processes.
- Differential diagnosis should distinguish between infectious causes (bacterial, viral, fungal, protozoal, and helminthic) and non-infectious causes (drug-induced, autoimmune diseases, lymphoproliferative, and malignant conditions).
- Treatment depends on the underlying cause and may include antibiotic, antiviral, and antiparasitic therapies, as well as surgical intervention or oncological management when indicated.

Part III

"Classical" Sexually Transmitted Diseases (STD)

13 Chancroid (Ulcus Molle)

Abstract

Chancroid, attributed to the bacterium *Haemophilus ducreyi*, is a painful sexually transmitted disease that presents with characteristic ulcers and may lead to lymphadenopathy. Transmission occurs through sexual contact and necessitates the presence of microlesions for the disease to manifest, potentially facilitating the entry of HIV. Chancroid is prevalent worldwide, particularly in tropical regions, and is more frequently reported in males. Clinical manifestations can range from superficial ulcers to more advanced forms, such as gangrenous ulcers associated with soft chancres. Diagnosis is contingent upon the detection of the pathogen, as symptoms may mimic those of other infections. The primary treatment involves antibiotic therapy, administered judiciously to avert the emergence of antibiotic resistance. Preventative measures include consistent condom usage and regular screening of sexual partners. Additionally, affected individuals are advised to undergo testing for HIV and syphilis.

13.1 Background

Chancroid is a classical sexually transmitted disease exclusively contracted through sexual intercourse. It causes painful ulcers that may merge to form a larger lesion with a granulomatous base. In approximately 50% of affected females, inguinal lymphadenopathy is also present.

13.2 Pathogen

The causative agent of this sexually transmitted infection is *Haemophilus ducreyi*, a gram-negative rod-shaped bacterium. When arranged linearly, these rods visually resemble long threads and may cluster in shapes reminiscent of fish. Humans are the

I. Mylonas, *Sexually Transmitted Diseases*,
https://doi.org/10.1007/978-3-031-78204-6_13

sole reservoir for this pathogen. The disease manifests only in the presence of microlesions on skin or mucous membranes, as intact skin serves as a effective barrier against penetration. Notably, the prepuce may contribute to increased susceptibility to the infection, with noncircumcised men exhibiting higher rates of disease manifestation.

The ulceration serves as a potential entry point for other pathogens, including HIV, due to the resultant tissue damage.

13.3 Epidemiology

Chancroid is a globally prevalent disease, affecting men at approximately double the rate observed in women. The prevalence of the disease demonstrates significant geographic variability. While it is uncommon in Europe and the United States, the pathogen is more prevalent in Africa, Asia, and Latin America. In various geographical areas, the incidence of chancroid has been observed to exceed that of syphilis. The disease has become endemic in certain regions, including the Indian subcontinent, Southeast Asia, tropical Africa, and specific regions of South America.

In Europe and the United States, the incidence of chancroid is low, ranging from 0.0% to 3% in the EU/EEA among patients with genital ulcers. From 1950 to 2021, nearly two million cases were documented in the United States. Nevertheless, the infection remains significantly prevalent in Africa, Asia, and Latin America, where it is a major cause of sexually transmitted ulcers. The prevalence in Africa ranges from 1% to 56% among patients with genital ulcers, depending on the country and demographic. Current specific figures for Asia and Latin America are not available. In Europe, most cases arise among long-distance travelers to Southeast Asia, although smaller regional outbreaks can occur.

13.4 Clinical Manifestation

13.4.1 Gynecology

Existing lesions in the external genital area allow the penetration of Haemophilus ducreyi. Following a 3- to 7-day incubation period, a small papule develops on an erythematous base at the entry site. Initially, the papule is painless, often leading to underreporting by the patient. The papule later progresses into a pustule, which subsequently ulcerates.

The ulcer is typically shallow. However, if left untreated, it may extend into more profound layers of tissue (Fig. 13.1). A bright red inflammatory rim surrounds the ulcer, which features a soft, irregular border and a distinct double edge characterized by undermining and a floating appearance due to acute, progressive

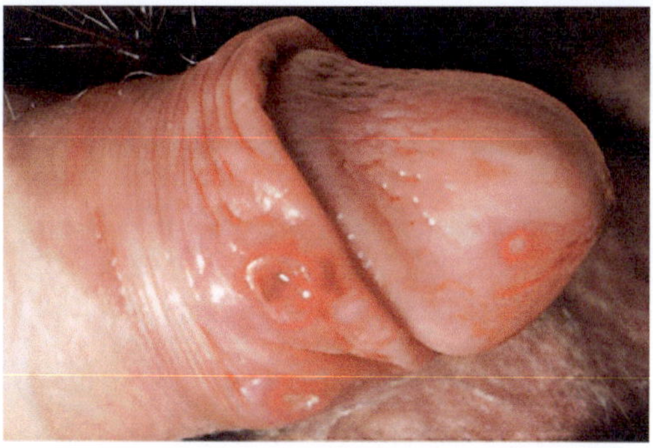

Fig. 13.1 Chancroid in a male patient (Zangerle et al. 2018). The hypertrophic borders of the chancre is clearly visible

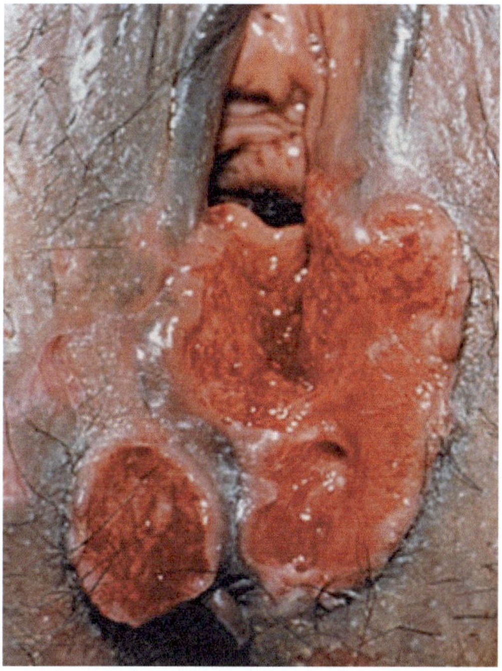

Fig. 13.2 Extensive and painful genital ulcers, that were classified as soft chancre. In such cases, a consequent differential diagnosis is necessary. (Leal Passos 2018)

inflammation (Fig. 13.2). The base exhibits a grayish-yellow color and vascularized granulation tissue, with new vessels forming that may lead to contact bleeding.

The ulcer is associated with significant pain and distinguishes itself from syphilitic primary lesions due to its soft edges. The size, number, and distribution of ulcers may vary widely.

In females, the labia, periurethral area, and posterior commissure are commonly affected (Fig. 13.2). While the vagina is less frequently involved, the cervix is often affected. Coexisting lesions are frequently noted in proximity, often merging. Isolated urethritis is rare.

Chancroid is classified into several types:

- **Transient ulcus molle**: Characterized by a small, rapidly healing ulcer followed by inflammatory lymphadenopathy.
- **Ulcus molle elevatum**: Displays an elevated ulcer due to excessive granulation; surgical removal of excess tissue may be warranted.
- **Ulcus molle folliculare**: A rare form resulting from autoinoculation, typically affecting the rima ani and labia majora, leading to ulcer formation.
- **Ulcus molle gangrenosum**: Exhibits rapid necrosis, often due to mixed bacterial infections, potentially resulting in complete penile involvement.
- **Ulcus molle serpiginosum**: A rare, rapidly progressing variant, presenting with a serpentine appearance that extends quickly to the abdomen and thighs.

In approximately 50% of cases, the disease is confined to the genital area. In the absence of antibiotic treatment, unilateral, often inguinal lymphadenitis develops, progressing to lymph node swelling (bubo) within 10–20 days. The inguinal region is predominantly affected, with the involved lymph nodes typically being inflammatory, red, soft, and fluctuating upon palpation. In approximately 50% of cases, perforation occurs with subsequent pus leakage. Following the formation of an abscess in the lymph nodes, fistulous tracts may develop, often with associated scars. There is no evidence of dissemination beyond local areas; however, rare cases may involve other regions such as the anal area or oral mucosa.

In the absence of treatment, chancroid may lead to a chronic course, resulting in fistulas and their associated scars.

13.4.2 Pregnancy

General patient conditions may deteriorate, accompanied by subfebrile temperatures. There are no documented cases of specific complications during pregnancy or maternofetal transmission related to chancroid. Information regarding the disease's frequency and significance during the puerperium or breastfeeding is also limited. Current consensus suggests that the probability of newborn infection is low. However, should treatment become necessary, it is imperative that adjustments to the approved medication be made based on the child's weight.

13.5 Diagnosis

The ulcer base typically harbors a limited number of pathogens. The objective of sampling is to obtain tissue rather than pus. Although medical history and characteristic clinical presentations suggest an infection caused by *Haemophilus ducreyi*, definitive diagnosis is established through pathogen detection.

13.5.1 Histopathology

Histologically, the ulcer is characterized by three distinct zones: superficial necrosis, an edematous corium layer rich in blood vessels, and a deep zone of inflammatory infiltrate. While this morphology aids in differentiation from other ulcerative conditions, biopsy has diminished in its significance for diagnosis.

13.5.2 Microscopy

In direct microscopic examination, the bacteria may not be readily detectable due to their low quantities and the inadequacy of Gram staining for effective visualization. Specific antibodies for immunofluorescence assessment remain limited to a handful of specialized laboratories. The bacterium *Haemophilus ducreyi* can be visualized effectively using methylene blue or Giemsa stains, with an increased yield observed with acridine orange staining, multiplied by a factor of 10; however, the smear's sensitivity and specificity remain low.

13.5.3 Microbiology

For cultural analysis, excised tissue must be transported in a specific medium. Immediate initiation of cultivation is paramount to preserve pathogen viability.

13.5.4 Serological and Molecular Biological Methods

Immunofluorescence tests and enzyme immunoassays are impractical for antigen detection. However, specialized laboratories may offer pathogen detection via polymerase chain reaction (PCR) methodologies.

Cultural evidence remains the most significant confirmation of infection with *Haemophilus ducreyi*.

13.6 Treatment

Initial therapy comprises antibiotic treatment with ceftriaxone and azithromycin; alternatives include ciprofloxacin, erythromycin, spectinomycin, or cotrimoxazole (Table 13.1). Notably, sulfonamide resistance has been documented in Thailand and Kenya, while tetracyclines and ampicillin are now limited in efficacy due to resistance emergence.

Therapeutic success is expected to manifest within 3–7 days, negating the need for subsequent tests to confirm treatment efficacy.

Table 13.1 Treatment options for chancroid (*ulcus molle*)

Therapy	Medications	Dosage	Duration
Recommendation	Ceftriaxone	250 mg intramuscularly, single dose	Single dose
	Azithromycin	1 g orally, single dose, potentially repeated	Single dose
Alternative	Ciprofloxacin	500 mg orally twice daily	3 days
	Erythromycin	500 mg orally four times daily	7 days or until healing
Older recommendations	Co-trimoxazole	960 mg orally twice daily	7–10 days
	Spectinomycin[a]	2 g intramuscularly, single dose	Single dose
Pregnancy[b]	Erythromycin ethylsuccinate	400 mg orally four times daily	7 days
	Erythromycin ethylsuccinate	800 mg orally four times daily	14 days
Bubo	Azithromycin	1 g orally, single dose	Single dose
	Ceftriaxone	250 mg intramuscularly, single dose	Single dose
	Erythromycin	500 mg orally or intravenously four times daily	7–14 days
Local treatment	Syndet[a] washing gel	2–3 times daily	Several weeks
	Polyhexanide (compresses)	1–2 times daily locally	7–10 days
	Chlorhexidine digluconate 1% cream	1–3 times daily locally	7–10 days
	Quinolinol sulfate 0.1% solution	1–3 times daily locally	7–10 days
	Triclosan 2% cream	2 times daily locally	7–10 days
	Potassium permanganate solution concentrate 1%	1–2 times daily locally	7–10 days

[a]Ulcer Care: Regardless of drug treatment, the affected areas should be regularly cleaned with soap to keep ulcers dry and clean, supporting healing and reducing the risk of secondary infections

[b]Spectinomycin: Accessibility might be limited. Verify availability before prescribing. Consider international pharmacy procurement if needed

[c]Erythromycin ethylsuccinate: Although similar efficacy to erythromycin is assumed, specific studies confirming this are lacking. Due to superior tolerability, erythromycin ethylsuccinate is regarded as the preferred treatment option in pregnancy

In conjunction with antibiotic therapy, disinfectant compresses containing quinosol or potassium permanganate may be applied. For buboes, puncture and drainage may provide effective relief, with procedures repeated if necessary; however, extensive incisions in bubo cases are discouraged.

In instances of coexisting HIV infection, an extended duration of therapy may be necessary, as healing may prove more difficult in this population.

13.7 Differential Diagnosis

The differential diagnosis for anogenital ulceration encompasses granuloma inguinale, syphilis, and herpes simplex virus types I and II. Accurate differentiation is vital, as these conditions may present similarly but necessitate distinct therapeutic approaches. A rare but possible cause for such ulcerations is HIV/AIDS, which, due to its immunosuppressive effects, may predispose individuals to anogenital ulcers.

13.8 Prevention

Following infection with *Haemophilus ducreyi*, immunity to subsequent infections does not develop. Notification requirements exist primarily in cases of frequent occurrences with suspected epidemiological connections. Clinical monitoring is advised for all patients post-therapy. Particularly for HIV-positive individuals, close observation is imperative due to slower recovery rates. Consideration of the following factors may be necessary in the event of treatment failure:

- Antibiotic resistance.
- Alternative causes of ulcerative disease.
- Reinfection.
- Unknown immunodeficiency.

Consistent use of condoms during intercourse is recommended as a preventive measure against bacterial transmission. Prophylactic treatment may also be considered for women with infected partners. Co-occurring infections with *Treponema pallidum* or *Neisseria gonorrhoeae* should be ruled out. Patients diagnosed with chancroid should undergo testing for HIV and syphilis, with a follow-up test scheduled for 3 months post-initial testing.

Key Points

- Chancroid, a sexually transmitted disease caused by *Haemophilus ducreyi*, is exclusively transmitted through sexual intercourse.
- The painful ulcers are often confluent, with inguinal lymphadenopathy occurring in approximately 50% of affected females. The disease arises from microlesions on the skin or mucosa, with noncircumcised men being more susceptible.
- Chancroid exhibits global prevalence, with varying incidence rates. Clinical manifestations differ in women, and distinct variants—including transient, elevatum, folliculare, gangrenosum, and serpiginosum—exist. The incubation period generally spans 3–7 days.
- Lymphadenitis may develop in the absence of antibiotic treatment, yet no specific complications during pregnancy or lactation have been reported.
- Diagnosis relies on clinical presentation and pathogen detection through microscopy and microbiological cultures.
- Antibiotic therapy remains the primary treatment, with consideration for resistance development.
- The application of local disinfectant compresses and, if necessary, bubo drainage is recommended.
- Differential diagnosis should include other infectious diseases associated with anogenital ulcerations.
- Immunity does not develop post-infection, necessitating preventative measures. Condom use provides protection against HIV and syphilis transmission, and testing for these infections, with a repeat evaluation at 3 months, is advisable.

Gonorrhea

14

Abstract

Gonorrhea, caused by *Neisseria gonorrhoeae*, can impact the urogenital tract, anorectal region, pharynx, and eyes. If left untreated, complications such as disseminated infection, septic arthritis, endocarditis, and pelvic inflammatory disease may occur. The incidence of gonorrhea is increasing in many countries, although reporting rates have fluctuated due to factors including the availability and utilization of healthcare services and socioeconomic conditions. Diagnosis of gonorrhea can be achieved through microscopy, culture, or molecular methods. The standard treatment regimen are according to local resistance profile and national guidelines. The escalating challenge of antibiotic resistance complicates the management of this infection. Prompt initiation of treatment is essential to prevent further transmission and associated complications. Preventive measures for gonorrhea include the adoption of safe sex practices, consistent condom use, and regular screenings for sexually transmitted infections.

14.1 Background

Although gonorrhea may appear negligible in many countries, estimates suggest that the incidence is increasing in various world regions. Infection with Neisseria gonorrhoeae usually occurs in the urogenital tract, but it can also appear in the anorectal, pharyngeal, or conjunctival areas. In the absence of timely treatment, complications such as disseminated gonococcal infection, septic arthritis, endocarditis, myocarditis, and meningitis may arise. In females, inflammation of the upper genital tract may occur. Neonatal conjunctivitis, also referred to as ophthalmia neonatorum, can develop during the neonatal period and within the first year of life as a consequence of infection.

I. Mylonas, *Sexually Transmitted Diseases*,
https://doi.org/10.1007/978-3-031-78204-6_14

14.2 Pathogen

Neisseria gonorrhoeae is a gram-negative, spherical bacterium classified in the genus Neisseria. It belongs to a small group that includes *Neisseria meningitidis*, *Neisseria mucosa*, *Neisseria sicca*, *Neisseria flava*, and *Neisseria cinerea*, as well as several nonpathogenic bacteria. Gonococci require specific conditions for optimal growth, characterized by low temperatures, reduced humidity, and minimal light exposure. These bacteria multiply through binary fission, leading to the tendency of sibling cells to adhere, often resulting in the appearance of diplococci or clusters in microscopic preparations.

Gonococci primarily associate with the cylindrical epithelium. Infection may extend beyond the urethra to include the Bartholin glands, cervix uteri, salpinx, and peritoneum in women. The multilayered squamous epithelium of the vagina is generally resistant to infection, except in prepubescent girls, in whom keratinization of epithelial cells has not yet occurred due to insufficient estrogen levels.

The pathogen is internalized into host cells via active endocytosis. Intracellular gonococci stimulate a nonspecific immune response by inducing the release of cytokines in response to the endotoxin present in the pathogen. These cytokines have a chemotactic effect on various inflammatory cells, which subsequently migrate to the site of infection. The recruited inflammatory cells exert a detrimental influence on tissue integrity, leading to increased permeability and facilitating the entry of additional pathogens into mucosal layers. In instances of persistent infection, localized inflammation may result in significant tissue damage that the body struggles to repair. Following an acute infection, damaged tissue is often replaced by connective tissue scars.

Autoinoculation can lead to rectal infections stemming from the urethra or female genital tract. In rare cases, conjunctival infection may occur if pathogenic microorganisms are transmitted, particularly affecting newborns during delivery, leading to purulent conjunctivitis. Additionally, the pathogens may be transmitted to the throat through contact transmission. In rare instances, gonococci may evade mucosal barriers and disseminate to skin and joints. Pregnant women are particularly at risk for systemic spread owing to partially compromised immune defenses.

Despite an intact immune response, infections seldom resolve spontaneously; they often become chronic, with persistent but attenuated purulent inflammation.

14.3 Epidemiology

Gonococci are *exclusively found* in humans and are highly infectious, transmitted through direct contact with mucous membranes during sexual intercourse or childbirth. The probability of infection following a single sexual encounter is estimated to be between 20% and 50% for males and between 60% and 90% for females. Outside of human hosts, these pathogens have a short life span.

The incidence and epidemiology of gonorrhea in Europe exhibit a complex pattern shaped by numerous factors, including healthcare accessibility and socioeconomic conditions:

- **Global Prevalence:** In 2020, the World Health Organization (WHO) estimated 82.4 million new infections with *Neisseria gonorrhoeae* among adults aged 15–49 years. In 2016, the global prevalence of urogenital gonorrhea was estimated at 0.9% in women and 0.7% in men, corresponding to approximately 30.6 million cases worldwide. The global incidence rate in 2016 was calculated at 20 per 1000 women and 26 per 1000 men, totaling 86.9 million new cases.
- **Regional Prevalence and Incidence:** Among women, the highest prevalence was observed in the WHO African Region (1.9%), followed by the Region of the Americas (0.9%) and the Western Pacific Region (0.9%), with the lowest prevalence in the European Region (0.3%). Among men, the highest prevalence was found in the WHO African Region (1.6%), followed by the Americas (0.8%) and the Western Pacific (0.7%), and the lowest in Europe (0.3%). The highest incidence was recorded in the WHO African Region, the Americas, and the Western Pacific, while the lowest was in the European Region.
- **European Union/European Economic Area (EU/EEA):** In 2019, 117,881 confirmed cases of gonorrhea were reported by 28 EU/EEA member states (including the UK), reflecting an overall reporting rate of 31.6 cases per 100,000 population. In 2021, 27 EU/EEA countries reported 46,728 confirmed cases, corresponding to a reporting rate of 13.7 cases per 100,000 inhabitants. A rising trend in reporting rates was noted between 2012 and 2019, followed by a decline in the initial year of the COVID-19 pandemic (2020). However, reporting rates increased again in 2021, surpassing 2019 levels. In 2022, confirmed gonorrhea infections in Europe reached a record high of 70,881 cases in the EU (excluding the UK).
- **The United States:** In 2020, the Centers for Disease Control and Prevention (CDC) reported a total of 677,769 cases of gonorrhea, making it the second most commonly reported notifiable sexually transmitted disease.
- **Canada:** As of 2018, gonorrhea was the second most commonly reported STD in Canada, with a reported incidence rate of 70.2 per 100,000 among men compared to 40.6 per 100,000 among women in 2015.
- **The United Kingdom:** In England, 82,592 diagnoses of gonorrhea were reported in 2022, representing a 50.3% increase compared to the previous year.

Gonorrhea is particularly prevalent in developing countries, with the majority of cases reported among individuals involved in commercial sexual activities. The inflammatory changes in mucosal membranes may facilitate the acquisition and transmission of HIV, as the number of viral particles in semen is significantly elevated in individuals with gonorrhea. The incidence of neonatal conjunctivitis resulting from gonococcal infection is estimated to range from 1% to 5%.

Gonorrhea presents a considerable public health challenge worldwide, characterized by high incidence and prevalence rates, especially within certain regions, populations, and age groups. Rates have been on the rise in numerous countries in recent years.

14.4 Clinical Manifestation

14.4.1 Gynecology

The clinical syndrome of gonorrhea is contingent upon the stage and severity of the infection.

Clinical Stages

- **Lower Gonorrhea:** The infection remains localized within the vulvovaginal and cervical regions.
- **Upper Gonorrhea:** In upper gonorrhea, the infection ascends through the cervical canal, potentially infecting the endometrium and fallopian tubes, and may reach the peritoneal space.
- **Extragenital Manifestations:** The infection can disseminate to other organs outside the genital tract by various mechanisms: as a primary predilection site, via autoinoculation, during the peripartum period, or through hematogenous spread.

14.4.1.1 Lower Gonorrhea

The principal symptom of gonorrhea in women is severe purulent inflammation of the cervix, typically presenting 2–7 days after initial infection (Fig. 14.1). Concurrent urethritis is observed in approximately 70–80% of infected individuals (Fig. 9.1). *Neisseria gonorrhoeae* is the primary agent responsible for cervicitis.

Cervical infection is characterized by the presence of *creamy, foul-smelling, yellowish-green purulent genital discharge*. Redness of the cervix and/or urethra may occur as an ionflammation result of the infection. Additionally, inflammation of the Bartholin's or Skene's glands may be seen. In cases of simultaneous secretion accumulation, a Bartholin's pseudo-abscess—ranging in size from that of a cherry to a chicken egg—may develop, leading to significant pain and impairing the patient's ability to sit or walk. Vulvitis may accompany the infection.

Gonococci can similarly infect the urogenital tract of prepubertal girls, although transmission through nonbiological means such as laundry, towels, toilet seats, or toys has not been demonstrated.

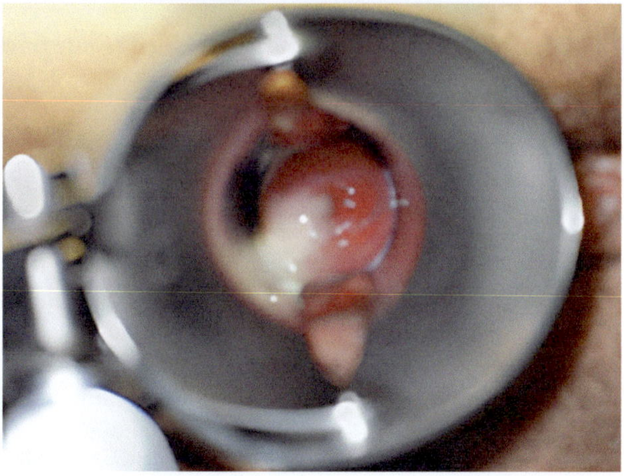

Fig. 14.1 Gonococcal cervicitis with profuse cervical discharge (Mylonas 2016)

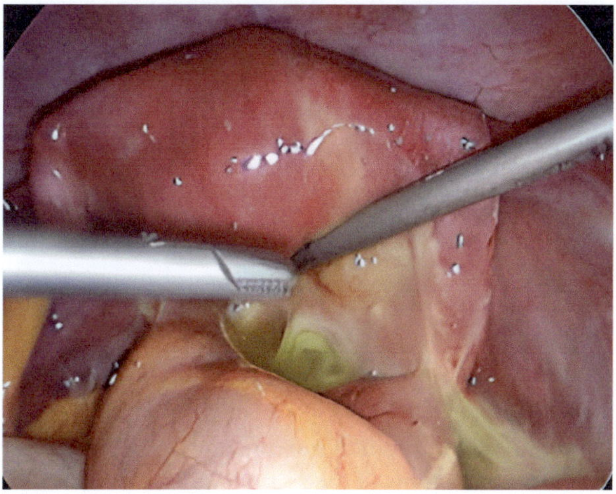

Fig. 14.2 PID secondary to ascending gonococcal infection (upper gonorrhea), characterized by creamy, yellow-greenish exudate (Mylonas 2016)

14.4.1.2 Upper Gonorrhea

An ascending infection may result in involvement of the endometrium, fallopian tubes, and ovaries. Infection of the endometrium typically manifests as metrorrhagia, although the endometrium is usually only temporarily infected. The presence of bleeding disorders may indicate endometritis; however, approximately 50% of women remain asymptomatic.

The infection can extend to the peritoneum via the fallopian tubes, leading to pelvic inflammatory disease (Fig. 14.2). Symptoms of PID may include cervical pain, adnexal swelling, and fever. These clinical features have become less common during the past decades. However, the rising incidence of gonorrhea indicates that a greater occurrence of gonorrhea-related PID should be expected.

A significant concern is that prolonged tissue damage may occur, leading to scarring. In narrow mucosal passages, such as the urethra or fallopian tubes, this scarring can result in narrowing or complete obstruction due to the development of strictures.

Obstructions in the fallopian tubes may result in significant long-term consequences, including infertility, ectopic pregnancies, and chronic lower abdominal pain. Gonococcal PID is present in approximately 40% of cases, although detection at the cervix is successful in only 60% of cases. As the pathogen ascends from the fallopian tubes into the abdominal cavity, it may disseminate further to the perihepatic region. Perihepatitis, also known as *Fitz-Hugh–Curtis syndrome*, results from an existing infection and is characterized by delicate adhesions between the liver capsule and adjacent abdominal organs, particularly the parietal peritoneum. Simultaneous identification of the pathogen in cases of acute gonococcal perihepatitis occurs in less than 10% of cases.

Subsequent complications may include:

- Urethral stricture, particularly in the context of multiple infections.
- Male sterility, especially following epididymitis.
- Female sterility, particularly after PID.
- Increased likelihood of ectopic pregnancy.
- Chronic lower abdominal pain.

14.4.1.3 Urethritis

A prominent symptom of gonorrhea is severe, painful inflammation of the urethra, leading to symptoms of urethritis (Chap. 9). Pus may be visibly discharged from the urethral opening (Fig. 9.1). Infection of the Bartholin glands is common in women and is associated with significant pain (Fig. 4.2, page 56). Over a span of days to weeks, the inflammatory response may contain microbial proliferation and facilitate the resolution of inflammatory symptoms.

In men, this stage is characterized by the presence of copious amounts of pus in the urethra overnight, typically expelled at the urethral orifice in the early morning prior to urination. The urethral opening may display redness indicative of inflammation. *Neisseria gonorrhoeae* may also cause epididymitis, presenting as unilateral testicular pain without discharge or dysuria. Upon examination, the epididymis may be enlarged and tender. In some cases, fever may also be present.

Urethral involvement may cause intense, burning pain during urination, potentially progressing to tenesmus if bacterial cystitis is also present. Although urethritis can occur in women, the symptoms are typically less pronounced than in men.

14.4.2 Other Sites of Manifestation

14.4.2.1 Pharyngitis Associated with Pharyngeal Gonorrhea

Pharyngitis (Chap. 10) associated with pharyngeal gonorrhea may result from orogenital exposure and is typically characterized by mild or absent symptoms. In only 5% of cases, pharyngeal gonorrhea presents as the sole infection. In patients with urogenital gonorrhea, a concurrent pharyngeal infection can be identified in approximately 8–20% of cases.

Clinical findings may include erythema and mucopurulent exudate in the throat, along with potential mucosal swelling. Patients commonly report difficulty swallowing. In rare instances, regional lymph node enlargement in the neck may also be identified. To prevent the spread of gonococcal infection to other body parts, prompt and adequate treatment is essential.

14.4.2.2 Rectal Gonorrhea—Proctitis

In women, perianal infections may arise from existing genital or anal infections, subsequently leading to anorectal infection. It is estimated that approximately 50% of women with genital gonococcal infections also exhibit rectal mucosa contamination. In MSM, isolated rectal infections occur in about 40% of cases, whereas this is rare in women, at approximately 5%.

Most rectal infections in women are asymptomatic or subclinical, while approximately two-thirds of men report symptoms. Possible symptoms may include hemorrhoid-like discomfort and proctitis.

Symptoms indicative of rectal infection may include:

- Anal itching.
- Rectal pain.
- Diarrhea with tenesmus.
- Pain during bowel movements.
- Feeling of fullness or constipation.
- Mucopurulent discharge or stool deposits.

Proctoscopy often reveals mucosal bleeding, tenderness, and purulent deposits. Asymptomatic rectal gonorrhea serves as a reservoir for further infections.

Differentiating pronounced rectal gonococcal infections from pelvic inflammatory disease (PID) can be challenging in women.

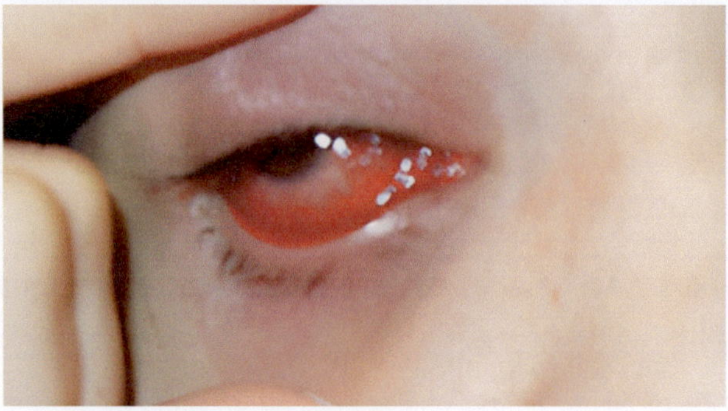

Fig. 14.3 Ophthalmoblennorrhea gonorrhoica (Mylonas 2016)

14.4.2.3 Ophthalmoblennorrhoea Gonorrhoica

Pathogens are typically transmitted to the eye via autoinoculation during the presence of genital gonorrhea or during childbirth.

14.4.2.3.1 Ophthalmoblennorrhoea Adultorum

Typically affects *one eye* and involves acute purulent infection characterized by burning and itching (Fig. 14.3). Ophthalmoblennorrhea may be associated with keratitis, eyelid edema, and discharge of yellowish-green purulent material. Patients frequently have difficulty opening their eyelids due to associated pain. Corneal ulcerations may develop, and, if untreated, lead to blindness. Due to the acute presentation, ophthalmoblennorrhea adultorum is often the first sign of a gonococcal infection.

14.4.2.3.2 Ophthalmoblennorrhoea Neonatorum

The risk of intrapartum infection of the newborn is estimated to be approximately 30–50%. Acute purulent conjunctivitis affecting *both eyes* typically occurs within the first 5 days postnatally. In the nineteenth century, over 50% of blindness cases were attributed to ophthalmoblennorrhea neonatorum.

14.4.2.4 Disseminated Infections

Disseminated infections arise in approximately 1–3% of adult patients with gonorrhea, with women being more frequently affected than men. A disseminated gonococcal infection typically presents as a triad of symptoms:

- Acute polyarthritis.
- Skin rash.
- Fever spikes.

The wrists and ankles are the most commonly affected joints, along with the fingers and toes. In approximately 50–75% of cases, patients present with skin symptoms and episodic fever.

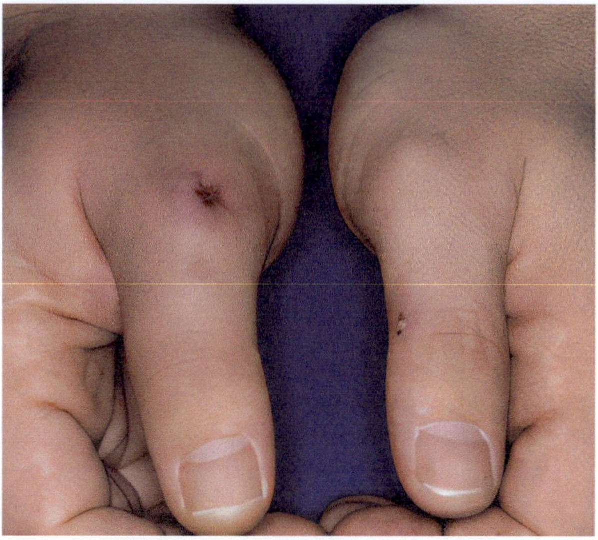

Fig. 14.4 Disseminated gonococcal infection (Buder and Lautenschlager 2022)

Acute arthritis often initially presents with tenosynovitis and arthralgia, with characteristic joint inflammation and effusion developing later in approximately 30–40% of affected patients. Oligoarticular or monoarticular arthritis—referred to as gonococcal monoarthritis—most commonly involves large joints, particularly the knee, and may arise suddenly, sometimes progressing from a polyarticular pattern. If left untreated, disseminated gonococcal infection (DGI) can advance to septic arthritis, predominantly affecting the elbows, wrists, knees, and ankles.

Characteristic skin manifestations of DGI typically include small, fluid-filled lesions that begin as vesicles and may evolve into pustules. Additional cutaneous findings can include bullae, petechiae, and necrotic lesions, frequently localized on the skin overlying joints or on distal extremities (see Fig. 14.4). These lesions often fluctuate in appearance and may regress as the infection progresses or resolves.

Disseminated infection carries the risk of severe systemic complications, such as bacterial endocarditis, perihepatitis (Fitz-Hugh–Curtis syndrome), osteomyelitis, meningitis, and myocarditis. Ocular involvement is an important but less common manifestation and may present as conjunctivitis, iridocyclitis, scleritis, or iritis. Patients with ocular involvement often experience redness, pain, photophobia, blurred vision, and tearing. If untreated, these inflammatory eye conditions can lead to complications, such as corneal ulceration or permanent vision impairment.

Patients with disseminated gonorrhea often do not exhibit urogenital symptoms.

14.4.3 Pregnancy

The clinical presentation of gonorrhea during pregnancy differs significantly from that in nonpregnant women due to the hormonal and physiological changes of gestation. These changes create a distinct environment that affects both susceptibility to infection and the manifestation of disease.

Hormonal fluctuations, especially elevated estrogen and progesterone levels, alter the vaginal mucosa by increasing its permeability and causing loosening. This predisposes pregnant women to gonococcal vaginitis, a condition less commonly seen in nonpregnant women. Progesterone also modulates the immune response, often suppressing inflammation, which may result in many pregnant women remaining asymptomatic or exhibiting only mild, nonspecific symptoms that can be mistaken for normal pregnancy-related changes.

Ascending infection leading to salpingitis is considerably less frequent during pregnancy compared to nonpregnant women. This reduced risk is attributed to protective mechanisms, such as the formation of dense cervical mucus that acts as a barrier, and anatomical changes after the first trimester that block bacterial migration into the upper genital tract. When salpingitis does occur, it generally presents early in pregnancy, often in women with preexisting infection at conception or shortly thereafter.

Untreated gonorrhea in pregnancy can lead to serious complications, such as septic abortion, particularly during the first trimester when the risk of ascending infection is highest. The infection can cause chorioamnionitis, premature rupture of membranes, intrauterine infection, and fetal loss, all of which contribute to significant maternal morbidity.

Pregnant women have an increased susceptibility to cervical gonorrhea, with risk estimates suggesting a fivefold rise compared to nonpregnant women. This heightened vulnerability is linked to pregnancy-induced changes in immunity, altered vaginal pH, and increased glycogen content, which promote bacterial colonization and growth.

Maternal gonorrhea is strongly associated with adverse birth outcomes. It increases the risk of low birth weight infants through mechanisms, such as intrauterine growth restriction. Additionally, it contributes to small-for-gestational-age births and preterm delivery. Untreated infection during pregnancy raises the likelihood of premature birth, prelabor rupture of membranes, and chorioamnionitis.

Postpartum complications related to gonorrhea include endometritis and myometritis, which are significant causes of postpartum morbidity. The risk of these infections is especially high following cesarean section due to surgical disruption of anatomical barriers. Puerperal sepsis resulting from ascending gonococcal infection can be life-threatening if not promptly managed.

The risk of intrauterine transmission is often heightened by premature rupture of membranes and premature birth.

14.4.4 Neonatology

Vertical transmission of gonorrhea during vaginal delivery remains a major concern. Approximately 30–35% of infants born vaginally to infected mothers develop gonococcal conjunctivitis or test positive for the organism. Even cesarean delivery does not entirely eliminate transmission risk if membranes rupture before the procedure. Neonatal complications include ophthalmia neonatorum, which can rapidly progress to corneal ulceration and blindness without timely treatment.

In the neonatal period and the first year of life, gonorrhea can cause neonatal conjunctivitis (ophthalmoblennorrhea neonatorum). The infection typically manifests within 2–5 days postnatally (Fig. 14.5). Prompt diagnosis and treatment are crucial, as untreated conditions may lead to perforation of the eyeball and blindness.

It is estimated that nearly all new cases of gonorrhea in individuals older than one year are attributed to sexual abuse.

Ophthalmoblennorrhea neonatorum is characterized by hyperacute, highly purulent infection acquired during birth. The infection commonly presents as bilateral conjunctivitis, accompanied by severe eyelid swelling and chemosis, indicative of inflammatory conjunctival swelling. Severe purulence can lead to corneal ulceration, perforation, and secondary glaucoma. Absent treatment may result in scarring and vision deterioration, potentially leading to complete blindness.

Neisseria gonorrhoeae **is the most common causative agent of ophthalmia neonatorum.**

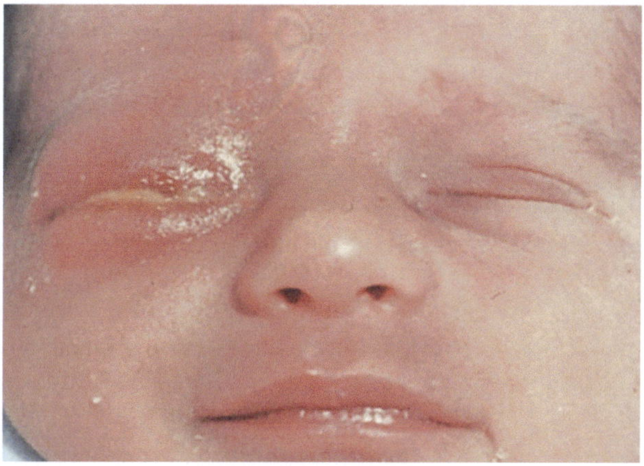

Fig. 14.5 Gonoblennorrhea in a neonate (Zangerle et al. 2018)

Approximately 35% of neonates with ophthalmia neonatorum also develop concurrent pharyngeal gonococcal infection, resulting from inadvertent inoculation of the oropharynx during passage through an infected birth canal. In addition to ocular involvement, isolated cases of gonococcal urethritis, vaginitis, or proctitis have been reported in neonates, all attributable to vertical transmission at delivery. Compared to the severe purulent inflammation characteristic of conjunctival infection, mucosal reactions at these nonocular sites are generally milder, presenting with low-grade erythema, minimal exudate, and limited discomfort.

Although uncommon, gonococcal pneumonia can develop within the first weeks of life, typically manifesting as tachypnea, cough, and diffuse infiltrates visible on chest radiography. This serious complication often follows unrecognized mucosal colonization. Other severe neonatal manifestations include sepsis—marked by fever or hypothermia, lethargy, and poor feeding; arthritis—characterized by joint swelling and restricted movement; and meningitis—indicated by signs, such as bulging fontanelle, irritability, and seizures. Localized scalp infections may also occur at sites of electrode placement or caput succedaneum, presenting as erythematous nodules that can ulcerate and necessitate systemic antibiotic therapy.

14.5 Diagnosis

The clinical diagnosis of gonorrhea is complicated by the presence of nonspecific symptoms. Infections with *Chlamydia trachomatis*, *Trichomonas vaginalis*, *Candida albicans*, and a wide range of other pathogens can produce similar or even identical symptoms. These pathogens may coexist with *Neisseria gonorrhoeae* within the female genital tract.

The diagnosis of gonorrhea relies on clinical symptoms and the culture-based detection of the pathogen. A comprehensive medical history can enhance targeted sampling efficiency, thus improving detection rates. The likelihood of detecting *Neisseria gonorrhoeae* is highest in smears taken from the mucous membranes that are primarily infected. In women, it is advisable to sample both the cervix and the urethra. In men, a urethral swab is sufficient for diagnosis. It is recommended that patients abstain from urination for a minimum of 4 h prior to urethral swab collection, with the optimal time for sample collection occurring before the first urination of the morning. The sensitivity of the test significantly increases when swabs are also obtained from the rectal and pharyngeal mucosa.

Diagnosing disseminated gonococcal infection is particularly challenging due to the intermittent nature of bacteremia. Detection of gonococci in the blood is only possible in 20–30% of cases, while diagnosis via joint punctate or skin biopsies is successful in 50% of cases. In the majority of cases (up to 80%), detection using genital swabs is effective. However, most patients with disseminated gonococcal infection do not present with urogenital symptoms.

14.5.1 Microscopy

If a gonococcal infection is suspected, a microscopic preparation of pus from the urethra, cervix, or other sites of infection should be evaluated. Following staining with methylene blue, the spherical or coccoid-shaped bacteria appear bright blue, displaying a characteristic diplococcus shape reminiscent of a bread roll or coffee bean. Typically, these pairs of bacteria are observed closely clustered, both extracellularly and intracellularly (Fig. 14.6). While the morphological characteristics of host cells and the bacteria may not be as clearly defined in Gram stains, red-colored diplococci can still be identified as gram-negative bacteria.

The microscopic identification of intracellular gram-negative gonococci in methylene blue and Gram stains provides enough evidence to diagnose a gonococcal infection. However, definitive proof of infection can only be established through microbiological cultures, as nonpathogenic species of *Neisseria* can also be present.

14.5.2 Microbiology

Due to the sensitivity of gonococci to light, cold, and dryness, rapid processing is recommended using specialized media and culture systems. Cultivation occurs on Thayer–Martin selective culture medium under high humidity (90–100%) and at a temperature of 35–36 °C in an atmosphere enriched with 4–6% CO_2. For cases of

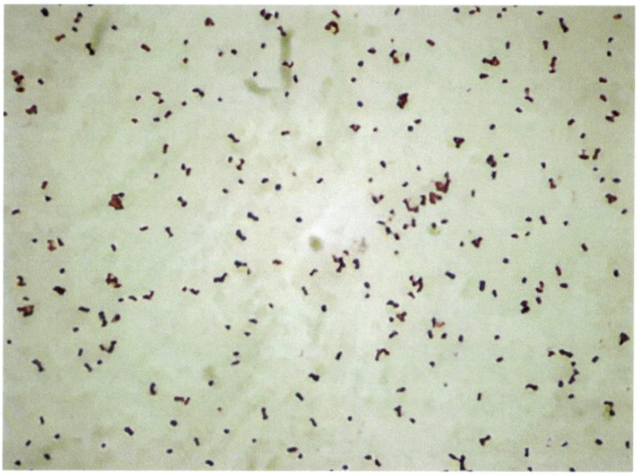

Fig. 14.6 Characteristic morphology of diplococci (Mylonas 2016)

disseminated infections sourced from blood, synovial fluid, or skin lesions, cultural detection of the pathogen is significantly less successful. *It is critical to perform resistance testing due to the increasing prevalence of multi-resistant strains.*

14.5.3 Serological and Gene Amplification Methods

Contemporary molecular-biology techniques—such as nucleic acid amplification tests (NAATs)—target pathogen-specific gene sequences to detect *Neisseria gonorrhoeae* directly from clinical specimens. Although NAATs can achieve sensitivities and specificities exceeding 95%, their high cost, technical complexity, and the need for specialized laboratory infrastructure have limited routine use in many settings. Early PCR-based assays suffered from cross-reactivity with commensal Neisseria species, but modern, highly specific probes (including transcription-mediated amplification and strand-displacement amplification platforms) now underpin most firstline diagnostic algorithms in tertiary and reference laboratories.

Matrix-assisted laser desorption/ionization time-of-flight mass spectrometry (MALDI-TOF MS) has recently emerged as a rapid, accurate method for identifying bacterial pathogens—including *N. gonorrhoeae*—directly from culture isolates. By analyzing peptide mass fingerprints of bacterial proteins, MALDI-TOF MS distinguishes pathogenic gonococci from nonpathogenic Neisseria species within minutes, with accuracy comparable to molecular assays and at lower per-sample cost once the instrument is in place. Its adoption in clinical microbiology laboratories is expanding, facilitating both species identification and preliminary strain typing for epidemiologic investigations.

The detection of the pathogen is indicative of a gonococcal infection. Microbiological diagnosis, including resistance pattern analysis, is highly recommended due to increasing resistance and the need for an adequate choice of effective antibiotics.

14.6 Treatment

14.6.1 General

The management of gonococcal infection has become increasingly complex and variable in recent years (Fig. 14.7). Due to the rising prevalence of antibiotic resistance, most international guidelines and recommendations since 2014 have

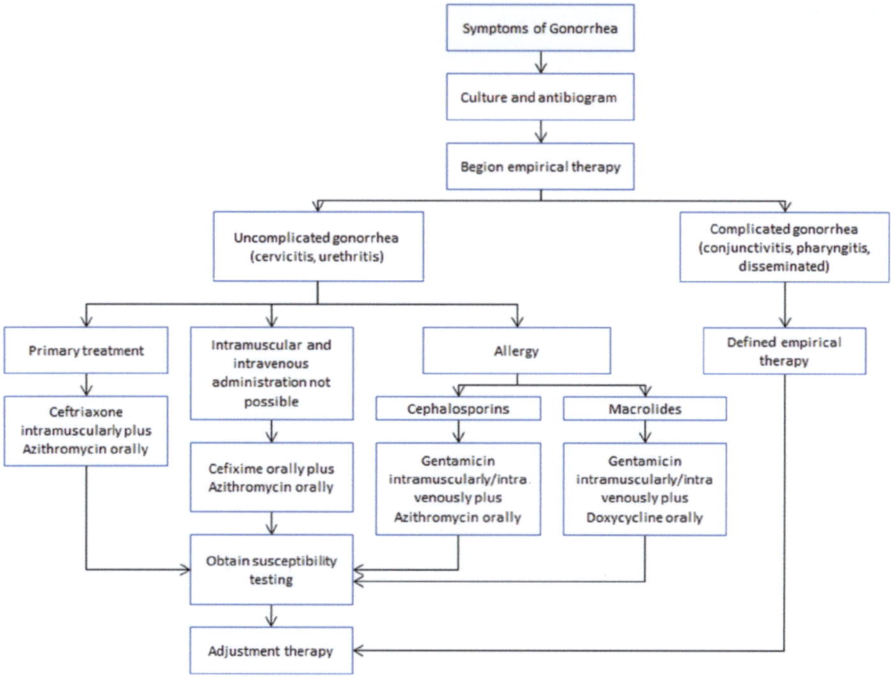

Fig. 14.7 Protocol for managing gonorrhea. (Courtesy of I. Mylonas)

advocated for the administration of a cephalosporin (particularly ceftriaxone) in conjunction with a macrolide (azithromycin) as the recommended treatment according to WHO (Table 14.1). This combination has remained in practice in some countries, despite anticipated increases in azithromycin resistance, which is projected to increase fivefold within 10 years. Consequently, various international recommendations, including those from the CDC, have emerged in response to this situation, leading to a reduction in the general recommendation of the ceftriaxone–azithromycin combination therapy.

To prevent further complications, it is crucial to initiate treatment as soon as possible.

In countries wherethe double antibiotic treatment has been dismissed for uncomplicated infections, a single dose of ceftriaxone is typically recommended.

Table 14.1 Treatment options for uncomplicated gonococcal infection in nonpregnant patients

Indication	Medication	Dosage	Duration
Recommendation[a]	Ceftriaxone	1 g intramuscularly/intravenously, single dose	Single dose
	Plus		
	Azithromycin	2 g orally, single dose	Single dose
Alternative[b]	Cefixime	800 mg orally, single dose	Single dose
	Plus		
	Azithromycin	2 g orally, single dose	Single dose
Alternative[c]	Cefixime	400 mg orally, single dose	Single dose
	Ciprofloxacin	500 mg orally, single dose	Single dose
	Ofloxacin[d]	400 mg orally, single dose	Single dose
	Levofloxacin	500 mg orally, single dose	Single dose
	Azithromycin	2 g orally, single dose	Single dose
Cephalosporin allergy or resistance[e]	Gentamicin	240 mg intramuscularly/intravenously, single dose	Single dose
	Plus		
	Azithromycin	2 g orally, single dose	Single dose
Macrolide allergy or resistance[e]	Gentamicin	240 mg intramuscularly/intravenously, single dose	Single dose
	Doxycycline	100 mg orally, twice daily	7 days
Fluoroquinolone regimen[e]	Ciprofloxacin	500 mg orally, single dose	Single dose
	Plus		
	Azithromycin	2 g orally, single dose	Single dose

[a]Most common recommendations (based on WHO)
[b]If intramuscular administration is contraindicated, and intravenous administration not possible
[c]Only with previously confirmed susceptibility
[d]As a racemate, generally lower efficacy. Levofloxacin (L-racemate) should be preferred as an alternative
[e]In case of allergy or resistance and without further alternatives

Uncomplicated gonococcal infections of the urethra, cervix, rectum, and pharynx should be treated as follows:

- A single dose of 500 mg ceftriaxone administered intramuscularly (1 g intramuscularly for patients weighing ≥150 kg).
- If ceftriaxone is unavailable, a single oral dose of 800 mg cefixime may be used.
- If a chlamydial infection cannot be ruled out, treatment with doxycycline 100 mg orally twice daily for 7 days is recommended.
- For patients allergic to doxycycline, a single dose of 1 g azithromycin should be administered if a chlamydial infection is suspected.
- Patients with a known allergy to cephalosporins (including ceftriaxone) should receive 240 mg gentamicin intramuscularly in a single dose, along with 2 g azithromycin orally in a single dose.

In the case of disseminated gonococcal infection (DGI) with arthritis, a longer course of parenteral antibiotics is necessary. Initially, DGI with gonococcal arthritis is treated with intravenous or intramuscular antibiotics (e.g., ceftriaxone 1 g administered intramuscularly or intravenously every 24 h, ceftizoxime 1 g administered intravenously every 8 h, or cefotaxime 1 g administered intravenously every 8 h). The treatment regimen should continue for 24–48 h after symptom resolution, after which it may be shifted to oral therapy for at least 7 days based on antimicrobial sensitivity test results.

Following successful therapy, additional cultures ("proof of cure") are not required.

If symptoms persist beyond 7 days, it is advisable to *collect samples for cultural examination and antimicrobial sensitivity testing*. Patients should refrain from sexual activity throughout the treatment period to prevent the transmission of infection to sexual partners.

14.6.2 Pregnancy

In recent years, several international health organizations have *endorsed the following treatment options* for uncomplicated gonorrhea during pregnancy:

- A single intramuscular dose of 500 mg ceftriaxone, which should be avoided during the first trimester and replaced with other cephalosporins.
- A single oral dose of 800 mg cefixime.
- A single intramuscular dose of 2 g spectinomycin, contingent on its availability. If necessary, this medication can be obtained from international pharmacies. Should penicillin-resistant gonococci be identified, the spectinomycin dosage may be doubled.
- If a cephalosporin allergy exists, the recommended treatment is a single intramuscular dose of 240 mg gentamicin, along with 2 g azithromycin administered orally as a single dose.

Azithromycin should not be given alone. The combined administration of ceftriaxone and azithromycin is still considered the standard in some guidelines, despite ongoing concerns about resistance development and challenges associated with administration during pregnancy.

Given the stringent indications for azithromycin in most countries, its use during pregnancy should follow a comprehensive risk assessment and ideally be deferred until after the first trimester (in some countries (i.e., Switzerland), only after the 20th week of pregnancy).

Previous recommendations for erythromycin or cefpodoxime treatment have been replaced by current guidelines due to the emergence of resistance. Local antibiotic treatment of conjunctivitis with erythromycin remains a viable option, although it is neither recommended nor commonly used in practice.

14.6.3 Special Cases

The treatment of pharyngeal gonococcal infections presents greater challenges compared to urogenital or rectal infections (Table 14.2). Only a limited number of antibiotics have demonstrated reliable efficacy in eliminating these infections. The CDC (Centers for Disease Control and Prevention in the United States) recommends administering a single intramuscular dose of 125 mg ceftriaxone or a single oral dose of 500 mg ciprofloxacin. In cases of resistance to fluoroquinolones, cefotaxime (500 mg or 1 g administered intramuscularly) is the preferred alternative.

Oral alternatives to cefixime cannot yet be recommended due to insufficient data regarding cefpodoxime. Additionally, a single dose of 1 g cefuroxime axetil is considered suboptimal.

If a patient has a known allergy to penicillin, the administration of spectinomycin (2 g intramuscularly) is advised. While spectinomycin is not commercially available in some countries, it may be obtained from international pharmacies. Alternatively, ciprofloxacin (500 mg orally) or azithromycin (2 g orally as a single dose) can be considered after a resistance test.

Patients diagnosed with ascending or disseminated gonococcal infections should be treated in a hospital setting (Table 14.2). In cases of complicated gonorrhea, the recommended duration of treatment is between 7–28 days, depending on the specific symptoms exhibited. Intravenous therapy should be administered for the first 7 days, after which a transition to oral medication can occur, either cefixime (2 × 400 mg) or, in the event of a negative resistance test, ciprofloxacin (2 × 500 mg). This transition should take place 24–28 hours after symptoms have improved. Postgonococcal urethritis (mixed infection) may occur following treatment, necessitating a culture to be performed 4–7 days after the completion of therapy.

It is essential that sexual partners are examined and treated as well.

Ophthalmoblennorrhea adultorum, associated with gonorrhea, is an acute emergency that requires immediate intervention. This severe eye infection can lead to significant complications and permanent damage if not addressed promptly. Timely initiation of antibiotic therapy is crucial (Table 14.2), along with the irrigation of the eye with copious amounts of a 0.9% saline solution.

Ophthalmoblennorrhea adultorum is considered an acute emergency!

Table 14.2 Management of complicated gonococcal infections

Site of infection	Indication	Medication	Dosage	Duration
Disseminated	First choice	Ceftriaxone[a]	1 g once daily intramuscularly or intravenously	2–3 days
		Cefixime	400 mg orally twice daily	7 days
		Ciprofloxacin	500 mg orally twice daily	7 days
		Levofloxacin	500 mg orally twice daily	7 days
	In meningitis	Ceftriaxone[a]	1 g twice daily intramuscularly or intravenously	14 days
	In endocarditis	Ceftriaxone[a]	1 g once daily intramuscularly or intravenously	28 days
Conjunctivitis in adults	First choice	Ceftriaxone[a]	1 g once daily intramuscularly	3 days
	Alternative[b]	Azithromycin	2 g orally	Single dose
		Doxycycline	100 mg orally twice daily	7 days
		Ciprofloxacin	250 mg orally twice daily	3 days
Pharyngeal	First choice	Ceftriaxone[a]	1 g intramuscularly or intravenously	Single dose
		Azithromycin	1.5 g orally	Single dose
	Alternative[c]	Ciprofloxacin	500 mg orally once	Single dose
		Ofloxacin[d]	400 mg orally once	Single dose
		Azithromycin	2 g orally once	Single dose

[a]Until receipt of the antibiogram
[b]In case of contraindication to ceftriaxone (e.g., allergy)
[c]Only with previously proven susceptibility
[d]As a racemate, generally less effective. Levofloxacin (L-racemate) is preferred as an alternative

Newborns exhibiting ophthalmoblennorrhea neonatorum or suspected gonococcal infections should receive ceftriaxone in a single dose of 25–50 mg/kg body weight, administered intravenously or intramuscularly, with the total dose not exceeding 125 mg. Local treatment with erythromycin is also a viable option. It is advisable to avoid the use of quinolones in children due to the potential risk of joint cartilage damage.

In the event of a diagnosis of genital gonorrhea, it is recommended that all sexual partners who engaged in sexual intercourse within the preceding 60 days be tested and treated if indicated. If the last sexual encounter occurred more than 60 days prior, the individual's most recent sexual partner should be informed and tested.

14.7 Differential Diagnosis

In the differential diagnosis of gonorrhea, careful consideration is required to distinguish it from other conditions presenting similar symptoms. Urethritis caused by organisms such as *Chlamydia trachomatis* should be noted for its shared manifestations, including dysuria and discharge. Trichomoniasis, often leading to vaginal or urethral irritation, must also be considered. Additionally, bacterial vaginosis, characterized by abnormal discharge, should be excluded via microscopic examination. Viral infections, such as herpes simplex virus, can produce genital lesions that may mimic the symptoms of gonorrheal infections. Lastly, noninfectious factors such as chemical irritation from personal hygiene products or mechanical irritation due to foreign objects should be taken into account.

14.8 Prevention

Given that young, unmarried individuals and sex workers are at higher risk for gonorrhea, educating these populations on preventive measures is crucial. Consistent and correct use of condoms during sexual intercourse provides a reliable and effective method for preventing the transmission of this infection.

A follow-up visit is recommended to assess adherence to treatment and evaluate the reduction of symptoms. In most countries, a repeat examination to assess treatment efficacy is not routinely recommended.

The administration of a 1% solution of Argentum nitricum (silver nitrate) into the conjunctival sac of newborns is still regarded as a recommended prophylactic measure for preventing ophthalmia neonatorum (blennorrhea) caused by gonococci. Although this intervention can cause chemical conjunctivitis in approximately 10% of cases—mimicking bacterial blennorrhea—this side effect is considered acceptable since it is temporary and does not result in lasting harm. Despite the World Health Organization's (WHO) continued endorsement of this cost-effective prophylactic measure, Credé prophylaxis is no longer prescribed or performed in most countries.

Requirements for a repeat examination include:

- **Persistent symptoms.**
- **Reexposure.**
- **Detection of antibiotic resistance.**
- **Pharyngeal or disseminated gonorrhea.**

Key Points

- Infection with *Neisseria gonorrhoeae* predominantly occurs in the urogenital tract but can also manifest in the anorectal, pharyngeal, or conjunctival regions.
- Untreated gonorrhea can lead to severe complications, including disseminated gonococcal infection, septic arthritis, endocarditis, myocarditis, and meningitis.
- The pathogen can cause neonatal conjunctivitis (ophthalmia neonatorum) in newborns.
- Gonorrhea is highly infectious and spreads through direct mucous membrane contact during sexual intercourse or childbirth.
- WHO estimated 82.4 million new infections among adults aged 15–49 in 2020, highlighting gonorrhea as a significant global health issue with increasing incidence in many countries.
- Inflammation resulting from gonorrhea can enhance the risk of HIV transmission.
- Lower gonorrhea primarily affects the vulvovaginal and cervical areas, often resulting in severe purulent cervicitis and concurrent urethritis in women.
- Upper gonorrhea can ascend through the cervical canal, potentially affecting the endometrium, fallopian tubes, and peritoneal space, which can lead to pelvic inflammatory disease (PID) and long-term complications, such as infertility.
- Extragenital manifestations may spread to other organs via autoinoculation, peripartum transmission, or hematogenous spread, resulting in complications like urethral stricture and sterility.
- During pregnancy, gonorrhea elevates the risk of cervical infection, premature birth, and low birth weight, and may worsen conditions like arthritis and tenosynovitis.
- Neonatal gonorrhea can lead to severe conjunctivitis (ophthalmoblennorrhea neonatorum) shortly after birth, with a significant risk of blindness if left untreated; it remains the leading cause of ophthalmia neonatorum.
- Diagnosis is based on clinical symptoms and the cultural detection of the pathogen, with a detailed medical history aiding in targeted sampling and detection rates. Ideally, a urethral swab should be collected before the first urination of the morning, with no urination occurring for at least 4 h prior.
- Diagnosing disseminated gonococcal infection is particularly challenging due to intermittent bacteremia; detection can be achieved through vaginal swabs, blood samples, joint punctates, or skin biopsies.
- Definitive proof of infection is only obtained through microbiological cultures.
- Resistance testing is essential due to the increasing prevalence of multiresistant strains.

(continued)

- Recommended therapies for uncomplicated gonorrhea in pregnancy include ceftriaxone, cefixime, and spectinomycin, with azithromycin considered only after comprehensive risk assessment; cephalosporin use should be avoided during the first trimester.
- Education and proper condom usage are recommended preventive measures.
- Follow-up visits should assess treatment adherence and symptom reduction, with repeat examinations required for persistent symptoms, reexposure, detection of antibiotic resistance, or specific forms of gonorrhea.

Lymphogranuloma Venereum (LGV) 15

Abstract

Lymphogranuloma venereum (LGV) is a rare, predominantly sexually transmitted disease caused by *Chlamydia trachomatis* serotypes L1–L3. The clinical presentation encompasses three stages: the primary lesion, lymphadenopathy of the inguinal lymph nodes, and a chronic phase that may result in elephantiasis. Men who have sex with men (MSM) and individuals living with HIV are at increased risk. Diagnosis is typically confirmed through polymerase chain reaction (PCR) testing for specific chlamydia serotypes, with serological testing serving as a supportive measure. The first-line treatment involves a 21-day course of doxycycline. Screening and treatment of sexual partners is crucial for prevention. Differential diagnosis must also consider other etiologies for genital ulcers and proctitis.

15.1 Background

Lymphogranuloma venereum (LGV), also referred to as lymphogranuloma inguinale (LGI), is characterized as a rare, sexually transmitted infection. The incidence is approximated at one case per one million individuals annually in developed countries. Recent years have witnessed localized outbreaks primarily among men who have sex with men (MSM), though instances of heterosexual transmission have been documented in Europe.

15.2 Pathogen

The causative agent of Lymphogranuloma venereum (LGV) is specific strains of the bacterium *Chlamydia trachomatis*, namely, serotypes L1, L2, and L3. These strains differ from the common serotypes that cause nongonococcal urethritis and

I. Mylonas, *Sexually Transmitted Diseases*,
https://doi.org/10.1007/978-3-031-78204-6_15

cervicitis. *Chlamydia trachomatis* is a gram-negative bacterium belonging to the Chlamydiaceae family. It has two forms: the elementary body (EB), which is infectious and can survive outside host cells, and the reticulate body (RB), which is noninfectious and replicates within host cells before transforming back into EBs for infecting new cells (Chap. 17).

Unlike serotypes A–K of *Chlamydia trachomatis*, which typically remain localized to mucous membranes, the group L exhibit invasive characteristics, disseminating through connective tissue and regional lymph nodes. Currently, the specific infectivity and reservoir of these pathogens remain undefined.

Chlamydia trachomatis L1–L3 is an invasive and lymphogenic pathogen.

15.3 Epidemiology

Globally, *Chlamydia trachomatis* serotypes L1–L3 account for approximately 1–2% of genital ulcerations. LGV is endemic in regions including Asia, Africa, South America, and the southeastern United States, but predominantly occurs within MSM populations in Europe and the United States, often co-occurring with HIV infections. The prevalence of LGV varies across global regions, with an estimated 2.5 million cases reported annually.

A distinguished increase in LGV cases in Europe has been observed, especially in Western Europe, although the overall prevalence remains relatively low. Isolated outbreaks have been reported in the United States among MSM, while the prevalence of LGV in Asia is recognized as low due to limited data. In Africa, certain areas report higher prevalence rates, reaching up to 6% in West and East Africa. The United Kingdom has documented a surge in LGV cases, particularly among MSM, revealing a prevalence rate of approximately 1–2% within this demographic. Conversely, Scandinavia reports only sporadic cases, and data availability in Latin America remains inconsistent, with no reliable prevalence estimates.

Furthermore, in 2021, the European Union reported a total of 1124 LGV cases, with a temporary decline during the COVID-19 pandemic. The disease predominantly affects individuals in high-risk groups, including seamen, MSM, and sex workers. Men are disproportionately affected, with a risk that is two to eight times higher than that of women. Among identified risk factors are low socioeconomic status and inadequate hygiene conditions, with higher incidences of anal lesions reported in MSM. Variability in incidence and prevalence rates of LGV has emerged from different epidemiological studies, where asymptomatic cases have been documented alongside symptomatic ones, particularly noted in the Netherlands.

Lymphogranuloma venereum (LGV), caused by *Chlamydia trachomatis* serotypes L1–L3, predominantly affects MSM, with varying global prevalence, higher rates in Africa and Western Europe, and significant risk factors including HIV co-infection, low socioeconomic status, and poor hygiene.

15.4 Clinical Manifestation

15.4.1 Gynecology

The clinical progression of lymphogranuloma venereum is categorized into three distinct stages.

15.4.1.1 Stage I

Stage I represents the primary infection, characterized by a small inflammatory papule on an erythematous base in the external genital area. This papule evolves rapidly to a papulovesicular and papulopustular efflorescence, which may ultimately ulcerate. In females, lesions can manifest on the vulva, vagina, and cervix. The primary lesion is typically painless, often remaining unnoticed. Spontaneous healing generally occurs within 10–14 days, leading patients to forgo medical consultation. Rarely, pharyngeal symptoms can present, alongside potential cervical lymphadenopathy.

15.4.1.2 Stage II

Following the primary lesion, approximately 2–3 weeks later, the infection disseminates via the lymphatic system. This results in the inflammatory swelling of the inguinal lymph nodes (bubo), frequently unilateral (Fig. 15.1). Infected inguinal lymph nodes may coalesce and adhere to the skin, yet retain mobility. Clinically, the inguinal region appears erythematous. Abscess formation is common within the lymph nodes, which may perforate, leading to fistula formation and subsequent scarring. If the primary lesion is situated in the vagina or rectum, perirectal and paraaortic lymph nodes may also be implicated. The formation of these buboes might be accompanied by systemic symptoms, such as malaise, appetite loss, weight reduction, and low-grade fever. Additional manifestations may include rheumatic symptoms and exanthema. In rare instances, complications like meningoencephalitis, hepatosplenomegaly, arthralgia, or conjunctivitis can arise due to the infection's lymphatic spread.

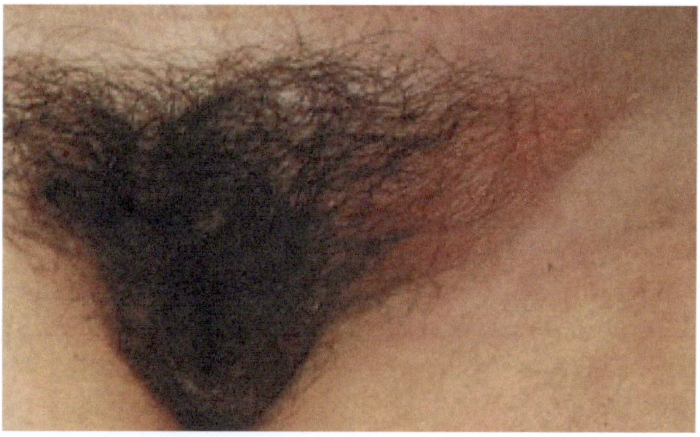

Fig. 15.1 Lymphadenopathy in lymphogranuloma inguinale (Abeck 2005)

15.4.1.3 Stage III

Elephantiasis genitoanorectalis ulcerosa was historically classified as a distinct clinical entity. This stage is characterized by fibrosis and strictures within the genitoanal region. A major complication includes the development of elephantiasis affecting the external genitalia and rectum. The clinical implications differ based on whether the disease presents in the genital or anal area.

Untreated, elephantiasis can lead to chronic ulcerative conditions of the external female genitalia (esthiomas) and "frozen pelvis syndrome." Genital elephantiasis typically initiates on the genitals, resulting in persistent ulcerations and lymphatic stasis. While some changes might be localized, such as those affecting the urethra or clitoris, the majority of cases involve extensive labial changes characterized by enlargement and papillomatous or vesicular alterations (Fig. 15.2). Urethral strictures and the formation of genitoanal or urogenital fistulas may also occur. In rectoanal involvement, the swelling of perirectal lymph nodes results in thickening, hardening, and narrowing of the rectum, with ulcerations detectable via proctoscopy. Perianal and perirectal fistulas may form, and after a prolonged clinical course, the effusion from fistula openings may diminish, resulting in a persisting nonhealing state referred to as fistula sicca.

The clinical manifestations of this disease include genital ulcers, lymphadenopathy, and proctitis.

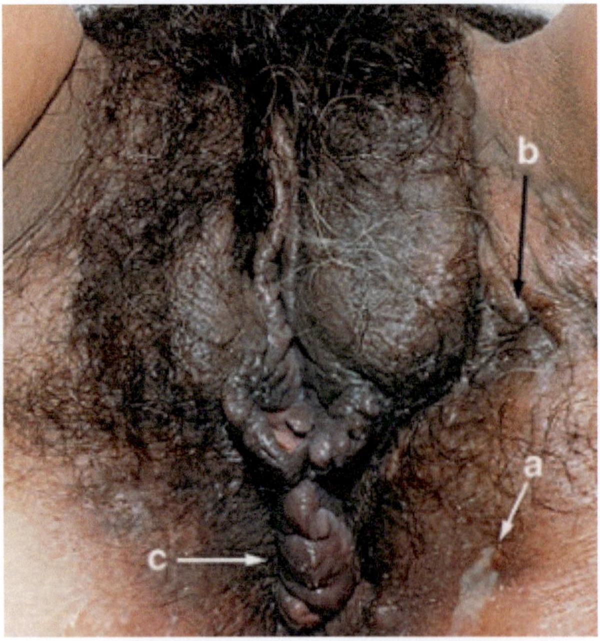

Fig. 15.2 Case of LGV with esthiomene, marked by vulvar edema, pus-filled fistulas, and contractions indicative of chronic genitorectal syndrome (Leal Passos et al. 2018). (**a**) a fistula discharging pus; (**b**) drained and healed fistulas with contractions; (**c**) rectal narrowing with stenosis

15.4.2 Pregnancy

The available evidence does not indicate that the pathogen is transmitted to the fetus or newborn. Although data on transmission frequency, clinical significance, and outcomes in neonatology are limited, neonatal infection seems improbable. However, systemic infections caused by *Chlamydia trachomatis* could result in conjunctivitis and pneumonia in neonates (Chap. 17). Continuous monitoring and potential treatment for both the pregnant individual and the newborn are warranted.

15.5 Diagnosis

Diagnosis involves detecting *Chlamydia trachomatis* serotypes L1–L3. Specimens may be obtained from ulcerations and aspirated fluid from buboes. For predominantly rectal manifestations, anorectal swabs can be collected, ideally under proctoscopic guidance.

Modern laboratory diagnostics typically employ a two-step process:

1. Initial molecular testing for *Chlamydia trachomatis* via PCR serves as a screening tool when clinical suspicion arises. Although a majority of commercially available tests are not authorized for nongenital specimens, numerous studies indicate their utility in such contexts.
2. Upon identifying *Chlamydia trachomatis*, a secondary PCR analysis targeting specifically serotypes L1–L3 is undertaken. In instances where molecular testing is unavailable, serological diagnosis may also be considered. A high titer of IgA anti-MOMP antibodies (major outer membrane protein) in patients exhibiting characteristic symptoms can substantiate a suspected diagnosis. Conversely, the significance of titers, irrespective of their magnitude, in asymptomatic patients remains ambiguous and requires further elucidation.

15.6 Treatment

Despite limited data, doxycycline administered orally at a dose of 100 mg twice daily for 21 days is recommended as the first-line therapy for LGV. This recommendation is supported by evidence from numerous case reports that demonstrate favorable clinical responses to doxycycline treatment.

As an alternative, erythromycin (500 mg orally four times daily) may be prescribed for a period of 21–28 days, particularly for patients unable to tolerate doxycycline or in certain clinical scenarios (refer to Table 15.1). Although azithromycin has been suggested as a possible treatment option, the therapeutic evidence supporting its effectiveness remains insufficient, and it is not routinely recommended. Historically, sulfonamides have shown some efficacy in treating LGV. However, they are no longer advised due to the availability of more effective and safer treatments.

Table 15.1 Treatment options for lymphogranuloma venereum (LGV)

Indication	Medication	Dosage	Duration
Recommendation	Doxycycline	100 mg orally twice daily	21 days
	Erythromycin	500 mg orally four times daily	21–28 days
Older recommendations	Co-trimoxazole	160/800 mg orally twice daily	21–28 days
	Ciprofloxacin	500 mg orally twice daily	21–28 days
	Azithromycin	1.5 g orally	Day 1, 8, 15 (and 22)
Pregnancy[a]	Erythromycin Ethylsuccinate	400 mg orally four times daily	21-28 days
	Erythromycin	500 mg orally four times daily	21–28 days
	Azithromycin	1.5 g orally	Day 1, 8, 15 (and 22)

[a]During pregnancy, erythromycin ethylsuccinate is preferred due to its presumed efficacy; however, data on its use in this population remain limited. Compared to erythromycin formulations, azithromycin has stricter indications during pregnancy and should be avoided unless absolutely necessary

In cases where buboes are fluctuant, aspiration through *intact skin* may alleviate symptoms. Surgical excision is typically *discouraged* due to the potential for chronic sinus formation. Patients with fibrotic changes or fistulas usually do not demonstrate clinical improvement with extended antibiotic therapy; thus, reconstructive surgery should be considered in these instances.

The recommended course of treatment is doxycycline or erythromycin for a period of 21 days. Azithromycin represents an alternative option. The use of sulfonamides is not advised.

15.7 Differential Diagnosis

The primary differential diagnoses for lymphogranuloma venereum (LGV) comprise sexually transmitted diseases presenting with genital ulcers, including syphilis, herpes simplex, chancroid, and donovanosis (granuloma inguinale). Additionally, conditions associated with lymphadenopathy or proctitis, such as Adamantiades–Behçet's disease, Crohn's disease, and colitis, should also be evaluated. Further differential considerations include fixed drug reactions and psoriasis.

Stage II inguinal lymphadenopathy presents challenges in differential diagnosis due to overlapping symptomatology, particularly with syphilis, genital herpes, and granuloma inguinale. Other infectious diseases, such as tuberculosis or neoplastic conditions (e.g., Hodgkin's disease), must also be considered.

15.8 Prevention

Sexual partners of individuals diagnosed with chlamydia or lymphogranuloma venereum (LGV) should undergo screening and receive appropriate treatment if they have been in contact with the infected person within the preceding 3 months. This measure is crucial to prevent reinfection and halt further transmission of the infection within the population. Retesting of the patient following treatment is generally not recommended in most clinical guidelines, provided that the prescribed therapy has been correctly administered for the full duration of 21 days as per the standard treatment protocol.

Individuals diagnosed with lymphogranuloma venereum should additionally be tested for HIV, hepatitis B, hepatitis C, and syphilis.

Key Points

- Lymphogranuloma venereum is a rare disease, predominantly caused by *Chlamydia trachomatis* serotypes L1–L3.
- The condition is particularly prevalent among men who have sex with men (MSM) and individuals living with HIV.
- *Chlamydia trachomatis* L1–L3 functions as an invasive and lymphogenic pathogen, with additional variants, such as L2b, having been identified.
- Clinical manifestations include genital ulcers, lymphadenopathy, and proctitis.
- Diagnosis is achieved through PCR testing for chlamydia serotypes and supportive serological assays.
- Recommended treatment consists of doxycycline or erythromycin for 21 days, with azithromycin as an alternative while sulfonamides are not advised.
- Differential diagnosis should encompass other sexually transmitted infections, such as syphilis, herpes, chancroid, and granuloma inguinale, alongside conditions presenting with lymphadenopathy or proctitis.
- Following treatment, monitoring for potential coinfections with HIV, hepatitis B, hepatitis C, and syphilis is recommended.

Syphilis (Lues) 16

Abstract

Syphilis is an infectious disease characterized by alternating clinically conspicuous and inconspicuous stages, and it is caused by the pathogen Treponema pallidum. The primary mode of transmission is sexual intercourse. Symptoms may include ulcers, skin rashes, and neurological complications. Without treatment, significant complications such as organ damage and cardiovascular issues may occur. Congenital syphilis can result in life-threatening health complications in unborn children. Timely diagnosis and treatment are of critical importance. Various diagnostic techniques are available for identifying the infection. Penicillin is the preferred drug, particularly during pregnancy. Alternative drugs, such as doxycycline or ceftriaxone, are used only in exceptional cases due to their reduced efficacy. Pregnant women with a penicillin allergy should undergo desensitization. Treatment initiation during pregnancy must not be delayed.

16.1 Background

Syphilis is a chronic, systemic infection caused by the spirochete bacterium *Treponema pallidum*. This sexually transmitted infection has a complex natural history characterized by distinct stages: primary, secondary, latent, and tertiary syphilis, each with unique clinical manifestations. Despite its historical significance as one of the oldest documented infectious diseases, syphilis persists as a substantial public health challenge worldwide. The incidence has surged in recent years, particularly among high-risk populations, necessitating ongoing surveillance, improved diagnostic methods, and effective treatment strategies. Untreated syphilis can result in severe neurological, cardiovascular, and multi-organ complications, rendering early detection and management imperative.

I. Mylonas, *Sexually Transmitted Diseases*,
https://doi.org/10.1007/978-3-031-78204-6_16

Syphilis is characterized as a cyclical infectious disease where clinically conspicuous and inconspicuous stages alternate, leading to considerable variability in symptoms.

16.2 Pathogen

The pathogen responsible for syphilis, *Treponema pallidum*, belongs to the family Spirochaetaceae and the genus Treponema. This genus comprises four human pathogens (Chap. 26) and at least six nonpathogenic strains:

- *T. pallidum* ssp. *pallidum*: Syphilis (Lues venereum).
- *T. pallidum* ssp. *endemicum*: Nonvenereal endemic syphilis.
- *T. pallidum* ssp. *pertenue*: Yaws.
- *T. carateum*: Pinta.

The bacterium *Treponema pallidum* subspecies *pallidum* is a highly motile spirochete characterized by six to fourteen coils, exhibiting a distinctive "corkscrew" motility. Once outside the host organism, the spirochetes perish rapidly.

16.3 Epidemiology

The bacterium *Treponema pallidum* ssp. *pallidum* is exclusively pathogenic to humans and has a global distribution. The predominant mode of transmission, constituting over 95% of cases, is sexual intercourse. Isolated instances of transmission through blood transfusions, kissing, or accidental inoculation have been documented; however, these routes are considered rare.

The incubation period is contingent upon the infectious dose and typically spans 2–10 weeks, with an average duration of 3 weeks. In animal models, such as rabbits, merely four spirochetes can induce infection. The risk of transmission during sexual intercourse is estimated to be between 40% and 60%, signifying that syphilis is highly infectious. Following infection, the microorganisms proliferate at the site of entry, demonstrating a proclivity for rapid dissemination and a pronounced tropism for endothelial cells within small blood vessels.

The advent of penicillin and its subsequent industrial production prompted a decline in syphilis cases after World War II. In 1945, the incidence of syphilis in North America was approximately 66 cases per 100,000 inhabitants. However, this decreased significantly in subsequent years, resulting in an incidence of around four cases per 100,000 inhabitants. A comparable decline was evidenced in Europe.

- **Global Epidemiology of Syphilis**: Over recent decades, syphilis has witnessed a troubling rise in global incidence. Global cases surged from 8.8 million in

1990 to 14.one million in 2019. This trend is mirrored in the global age-standardized incidence rate (ASIR), which increased from 160.03 to 178.48 per 100,000 population during this period. The estimated annual percentage change (EAPC) in ASIR was 0.16 (95% CI: 0.07–0.26), indicating a statistically significant increase over time, predominantly among males, while the rate decreased among females. The incidence peaked for both genders between ages 20 and 30. Despite this rising prevalence, the global age-standardized death rate and disability-adjusted life year (DALY) rates for syphilis have declined from 1990 to 2019.

- **Epidemiology in Europe**: Syphilis remains a significant public health concern in Europe. In 2021, 25,270 confirmed cases of syphilis were recorded across 28 EU/EEA countries, yielding a notification rate of 7.0 per 100,000 population. Notably, the gender disparity is marked; men were nine times more likely to be infected than women, with the highest rates evident in men aged 25–34 years. Among cases with known transmission categories, a substantial proportion (77%) involved men who have sex with men (MSM). Alarmingly, notifications of syphilis among MSM rose by 87% between 2015 and 2021, highlighting an escalating public health challenge.
- **Epidemiology in the United States**: In the United States, syphilis infections have steadily increased since the 1980s and 1990s, predominantly among MSM. In 2016, over 52% of the 27,814 reported syphilis cases were attributed to MSM. The highest rates of primary and secondary syphilis occurred among men aged 20–34 years, particularly in the Western regions and among men of color. This persistent trend poses a significant public health challenge, as emphasized by the Centers for Disease Control and Prevention (CDC).
- **Epidemiology in Asia**: Asia presents a diverse landscape concerning syphilis prevalence. In 1995, South and Southeast Asia recorded the highest global prevalence, with an estimated 12 million cases. In recent years, large populations in countries such as China and India have contributed to an increasing incidence of syphilis. Nonetheless, the scale of population sizes may render the rising trend less pronounced on a per capita basis. Regional variations are significant, with prevalence rates generally ranging from 10% to 30%.
- **Epidemiology in Africa**: Sub-Saharan Africa bears a disproportionate burden of syphilis, exhibiting the highest age-standardized incidence rates, particularly in Central and Southern sub-Saharan Africa. Syphilis significantly contributes to perinatal deaths in the region, accounting for approximately 20% of these fatalities. Factors such as economic instability, inadequate medical treatment facilities, and ineffective disease prevention strategies have exacerbated the spread of syphilis in many parts of Africa.

The incidence of diaplacental *congenital infection* has declined significantly. While it is exceedingly rare for an infected pregnant woman to be treated in developed countries, it is not uncommon in lower-income nations. In Africa, the estimated prevalence of pregnant women testing positive for syphilis ranges between

0.5% and 20%, with approximately 25% of newborns believed to succumb to congenital syphilis. The prevalence rates in Southeast Asia are similarly high.

- **Global Epidemiology of Congenital Syphilis**: Congenital syphilis poses a substantial public health issue worldwide, significantly contributing to infant mortality and morbidity. In 2013, the World Health Organization (WHO) reported that 1.9 million pregnant women were infected with syphilis globally. Among these cases, 66.5% experienced adverse fetal effects without timely intervention. Congenital syphilis accounts for an estimated 305,000 perinatal deaths annually worldwide, with approximately 520,000 adverse fetal outcomes attributed to congenital syphilis each year. This incidence surpasses that of congenital HIV infection, with approximately half of the stillbirth rate in regions with high syphilis prevalence attributable to this infection alone.
- **Epidemiology in Europe**: In 2021, 55 confirmed cases of congenital syphilis were reported by 11 out of 24 EU/EEA countries contributing data. The following year saw 69 confirmed cases reported from 14 EU/EEA countries, while 11 other countries reported no cases. This increase in congenital syphilis notifications within the EU/EEA follows a decrease in 2020. Despite annual fluctuations, national notification rates have remained consistently low across most EU/EEA countries from 2012 to 2022, with five countries reporting no vertical transmission events during this period.
- **Epidemiology in the United States**: The incidence rates of maternal and congenital syphilis in the United States alarmingly rose between 2017 and 2022, escalating from 87.2 to 280.4 per 100,000 live births. This more than 2.5-fold increase underscores a pressing public health challenge requiring urgent attention and intervention.
- **Vertical Transmission Rates**: Vertical transmission of syphilis remains a critical concern in various regions. A study conducted in Brazil documented a vertical transmission rate of 65.8%, with 52 newborns affected by congenital syphilis. In France, between 2011 and 2018, 27.3% of infants diagnosed with congenital syphilis were stillborn.

It is estimated that approximately one million pregnancies worldwide are adversely affected by maternal syphilis. The estimates suggest around 270,000 children are born with congenital syphilis, approximately 460,000 pregnancies result in miscarriage or perinatal fetal death, and about 270,000 premature births occur. These figures significantly exceed those associated with other neonatal infections, including HIV and tetanus, which account for 540,000 and 300,000 cases per year, respectively.

16.4 Clinical Manifestation

Clinically, a distinction is made between acquired syphilis (*syphilis acquisita*) and congenital syphilis (*syphilis connata*).

Acquired syphilis manifests as a cyclical infectious disease, alternating between clinically conspicuous and inconspicuous stages (Table 15.1). The typical symptoms of untreated syphilis now occur less frequently in industrialized countries.

While a syphilis infection may resolve spontaneously after the primary lesion has healed, it can also develop into a chronic systemic disease. In the absence of treatment, approximately 20% of infected individuals will experience late complications within 15–20 years, with cardiovascular manifestations being the most prevalent.

16.4.1 Gynecology

16.4.1.1 Early Syphilis or Primary Syphilis (Lues I)

Approximately 3 weeks after infection, the characteristic primary lesion, known as chancre, becomes evident. This efflorescence typically manifests on the external genitalia. In females, the most common sites include the labia and vulva (Fig. 16.1), while the cervix is less frequently affected. In males, the chancre usually appears on the coronary sulcus, the inner preputial fold, and the shaft of the penis. Occasionally, the chancre may also present at other sites such as the oral mucosa or anal area.

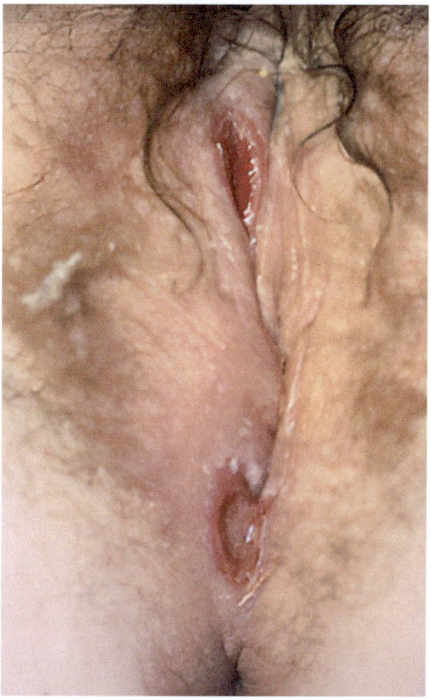

Fig. 16.1 Primary lesion of a syphilis infection (Mendling 2006). The soft but well-defined margins of the ulcer are characteristic

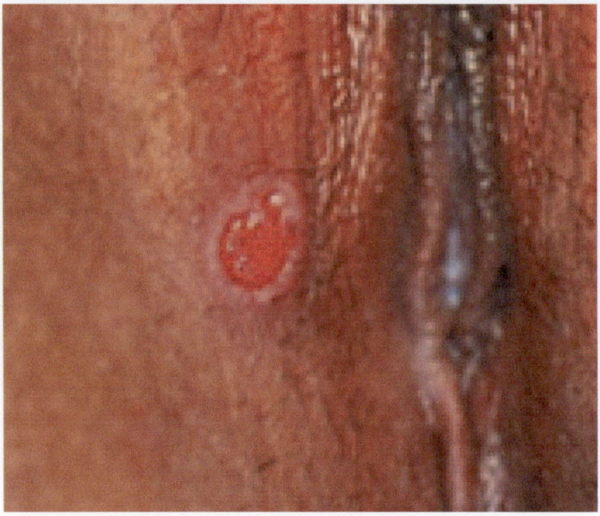

Fig. 16.2 A hard chancre on the vulva with characteristic base and wall hypertrophy of the ulcer (Leal Passos et al. 2018)

The presence of individual papules or a painless, hardened ulcer, coupled with painless swelling of the inguinal lymph nodes bilaterally, indicates primary syphilis. The typical primary chancre begins as a single painless papule that subsequently transforms into a painless indurated ulcer at the site of entry (Fig. 16.2). In approximately 30% of cases, additional lesions may develop. Furthermore, the inguinal lymph nodes exhibit a painless, rough, and well-defined swelling. The ulcer usually heals on its own within about 3 to 6 weeks, although lymphadenopathy may linger for a longer period.

Patients may overlook the papules, particularly since they may heal spontaneously.

16.4.1.2 Secondary Syphilis (Lues II)

Secondary syphilis typically develops approximately 9–12 weeks after the initial infection. During this stage, general symptoms such as fever, weight loss, and profound malaise may occur. Approximately 50% of patients report severe headaches, historically recognized as one of the earliest manifestations of syphilis.
Additional systemic symptoms associated with secondary syphilis include:

- Fatigue
- Loss of appetite
- Mild fever
- Myalgias
- Polyarthritic pain (commonly affecting bones, such as the femur, tibia, and humerus)

Patients may overlook papular lesions during this stage, as they often heal spontaneously.

Skin and Mucous Membrane Involvement: Discerning between the primary and secondary stages can be challenging, as approximately 30% of individuals may still exhibit the primary chancre at the onset of secondary syphilis. During this stage, the skin and mucous membranes are involved in 80% of cases. The nature and extent of skin and mucosal reactions depend on the antigen burden (spirochete load) and the intensity of the host's immune response. The most common skin manifestations include:

- Macular (Fig. 16.3), maculopapular, papular, or annular eruptions.
- Rarely, nodular and pustular lesions may develop.
- Vesicular eruptions are a hallmark feature of congenital syphilis.
- Other dermatological symptoms include:
- Palmoplantar syphilis (involving palms and soles).
- Condylomata lata (moist, wart-like lesions found in genital or perianal regions) (Fig. 16.4).
- Mucous membrane plaques on the tongue.

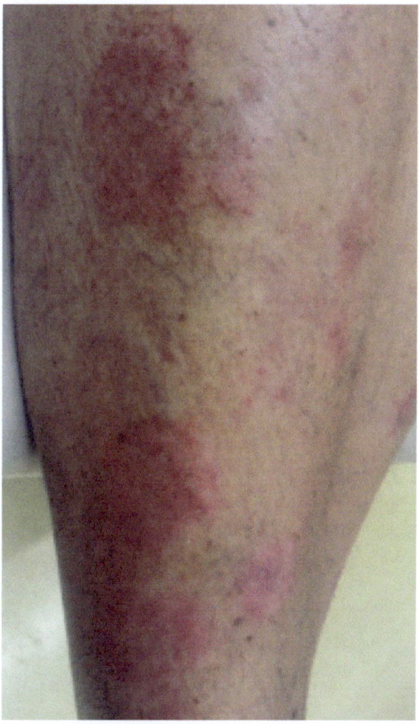

Fig. 16.3 Secondary syphilis presenting with a skin rash on the lower extremities (Mylonas 2016)

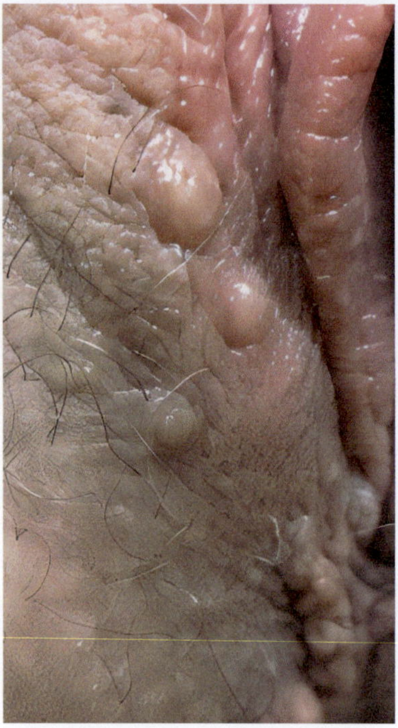

Fig. 16.4 Incipient condylomata lata in a patient with secondary syphilis (Mylonas 2016)

- Angina syphilitica (syphilitic tonsillitis).
- Specific alopecia (moth-eaten hair loss).
- Syphilitic leukoderma (patchy depigmentation of the skin).

Systemic Dissemination: In the absence of treatment, *Treponema pallidum* can disseminate further, leading to involvement of additional organs such as:

- Liver: Syphilitic hepatitis.
- Kidneys: Glomerulonephritis or acute nephrotic syndrome.
- Generalized lymphadenopathy (polyscleradenitis) is commonly observed during this stage.

Course and Duration: The secondary stage of syphilis typically lasts for 1–2 years. Clinical manifestations, including skin symptoms, may resolve spontaneously without significant consequences after a single occurrence; however, recurrences are common. These recurrent episodes tend to diminish in severity over time as the disease progresses.

Severe forms of syphilis, labeled as syphilis maligna, are especially prevalent in immunocompromised individuals. Along with the previously mentioned general symptoms, ulcerations of the skin may also occur.

16.4.1.3 Latent Syphilis (Lues Latens Seropositiva)

Following the initial manifestations of early syphilis, a clinically asymptomatic phase, termed **latent syphilis**, ensues. During this stage, approximately 40% of cases involve the central nervous system, leading to persistent dissemination of *Treponema pallidum*. Remarkably, even before the availability of antibiotics, spontaneous self-resolution occurred in nearly half of those diagnosed with syphilis.

Latent syphilis is divided into two stages based on the duration since initial infection:

- **Early Latent Syphilis:** Refers to the asymptomatic phase occurring within the first year of infection.
- **Late Latent Syphilis:** Refers to the asymptomatic phase persisting beyond 1 year of infection.

While patients in either stage may exhibit no clinical symptoms, this is not universally the case, as variability in disease progression exists among individuals.

16.4.1.4 Late Syphilis and Neurosyphilis

Tertiary syphilis is now rarely encountered due to improvements in early diagnosis and treatment. The latent phase of syphilis typically progresses slowly, primarily affecting the aorta and the central nervous system (CNS). Asymptomatic neurosyphilis refers to the involvement of *Treponema pallidum* within the CNS without clinical symptoms. In untreated individuals, symptomatic manifestations generally emerge approximately 2 years after the initial infection. The time frame from primary infection to the onset of symptomatic neurosyphilis varies widely, ranging from 5 to 40 years (see Table 16.1).

- **Symptomatic Neurosyphilis:** Symptomatic neurosyphilis is categorized into two primary forms: parenchymatous and meningovascular.
  - **Meningovascular Neurosyphilis:** This form is associated with focal or generalized seizures, hemiplegia, and may present with aphasia.
  - **Parenchymatous Neurosyphilis:** This form includes neurological deficits, alterations in personality, and may progress to tabes dorsalis.
  - **Tabes dorsalis**, a late manifestation, is characterized by sensory ataxia, muscle weakness, loss of muscle tone, intense pain, and the presence of Argyll Robertson pupils. Cranial nerve involvement, dementia, tremors, dysuria, and areflexia may also be observed.
- **Cardiovascular Syphilis:** Cardiovascular syphilis primarily affects the cardiovascular system, with common complications, including aortic aneurysms, aortic valve insufficiency, and stenosis of the coronary arteries (see Table 16.1). These complications typically develop over 10–30 years following initial infection.
- **Gummata:** Gummata, though now rare, are characterized by destructive granulomas formed by nonspecific granulation tissue. These granulomas consist of

Table 16.1 Clinical manifestations of late syphilis

Manifestation	Symptoms	Time frame post-infection (years)
Cardiovascular syphilis	Aortic aneurysm, coronary artery stenosis, aortic valve insufficiency	10–30
Neurosyphilis	**Acute syphilitic meningitis:** Headache, meningeal irritation, sensory disturbances	<2
	Meningovascular neurosyphilis: Cranial nerve paralysis	5–7
	General paresis: Personality changes, headache, vertigo, vascular damage	5–7
	Tabes dorsalis: Dementia, fatigue, muscle weakness, intense tremor, pain, dysuria, ataxia, Argyll Robertson pupils	10–20
Gummata	Monocytic infiltrates with tissue destruction	1–46

central necrosis surrounded by mononuclear cells, epithelioid cells, and fibroblasts. Treponema pallidum organisms may still be identified within these lesions.

In cases of osteomyelitis, hepatitis, chorioretinitis, or neurological symptoms, it is essential to rule out syphilis infection.

16.4.1.5 Reinfections

Reinfection with syphilis is possible even after previous successful treatment. It is important to understand that existing antibodies do not confer protection against reinfection. The presence of syphilis antibodies in the form of a serum scar does not imply immunity against *Treponema pallidum* ssp. *pallidum*.

16.4.2 Pregnancy

16.4.2.1 Congenital Syphilis (Lues Connata)

Congenital syphilis arises when the infection in a pregnant woman is unrecognized and untreated in a timely manner (Table 16.2). The pathogen can be transmitted to the fetus at any point through the placenta. The likelihood of fetal infection is particularly high in cases of early maternal syphilis. Early pregnancy infections can lead to miscarriage, stillbirth, and premature birth.

The timing of maternal infection significantly influences the severity of the infant's condition. In the absence of miscarriage or stillbirth, most infants are born asymptomatic and appear healthy.

However, clinical manifestations of congenital syphilis in infected newborns may become evident between the second and twelfth weeks of life, presenting as skin symptoms (Table 16.2). In the majority of cases, maculopapular rash and

Table 16.2 Clinical manifestations of congenital syphilis

Time of manifestation	Symptoms
Early manifestation < 2 years after birth	— Fulminant disseminated infection — Mucocutaneous lesions — Pemphigus syphiliticus — Parrot furrows — Coryza syphilitica — Pneumonia alba — Hepatosplenomegaly — Anemia
	— Neurosyphilis — Osteochondritis syphilitica
Late manifestation (syphilis connata tarda) >2 years after birth	— Lymphadenopathy — Anemia — Condylomata — Neurosyphilis — Hepatosplenomegaly — Recurrent arthropathies — Rare mesaortitis luica — Hutchinson's triad with: Sensorineural hearing loss, keratitis parenchymatosa, Hutchinson's teeth (barrel teeth) — Bone diseases and deformities — Sabre tibia — Saddle nose

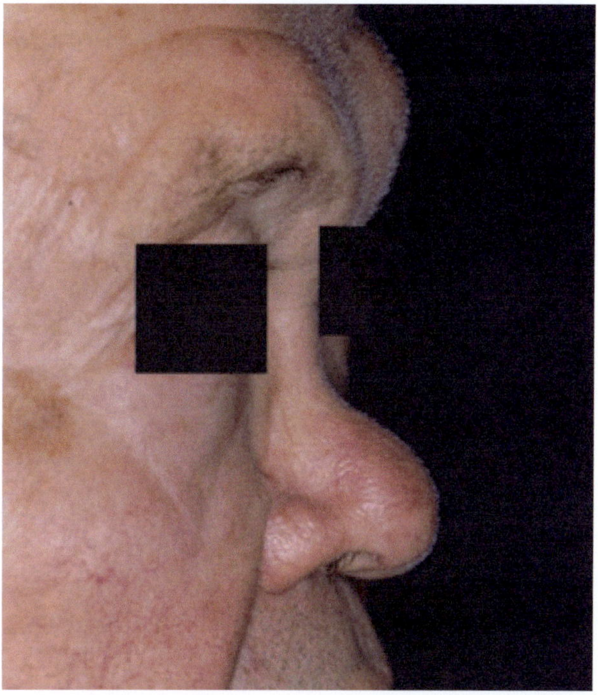

Fig. 16.5 "Saddle nose" deformity in congenital syphilis infection (Geusau 2022)

syphilides develop on the palms of the hands and soles of the feet, with a potential progression to pemphigus syphiliticus, characterized by blistering. The initial presentation may also include a bloody, mucous nasal discharge (coryza syphilitica), observed up to 2 years of age. If untreated, the infection may spread to the nasal skeleton, leading to deformity (referred to as "saddle nose" in Fig. 16.5).

Other organs may also become involved at this stage, with possible manifestations including hepatosplenomegaly, pneumonia, and osteochondritis. Meningitis can progress to hydrocephalus.

If congenital syphilis remains inadequately treated, late manifestations resembling the tertiary stage of *syphilis acquisita* may develop after several years. The most common causes of mortality in young children are pulmonary hemorrhage, hepatitis, and superinfections.

16.4.2.2 Late Congenital Syphilis (Syphilis Connata Tarda)

The late manifestations of congenital syphilis (*syphilis connata tarda*), occurring after the second year of life, typically emerge long after birth during infancy or later. These manifestations often present as the Hutchinson triad, which includes:

- Keratitis parenchymatosa (Fig. 16.6).
- Sensorineural hearing loss.
- Dental changes, characterized by crescent-shaped indentations on the incisors and a barrel-shaped appearance of the teeth (Fig. 16.7).

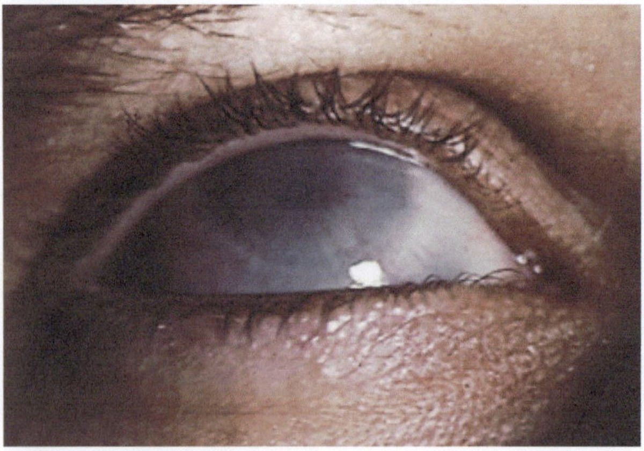

Fig. 16.6 Syphilis connata, characterized by keratitis parenchymatosa, is a component of the Hutchinson triad (Zangerle et al. 2018)

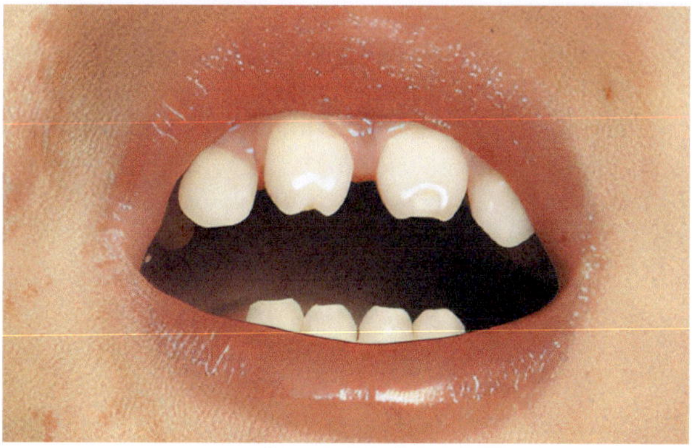

Fig. 16.7 Barrel-shaped teeth associated with congenital syphilis infection (Geusau 2022)

In addition, inflammatory periosteal thickening of the tibiae, known as "saber legs," can occur (Table 16.2).

The Hutchinson triad is a constellation of three clinical manifestations: keratitis parenchymatosa, sensorineural hearing loss, and tooth changes (crescent-shaped indentations on the incisors, barrel-like shape).

16.5 Diagnosis

A variety of examination methods are available to detect syphilis infection. Direct detection via dark-field microscopy is only feasible on primary lesions or lesions present in the secondary stage. Serological examinations are of particular importance in the diagnosis of syphilis following the healing of these lesions.

16.5.1 General

16.5.1.1 Methods of Detection

The diagnosis of syphilis is achieved through two primary methods: direct and indirect.

- **Direct Methods**
  - **Microscopic Examination**:
    - **Dark-Field Microscopy**: This technique identifies *Treponema pallidum* by examining fluids or smears from lesions, allowing for observation of the characteristic morphology and motility of the spirochetes.
    - **Direct Fluorescence Antibody (DFA) Test**: This test detects antigens of *T. pallidum* and serves as an alternative to dark-field microscopy, without requiring the presence of motile treponemes.

  - **Histological Examination**: This method identifies *T. pallidum* in tissue sections using specific staining techniques.
  - **Nucleic Acid Amplification Techniques**: These methods detect *T. pallidum* in clinical specimens. Although promising, they have not yet been standardized for routine use.
- **Indirect Methods**
  - **Nontreponemal Tests**:
    - **Rapid Plasma Reagin (RPR) Test** and **Venereal Disease Research Laboratory (VDRL) Test**: These tests detect IgM and IgG antibodies against cardiolipin, a substance released following cell damage during infection.
  - **Treponemal Tests**:
    - **Qualitative and Quantitative Tests**: These tests measure antibody titers that typically increase with active disease and decrease with successful therapy. Serum is generally the preferred test material, although plasma can also be used for certain nontreponemal serological tests.
    - **Cerebrospinal Fluid (CSF)**: This is utilized for diagnosing neurological syphilis, particularly in cases of congenital and tertiary syphilis.

16.5.1.2 Syphilis Screening Strategy in Pregnant Women

The World Health Organization (WHO) has established recommendations for syphilis screening strategies in pregnant women, based on the prevalence of the disease in the area.

- **Low Prevalence Areas (Less Than 5%)**: Use the rapid syphilis test (RST) to screen pregnant women. This approach is recommended over a single on-site RPR test.
- **High Prevalence Areas (5% or More)**:
  - **On-Site Rapid Syphilis Test**: A dual test for HIV and syphilis should be conducted. If positive, administer the first treatment dose immediately.
  - **Follow-Up RPR Test**: If the RPR test is positive, initiate treatment based on the duration of syphilis. A series of tests and treatments is recommended rather than relying on a single RST or RPR test conducted on-site.

The diagnosis of syphilis involves a variety of methodologies, including both direct and indirect methods. Direct methods include microscopic examination and histological staining, whereas indirect methods involve serological tests and molecular techniques. Direct methods focus on identifying Treponema pallidum through microscopic or molecular approaches, while indirect methods detect antibodies produced in response to the infection. The World Health Organization (WHO) has issued guidelines to inform screening strategies for pregnant women, emphasizing tailored approaches based on regional prevalence to ensure timely and effective treatment.

16.5.1.3 Direct Pathogen Detection

16.5.1.3.1 Dark-Field Microscopy

Direct pathogen detection from the transudate of a primary lesion or from lesions in the secondary stage is achieved using dark-field microscopy. The collection of examination material is critical. The lesions should be carefully cleaned using a swab moistened with saline solution, followed by meticulously dabbing the surface with a second swab to avoid bleeding from the lesion. The resulting exudate can then be obtained by gently squeezing out fluid from deeper skin layers and applying it to a microscope slide. However, dark-field microscopy has become less common, with only specialized laboratories continuing to utilize this method.

A negative result does not rule out infection, as the detection limit is approximately 10^5 spirochetes/mL.

16.5.1.3.2 Molecular Biological Methods

The sensitivity of molecular biological methods varies significantly, with some demonstrating a sensitivity as low as 40%, while others can achieve up to 100%. Pathogen detection from tissue biopsies is feasible using PCR, but this test is currently employed only for specific purposes, as serological detection is generally more informative and cost-effective.

16.5.1.4 Antibody Detection

A systematic approach is currently utilized to diagnose syphilis infection (Fig. 16.8). Detection of specific antibodies against *Treponema pallidum* ssp. *pallidum* serves as a serological screening test. Tests such as the TPHA (*T. pallidum* hemagglutination test), TPPA (*T. pallidum* particle agglutination test), or Tp-ELISA (T. pallidum enzyme-linked immunosorbent assay) may be employed.

If the initial test result is negative, further examinations may be considered unnecessary if there is no clinically justified suspicion of early infection. In such cases, weekly testings are performed until a syphilis infection can be reliably excluded. The TPHA test typically becomes positive (reactive) approximately 2 weeks after infection and remains reactive throughout the course of the disease. Interpretation of titer data provides indirect insight into the activity of the infection. Following treatment or resolution of syphilis, the test remains positive for life, a phenomenon commonly referred to as a "serum scar[1]."

[1] Following resolution by effective therapy or spontaneous clearance, treponemal assays such as TPHA remain persistently reactive lifelong because treponemal-specific immunoglobulins are sustained indefinitely after infection regardless of therapeutic outcome, the assays cannot distinguish active infection from previously treated or resolved disease, and seroreversion is uncommon—particularly after late-stage syphilis—resulting in most patients maintaining a stable, low-titer serological scar.

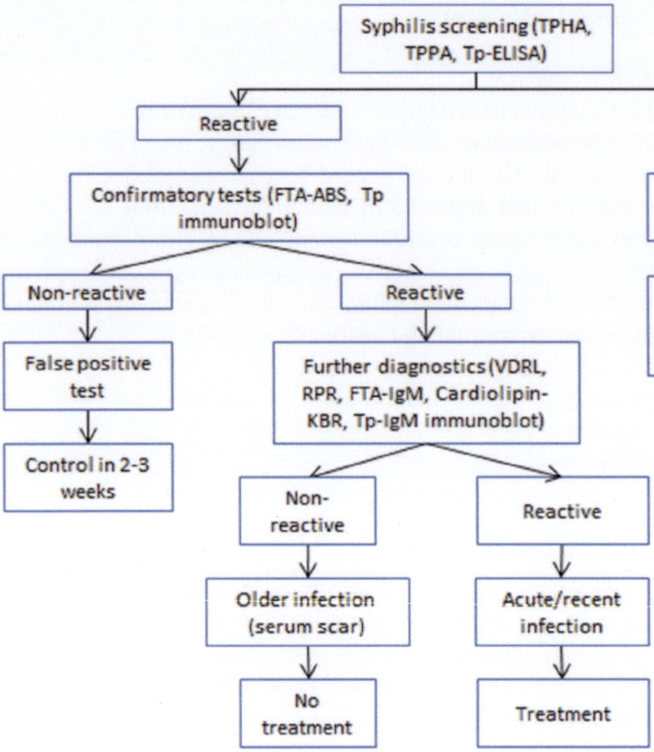

Fig. 16.8 Diagnostic approach for syphilis. (Courtesy of I. Mylonas)

The FTA-ABS (fluorescent Treponema Antibody Absorption) test is regarded as a confirmatory test for questionable (weakly reactive) or positive (reactive) results from the TPHA. The VDRL test and RPR test typically become positive 5–6 weeks after infection. However, the VDRL test may yield false-positive results in cases of infectious mononucleosis, tuberculosis, leprosy, malaria, and other diseases, including collagenoses, rheumatic diseases, liver diseases, carcinomas, pregnancy, and vaccinations. These nonspecific positive results can be clarified through treponema-specific tests.

Although the VDRL test is not suitable for detecting recent infection, it is useful for monitoring treatment. When an adequate dosage of antibiotics is administered, a reduction in the titer of three to four levels is expected. Nevertheless, the FTA-ABS-IgM test or the Tp-IgM ELISA is recommended to monitor the efficacy of the treatment.

Currently available serological tests for antibody detection cannot differentiate between human treponematoses, including venereal syphilis, endemic syphilis, yaws, and pinta.

16.5.1.5 Diagnostics During Pregnancy

It is not universally the case that a typical "primary focus" (primary lesion) on the labia and/or vulva develops following infection with *Treponema pallidum* ssp. *pallidum*. In contrast, patients with early latent syphilis and late latent syphilis are generally asymptomatic, although exceptions do occur. Therefore, pregnant women should undergo serological testing for syphilis antibodies during the first trimester in accordance with maternity guidelines.

16.5.1.6 Diagnosis of Congenital Syphilis

The serological approach for diagnosing newborns of untreated mothers, with confirmed infection by *Treponema pallidum* ssp. *pallidum* before or during pregnancy, does not differ from the serological diagnosis of infections during pregnancy. The determination of antibodies in umbilical cord blood at birth is not recommended, as these antibodies may be passively transferred to the child.

16.5.2 Screening Strategies

16.5.2.1 Syphilis Screening According to the "Classic Algorithm"

Conventional syphilis screening algorithms are based on the "normal" or traditional approach, which involves the use of nontreponemal tests such as rapid plasma reagin (RPR) or Venereal Disease Research Laboratory (VDRL) as initial screening tests, followed by confirmation by treponemal tests such as TPPA or enzyme immunoassay (EIA).

The conventional method for screening for syphilis, as outlined in the standard algorithm, is as follows:

- The preliminary screening test is: A nontreponemal test, such as the rapid plasma reagin (RPR) or Venereal Disease Research Laboratory (VDRL) test, is employed to identify the presence of antibodies against cardiolipin, which are generated during a syphilis infection.
- The confirmatory test is: In the event that the preliminary test result is positive, a treponemal test, such as TPPA or EIA, is performed to confirm the presence of specific antibodies to *Treponema pallidum* and to establish a definitive diagnosis. Treponemal tests are typically more specific, but may be costlier and more time-consuming than nontreponemal tests.
- The standard algorithm assumes that a positive nontreponemal test indicates the presence of antibodies against cardiolipin, which may indicate a possible syphilis infection. A positive treponemal test then serves to confirm the presence of antibodies against *Treponema pallidum*, thereby indicating the presence of a syphilis infection.

It must be emphasized that screening algorithms and clinical guidelines for syphilis vary by region and practice; therefore, local public health authorities' recommendations and institutional protocols should be followed to ensure appropriate and accurate syphilis screening.

16.5.2.2 Syphilis Screening According to the "Reverse Algorithm"

The term "reverse algorithm" refers to a diagnostic approach in which treponemal tests are employed as the initial screening test, followed by nontreponemal tests for confirmation if the initial test is reactive (Fig. 16.8).

> **This approach has become the standard methodology in screening programs in developed countries.**

Historically, nontreponemal tests, such as the RPR (rapid plasma reagin) test or the VDRL (Venereal Disease Research Laboratory) test, have been employed to screen for syphilis, with treponemal tests, such as TPPA or the enzyme immunoassay (EIA), serving as the confirmatory step. In recent years, however, the inverse algorithm has gained popularity as an alternative approach.

In the "reverse" algorithm, an initial screening is performed with a treponemal test that detects specific antibodies against *T. pallidum*. In the event that the treponemal test is found to be reactive, this indicates the presence of antibodies against T. pallidum in the patient's blood. Nevertheless, this does not necessarily indicate an active infection or recent exposure. In such instances, a nontreponemal test is conducted subsequently to substantiate the infection. This is typically accomplished through the use of the RPR or VDRL test, which quantifies the concentration of antibodies directed against cardiolipin.

The reverse algorithm offers several advantages, including simplicity, cost-effectiveness, and convenience. This approach allows for a more rapid evaluation and identification of active syphilis cases, while also helping to minimize the number of unnecessary confirmatory tests for false-positive treponema results. It is important to note that specific testing algorithms and guidelines may vary by region and care provider. Therefore, it is essential to adhere to the recommendations of the local health department with regard to syphilis screening and diagnosis.

16.5.2.3 World Health Organization (WHO)

The World Health Organization (WHO) has issued recommendations for a syphilis screening strategy in pregnant women. Furthermore, the WHO has proposed screening strategies that are primarily employed in countries or regions with inadequate infrastructure.

- The rapid syphilis test (RST) is a diagnostic test. The test detects antibodies against the bacterium *Treponema pallidum* in the blood. The test is rapid and straightforward, allowing for on-site implementation and providing results within a few minutes.
- The RST is typically based on immunochromatographic technology, in which specific antibodies against T. pallidum are bound to a test strip. Upon contact with the test strip, a visible line or color change will occur in the sample,

indicating the presence of antibodies indicative of syphilis in the blood, serum, or plasma. This signifies a positive test result.
- The RST offers several advantages, particularly in the context of screening pregnant women or in areas with limited resources.
- The test is rapid, with results available within a few minutes, thereby facilitating prompt decision-making.
- The test is relatively simple to perform. The RST does not necessitate the use of complex laboratory equipment or the acquisition of specialized training to perform.
- The test is portable, facilitating its use in remote areas or in mobile health services where access to laboratory facilities is limited. The RST is portable and can be utilized in remote areas or in mobile health services where access to laboratory facilities is limited.
- Additionally, the test is cost-effective. The RST is typically less expensive than other laboratory tests, thereby enabling syphilis screening programs to be carried out cost-effectively.
- Although the RST is rapid and provides an immediate diagnosis, further laboratory tests are often required to confirm positive RST results and to determine the infection status more accurately. Subsequent tests typically include treponema tests such as the TPPA or the enzyme immunoassay (EIA).
- It is recommended that:
  – In areas with a low prevalence of syphilis (less than 5%), the rapid syphilis test (RST) should be employed for screening pregnant women in lieu of a single on-site RPR test.
  – In areas with a high prevalence of syphilis (5% or more), it is recommended that an on-site rapid syphilis test (a dual test for HIV and syphilis) be performed, that a first dose of treatment be administered if the result is positive, and that an RPR test be conducted. If the RPR test is positive, the recommended course of action is to administer treatment according to the duration of syphilis. A series of tests and treatments is recommended instead of a single RST or RPR test on site.

Without a defined screening algorithm, it is important to carefully consider local resources, recommendations, and conditions to ensure the most appropriate selection is made.

16.6 Therapy

16.6.1 Gynecology

Penicillin G, a β-lactam antibiotic, remains the drug of choice for treating syphilis (Table 16.3). Alternative treatments typically include antibiotics such as doxycycline or ceftriaxone. Although tetracycline is no longer manufactured or marketed in most countries, older guidelines still list it as a potential treatment option.

Table 16.3 Treatment options for syphilis. IU = International Units

Indication	Recommendation	Medication	Dosage	Duration
Lues I and II	Recommendation	Benzathine benzylpenicillin	2.4 million IU intramuscularly	Single dose
	Alternative	Ceftriaxone	1 g/day intravenously	10 days
	Bleeding disorder	Ceftriaxone	1 g/day intravenously	10 days
		Doxycycline	100 mg orally twice daily	14 days
	Allergy	Doxycycline	100 mg orally twice daily	14 days
Lues latens	Recommendation	Benzathine benzylpenicillin	2.4 million IU intramuscularly	On day 1, 8, and 15
	Alternative	Ceftriaxone	1 g/day intravenously	10 days
	Allergy	Doxycycline	100 mg orally twice daily	28 days
Lues III	Recommendation	Benzylpenicillin (penicillin G)	4 million IU intravenously six times per day	14 days
	Alternative	Ceftriaxone	2 g/day intravenously	14 days
Lues IV (neurosyphilis)	Recommendation	Benzylpenicillin (penicillin G)	4 million IU intravenously six times per day	14 days
	Alternative	Procaine benzylpenicillin plus	2.4 million IU/day intramuscularly	14 days
		Probenecid	500 mg orally four times per day	14 days
	International pharmacy	Clemizole penicillin G[a]	1 million IU/day intramuscularly	21 days
Older medications		Erythromycin[b]	500 mg orally four times per day	14–21 days
		Erythromycin lactobionate[b]	500 mg intravenously 4 times per day	14 days
		Tetracycline[c]	500 mg orally 4 times per day	14 days
		Procaine Benzylpenicillin[d]	0.6 million IU/day intramuscularly	14–21 days
Congenital syphilis	Infants and young children	Penicillin G	100,000–150,000 IU/kg/day intravenously	14 days
		Ceftriaxone	75 mg/kg/day intramuscularly or intravenously	14 days
	School-age children	Penicillin G	200,000–300,000 IU/kg/day divided into 3 doses	14 days
		Ceftriaxone	0.25–0.5 g/day intramuscularly or intravenously	14 days

(continued)

Table 16.3 (continued)

Indication	Recommendation	Medication	Dosage	Duration
Jarisch–Herxheimer reaction		Prophylaxis with prednisolone	1 mg/prednisolone equivalent/kg orally	Prophylactic
Granulomas		Pretreatment with prednisolone	25–50 mg/day	1–2 weeks

[a]Clemizole penicillin G has the best penetration into the cerebrospinal fluid among all penicillins. However, it is not available in many countries. It may be possible to order it from an international pharmacy

[b]Erythromycin therapy is no longer recommended due to the prevalence of resistance

[c]The previously commonly used tetracycline therapy is currently not possible as tetracycline is no longer commercially available. If needed, a similar antibiotic like doxycycline should be used, or an attempt can be made to obtain it from an international pharmacy

[d]Procaine benzylpenicillin is not indicated for the treatment of syphilis due to its low benzathine penicillin concentration. However, it has been found to be effective when administered (USA 1999). The duration and continuous administration of the treatment are crucial factors to consider

In recent years, manufacturers worldwide have faced prolonged and unclear production delays and supply bottlenecks. As a result, the World Health Organization (WHO) has recommended considering treatment with ceftriaxone (not in the first trimester) as a possible, though not optimal, substitute drug.

The duration and dosage of antibiotic therapy depend on the stage of the disease.

In congenital syphilis, lues III, and neurosyphilis, a higher dose of penicillin G is necessary and that a minimum treatment duration must be maintained.

An alternative treatment option is clemizole penicillin. However, this is no longer commercially available in many countries, necessitating the ordering of the medication from international pharmacies. Syphilis is only treated orally in exceptional cases.

Although antibiotic treatment can eliminate the pathogen, it cannot reverse organ damage that has already occurred.

16.6.2 Therapy During Pregnancy

16.6.2.1 General

Given that penicillins remain the most effective drugs against treponema, desensitization is carried out during pregnancy if there is a history of penicillin allergy (Table 16.4). A sensitivity test is often not conducted due to the urgent indication for treatment.

The structural similarity of amoxicillin to penicillin, its safety during pregnancy, and high bioavailability have led to several case reports demonstrating a positive therapeutic effect. Cefixime is currently under investigation as a potential alternative to penicillin in pregnant women with syphilis. Nevertheless, neither of these options addresses the issue of penicillin allergies.

- The administration of ceftriaxone during the first trimester is contraindicated. Syphilis infections (first diagnoses) from the second trimester onward can be treated with approved medication if indicated.

Table 16.4 Management of syphilis during pregnancy. If diagnosed in the last trimester, therapy should be completed before delivery. If completion is not feasible, additional therapy to the newborn should be administered. IU = International Units

Stage	Trimester	Recommendation	Dosage and duration	Penicillin allergy
Early syphilis	I	Benzathine benzylpenicillin	2.4 million IU intramuscularly, single dose	Desensitization followed by penicillin therapy
	II and III	Benzathine benzylpenicillin	2.4 million IU intramuscularly, single dose	Ceftriaxone 2 g intravenously once daily for 14 days
Late syphilis	I	Benzathine benzylpenicillin	2.4 million IU intramuscularly, on day 1, 8, 15	Desensitization followed by penicillin therapy
	II and III	Benzathine benzylpenicillin	2.4 million IU intramuscularly, on day 1, 8, 15	Ceftriaxone 2 g intravenously once daily for 14 days
Neurosyphilis[a]	I	Penicillin G	18–24 million IU/day intravenously, 3–four million IU every 4 h	Desensitization followed by penicillin therapy
	II and III	Penicillin G	18–24 million IU/day intravenously, 3–4 million IU every 4 h	Ceftriaxone 2 g intravenously once daily for 14 days

If diagnosed in the last trimester, therapy should be completed before delivery. If completion is not feasible, additional therapy should be administered to minimize transmission to the newborn

[a]For neurosyphilis, high-dose penicillin G therapy is recommended. Alternative treatment with procaine benzylpenicillin 2.4 million IU/day intramuscularly plus probenecid 500 mg orally four times daily for 14 days is currently only documented in case reports

- As a precautionary measure, the treatment can be repeated 1–2 months before the expected date of delivery at the same dosage and duration.
- It is recommended that therapy in the third trimester be completed before the birth, as otherwise the newborn should be treated.

> **It is recommended that alternative medications be administered only in exceptional cases. The use of ceftriaxone is contraindicated during the first trimester of pregnancy.**

16.6.2.2 Special Features

In cases of penicillin allergy during pregnancy, some guidelines recommend administering ceftriaxone intravenously instead of undergoing desensitization. This recommendation conflicts with international data and guidelines and lacks scientific substantiation. Despite these discrepancies, international guidelines continue to advocate for desensitization based on scientific evidence. Therefore, it is prudent to view these guidelines with caution, as they do not align with international recommendations, and the rationale presented is inadequate.

16.6.2.2.1 Penicillin Allergy and Desensitization

The prevalence of penicillin allergies is approximately 8–10% in the United States and Western Europe, while data on prevalence in developing countries is lacking. In about 10–15% of individuals with penicillin allergies, the reaction is IgE-mediated, which can lead to symptoms such as urticaria, angioedema, bronchospasm, or hypotension. Reexposure to penicillin in such individuals can be fatal. It is recommended that the desensitization process occur in an inpatient setting, as approximately one-third of patients may experience an allergic reaction, which, although usually mild, requires immediate medical attention.

The desensitization process typically lasts between 4 and 12 h, after which the full therapeutic dose of penicillin and other β-lactam antibiotics can be safely administered. If penicillin is needed again in the future, the desensitization process must be repeated, as the tolerant state is lost after 24–36 h.

In pregnant patients with documented penicillin hypersensitivity, parenteral ceftriaxone has been used as an alternative regimen, typically administered as a 14-day intravenous course during pregnancy. Syphilis is most commonly identified by positive serological assays in accordance with established antenatal guidelines at the time of initial booking (first trimester). Administration of ceftriaxone during the first trimester is discouraged owing to limited pharmacokinetic and safety data from regulatory approvals; however, deferring therapy until the second trimester is not recommended because prompt antimicrobial intervention is required. Ceftriaxone, as a β-lactam antibiotic, should be prescribed with caution in individuals with penicillin allergy, and specialist infectious disease or obstetric consultation is advised to determine the safest therapeutic approach.

In cases of penicillin allergy, alternative antibiotic treatments may be considered. Erythromycin is not a viable therapeutic option during the early months of pregnancy due to its pharmacodynamic properties, including limited placental permeability and contraindications in the first trimester. Meanwhile only the European USTI guidelines recommend azithromycin. However, it has limited approval for use during pregnancy and should generally be avoided. The administration of tetracyclines is contraindicated throughout pregnancy.

Ceftriaxone is commonly delivered by intravenous infusion in an inpatient setting for practical and economic reasons; patient adherence is a recognized concern because penicillin desensitization typically requires a shorter hospital stay than continuous 14-day IV therapy. When given intramuscularly, historical guidelines have recommended a minimum treatment duration of 10 days. It should be noted that missed daily doses may compromise therapy efficacy and, in some protocols, necessitate restarting the entire treatment course; therefore, treatment planning should include measures to maximize adherence.

It is very important to start treatment immediately during pregnancy.

16.6.2.2.2 Jarisch–Herxheimer Reaction

The Jarisch–Herxheimer reaction is a transient physiological response to the treatment of certain infections, including syphilis, with antibiotics. This reaction typically manifests shortly after treatment initiation and may present with symptoms such as fever, chills, headache, muscle aches, as well as a temporary exacerbation of preexisting symptoms. It is regarded as an immune system response to the destruction of bacteria and usually resolves within a few hours to 1–2 days.

In cases of secondary syphilis with a high pathogen load, the likelihood of experiencing a Jarisch–Herxheimer reaction during treatment increases. Prophylaxis can be initiated with a single oral dose of 1 mg of prednisolone per kilogram of body weight, administered 30 min prior to the commencement of therapy.

16.7 Differential Diagnosis

When diagnosing syphilis, it is crucial to consider differential diagnoses, as the symptoms can resemble those of numerous other infections and conditions. Significant pathogens causing genital ulcerations that should be included in the differential diagnosis include *Herpes simplex virus* types I and II, *Chlamydia trachomatis*, *Haemophilus ducreyi*, *Calymmatobacterium granulomatis*, and human immunodeficiency virus/acquired immunodeficiency syndrome (HIV/AIDS). Additionally, noninfectious causes such as Adamantiades–Behçet disease, balanitis/

balanoposthitis, molluscum contagiosum, HPV-induced condylomata lata, candidosis, scabies, fixed drug exanthema, and primary genital herpes should also be considered.

Syphilis is often referred to as the "great chameleon" of medicine due to its ability to cause a variety of symptoms that can easily be mistaken for those of other diseases. This capacity for mimicry renders diagnosis particularly challenging.

16.8 Prevention

16.8.1 Preventive Measures

Safer Sex and Barrier Methods

- **Condoms:** Correct and consistent use during vaginal, oral, and anal intercourse is strongly recommended to reduce transmission risk.
- **Dental Dams:** Use is advised as a barrier method during orogenital contact to prevent infection.

Regular Testing for High-Risk Groups

- **Populations:** MSM, transgender women (TGW), sex workers, and people living with HIV should undergo serological testing every 3 months.
- **Partners of Syphilis Cases:** Immediate testing upon notification of an index infection is mandatory; a follow-up test after 2–6 weeks may be considered to detect seroconversion.

Education and Health Literacy

- **Sexual Health Education:** Comprehensive information on transmission routes (direct contact with ulcers or exudates), clinical stages (primary to tertiary syphilis), and late complications (cardiovascular syphilis, neurosyphilis, and gummatous lesions) should be provided.
- **Partner Management:** Identification, notification, and concurrent testing and treatment of sexual contacts are essential components to interrupt transmission chains.

Hygiene Measures in Clinical Settings

- **Standard Precautions:** Strict adherence to hand hygiene, use of disposable gloves, and sterile instruments is mandatory.
- **Disinfection:** Surfaces and instruments exposed to lesions must be disinfected immediately using agents with proven efficacy against *Treponema pallidum*.

16.8.2 Pregnancy and Congenital Syphilis

Early and accurate syphilis screening during pregnancy is critical to preventing adverse outcomes such as stillbirth, preterm birth, and congenital infection. International guidelines consistently recommend universal serologic testing at the initial prenatal visit (Table 16.5), irrespective of individual risk factors, to enable early detection of both primary and latent infections. In regions with high syphilis prevalence, repeat screening during the third trimester and at delivery is advised to identify new infections acquired after the initial test. Where resources are constrained, risk-based retesting—focusing on women with new sexual partners, substance use, or HIV co-infection—is considered an effective alternative. The use of point-of-care dual HIV/syphilis rapid tests has improved screening coverage by providing immediate results and enabling same-day treatment, especially in low- and middle-income countries.

Table 16.5 Screening recommendations for syphilis during pregnancy

Organization/ authority (year)	Initial screening	Repeat testing third trimester	Repeat testing at delivery	EACS criteria/ notes
ACOG (USA, 2024)	Universal	Universal	Universal	Abandonment of risk-based approach. Three mandatory tests in some jurisdictions (e.g., NY from 05/2024); clinics must align workflows accordingly
ASHM (Australia, 2024)	Universal, at first antenatal booking	Risk-based (new partner, multiple partners, comorbid STDs)	If untested or unclear prenatal status	Repeat third trimester only for women with risk factors; point-of-care dual tests preferred; quarterly STD screens only for those on doxycycline
BASHH/IDPS (UK, 2024)	Universal	Recommended, especially if risk factors apply	If no result prior to delivery	≥1 new partner or ≥1 STD in past 6 months triggers repeat; third test required if no result before birth

(continued)

Table 16.5 (continued)

Organization/ authority (year)	Initial screening	Repeat testing third trimester	Repeat testing at delivery	EACS criteria/ notes
Brazil MoH (2023)	Universal, first visit	Universal	If positive during pregnancy	Accepts rapid POC dual tests; repeat at delivery only for women with positive or missing prenatal results
CNGOF (France, 2023)	Universal, at first prenatal test	Universal	If no prenatal test	Mandates three tests: early pregnancy, third trimester, and delivery; uses rapid dual syphilis/HIV tests in maternity wards
EKSI (Switzerland, 2025)	Universal, ideally at first presentation	Risk-adapted (drug use, new partners)	If no first trimester screen or positive tests	Point-of-care dual tests recommended; guidelines under development aligned with EACS/ÖAG
Germany (2023)	Universal (Maternity Directive)	Repeat if symptoms or risk factors; MSM partners ≥2×/year	–	Risk criteria: ≥10 male partners in 6 months or recurrent STDs. Non-nominal reporting
Kenya MoH/ NASCOP (2022)	Universal, first ANC visit	Universal in high-prevalence counties; risk-based elsewhere	If no prenatal syphilis screening	Part of PMTCT package; uses rapid dual tests; repeat third trimester universal where prevalence is high
NZSHS/ NZMOH (New Zealand, 2020)	Universal at booking	Risk-based (new partner, STD history, substance use)	If no prior screening	Antibiotic resistance concerns acknowledged; quarterly STD screening mandated only for women on doxycycline prophylaxis

(continued)

Table 16.5 (continued)

Organization/ authority (year)	Initial screening	Repeat testing third trimester	Repeat testing at delivery	EACS criteria/ notes
SEGO (Spain, 2022)	Universal at antenatal booking	Universal	If no prior test	Requires testing in first and third trimester; delivery testing optional if rapid test unavailable during pregnancy
SOGC (Canada, 2024)	Universal, ideally at first prenatal visit	Recommended for women with new partners or other STD risk factors	If no prior/ inadequate testing	Canadian criteria mirror EACS: ≥2 bacterial STDs in past 3 years, ≥5 partners in 6 months, new partner, HIV/ PrEP use, substance use, or high incidence region
South Africa NDoH/RSPH (2024)	Universal, booking	Universal	If no prior test or positive in pregnancy	Integrated with HIV PMTCT programs; point-of-care syphilis/HIV dual testing at delivery in high-burden settings
USPSTF (USA, 2025)	Universal, as early as possible	No formal recommendation (evidence gap)	–	Grade A recommendation; high benefit–risk ratio. Refers to CDC/ACOG for operational details
WHO (2025)	Universal, ideally before end of first trimester	Universal in high burden settings; risk-adapted where resources limited (dual tests preferred)	If no prior testing	Repeat indicated in high-prevalence areas; otherwise risk-adapted based on new partners, substance use, or HIV infection

The World Health Organization (WHO) has issued comprehensive guidelines for the screening and management of syphilis during pregnancy:

- Syphilis screening is recommended at the initial prenatal visit, during the third trimester, and at delivery.
- Upon a positive test result, a thorough medical history must be obtained.
- Diagnostic evaluation should determine the stage of infection.
- In asymptomatic cases, confirmation of adequate prior treatment is essential.
- If treatment history is uncertain or if there is a fourfold increase in antibody titers, repeat treatment is mandatory.
- Treatment regimens depend on disease stage; for recent infections within 1 year, two doses of benzathine penicillin G are recommended to protect the fetus.
- When a viable fetus is present, detailed fetal anatomical assessment via ultrasound should be performed.
- The initial dose of benzathine penicillin G should be administered at birth, with continuous fetal monitoring for 24 h thereafter.
- If fetal risk indicators or anomalies are detected, early delivery should be considered, followed by appropriate neonatal therapy prior to the estimated due date.
- Prenatal diagnostic procedures may be considered during the third trimester as indicated.
- Neonatology services should be notified at birth to ensure timely and appropriate neonatal evaluation.
- Histopathological examination of the placenta is recommended to assist in diagnosis and management.

16.8.3 Antibiotic Preventive Strategies: Doxycycline Post-Exposure Prophylaxis (DoxyPEP)

Definition: Doxycycline post-exposure prophylaxis (DoxyPEP) involves administering 200 mg of doxycycline within 72 h after unprotected sexual intercourse to prevent bacterial sexually transmitted infections (STDs), such as syphilis, chlamydia, and gonorrhea.

Efficacy: Clinical trials have demonstrated high efficacy of DoxyPEP against syphilis. The French IPERGAY study reported a 73% risk reduction; the US DoxyPEP study found reductions of 87% in PrEP users and 77% in HIV-positive individuals; the DOXYVAC trial observed reductions between 79% and 87%. A large cohort study from California confirmed these findings with an 80% decrease in syphilis infections. Therefore, DoxyPEP is highly effective against syphilis (73–87%) and chlamydia (70–89%). Its effectiveness against gonorrhea is moderate (43–57%) and depends on local antibiotic resistance patterns.

Target Population: Primarily effective in men who have sex with men (MSM) and transgender women (TGW).

- Strongly recommended for HIV-positive individuals and PrEP users within these groups.
- The CDC recommends DoxyPEP for MSM and TGW with at least one bacterial STD diagnosed in the previous 12 months.
- Efficacy is limited in cisgender women; a Kenyan study showed no significant effect in women, likely due to low adherence.
- A Japanese study involving sex workers documented a 67% reduction in STDs with daily doxycycline use.
- Data remain inconclusive for non-pregnant women of reproductive age.
- Use during pregnancy is restricted due to potential fetal risks and developmental concerns.

Dosage: The recommended dose is a single 200 mg dose of doxycycline, ideally within 24 h and no later than 72 h after unprotected intercourse. No more than one dose should be taken within 24 h.

Prescription Practices: Doxycycline is prescription-only in most European countries. Coverage varies widely: in the United Kingdom, DoxyPEP is available through the NHS, while in many other countries patients must cover costs for off-label use themselves.

Monitoring and Follow-Up: All guidelines emphasize the need for regular STD screening every 3–6 months alongside ongoing risk assessment. Community pharmacies are being considered as potential dispensing sites.

Current Guidelines and Recommendations

- **USA (CDC, 2024):** The Centers for Disease Control and Prevention recommend DoxyPEP for MSM and TGW who have had at least one bacterial STD within the past year. The suggested dosage is 200 mg doxycycline within 72 h after unprotected sex. Studies document over 70% reduction in syphilis and chlamydia infections, with approximately 50% reduction in gonorrhea.
- **United Kingdom (BASHH, June 2025):** The UK was among the first countries to publish national guidelines on DoxyPEP. The British Association for Sexual Health and HIV (BASHH) recommends DoxyPEP primarily for MSM and TGW at increased risk for syphilis. Studies demonstrated an 80% reduction in syphilis cases. The recommended dose is 200 mg within 24–72 h following intercourse.
- **European/EU Perspectives:** European institutions Europe recognize DoxyPEP's individual effectiveness but express concerns about antibiotic resistance and broader population impacts; the WHO is preparing guidelines expected in June 2025. Belgium restricts DoxyPEP to research settings, though around 10% of MSM use it informally, with willingness decreasing after antibiotic resistance information. Germany maintains a restrictive policy, recommending DoxyPEP only after individual risk assessment for MSM and TGW with specific risk factors, with patients covering costs due to off-label use. France, supported by strong clinical trial evidence (IPERGAY and DOXYVAC), reports significant reductions in syphilis and chlamydia incidence. Italy documents an 80% reduction in bacterial STDs among MSM with HIV or on PrEP, but therapy acceptance

is low. The Netherlands takes a cautious stance due to resistance concerns despite informal use among MSM. Austria follows case-by-case recommendations aligned with EACS guidelines, without routine STD PEP endorsement, emphasizing individualized risk-benefit analysis. Switzerland advises against routine use due to safety and resistance issues, supporting case-by-case use and ongoing studies evaluating efficacy in high-risk groups. In Spain, informal DoxyPEP use occurs within the GBMSM community despite no official recommendations and limited professional support.

- **South and Latin America:** Comprehensive research and implementation efforts on DoxyPEP are actively ongoing in South and Latin America. The HPTN 113 study, conducted in Lima (Peru), Rio de Janeiro (Brazil), and Buenos Aires (Argentina), targets young MSM and nonbinary individuals enrolled in existing PrEP programs. Peru, Brazil, and Argentina already possess established PrEP infrastructures for key populations and are now expanding their prevention strategies by incorporating DoxyPEP to enhance protection against syphilis and other bacterial STDs.
- **Asia-Pacific:** Australia has developed detailed consensus guidelines through the Australasian Society for HIV Medicine (ASHM), recommending DoxyPEP primarily for gbMSM at high risk, with emphasis on regular reassessment of indication. New Zealand adopts a cautious stance, recognizing DoxyPEP's efficacy while prioritizing antibiotic resistance monitoring and requiring quarterly multisite STD screening. In Japan, ongoing research—including a study among sex workers demonstrating a 67% reduction in bacterial STDs with daily doxycycline prophylaxis—reflects growing interest, although national guidelines have yet to be finalized. South Korea, Taiwan, and the Philippines are closely monitoring these developments, engaging in expert discussions but have not issued formal recommendations to date.
- **Africa:** South Africa leads the continent in DoxyPEP adoption, recommending its use for high-risk MSM within specialized sexual health clinics that integrate antimicrobial resistance surveillance. Although other African countries have not yet established formal DoxyPEP guidelines, many are strengthening STD surveillance systems. Countries with established PrEP programs—such as Kenya and Uganda—are considered likely early adopters pending local research outcomes and guideline development.
- **Upcoming WHO Developments**: The WHO plans comprehensive guidelines on doxycycline prophylaxis for STD prevention in 2025. The Guideline Development Group met virtually on June 25–26, 2025 to develop evidence-based recommendations targeting MSM and transgender persons. Updated STD guidelines including targeted screening recommendations were published in July 2025.

16.8.4 Additional Infection Risks and Reporting Obligations

Reinfection Risk: No immunity develops after syphilis infection, allowing reinfections. Repeat infections show weaker immune responses and higher RPR titers. Reinfections tend to be asymptomatic, complicating diagnosis and increasing transmission risk. Reinfection rates of 20–25% occur in high-risk groups, especially MSM and people with HIV.

Parenteral Transmission: Syphilis can rarely be transmitted via blood transfusion or needlestick injury when exposed to syphilitic lesions. Since donor screening and blood refrigeration were introduced, transfusion-related cases have become extremely rare. Risk to healthcare workers from needlesticks is very low but not zero. *Treponema pallidum* DNA may be present in some seropositive donors despite antibodies. Mandatory serological screening and refrigeration reduce transmission risk.

Breastfeeding Transmission: Syphilis is not transmitted through breast milk. Breastfeeding is only contraindicated if active breast chancres are present. The main concern is in utero transmission, which can occur as early as 17 weeks gestation with high rates in primary and secondary syphilis. Maternal syphilis also increases HIV mother-to-child transmission risk.

Reporting Obligations: Syphilis is routinely notifiable in most countries worldwide. Both acquired and congenital cases require timely reporting, often within days. Non-nominal systems protect confidentiality while enabling surveillance. Laboratories and healthcare providers must report confirmed or suspected cases, focusing on early infectious stages. Surveillance supports partner notification and treatment to prevent further spread.

Reporting to local authorities is mandatory in several countries.

Key Points

- Syphilis is an infectious disease characterized by a cyclical course.
- The pathogen, *Treponema pallidum*, is a motile spirochete.
- The primary mode of transmission is through sexual intercourse.
- The incubation period is approximately 3 weeks.
- If left untreated, syphilis can lead to chronic systemic diseases.
- Symptoms of syphilis may vary and manifest in different stages.
- The initial presentation of primary syphilis involves a painless ulcer on the genitalia.
- Secondary syphilis manifests through the emergence of skin rashes and associated symptoms, such as fever and weight loss.
- Latent and late syphilis may affect various organs, including the nervous and cardiovascular systems.
- Congenital syphilis occurs when the infection is not recognized and treated promptly, potentially leading to a range of cutaneous symptoms and other organ involvement in the newborn.
- Late manifestations of congenital syphilis can develop long after birth, resulting in complications such as hearing loss and dental changes.

(continued)

- Differentiating between direct and indirect diagnostic procedures is essential.
- Direct detection methods include dark-field microscopy, direct fluorescent antibody testing, histological examination, and nucleic acid amplification techniques like polymerase chain reaction (PCR) utilized for congenital syphilis detection.
- Indirect detection methods encompass nontreponemal tests (e.g., RPR, VDRL) and treponemal tests (e.g., TPPA, EIA).
- Penicillin G remains the drug of choice for treating syphilis, with alternatives like doxycycline or ceftriaxone being less favorable.
- The Jarisch–Herxheimer reaction is a temporary reaction to antibiotic therapy; the duration and dosage of treatment vary based on disease stage.
- Therapy must be initiated promptly during pregnancy, with desensitization recommended for pregnant women with penicillin allergies.
- The most effective prevention strategy is through education and the use of condoms to avoid syphilis infections.
- Regular examinations for pregnant women are recommended for early diagnosis and treatment; partner treatment adherence is also crucial. Reporting obligations for syphilis vary by country or region.

Part IV

Other Sexually Transmitted Diseases

Chlamydia Trachomatis 17

Abstract

Chlamydia trachomatis infection is recognized as the most prevalent bacterial infection transmitted sexually across the globe, with a distinguished prevalence peak among individuals aged 15–24 years. An estimated 130 million new infections are documented annually worldwide. Clinical manifestations of the infection may vary, ranging from cervicitis accompanied by discharge to asymptomatic presentations. If left untreated, infections can result in significant complications, including endometritis, salpingitis, and pelvic inflammatory disease (PID), which can in turn lead to infertility and persistent abdominal pain. Pregnant individuals face heightened risks of premature rupture of membranes, chorioamnionitis, and premature labor. Diagnosis is achieved through polymerase chain reaction (PCR) testing. Treatment usually involves the administration of antibiotics, such as doxycycline, macrolides, or quinolones. The management of chlamydial infections in pregnant women is inherently more complex and necessitates careful evaluation. Screening for chlamydial infections is routinely conducted in numerous countries.

17.1 Background

17.1.1 Urogenital *Chlamydia trachomatis* Infection

Urogenital infection caused by *Chlamydia trachomatis* is one of the most common bacterial sexually transmitted infections (STIs) globally. The incidence and prevalence rates of genital *Chlamydia trachomatis* infections show significant variation, ranging from as low as 1% to as high as 40%, depending on the population studied and the region. This wide disparity in rates is influenced by factors, such as differences in healthcare access, screening programs, sexual behavior, and awareness about STIs.

I. Mylonas, *Sexually Transmitted Diseases*,
https://doi.org/10.1007/978-3-031-78204-6_17

Table 17.1 Risk factors for chlamydial infection

Risk factor	Description
Gender	– Higher prevalence in women (455/100,000), approximately 3.5 times higher than in men
Race and ethnicity	– Patient race does not appear to be associated with chlamydial infection – African American patients appear to be the most affected
Age	– Increased risk of infection at age < 25 years
Sexual behavior	– Multiple sexual partners
	– New sexual partner
	– New partner in the last 90 days
Sexual education	– No or little use of condoms
Sexually transmitted infection (STD)	– Patients with other STDs in their medical history or present at the time of examination
Clinical examination	– Abnormalities on vaginal examination, such as cervical discharge, cervicitis, or cervical ectopia

The development of a chlamydia infection is influenced by several risk factors, with unprotected sexual intercourse being the most significant. In particular, young adults under the age of 25 are disproportionately affected and represent a high-risk group due to increased sexual activity, a higher number of sexual partners, and lower rates of consistent condom use. The absence or inconsistent use of condoms significantly raises the risk of acquiring a *Chlamydia trachomatis* infection, as it facilitates direct transmission during sexual contact. Additionally, sociocultural factors, such as lack of education on STI prevention, limited access to sexual health services, and stigma surrounding STI testing, may further contribute to higher infection rates in certain populations. These considerations underscore the need for targeted prevention strategies, including public education campaigns, routine screening for high-risk groups, and promotion of consistent condom use (see Table 17.1 for risk factors).

Infection with *Chlamydia trachomatis* can result in various diseases (Table 17.2). In women, one of the most serious consequences is pelvic inflammatory disease (PID), which can result in chronic pelvic pain, infertility, and ectopic pregnancies. In men, untreated chlamydia can lead to epididymitis, characterized by inflammation of the epididymis, which may cause pain and swelling. Both genders can experience reactive arthritis, an inflammatory response that affects the joints, urethra, and eyes. Additionally, *Chlamydia trachomatis* can increase the risk of acquiring and transmitting HIV. In newborns, maternal infection during pregnancy can lead to complications such as conjunctivitis and pneumonia.

Table 17.2 Diseases caused by *Chlamydia trachomatis*

Disease	Symptoms
Pelvic inflammatory disease	– Infertility (approximately 20%)
	– Chronic pelvic pain (approximately 18%)
	– Extrauterine pregnancy (approximately 6%)
	– Peritonitis and perihepatitis (Fitz-Hugh–Curtis syndrome)
	– Ascites with right-sided upper abdominal pain, nausea, and vomiting
Cervicitis	– Often only nonspecific symptoms
	– Mucopurulent discharge from the cervix (less than with gonorrhea)
	– Frequently increased and foul-smelling discharge, especially with additional infection of other pathogenic germs (e.g., bacterial vaginosis)
	– Contact bleeding during sexual intercourse
	– Only a small proportion is associated with pronounced cervicitis
Trachoma	– Most common cause of blindness in less developed countries
	– Purulent conjunctivitis approximately 1 week after initial infection
	– Chronic infections lead to scarring, which can result in eyelid changes (entropion), mechanical damage to the cornea, and blindness
Nongonorrheal urethritis	– Purulent, painful urethritis
	– Possible complications: Urethral stricture, male sterility after epididymitis, female sterility after PID, pharyngitis after oral sex, proctitis after anal sex or as a smear infection in women
Lymphogranuloma venereum	– Beginning with a painless ulcer in the genital region
	– Swelling of the regional lymph nodes
Reactive arthritis	– Can occur after about 4 weeks, especially in men
	– Accompanied by urethritis and conjunctivitis (Reiter's syndrome)
Inclusion body conjunctivitis	– Benign infection, often after exposure to pathogens in swimming pools
	– Newborn infection during birth
	– Usually heals spontaneously within 6 months
	– In rare cases, trachoma-like clinical pictures develop
Peripartum transmission	– Peripartum transmission in approximately 36–60% of infected mothers
	– Inclusion conjunctivitis in approximately 18% of infected infants
	– Pneumonia in approximately 16% of infected infants
	– Approximately 50% prevalence of maternal bacterial vaginosis
	– Increased peripartum mortality

17.2 Pathogen

Chlamydiae are categorized as obligate intracellular bacteria. The current taxonomic framework classifies the Chlamydiaceae family into several categories, including:

- *Chlamydia trachomatis*, *Chlamydia muridarum*, and *Chlamydia suis.*
- *Chlamydophila psittaci*, *Chlamydophila abortus*, *Chlamydophila caviae*, *Chlamydophila felis*, *Chlamydophila pecorum*, and *Chlamydophila pneumoniae.*

- Additional genera, such as Simkania and Waddlia. The medical significance of these additional bacteria remains ambiguous.

Chlamydia trachomatis is marked by a unique biphasic developmental cycle, which incorporates two morphologically distinct forms:

- **Elementary Bodies (EBs):**
  - **Infectious Form:** EBs represent the extracellular, infectious form of *C. trachomatis.*
  - **Size:** Typically measuring approximately 0.3 μm in diameter.
  - **Characteristics:** EBs are metabolically inactive and remarkably adapted for survival outside host cells. They possess a rigid outer membrane, primarily composed of the major outer membrane protein (MOMP), which is crucial for binding to and entering host cells.
- **Reticulate Bodies (RBs):**
  - **Noninfectious Form:** RBs constitute the intracellular, noninfectious form.
  - **Size:** Ranging from approximately 0.5–1.0 μm in diameter.
  - **Characteristics:** RBs are metabolically active and replicate within a membrane-bound vacuole in host cells, termed an inclusion. They undergo binary fission before reverting to EBs, which are subsequently released to infect new cells.

Chlamydia trachomatis is categorized into several serotypes, each associated with distinct clinical manifestations. The classification of serotypes is based on their antigenic properties and the specific diseases they induce.

- **Serotypes A–C:** Primarily associated with trachoma, a chronic ocular infection. Trachoma typically begins with conjunctival and corneal inflammation, which, if untreated, may result in scarring, trichiasis (inward turning of eyelashes), and ultimately, blindness. This is a significant cause of preventable blindness globally, predominantly affecting children in regions with inadequate sanitation and limited healthcare access.
- **Serotypes D–K:** Linked to urogenital infections in both men and women. In men, these serotypes often result in nongonococcal urethritis (NGU), manifesting symptoms such as dysuria and urethral discharge. In women, infections can lead to urethritis and cervicitis. Untreated, the infection may ascend to the upper genital tract, causing pelvic inflammatory disease (PID), encompassing conditions such as endometritis, salpingitis, and pelvic peritonitis.
- **Serotypes L1–L3:** Associated with lymphogranuloma venereum (LGV), a sexually transmitted infection predominantly affecting the lymphatic system. LGV typically begins with a small, painless genital ulcer at the infection site, which may go unnoticed. Progression to the secondary stage is marked by painful regional lymphadenopathy and the formation of buboes, which may rupture and discharge. If left untreated, LGV can result in chronic inflammatory responses during the tertiary stage, leading to strictures and fistulas in the genital and anorectal regions.

17.3 Epidemiology

Chlamydia trachomatis is recognized as the most prevalent sexually transmitted bacterial infection worldwide.

17.3.1 Prevalence in Nonpregnant Women

- **General Overview:** The infection disproportionately affects individuals aged 15–24, with an estimated 130 million new *Chlamydia trachomatis* infections globally each year. The overall prevalence of *Chlamydia trachomatis* among adults aged 15–49 is approximately 4.2%.
- **Europe:** Europe exhibits a high incidence rate of *Chlamydia trachomatis* infections, particularly in Western European countries, where the prevalence among adults generally falls between 3% and 5%.
- **Scandinavian Countries:** Denmark, Finland, Iceland, Norway, and Sweden report the highest incidence rates of *Chlamydia trachomatis*, exceeding 250 cases per 100,000 population. In 2022, these countries collectively accounted for 57% of the chlamydia cases reported in the European Union/European Economic Area (EU/EEA).
- **United Kingdom:** The prevalence of chlamydia infection is notably high in the UK, with approximately 64% of diagnosed cases occurring among young adults aged 16–24, likely due to risky sexual behaviors. In 2007, the UK accounted for about 49% of the total number of chlamydia cases reported by all EU/EEA member states, with a notification rate of 201 per 100,000 population, the highest in Europe at that time.
- **United States:** Young adults in the United States experience particularly high incidence rates of *Chlamydia trachomatis*, with an estimated prevalence rate of 4.7% observed in women of childbearing age.
- **Asia:** The prevalence of *Chlamydia trachomatis* across Asia exhibits significant regional disparities. Some countries report prevalence rates exceeding 5%, while others average below 3%.
- **Africa:** High incidence rates are especially prevalent in sub-Saharan Africa, where certain regions report prevalence rates exceeding 10%, particularly among young women.
- **Latin America:** Data regarding *Chlamydia trachomatis* prevalence in Latin America is incomplete; however, the incidence is believed to be high, with significant variability observed between countries.

A prevalence rate exceeding 5% may also be observed in populations without apparent risk factors.

17.3.2 Prevalence in Pregnant Women

- **General Overview:** The prevalence of *Chlamydia trachomatis* among pregnant women shows considerable variation across different regions worldwide.
- **Europe:** The prevalence among pregnant women typically ranges from 2% to 6%, with countries like Germany and France exhibiting lower rates within this range.
- **Scandinavian Countries:** In Scandinavian countries, the prevalence among pregnant women is estimated to be between 2% and 4%.
- **The United Kingdom:** In the United Kingdom, the estimated prevalence rate among pregnant women is between 3% and 5%.
- **The United States:** The estimated prevalence rate among pregnant women in the United States is approximately 4.5%. Young pregnant women are particularly affected, showing higher prevalence rates in this demographic.
- **Asia:** The prevalence of *Chlamydia trachomatis* among pregnant women across Asia varies considerably, ranging from less than 2% to over 10%. Countries in Southeast Asia, including Cambodia, Indonesia, Laos, Malaysia, Myanmar, the Philippines, Singapore, Thailand, and Vietnam, report notably higher prevalence rates.
- **Africa:** Many African countries, particularly in sub-Saharan Africa, report exceedingly high prevalence rates in pregnant women, reaching 15% or more in some areas.
- **Latin America:** Data regarding the prevalence of *Chlamydia trachomatis* in pregnant women in Latin America is incomplete; however, estimates suggest a prevalence range of 2–8%, with higher rates more common in economically disadvantaged regions.

The prevalence of *Chlamydia trachomatis* among pregnant women is significantly higher in developing countries compared to industrialized nations. Current prevalence and incidence data for infected pregnant women remain unknown in many regions, with estimates ranging from 1% to 4%.

17.4 Clinical Manifestation

17.4.1 Gynecology

The clinical presentation of *Chlamydia trachomatis* infection can vary from the characteristic mucopurulent discharge from the cervix to nonspecific cervicitis (Fig. 17.1) and can even be completely asymptomatic. Acute inflammation of the cervix is often associated with purulent discharge, which may have a strong odor. In contrast, chronic or nonspecific cervicitis typically manifests with mild symptoms, such as minimal discharge or slight abnormal bleeding.

Possible forms of chlamydial infection include:

- Arthritis.
- Cervicitis (Chap. 7).
- Conjunctivitis.
- Perihepatitis (Fitz-Hugh–Curtis syndrome).
- Pelvic inflammatory disease (PID) (Chap. 8).
- Proctitis or proctocolitis (Chap. 11).
- Urethritis (Chap. 9).

Chlamydial infections have only a weak correlation with the severity of a cervicitis, with an estimated 70–80% of cases being clinically asymptomatic, which often results in misdiagnosis. The infection can result in endometritis and salpingitis due to the seeding of the internal female genital tract with bacteria. Peritoneal seeding may cause ascites and *perihepatitis* (Fitz-Hugh–Curtis syndrome), which is often clinically associated with right-sided upper abdominal pain (Fig. 17.2). Additionally, autoinoculation may result in conjunctivitis (Fig. 17.3).

Untreated cervical chlamydial infections are known to significantly increase the risk of PID (Chap. 8), with some studies reporting prevalence rates of up to 40%. Salpingitis caused by *Chlamydia trachomatis* may occur even in the absence of clinically manifest cervicitis (Fig. 17.1), leading to damage and scarring of the

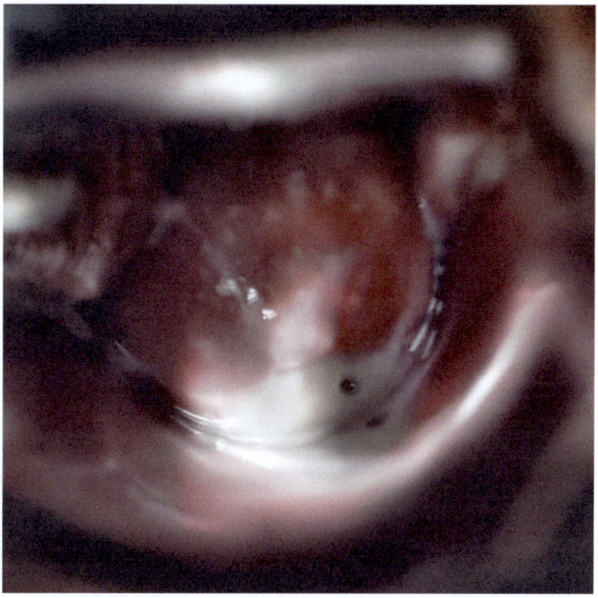

Fig. 17.1 Cervicitis induced by Chlamydia trachomatis (Mylonas 2016)

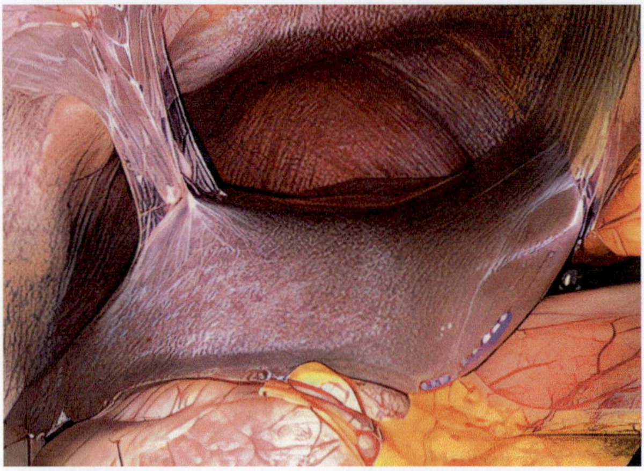

Fig. 17.2 Fitz-Hugh-Curtis syndrome. Surgical intervention does not significantly alleviate symptoms (Mylonas 2016)

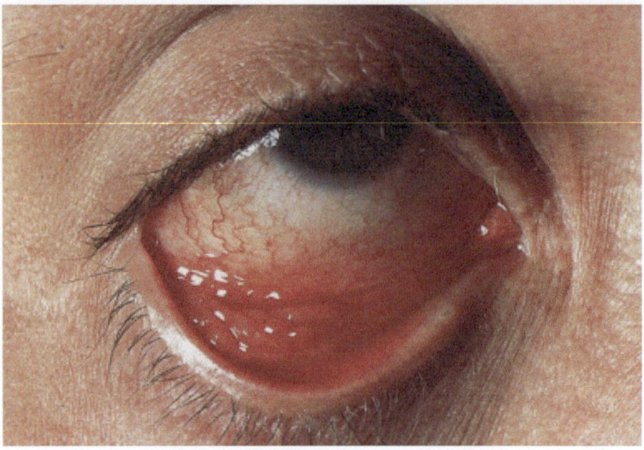

Fig. 17.3 Conjunctivitis caused by Chlamydia trachomatis (Zangerle et al. 2018)

fallopian tubes, particularly in cases of chronic or subclinical infections. A retrospective population-based cohort study conducted in Sweden and Norway revealed an elevated risk of PID among women who tested positive for *Chlamydia trachomatis*. Additionally, the risk of PID was found to be increased in individuals who suffered reinfection (Fig. 17.4).

The most prevalent complications of a PID include infertility (approximately 20%), chronic abdominal pain (approximately 18%), and extra-uterine pregnancy (approximately 6%).

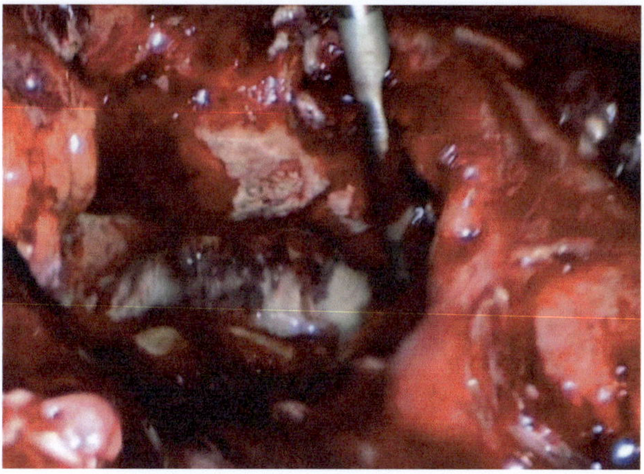

Fig. 17.4 Acute pelvic inflammatory disease with detection of Chlamydia trachomatis from the fallopian tubes (Mylonas 2016)

17.4.2 Pregnancy

Despite the conflicting results of various studies, there is an observed increase in the incidence of premature rupture of membranes, chorioamnionitis, premature birth, low birth weight, and consequent perinatal morbidity and mortality among pregnant women with chlamydial infections.

Pregnancy-related complications associated with infection include:

- Chorioamnionitis, premature rupture of membranes, premature birth, low birth weight, miscarriage, and spontaneous abortion. These complications may be exacerbated by endometritis, an infection of the inner lining of the uterus.
- Pregnant women with chlamydial infections have been found to have nearly twice the prevalence of bacterial vaginosis (Chap. 35), which is also linked to premature birth.
- Late postpartum endometritis.

Routine screening for *Chlamydia trachomatis* during pregnancy is considered standard care in many countries. It is recommended that this screening should be performed during the initial maternity examination and, if necessary, again between the 30th and 34th week of pregnancy.

17.4.3 Neonatology

Peripartum transmission of *Chlamydia trachomatis* occurs in approximately 36–60% of infected mothers. About 18% of infants born to infected mothers develop a inclusion conjunctivitis, while approximately 16% present with pneumonia. Otitis media, or inflammation of the nasopharynx, may also occur. These transmission routes can lead to increased perinatal morbidity and mortality.

Any conjunctivitis in an infant under 30 days of age should be presumed to be of chlamydial origin.

17.5 Diagnosis

Accurate and timely diagnosis of *Chlamydia trachomatis* is essential to prevent complications and curb the spread of infection.

Nucleic Acid Amplification Tests (NAATs): NAATs are regarded as the diagnostic standard for *Chlamydia trachomatis* because superior sensitivity and specificity are provided by these assays. Multiple specimen types may be tested: urine samples are particularly useful in males and are commonly employed in screening programs for both sexes; endocervical swabs are frequently obtained from women, especially when acute symptoms are present; vaginal swabs, including self-collected specimens, have been demonstrated to be effective and convenient though availability remains limited in some countries; urethral swabs are employed for diagnosing infections in males; and rectal and pharyngeal swabs are indicated for detection of extragenital infection.

Diagnosis of *Chlamydia trachomatis* predominantly relies on NAATs due to their superior sensitivity and specificity.

Cell Culture: When demonstration of organism viability is required, for example, in medicolegal contexts, *Chlamydia trachomatis* may be cultivated in living cell monolayers by cell culture. This method is less sensitive than NAATs, is labor-intensive and time-consuming, and requires specialized laboratory infrastructure. Clinical guidance dictates that any conjunctivitis occurring in an infant younger than 30 days of age should be presumed to be of chlamydial origin until proven otherwise. Given assay performance characteristics, diagnosis of *C. trachomatis* is predominantly reliant upon NAATs.

Direct Fluorescent Antibody (DFA) Test: DFA testing is performed by allowing fluorescently labeled antibodies to bind chlamydial antigens in the specimen, permitting visual confirmation of the organism. DFA is less sensitive than NAATs and is highly dependent upon specimen quality and technician proficiency.

Enzyme-Linked Immunosorbent Assay (ELISA): ELISA detects chlamydial antigens in clinical specimens. Because a relatively straightforward protocol is required, ELISA may be applied to large-scale screening; however, it is less sensitive than NAATs and may produce false-positive results.

Serological Tests: Serological assays measure antibodies directed against *Chlamydia trachomatis* in serum and are useful for the diagnosis of chronic or invasive disease. These tests are unsuitable for routine diagnosis of acute urogenital infection because antibodies require time to develop and may persist after infection resolution.

Point-of-Care Testing: Rapid point-of-care assays that yield immediate results are valuable where laboratory access is limited; however, these tests generally exhibit lower sensitivity and specificity compared with NAATs. In women, cervical and vaginal swab specimens typically contain higher concentrations of *C. trachomatis* than urine; therefore, appropriate specimen selection should be ensured to maximize diagnostic yield.

In women, higher concentrations of *Chlamydia trachomatis* can be detected in cervical and vaginal swab samples than in urine, highlighting the importance of using appropriate specimen types for diagnosis.

17.6 Treatment

All infections caused by *Chlamydia trachomatis* must be treated with antibiotics at sufficient doses (Table 17.3). Given that the pathogens are intracellular and their multiplication cycle lasts 48–72 h, treatment is recommended to continue for at least 10–14 days.

Table 17.3 Therapeutic options for uncomplicated chlamydial infection outside of pregnancy

Indication	Medication	Dosage	Duration
Standard	Doxycycline	100 mg orally twice daily	7–10 days
	Azithromycin	1.5 g orally	Single dose[a]
Alternative	Levofloxacin	500 mg orally once daily	7–10 days
	Moxifloxacin	400 mg orally once daily	7–10 days
	Erythromycin	500 mg orally four times daily	7–10 days
	Erythromycin ethylsuccinate	400 mg orally four times daily	14 days
	Erythromycin ethylsuccinate	800 mg orally four times daily	7–10 days
Older medications	Clindamycin	300 mg orally four times daily	14 days
	Clarithromycin	500 mg orally twice daily	10 days
	Amoxicillin	500 mg orally three times daily	10–14 days

[a]Potentially repeated after 2–5 days

17.6.1 Gynecology

The standard treatment regimen includes the administration of doxycycline and azithromycin or a class III quinolone, such as levofloxacin (Fig. 17.5). Although ciprofloxacin has demonstrated some *in vitro* efficacy against Chlamydia, it is not recommended for treating infections. In cases of PID with concurrent chlamydial infection, an effective antibiotic should be selected for combination therapy (Sect. 8.6.1).

A single dose of azithromycin is often recommended for treating uncomplicated infections of the lower genital tract in adults. A dosage of 1, 1.5, or 2 g (depending on local guidelines) is advised. Further treatment with this medication may be necessary, as a lower response rate to azithromycin has been observed in cases of rectal infection compared to doxycycline.

Therapy for sexual partners is mandatory.

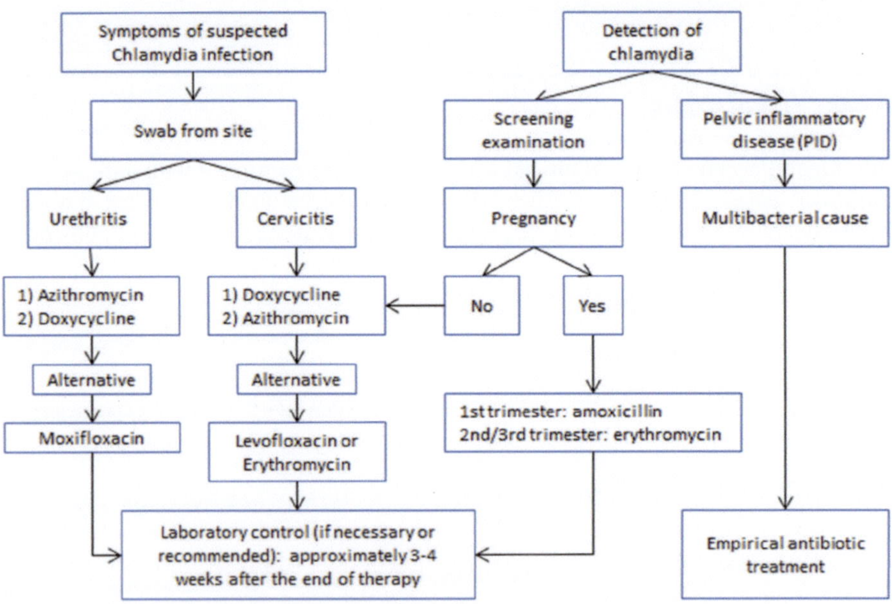

Fig. 17.5 Procedure for suspected Chlamydia trachomatis infection. (Courtesy of I. Mylonas)

17.6.2 Pregnancy

Tetracyclines and quinolones are contraindicated during pregnancy. Given the extensive scientific evidence supporting its efficacy and tolerability, oral erythromycin succinate is recommended at a dosage of 800 mg four times daily for a minimum of 7 days in many countries (Table 17.4). If intolerance occurs, the dose can be reduced by half, and the treatment duration doubled. Erythromycin estolate is contraindicated during pregnancy due to its risk of causing liver toxicity the fetus.

However, there has been irregular availability of erythromycin succinate, so it is advisable to verify the medication's availability before prescribing.

Guidelines in some regions permit the treatment of pregnant women with a single dose of azithromycin at 1.5 g. While both European and US approvals place stringent indications on this medication, azithromycin is only recommended during pregnancy under significant restrictions.

Table 17.4 Therapeutic options for uncomplicated chlamydial infection during pregnancy

Indication	Medication	Dosage	Duration
Standard	Erythromycin Ethylsuccinate[a]	400 mg orally four times daily	14 days
	Erythromycin Ethylsuccinate[a]	800 mg orally four times daily	7 days
Alternative	Amoxicillin	1000 mg orally three times daily	10–14 days
	Erythromycin[a]	500 mg orally four times daily	10–14 days
	Azithromycin[b]	1.5 g orally, single dose	Potentially repeated after 2–5 days
Newborns/ children	Erythromycin	50 mg/kg/day orally four times daily	21 days

[a]The availability of the medication should be verified before prescribing. It should not be administered during the first trimester

[b]Some national guidelines recommend azithromycin for treatment. However, according to approval data, this ketolide has very limited use compared to erythromycin and amoxicillin. Additionally, credible epidemiological evidence suggests that azithromycin, unlike erythromycin ethylsuccinate and amoxicillin, could be associated with adverse pregnancy outcomes. Therefore, numerous institutions have already adjusted their guidelines. For example, the CDC (United States) now recommends amoxicillin again as the primary treatment option

Key recommendations for treating *Chlamydia trachomatis* infection in pregnant women include:

- Treatment with erythromycin succinate should be initiated as soon as possible after diagnosis but not before the end of the 14th week of pregnancy to ensure the safety of both mother and fetus.
- If therapy is initiated during the first trimester, amoxicillin should be used for at least 10 days (Fig. 17.5).
- The efficacy of the treatment should be evaluated 3–4 weeks *after* therapy concludes.

Clinical evalations during recent decades have shown that treatment with amoxicillin is equivalent to that with erythromycin, contrary to theoretical concerns (i.e., intracellular localization of bacteria) raised in studies conducted in the 1980s. As a result, the American CDC guidelines now recommend amoxicillin treatment again.

17.6.3 Postpartum and Newborns

The treatment recommendations made during pregnancy should be applied analogously in the postpartum period or adjusted for sick newborns (erythromycin 40–60 mg/kg body weight/day for 14 days). Erythromycin is effective for treating conjunctivitis, with an efficacy rate of 80–90%. Azithromycin (20 mg/kg body weight/day for 3 or 5 days as a single daily administration) has demonstrated efficacy rates of up to 85%. Alternatively, azithromycin can be administered at 10 mg/kg body weight/day once weekly for 3 weeks. Recognition of the child's exposure during birth does not constitute an indication for prophylactic therapy; however, it does necessitate targeted monitoring of the newborn.

It is recommended that both the mother and child be examined at the earliest opportunity, ideally within six weeks of the conclusion of therapy.

17.7 Differential Diagnosis

Several diseases may present with symptoms similar to those of a *Chlamydia trachomatis* infection, necessitating consideration in the differential diagnosis:

- **Gonorrhea:** Caused by *Neisseria gonorrhoeae*, this infection often presents with urogenital symptoms analogous to those of *Chlamydia trachomatis*, including purulent urethritis, cervicitis, and proctitis.

- **Trichomoniasis:** Another sexually transmitted infection caused by the protozoan *Trichomonas vaginalis*, it can manifest with symptoms similar to those of Chlamydia, such as discharge and itching.
- **Bacterial Vaginosis (BV):** Characterized by an overgrowth of bacteria in the vagina, BV can lead to symptoms that resemble those of a chlamydial infection, including foul-smelling, watery discharge.
- **Mycoplasma Infections:** Infections caused by *Mycoplasma genitalium* or *Ureaplasma urealyticum* can also present symptoms similar to *Chlamydia trachomatis*.
- **Genital Herpes:** Caused by the herpes simplex virus (HSV), genital herpes is characterized by painful blisters in the genital area, which may sometimes be misdiagnosed as chlamydial ulcers.
- **Urethritis:** This condition can arise from various pathogens apart from *Chlamydia trachomatis*.
- **Pelvic Inflammatory Disease (PID):** It is crucial to differentiate between the various etiologies of PID, including appendicitis.

17.8 Prevention

Preventing *Chlamydia trachomatis* infections involves a multifaceted approach that combines public health initiatives, education, and individual behavioral changes. Key strategies for preventing chlamydial infections include:

- **Screening Programs:**
  - **Routine Screening:** Regular screening for sexually active individuals, particularly those under the age of 25, is recommended to identify and treat asymptomatic infections.
  - **Targeted Screening:** Focused on high-risk groups such as pregnant women, men who have sex with men (MSM), and individuals with multiple sexual partners.

Annual screening has been introduced in several countries for all sexually active women up to the age of 25. Furthermore, routine screening during pregnancy is recommended both nationally and internationally and has been incorporated into maternity guidelines in many countries, ideally conducted during the initial prenatal visit.

- **Partner Notification and Treatment:**
  - **Expedited Partner Therapy (EPT):** Prescribing medications to the sexual partners of infected individuals without requiring a medical examination to prevent reinfection and further transmission.

  - **Contact Tracing:** Health authorities assist in notifying, testing, and treating the sexual partners of individuals diagnosed with chlamydia.
- **Accessible Healthcare Services:**
  - **Testing Facilities:** Increasing the availability and accessibility of testing facilities, particularly in underserved areas.
  - **Affordable Treatment:** Ensuring treatment is affordable and accessible, including the provision of free antibiotics in some regions.
  - **Treatment Adherence:** Ensuring complete adherence to prescribed antibiotic regimens to effectively eradicate the infection.
  - **Medical Prophylaxis:** The prescription of eye infection prophylaxis with 1% silver nitrate (Credé prophylaxis) against gonococci and other pathogens is no longer mandatory. Nevertheless, as there are currently no superior alternatives available, this prophylaxis is still recommended or prescribed by law in numerous countries.
- **Sexual Health Education:**
  - **Awareness Campaigns:** Public health initiatives to raise awareness about chlamydia, its transmission, symptoms, and complications.
  - **Comprehensive Sex Education:** Education programs in schools and communities covering safe sex practices, the importance of regular testing, and effective contraceptive use.
  - **Condom Use:** Consistent and correct use of condoms during vaginal, anal, and oral sex significantly reduces the risk of chlamydia transmission.
  - **Community Engagement:** Engaging community leaders and influencers to reduce the stigma associated with sexually transmitted diseases (STD).
  - **Confidential Services:** Promoting confidential and nonjudgmental sexual health services to encourage individuals to seek testing and treatment.

To prevent *Chlamydia trachomatis* infection, it is recommended that children and adolescents receive proper education regarding sexually transmitted diseases and sexual hygiene. The consistent use of condoms offers a degree of protection against infection.

Key Points

- Urogenital *Chlamydia trachomatis* infection is a prevalent sexually transmitted bacterial infection worldwide, predominantly affecting young, sexually active individuals.
- It is estimated that over 130 million new infections occur globally each year, although these figures are likely underestimated.
- *Chlamydia trachomatis* are intracellular bacteria that can cause a variety of diseases.
- The multiple serotypes of *Chlamydia trachomatis* lead to diverse clinical manifestations.
- This pathogen is the most prevalent sexually transmitted bacterial infection, particularly among individuals aged 15–24.
- High incidence rates are reported in Europe and the United States; Africa is particularly affected.
- Pregnant women face an increased risk of complications, including premature rupture of membranes and premature birth.
- Diagnosis is typically made using polymerase chain reaction (PCR).
- Treatment generally involves antibiotics such as doxycycline, azithromycin, or levofloxacin.
- Management of pregnancy cases necessitates a critical assessment according to established guidelines.
- Partner therapy is obligatory in all cases.
- Screening for chlamydia during pregnancy is a standard practice.
- Adequate education about sexually transmitted diseases and condom use can contribute significantly to prevention efforts.

Condylomata Acuminata

18

Abstract

Condylomata acuminata, a condition resulting from infection by human papillomaviruses (HPV), presents predominantly as warts in the anogenital region. Multiple types of HPV have been identified, with types 6 and 11 primarily associated with genital warts. Conversely, high-risk types, such as HPV 16 and 18, are linked to the development of precancerous lesions. Transmission predominantly occurs through sexual contact; however, vertical transmission during childbirth has also been documented. Diagnosis is based on clinical evaluation, with biopsies used in certain cases. Treatment options depend on the specific symptoms observed. While the available treatments have proven effective, the virus cannot be eliminated. Preventive measures, including vaccination against specific HPV types in alignment with national vaccination guidelines, are recommended to thwart the onset of genital warts and precancerous lesions. Additionally, individuals are encouraged to limit sexual partners and utilize condoms to mitigate infection risk.

18.1 Background

Human papillomaviruses (HPV) infect the epithelial cells of skin or mucous membranes, leading to unregulated cellular proliferation. This process results in the formation of warts at the infection site; however, specific HPV types may induce malignant transformations.

In recent decades, substantial advancements in pathogenesis, diagnostics, and therapeutic approaches have emerged. Notably, the introduction of prophylactic vaccines targeting specific HPV types for the prevention of Condylomata acuminata and precancerous cervical lesions has significantly influenced contemporary medical practice. Moreover, HPV infections have been implicated in an increasing variety of malignancies, including vulvar, penile, and anal carcinoma.

I. Mylonas, *Sexually Transmitted Diseases*,
https://doi.org/10.1007/978-3-031-78204-6_18

While an HPV infection is a key prerequisite for carcinoma development, it is crucial to consider various other factors—both endogenous (e.g., immunosuppression, genetic predisposition) and exogenous (e.g., HIV, chlamydia infection, smoking)—to fully understand carcinoma manifestation. Enhanced monitoring of women affected by the disease is essential to facilitate early recognition and intervention for precancerous stages.

18.2 Pathogen

Condylomata acuminata are attributed to human papillomaviruses (HPV), which are classified as double-stranded DNA viruses (dsDNA) within the Papillomaviridae family, and are nonenveloped in structure. To date, over 150 HPV genotypes have been identified.

These viruses are associated with numerous diseases, and a range of benign skin conditions can arise from different HPV types (Table 18.1). Such conditions include verruca plana, verruca vulgaris, verruca plantaris, epidermodysplasia verruciformis, and genital warts (condylomata acuminata).

Furthermore, these viruses are recognized as principal etiological agents in various cancers, such as cervical, anal, vulvar, vaginal, and oropharyngeal carcinomas. Certain high-risk HPV types are correlated with an elevated risk of cancer development.

Table 18.1 Benign cutaneous conditions associated with different HPV types

HPV pathogens	Clinical manifestation
Verruca plana	– Flat, pinhead-sized, white to light brown, itchy warts with a smooth surface on the hands and face in children and adolescents – Common in immunosuppressed patients
Verruca vulgaris	– Pinhead to pea-sized, gray, hard warts with a fissured, hyperkeratotic surface on the back of the hands and feet, wrists, and face
Verruca plantaris	– Wide and flat, deep, painful warts on the balls of the toes and heels, less so on the soles of the feet in children – Transmission often occurs in bathing establishments
Epidermodysplasia verruciformis	– Rarely occurring, generalized, dysplastic, gray-white to yellow-brownish, scaly keratosis – Especially on the extremities in children with a genetic disposition – Often associated with immunodeficiencies – Malignant degeneration is possible after 10–20 years
Genital warts (condylomata acuminata)	– Wreath-shaped, pale to reddish, flat and pointed condylomas on the penis, vulva, cervix uteri, and in the anal region – Common in immunosuppressed and pregnant patients. Malignant degeneration is rare

- **HPV Subdivision.**
  - **Low-Risk HPV Types (LR Types):** Types 6 and 11 are predominantly associated with Condylomata acuminata.
  - **High-Risk HPV Types (HR Types):** These include the most prevalent genotypes, namely, types 16 and 18, with types 31, 33, 39, 45, and 59 also being significant.

Double or multiple infections with varying genotypes are common. Approximately 30–80% of the adult population is estimated to be infected with HPV. However, persistent infection occurs in only 10-30% of cases among women.

Most infections are transmitted through sexual contact with HPV-positive individuals, accounting for an estimated prevalence of approximately 70%. Additionally, transmission may arise through direct physical contact, with the potential inoculation of infectious material via small cutaneous lesions.

Only about 1% of sexually active adolescents exhibit condylomata.

18.3 Epidemiology

HPV constitutes a significant global health challenge and is recognized as the most prevalent sexually transmitted infection, primarily affecting individuals aged 15–24 years. The predominant mode of HPV transmission occurs through vaginal or anal intercourse, although oral–genital and genital–genital contact may also facilitate transmission. Studies of heterosexual couples indicate that the transmission rates from women to men exceed those from men to women.

The prevalence of HPV is markedly greater in developing nations, particularly across regions such as Africa and Asia, with young women exhibiting particularly high rates. In most developed countries, HPV prevalence is estimated at approximately 1–6% among women and 1–3% among men. An increasing trend in prevalence, notably in underdeveloped areas, suggests a potential rise in HPV-positive women to an estimated 17% by 2025.

- **Regions with High Cervical HPV Prevalence:**
  - Sub-Saharan Africa: 24%.
  - Latin America/Caribbean: 16%.
  - Eastern Europe: 14%.
  - South-East Asia: 14%.

- **Prevalence by Cytology:**
  - Normal Cytology: 2.8%.
  - Low-Grade Lesions: 21.7%.
  - High-Grade Lesions: 55–70%.
  - Cervical Cancer: 52.3–90%.

The annual incidence of anogenital warts is estimated at 160–289 cases per 100,000 individuals. The majority of HPV infections are self-limiting, with approximately 90% resolving within 2 years. For young women, HPV prevalence peaks between ages 20 and 24, whereas HPV prevalence in men remains steady through ages 50–60.

- **Prevalence and Incidence of Condyloma Acuminata (Genital Warts):**
  - **Worldwide:** The prevalence of condyloma acuminata ranges from 5% to 20% globally. While often asymptomatic, condyloma acuminata can adversely affect psychological well-being and diminish quality of life.
  - **United States:** An annual incidence of approximately 1% makes it one of the most prevalent sexually transmitted diseases, with reports indicating that prevalence may exceed 50%.
  - **International:** The variable prevalence indicates that HPV infections resulting in condyloma acuminata are at least as common in different countries, such as England, Panama, Italy, and the Netherlands, spanning both developed and developing regions.
  - **High-Risk Groups:** Older teenagers and young adults in their twenties represent the demographics at highest risk, with notable increases in prevalence documented over the past two decades.

Condyloma acuminata (genital warts), are exceedingly prevalent, with a global prevalence ranging between 5% and 20%. In the United States, the prevalence is estimated to exceed 50%, with an annual incidence rate of approximately 1%. The demographic groups at the highest risk of contracting this infection include young adults and older teenagers. Furthermore, there has been a substantial increase in prevalence over the past two decades.

HPV infections are frequently observed shortly following the commencement of sexual activity. The cumulative incidence of HPV infection among young women in the first year after their initial sexual intercourse is 28.5%, rising to nearly 50% within 3 years. Even women aged 18–25 with a single sexual partner may exhibit an infection rate of up to 15%. With two sexual partners, the incidence ascends to 22.3%, and in the case of more than three partners, it reaches 31.5%.

The precise mechanism of HPV transmission to the newborn remains unclear; vertical transmission during delivery is likely the predominant route. However, it is also conceivable for a pregnant woman to contract HPV prior to childbirth, as evidenced by HPV detection in the amniotic fluid of women with cervical HPV lesions.

Instances of newborns contracting HPV following cesarean delivery with an intact amniotic sac have been documented.

The risk of newborn HPV infection during vaginal delivery is estimated at one case per 231–400 births, although lower incidences (up to one case per 10,000 births) have been reported under specific circumstances. Nevertheless, comprehensive epidemiological studies for precise risk assessment are still required.

Socio-demographic factors, such as early marriages, elevated divorce rates, and lower levels of education, have been associated with a heightened prevalence of HPV. Research further indicates that the risk of infection escalates in individuals with a higher number of sexual partners, placing both women and men with multiple partners at increased risk of HPV infection.

18.4 Clinical Manifestation

18.4.1 Gynecology

The clinical presentation of condylomata acuminata is influenced by the predominant HPV types, particularly the low-risk types 6 and 11.

The clinical manifestation of condyloma acuminata is characterized by variable appearance, including wreath-shaped, pale to reddish, small- to medium-sized, cauliflower-like condylomas, some of which may exhibit pigmentation. The most common sites for these condylomas are the posterior commissure and the perianal area.

Typically, condylomata acuminata do not present with additional symptoms. However, localized itching or burning may occur in some individuals. The presence of these growths can be bothersome due to their appearance and size, despite the absence of visible condylomas not excluding the possibility of an HPV infection.

The absence of visible genital warts does not exclude the possibility of an HPV infection.

18.4.2 Pregnancy

In cases of extensive condylomata acuminata in the birth canal, there is a potential risk for the newborn to contract HPV during delivery. Nonetheless, the limited viral presence detected in condylomas suggests that the risk of transmission remains low. Therefore, a cesarean section is only warranted in rare circumstances. Currently, no reliable data is available to quantify the frequency of peripartum HPV transmission.

18.4.3 Neonatology

Laryngeal papillomatosis is one of the most common manifestations of HPV in newborns and infants. The initial manifestation is often a rough or hoarse change in voice, not easily discernible in newborns. Consequently, diagnosis is typically established at an average age of 6 years.

As the condition progresses, symptoms may include chronic coughing and shortness of breath. Difficulty swallowing and recurrent pneumonia may also arise. Papillomatosis can potentially extend to the nasopharynx, esophagus, and deeper airways.

At this time, cesarean delivery for maternal Condylomata acuminata is not recommended solely as a preventive measure against laryngeal papillomatosis. However, in instances of extensive Condylomata (Buschke-Löwenstein tumor) that could obstruct the birth canal, cesarean delivery may be warranted.

18.5 Diagnosis

The diagnosis of condylomata acuminata is primarily clinical. A biopsy may be performed for confirmation, particularly when lesions appear atypical, hardened, pigmented, or integrated with surrounding tissue (Fig. 18.1). Typically, condylomas are observed as pale to reddish lesions arranged in a ring formation (Fig. 18.2), displaying diverse morphological characteristics. Biopsies may also be warranted if there are uncertainties in diagnosis, if lesions do not respond to conventional therapy, or if they worsen under treatment.

Application of 3% acetic acid to the cervix (Fig. 18.3) or vulva (Fig. 18.4) can reveal subclinical infections by visualizing white spots. Subclinical infections may also be analyzed through DNA detection using hybridization or polymerase chain reaction (PCR).

Cervical lesions are typically identified via routine cervical cancer screening protocols. These screening guidelines vary across different countries and are determined by national recommendations. For women with abnormal screening outcomes, colposcopy followed by targeted biopsy remains the standard diagnostic approach for assessing lesions and invasive cervical carcinomas.

HPV testing is increasingly used alongside cervical cytology (Papanicolaou smear) screening programs for the early detection of intra-cervical neoplasia in numerous countries.

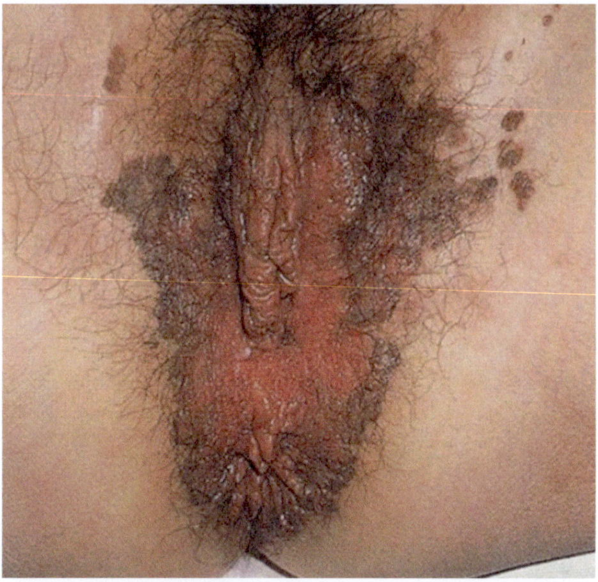

Fig. 18.1 Condylomata acuminata (pigmented) (Mylonas 2010)

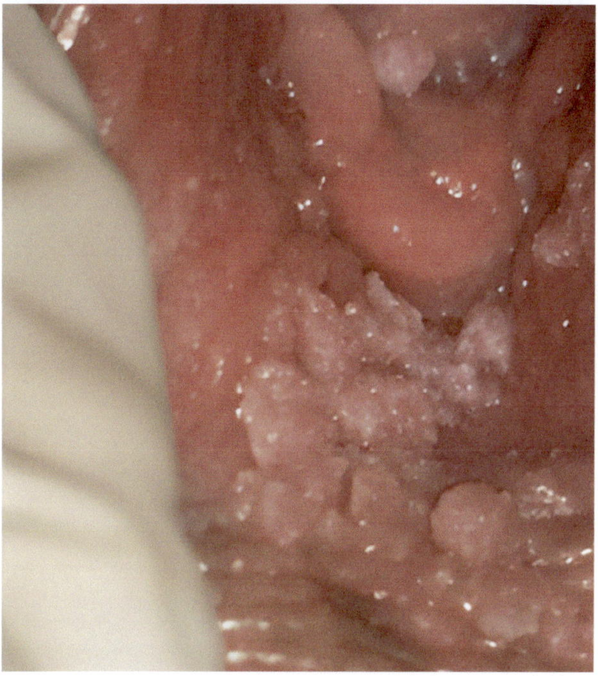

Fig. 18.2 Condylomata acuminata: The characteristic morphology of the condyloma is distinctly recognizable (Mylonas 2016)

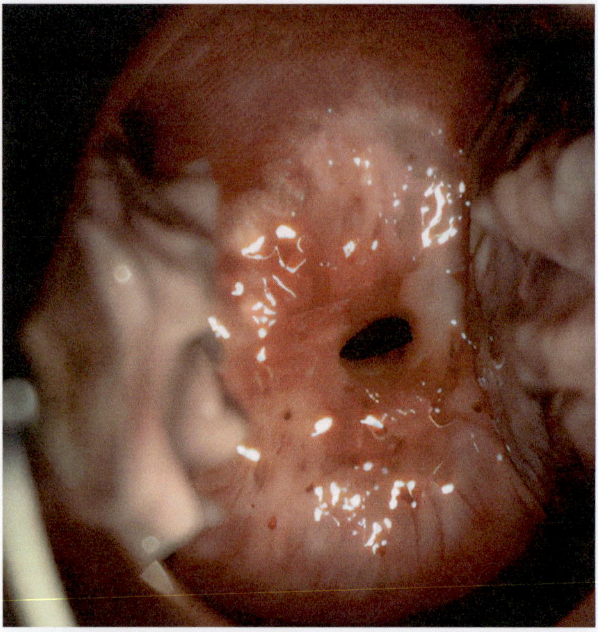

Fig. 18.3 Cervical intraepithelial neoplasia (CIN2) (Mylonas 2016)

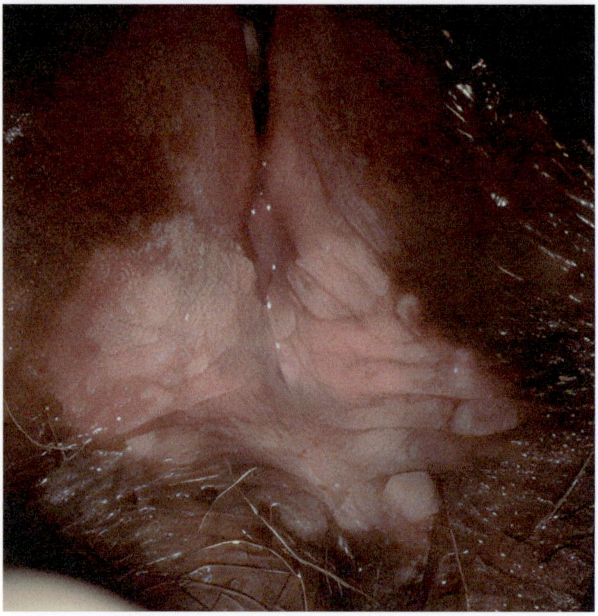

Fig. 18.4 Vulvar intraepithelial neoplasia (VIN2) (Mylonas 2016)

18.6 Treatment

The treatment approach focuses on managing the clinical manifestations of human papillomavirus (HPV) infection rather than directly targeting the underlying infection itself (Fig. 18.5). This approach is necessary because HPV infections are often self-limited, and the immune system can frequently clear the virus over time.

In most cases, spontaneous remission occurs, even without intervention, warranting a watch-and-wait strategy.

If spontaneous remission does not materialize, or if the patient experiences considerable discomfort, surgical excision of the condylomas may be necessary (Table 18.2). For smaller lesions, topical drug therapy might be considered.

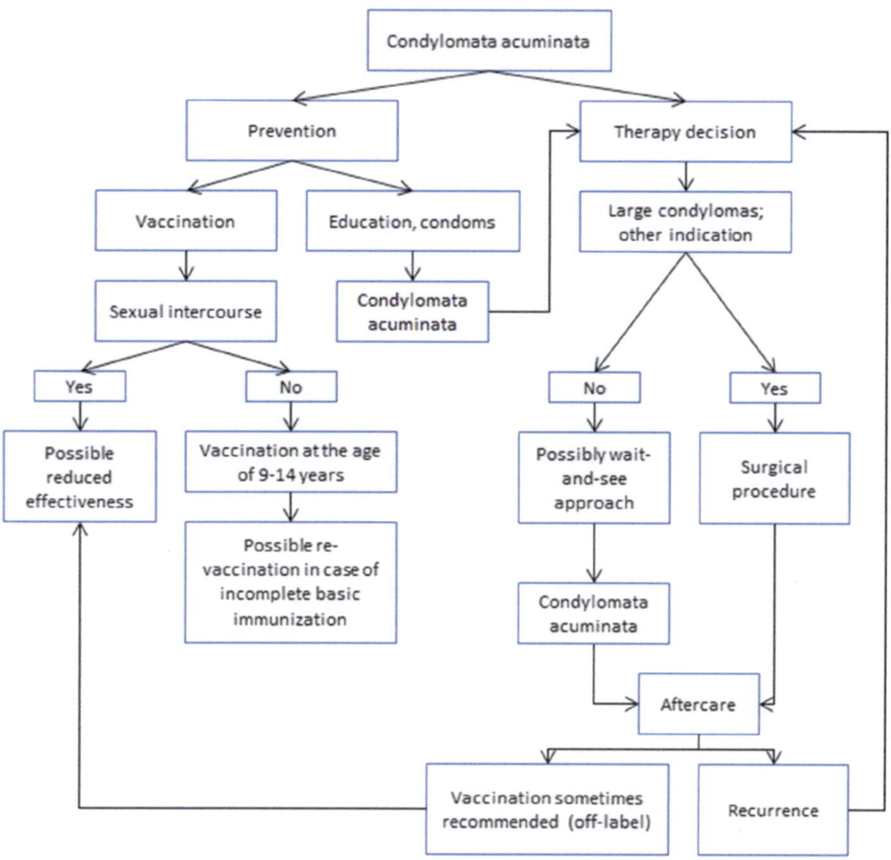

Fig. 18.5 Management protocol for condylomata acuminata. (Courtesy of I. Mylonas)

Table 18.2 Conservative management options for isolated condylomata acuminata (maximum treatable wart area: 10 cm^2)

Medication	Comments
Podophyllotoxin	– 0.5% solution applied with a cotton swab two times a day for 3 days – 0.15% cream applied with the finger two times a day for 3 days on genital warts followed by a 4-day break – Repeat for a maximum of four cycles – Maximum daily dose: 0.5 mL – Caution: Increased toxic effects when applied to overlapping skin due to strong absorption – Application only by a physician – Contraindication: Pregnancy, immunosuppression
Interferon β gel	– Local therapy after surgical removal: Five times a day for 4 weeks – Maximum treatable area: <10 cm^2 – Contraindication: Pregnancy, immunosuppression
Imiquimod (5% cream)	– Three times a week (at night) for a maximum of 16 weeks – Wash off the area with water 6–10 h later – Side effect: Flu-like symptoms may occur – Contraindication: Pregnancy, immunosuppression
Trichloroacetic acid 80–85% (local)	– Sparing application to lesions – Trichloroacetic acid is applied to the warts by the physician using an applicator, causing cell necrosis – Repeat after 2 weeks if necessary – Good results are achieved with small, nonkeratinized condylomata acuminata in mucosal areas – Safe use during pregnancy – Overdose: Neutralization with sodium carbonate – Side effect: Burning and pain
Sinecatechin or green tea catechins (10–15% ointment)	– Three times a day for up to 16 weeks – Mild local skin reactions (redness, itching, skin irritation, pain) – Contraindication: Pregnancy – Caution: Damage to condoms

However, in cases where Condylomata acuminata are recurrent or extensive, surgical interventions such as excision, electrosurgery, or laser therapy are also utilized (Table 18.3). It is important to emphasize that these treatment modalities are aimed at removing visible lesions and alleviating symptoms but do not eliminate the underlying HPV infection. The virus may persist in latent form within the host, and recurrence of lesions remains possible.

Preventative vaccination is recommended, ideally before the onset of sexual activity for young girls. A therapeutic vaccination is not available yet.

Table 18.3 Therapeutic options for large or extensive condylomata acuminata

Options	Comments
Surgical therapy	– Indications: Electrocautery or laser treatment is recommended for extensive or recurrent warts
	– Removal Techniques: Condylomata acuminata can be removed using scissors, sharp instruments, curettage, electrocautery, or CO_2/Nd:YAG laser
	– Anesthesia: Always required during these procedures
Liquid nitrogen (cryotherapy)	– Applied through the spray method, a cotton swab, or contact cryotherapy using a closed procedure with a cryoprobe (CO_2, N_2O, N_2)
	– Therapy should be repeated weekly or biweekly as needed
	– Caution: May cause deep necrosis, contraindicated for anal or urethral use
	– Complications: Initial local complications may arise following treatment
	– Recurrence: Recurrence rates are high, reaching up to 75%

It is important to begin treatment promptly to prevent the lesions from spreading or growing. Due to the high likelihood of recurrence, regular follow-up examinations are crucial. In instances of perianal lesions, a proctologic evaluation should be conducted, as approximately 50% of cases may reveal additional rectal infestations. In cases of severe infection, the possibility of concurrent HIV infection should be considered. Patients should also be encouraged to discuss the examination and potential treatment of their partners.

Management of cervical intraepithelial neoplasia (CIN), particularly CIN2 and CIN3, is primarily surgical, focusing on excising the affected areas via electrosurgery. For adenocarcinoma *in situ*, treatment generally involves conization or hysterectomy, whereas the management of cervical carcinoma is contingent upon the disease stage, tumor size, patient age, and fertility preservation desires. Surgical measures, including electrosurgical excision, radiation therapy, and chemotherapy, are employed based on national guidelines and recommendations.

Currently, there is no definitive treatment for laryngeal papillomatosis in children. Surgical interventions (such as endoscopic laser techniques) aim to eliminate HPV while preserving anatomical structures and ensuring airway patency. In severe cases, various medical treatment options (like antivirals or immunomodulators) may be utilized, although their efficacy remains to be fully established.

18.7 Differential Diagnosis

In the differential diagnosis of condylomata acuminata, it is important to consider other diseases that may present with similar symptoms. These include condylomata lata in syphilis, mollusca contagiosa, genital herpes, and seborrheic keratoses (Table 18.4).

Table 18.4 Differential diagnoses for condylomata acuminata

Differential diagnosis	Features
Condylomata lata (syphilis)	– Flat, weeping papules or plaques – Often in the genital or anal area – Can occur in combination with other syphilis symptoms
Genital herpes	– Grouped, painful blisters or ulcerations – Itching and burning – May be prone to recurrent episodes
Mollusca contagiosa	– Small, firm-elastic papules with a central dent – Common in children and immunocompromised patients – Can occur in the genital region
Papilloma	– Benign epithelial tumors – Often stalked or wart-like – Can occur in the genital area, but are rare
Seborrheic keratosis	– Benign, wart-like skin changes – Often brownish or blackish in color – Usually occur at an older age, rarely genital
Verrucae planae (flat warts)	– Flat, slightly raised papules – Often multiple and arranged in groups – Can occur in the genital area, but are rare
Verrucae vulgares	– Thickened squamous epithelium – Irregular, thickened surface – Frequently on hands and feet, rarely in the genital area

18.8 Prevention

18.8.1 General

The correct use of condoms can reduce the risk of HPV and HPV-associated diseases (e.g., genital warts, cervical cancer) by up to 70%. The only effective method of preventing genital HPV infections is by abstaining from sexual activity, which entails refraining from genital contact with another person. Individuals who are sexually active can reduce their risk by limiting the number of sexual partners or choosing a partner with few or no previous sexual partners. Additionally, counseling about HPV can be beneficial for patients.

18.8.2 Vaccination

The HPV vaccine is an effective means of prevention (Table 18.5). The vaccines are based on non-infectious, recombinant type-specific L1 capsid proteins in "viral-like particles" (VLP) as immunogens. The vaccines are not produced in cell cultures but rather with the assistance of genetically modified yeast or insect cells. Approval of the vaccines varies slightly, and most health authorities recommend using the same vaccine whenever possible. Different HPV vaccines offer immunity against varying numbers of HPV types:

- **Bivalent Vaccines**: Protect against two virus types, specifically HPV 16 and HPV 18.

Table 18.5 HPV vaccination strategies

Basics	Comments
General	– The HPV vaccination is a standard vaccination (routine vaccination) for girls/women and boys/men
	– Genital warts are mainly caused by the low-risk types 6 and 11. HPV 40, 42, 44, 54, or 61 occur less frequently
	– HPV vaccination is possible against the two high-risk types (double HPV vaccine—HPV types 16 and 18) and nine HPV vaccines (HPV types 6, 11, 16, 18, 31, 33, 45, 52, 58)
	– The complete vaccination series should be completed before the first sexual intercourse
	– Women and men over the age of 17 who have not yet received the HPV vaccine can still gain benefits from vaccination. However, its effectiveness is reduced in individuals who have already been exposed to HPV
Basic immunization	– **Girls:** Ages 9–14 years (dual and nine-dose HPV vaccine), two doses 6 months apart
	– **Boys:** Age 9–14 years with two doses 6 months apart
"Catch-up" vaccination	– **Girls:** Age > 13 years or > 14 years or if there is a vaccination interval of <6 or < 5 months between the first and second dose, a third vaccination dose is required (observe the information in the information for healthcare professionals)
	– **Boys:** Age 17 years

- **Tetravalent Vaccines**: Protect against four virus types—namely, HPV 6, 11, 16, and 18.
- **Nonavalent Vaccines**: Protect against nine virus types, including HPV 6, 11, 16, 18, 31, 33, 45, 52, and 58.

All vaccines demonstrate high efficacy in preventing HPV-specific cervical intraepithelial neoplasia. Clinical studies have shown that these HPV vaccines are highly effective in preventing CIN2, CIN3, and anal intraepithelial neoplasia (AIN), with efficacy rates exceeding 93%. The tetravalent HPV vaccine has similarly high efficacy (up to 80%) in preventing anogenital warts. It is anticipated that European approval of a nonavalent vaccine, targeting multiple HPV types, will be granted in the near future.

The vaccines have a preventive effect and are most effective when given before HPV infection, ideally before the first sexual intercourse. Despite suboptimal acceptance of vaccination in several countries, recent studies indicate that vaccination, particularly against the primary causes of genital warts (HPV 6 and 11), can reduce the incidence of these infections by up to 80%. In Australia, where vaccination is mandatory during school years, a reduction in genital warts was observed not only in vaccinated girls but also in unvaccinated boys, illustrating the "herd effect"[1].

[1] Herd immunity, also known as the "herd effect," arises when a substantial proportion of a population develops immunity to an infectious disease, either through vaccination or prior infection. This leads to a reduction in the overall transmission of the disease, indirectly protecting individuals who remain susceptible. Consequently, unvaccinated or non-immune individuals are less likely to be exposed to the disease, thereby decreasing their risk of infection.

Consequently, it can be concluded that vaccination against condylomata acuminata is highly effective. However, confirmation of its efficacy against cervical carcinomas will require long-term studies.

In healthy women over 30 years of age, the incidence of HPV infection is approximately 5%. For women with CIN1, the incidence increases to around 50%, while it is approximately 75% for CIN2, 95% for CIN3, and can reach up to 98% in those with cervical carcinoma.

18.8.3 Early Detection of Cervical Cancer

In several countries, new regulations have been implemented for the early detection of cervical cancer, utilizing HPV testing either as a replacement for the annual cytological smear (Papanicolaou test) or in conjunction with it. A crucial aspect of these programs is the introduction of a new clarification algorithm, which is designed to assist healthcare providers in effectively managing abnormal test results.

Cytological findings from Pap tests are carefully classified according to the 5-tier Papanicolaou scale, as well as the Munich nomenclature III for gynecological cytodiagnostics (see Table 18.6). These classifications enable clinicians to determine the most appropriate follow-up care for patients based on their test results, ensuring timely and effective interventions when necessary.

Key Points

- Human papillomaviruses (HPV) can cause warts and malignant changes and are associated with various types of carcinoma, including those affecting the vulva, penis, and anus.
- The development of carcinomas is influenced by additional factors, including endogenous (e.g., immunosuppression) and exogenous (e.g., smoking) factors.
- HPV are double-stranded DNA viruses belonging to the Papillomaviridae family, with over 150 genotypes classified into low-risk (LR, types 6, 11) and high-risk (HR, types 16, 18, 31, 33, 45, 59).

(continued)

- HPV infections are prevalent, yet only a minority of women experience persistent infection.
- HPV is primarily transmitted through sexual intercourse, with women exhibiting higher transmission rates than men.
- HPV infection is often self-limiting.
- It is possible for the virus to be transmitted from mother to child at birth, although this is a rare occurrence.
- HPV can manifest in various forms, including ring-shaped warts with pale to reddish coloration, which may vary in size and occasionally be pigmented. These lesions are most commonly observed in the area of the posterior commissure and perianal region.
- The symptoms of an HPV infection are typically mild, with localized itching or burning occasionally occurring.
- The risk of HPV transmission to newborns is low, which is why a cesarean section is rarely necessary. Laryngeal papillomatosis can manifest as an HPV-related condition in newborns and infants, although diagnosis is often delayed.
- Diagnosis is primarily clinical, with a biopsy required for atypical features.
- Subclinical HPV infections can be identified via acetic acid tests and HPV DNA detection tests.
- Screening for cervical cancer varies considerably between countries, with treatment options including a wait-and-see approach and surgical interventions.
- The most effective method of prevention is the administration of prophylactic HPV vaccination prior to the initiation of sexual activity. A variety of vaccines are currently available that protect against specific HPV types and reduce the incidence of genital warts.
- The use of condoms has been demonstrated to significantly reduce the risk of HPV infection.

Table 18.6 Nomenclature for gynecologic cytology, including Papanicolaou Classification, Bethesda System, American Classification, BSCC Guidelines, Munich Classification, and WHO Classification

Category	Papanicolaou Classification	Bethesda System	American Classification	BSCC Guidelines	Munich Classification	WHO Classification
1. Inadequate sample	Class 0: Inadequate or unsatisfactory	Unsatisfactory for evaluation	Unsatisfactory	Inadequate	Group 0: Insufficient material	Category 0: Specimen rejected/inadequate
Next steps	Repeat smear	Repeat smear	Repeat smear	Repeat smear	Repeat smear	Repeat smear
2. Negative for intraepithelial lesion or malignancy (NILM)	Class I: Normal	Negative for intraepithelial lesion or malignancy	NILM	Negative	Group I: Unsuspicious findings	Category 1: Normal
Next steps	Routine screening intervals	Routine screening intervals	Routine screening intervals	Routine screening intervals	Routine screening intervals	Routine screening
3. Atypical squamous cells	Class II: Atypical cells, reactive or repair	ASC-US	ASC-US	Borderline changes in squamous cells (BNA)	Group II: Limited protective value	Category 2: Infection or inflammation
		ASC-H	ASC-H	Severe dyskaryosis	Group III: Dubious findings	
Next steps		Colposcopy	Colposcopy	Colposcopy	Colposcopy	
4. Low-grade lesions (LSIL)	Class III: Mild dysplasia (CIN 1)	LSIL	LSIL	Low-grade dyskaryosis	Group IIp: Minor nuclear changes	Category 3: Squamous cell abnormality grade I
Next steps		Colposcopy if persistent	Colposcopy if persistent	Colposcopy if persistent	Colposcopy if persistent	
5. High-grade lesions (HSIL)	Class III: Moderate to severe dysplasia (CIN 2/3)	HSIL	HSIL	High-grade dyskaryosis (moderate)	Group IIIp: Immature cover cells	Category 4: Squamous cell abnormality grade II/III
				High-grade dyskaryosis (severe)	Group IV: Immediate preliminary stages	

Next steps		Colposcopy, biopsy, treatment	Colposcopy, biopsy, treatment	Colposcopy, biopsy, treatment	Differential colposcopy, therapy where necessary	Biopsy and treatment
6. Glandular abnormalities	Class III: Glandular atypia	AGC	AGC	Borderline changes in glandular cells	Group IIIg: Atypical glandular cells	Category 5: Glandular abnormality
		AIS	AIS	Glandular neoplasia	Group IIIe: Abnormal endometrial cells	Category 6: Adenocarcinoma in situ
Next steps		Colposcopy, further sampling	Colposcopy, further sampling	Colposcopy, endometrial sampling, biopsy if needed	Comprehensive diagnostics and follow-up	Comprehensive diagnostics and follow-up
7. Malignancy	Class V: Malignant cells	Squamous cell carcinoma, adenocarcinoma	Malignant cells	Glandular/ malignant neoplasia	Group V: Malignant cells (cancer)	Category 7: Malignancy
Next steps	Immediate diagnostic workup, staging, treatment	Immediate diagnostic workup, staging, treatment	Immediate diagnostic workup, staging, treatment	Biopsy, oncologic assessment, treatment planning	Comprehensive diagnostics and appropriate treatment	Immediate diagnostic workup, staging, treatment

AGC Atypical glandular cells, *AIS* Adenocarcinoma in situ, *ASC-H* Atypical squamous cells, cannot exclude high-grade squamous intraepithelial lesion, *ASC-US* Atypical squamous cells of undetermined significance, *BNA* Borderline nuclear abnormalities, *CIN* Cervical intraepithelial neoplasia, *HSIL* High-grade squamous intraepithelial lesion, *LSIL* Low-grade squamous intraepithelial lesion, *NILM* Negative for intraepithelial lesion or malignancy

Granuloma Inguinale

19

Abstract

Granuloma inguinale, also referred to as donovanosis, is a sexually transmitted disease caused by the bacterium *Calymmatobacterium granulomatis* (formerly *Klebsiella granulomatis*). It results in genital ulcers and predominantly affects men, especially in tropical regions. It is also associated with pregnancy and HIV infection. Common symptoms include painless ulcers that bleed easily, potentially leading to severe complications, including elephantiasis if untreated. Diagnosis is confirmed through microscopic examination for Donovan bodies. Treatment generally involves antibiotics, such as tetracyclines or trimethoprim-sulfamethoxazole. In cases of concurrent HIV infection, therapy must be adjusted accordingly. Preventive measures include the use of condoms, along with regular testing for coinfection.

19.1 Background

Granuloma inguinale, also known as Donovanosis or granuloma venereum, is an infectious venereal disease first documented in 1905 by tropical physician Charles Donovan. The disease induces ulcers in the genital region that typically bleed upon contact. Following the identification of the causative bacterium and the development of antimicrobial treatments, interest in Grnuloma inguinale declined until the late 1980s. However, recent years have witnessed a resurgence in research focusing on its role as a cofactor in HIV infections.

I. Mylonas, *Sexually Transmitted Diseases*,
https://doi.org/10.1007/978-3-031-78204-6_19

19.2 Pathogen

The pathogen responsible for granuloma inguinale, *Calymmatobacterium granulomatis*, is a gram-negative, encapsulated, nonmotile bacterium that replicates intracellularly. These pathogens reside within large mononuclear cells, forming identifiable structures known as Donovan bodies. Genetically, *Calymmatobacterium* species are closely related to *Klebsiella*, prompting the proposal of *Klebsiella granulomatis* as a more accurate nomenclature. Currently, there is no evidence of a host reservoir outside of humans.

19.3 Epidemiology

Transmission of the infection occurs primarily through sexual intercourse and nonvenereal contact. The incubation period may vary from a few days to 12 weeks. Granuloma inguinale exhibits a heterogeneous distribution globally, with endemic regions primarily in South Africa, parts of Southeast Asia, Caribbean islands, and Aboriginal areas in Central Australia. The prevalence of granuloma inguinale demonstrates regional disparities:

- In South Africa, the disease has historically shown a high incidence in rural KwaZulu-Natal. Although the rates are declining, cases continue to be reported in remote communities.
- Southeast Asia, particularly India, Papua New Guinea, and Indonesia, harbors endemic pockets where the disease accounts for approximately 10–15% of genital ulcer cases in some clinics. It is notably more prevalent in this region, contributing significantly to gender-specific ulcerative diseases, especially in Southeast Asia and India.
- In Central Australia, the disease is recognized among Aboriginal populations in the Top End region, with ongoing control efforts in place.
- The Caribbean Islands, including Grenada and neighboring islands, are also endemic regions, with travel-associated cases occasionally reported among visitors.
- Latin America, particularly Brazil, experiences higher incidence rates concentrated in northern and northeastern states, with an estimated rate of 2–5 cases per 100,000 population annually. The disease is more common in this region compared to many others.
- In the United States, approximately 80–120 cases are reported each year, predominantly among individuals from endemic regions or recent immigrants. In Europe, the incidence remains low overall, with most cases occurring among travelers returning from endemic areas.

The incidence of the disease in the male population is approximately ten times higher than in females. Pregnancy is believed to play a role in the manifestation of the condition among women.

19.4 Clinical Manifestation

19.4.1 Gynecology

Following an average incubation period of 7–10 days, a painless, pruritic, vesiculo-pustular papule or nodule typically forms, transitioning to a granulomatous lesion that exulcerates within days. The epidermis over these lesions is fragile and susceptible to bleeding with minimal mechanical stress. Lesions may manifest either singularly or in a recurrent pattern. The clinical presentation can vary significantly, with manifestations ranging from slight bleeding to ulcerative or verrucous changes. Hypertrophic and sclerotic skin changes may also occur (Fig. 19.1).

The ulcerations are generally painless, often leading patients to seek medical attention only when the condition is advanced.

In untreated cases, lesions may extend peripherally, creating large, reddish, "beet-shaped" ulcerogranulomatous areas. Hemorrhagic-purulent lesions may develop in the anogenital region and spread to the groin, though fluor vaginalis is rarely observed (Fig. 19.2).

Most patients demonstrate preserved general health, though secondary changes in the groin can be painful. Occasionally, the primary symptom may present as a palpable submucosal mass in the rectum. Primary infections may also occur in the face, throat, neck, mouth, or intestines. In these cases, palpation findings or

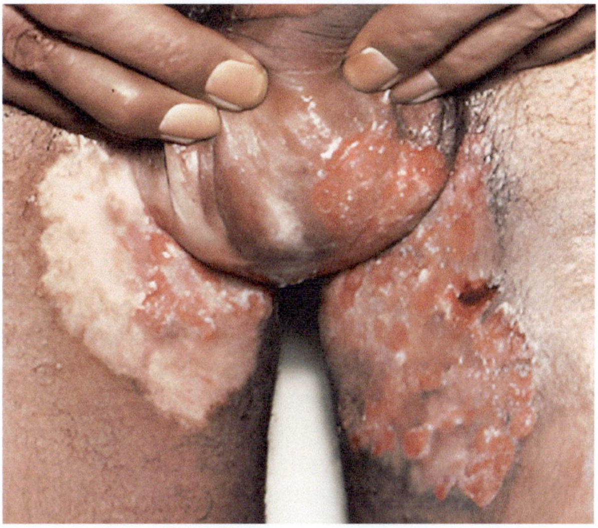

Fig. 19.1 Granuloma inguinale (Zangerle et al. 2018)

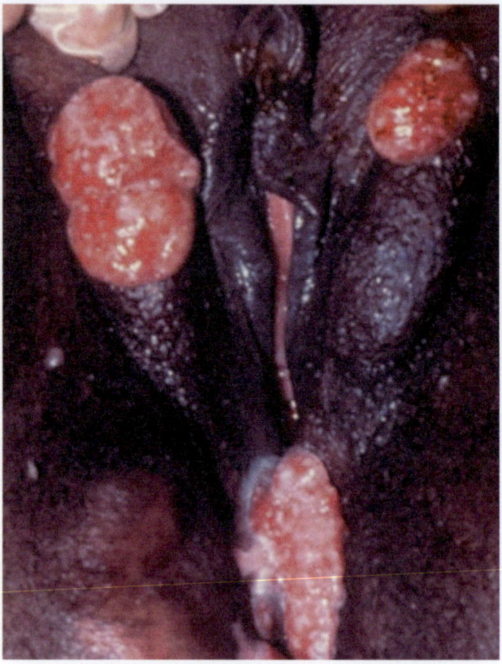

Fig. 19.2 Clinically, donovanosis can manifest in different forms, including ulcerative lesions with raised borders, vegetative lesions, or extragenital lesions (Leal Passos et al. 2018)

ultrasound examinations may reveal inflammation. In rare circumstances, systemic dissemination can lead to osteomyelitis.

As the disease advances, the inguinal area may exhibit swelling and tenderness originating from the subcutaneous tissue. Notably, the raised inguinal wall remains uninfiltrated, with no involvement of the lymph nodes - a phenomenon referred to as pseudobuboes. Without treatment, the infection may induce secondary obstruction of lymphatic vessels, resulting in elephantiasis of the labia or penis and scrotum.

Following healing, residual scarring may persist, which may, in select instances, lead to lymphatic congestion and severe cases of elephantiasis.

19.4.2 Pregnancy

In pregnant patients, granuloma inguinale (donovanosis) is most commonly manifested by one or more painless, beefy-red nodules or papules that ulcerate and gradually enlarge. Lesions are generally confined to the vulva, perineum, and adjacent inguinal folds rather than involving deeper genital tract structures. Because ulceration progresses insidiously and often lacks marked pain or systemic features, presentation is frequently delayed until lesions have coalesced into large, raised, friable ulcers with exuberant granulation tissue and everted, rolled margins.

Despite a high local bacterial load within ulcers, transplacental transmission of *Klebsiella granulomatis* has not been documented, and intrauterine or intrapartum neonatal infection has not been confirmed even when extensive vulvoperineal lesions are present at delivery. Consequently, the risk of congenital or perinatal transmission is considered negligible, and adverse obstetric outcomes such as miscarriage, preterm labor, or fetal growth restriction have not been causally linked to maternal donovanosis. The overall course of pregnancy has been reported to remain unaffected by the infection, and systemic dissemination attributable solely to granuloma inguinale has not been observed in the postpartum period.

Physiologic immunologic and vascular adaptations of pregnancy may alter local disease expression. Progesterone-mediated immune modulation within genital mucosa and changes in local cell-mediated immunity can facilitate more rapid lesion expansion and florid granulation. Increased pelvic blood flow and tissue edema may augment friability and bleeding. As a result, pregnant patients may present with larger, more vascularized ulcers than nonpregnant patients at a comparable disease stage.

Granuloma inguinale likely does not affect the course of pregnancy. The causative pathogen does not disseminate postpartum, even when the birth canal is involved.

19.5 Diagnosis

Examination of the external genitalia reveals ulcerating, purulent, or hemorrhagic lesions suggestive of infection (Fig. 19.3). A thorough assessment of the patient's ethnic background or the sexual history of partners associated with endemic areas is essential to establish epidemiological correlations.

Microscopic diagnosis of granuloma inguinale (donovanosis) is confirmed by demonstrating Donovan bodies—intracellular, gram-negative, encapsulated bacilli (approximately 1–2 μm) within the phagosomal vacuoles of macrophages and histiocytes—characterized by bipolar chromatin condensation and a distinctive "safety-pin" appearance.

Giemsa stain is the preferred initial method; organisms appear intensely basophilic with a clear halo suggesting a capsule. If Giemsa results are equivocal, Warthin–Starry silver staining provides enhanced contrast, while Wright stain yields blue bacilli outlined by pink capsules. Suitable specimens include Papanicolaou smears, tissue biopsies, impression smears, and material obtained post-curettage.

Morphologically, the bacilli are pleomorphic—ranging from straight rods to curved, dumbbell-shaped forms—with the bipolar granules most prominent in elongated organisms. Culture on HEp-2 cell monolayers (in RPMI 1640 medium supplemented with fetal calf serum and appropriate antibiotics) requires specialized reference-laboratory facilities and extended incubation periods.

Molecular assays, notably PCR targeting species-specific genes, offer superior sensitivity and specificity and are strongly recommended when microscopic findings are inconclusive or precise organism identification is critical.

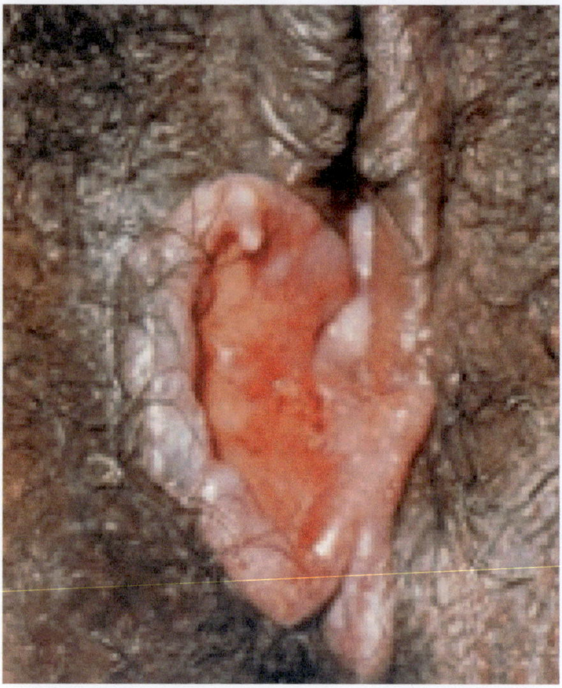

Fig. 19.3 Hypertrophic borders of skin lesion of donovanosis (Leal Passos et al. 2018)

Histopathological examination typically reveals scant epithelial cells, absence of Langhans-type giant cells, and a predominantly neutrophilic infiltrate. When available, electron microscopy can further confirm the diagnosis by visualizing the gram-negative cell-wall architecture and surrounding capsular material.

Recommended Diagnostic Algorithm

1. Perform rapid Giemsa or Wright staining for initial screening.
2. If findings are suggestive or unclear, apply Warthin–Starry silver stain and initiate PCR.
3. Reserve cell culture and electron microscopy for atypical presentations or definitive reference-laboratory confirmation.

Other bacterial superinfections can complicate preexisting ulcerated wounds and may lead to diagnostic misinterpretation.

19.6 Treatment

The causative pathogens exhibit sensitivity to tetracyclines, trimethoprim-sulfamethoxazole, fluoroquinolones, and macrolides. Effective treatment necessitates administering adequate doses over extended durations, as the pathogens reside intracellularly. Healing typically commences at the ulcer's periphery, progressing inward.

Doxycycline and trimethoprim-sulfamethoxazole are the preferred antibiotics. Alternative options include fluoroquinolones and macrolides, although data supporting their use remains limited. If patient symptoms do not improve within a few days of starting treatment, the addition of aminoglycosides (e.g., gentamicin 1 mg/kg intravenously every 8 h) may be considered as an adjunct therapy. Disinfectant compresses, such as those containing quinosol or potassium permanganate, may also be utilized.

- **First Choice:**
  - Azithromycin 1 g orally once per week on day 1, 8, and 15 or
  - Azithromycin 500 mg orally once daily for 21 days or until healing
- **Alternative Options:**
  - Co-trimoxazole 960 mg orally twice daily for 21–28 days or until healing or
  - Doxycycline 100 mg orally twice daily for 21 days or until healing or
  - Ciprofloxacin 500 mg orally twice daily for 21 days or until healing or
  - Erythromycin 500 mg orally four times daily for 21 days or until healing or
  - Clarithromycin 500 mg orally twice daily for 14 days or until healing or
  - Roxithromycin 300 mg orally once daily for 14 days or until healing
  - **Note:** Clarithromycin and roxithromycin have demonstrated positive effects; however, the currently available efficacy data remain limited.
- **Pregnancy:**
  - Erythromycin 500 mg orally/intravenously four times daily for 14–21 days or until healing
  - Azithromycin 1 g orally once per week on day 1, 8, and 15
  - Clarithromycin 250–500 mg orally twice daily for 14 days or until healing
  - **Note:** Azithromycin and clarithromycin should be used only after the first trimester and following a thorough evaluation, due to the potential risk of adverse effects.
- **Treatment Failure:**
  - Previously used antibiotic plus Gentamicin 1 mg/kg body weight intravenously three times daily until healing.

In the presence of concomitant HIV infection, the duration of treatment may need to be extended or simultaneous administration of aminoglycosides should be considered.

Spontaneous healing is unlikely without systemic treatment, and chronic infection may persist despite timely antibiotic intervention. Scarring may result from treatment, with recurrences possible between three and 18 months after what was previously considered successful antibiotic therapy. A subsequent clinical examination is therefore recommended. Additionally, sexual partners should be screened and treated if diagnosed within 60 days of the initial case.

A follow-up clinical examination is generally recommended three to six months after diagnosis. Many current guidelines, however, do not support repeat laboratory tests.

19.7 Differential Diagnosis

The differential diagnosis for granuloma inguinale includes genital herpes, lymphogranuloma venereum, pemphigus vegetans, primary or metastatic carcinoma, and syphilis.

19.8 Prevention

Given that the transmission of *Klebsiella granulomatis* predominantly occurs through sexual intercourse, the use of condoms constitutes an important preventive strategy. However, other potential nonvenereal transmission routes should also be considered.

Coinfections, including syphilis and HIV, are common and require serologic testing for those affected.

Prompt diagnosis allows for the commencement of suitable antibiotic treatment, with ulcerative lesions healing through scar formation. On the other hand, if left undiagnosed and untreated, there is a significant risk of progressing to elephantiasis, which carries a severe prognosis.

Key Points

- Granuloma inguinale (donovanosis, granuloma venereum) is a rare venereal disease caused by *Klebsiella granulomatis* (formerly *Calymmatobacterium granulomatis*).
- The disease is primarily transmitted through sexual intercourse or nonvenereal contact, with an incubation period varying from a few days to 12 weeks.
- Granuloma inguinale is most common in tropical and subtropical regions, occurring infrequently in Europe due to travel-related cases. Males are more frequently affected than females.
- Efflorescences are typically painless and itchy, potentially progressing to ulcerogranulomatous lesions. Lesions can vary in appearance and may be prone to bleeding.
- Current evidence suggests that the disease is not transmitted to fetuses or newborns, and it does not seem to affect pregnancy outcomes.
- Diagnosis involves clinical examination and identification of Donovan bodies using specific staining techniques.
- Antibiotic treatment typically includes tetracyclines, trimethoprim-sulfamethoxazole, or other comparable antibiotics.
- In patients with immunosuppression, treatment duration should be modified accordingly.

Genital Herpes (HSV-1 and HSV-2) 20

Abstract

Herpes simplex virus (HSV) infection is a common sexually transmitted disease, recognized as the etiologic agent of genital herpes. Two distinct types of herpes simplex virus have been identified: HSV-1 and HSV-2. Primary infections may lead to painful blisters and ulcers in the genital region, while recurrent infections are generally less severe. Accurate diagnosis can be challenging due to the variability in clinical presentation. Antiviral therapies, such as acyclovir, have been shown to alleviate symptoms and reduce the frequency of outbreaks. Caution is advised for pregnant women with genital herpes due to the potential for neonatal transmission during delivery. To reduce this risk, antiviral medication may be given during pregnancy, or a cesarean section may be recommended. Preventive measures, such as avoiding sexual contact during outbreaks and using condoms, can effectively decrease the spread of HSV.

20.1 Background

Herpes simplex virus type 2 (HSV-2) is primarily responsible for genital herpes, although increasing cases of genital infection due to HSV-1 have been reported. HSV infection ranks among the most prevalent sexually transmitted viral diseases worldwide. Approximately 75–90% of individuals with HSV-2 are unaware of their infection. Since 75% of those diagnosed with genital herpes —whether it is a primary infection or a recurrence—present with no or atypical symptoms, obtaining an accurate diagnosis can be challenging. The principal risk during pregnancy is the potential transmission of the virus to the fetus or neonate, which can lead to severe clinical outcomes.

I. Mylonas, *Sexually Transmitted Diseases*,
https://doi.org/10.1007/978-3-031-78204-6_20

20.2 Pathogen

Herpes simplex virus (HSV) is a member of the Herpesviridae family and is characterized by an enveloped, double-stranded DNA genome. Two distinct types exist:

- **HSV-1**: Traditionally associated with orolabial infections ("cold sores"), but capable of causing genital lesions.
- **HSV-2**: Primarily linked to genital herpes, yet also able to produce orolabial disease.

Both HSV-1 and HSV-2 establish lifelong latency in sensory nerve ganglia following primary infection. During latency, the viral genome persists within neuronal nuclei without producing infectious virions. Periodically, HSV can reactivate and travel down axons to the skin or mucosa, leading to symptomatic or asymptomatic viral shedding.

Mechanisms of latency and reactivation are fundamental to the pathophysiology of herpes simplex virus (HSV) infection. Following primary mucocutaneous infection, the virus invades sensory nerve endings and is transported retrogradely to neuronal ganglia, such as the trigeminal or sacral ganglia. Within these ganglionic

Table 20.1 Commonly recognized triggers for reactivation

Trigger	Impact on reactivation	Underlying mechanism
Advanced age	Increased recurrence frequency in elderly	Senescence of innate and adaptive immune compartments diminishes antiviral surveillance
Host genetic factors	Variable predisposition to relapse	Polymorphisms in immunomodulatory genes (e.g., TLRs, cytokine receptors) influence individual reactivation thresholds
Immunosuppression	Strong risk factor, especially in patients undergoing chemotherapy or corticosteroid therapy	Reduced T-cell responses and natural killer cell activity permit latent virus to reactivate
Intercurrent infections	Facilitates outbreaks during other illnesses	Immune resources diverted to fight concurrent pathogens lead to transient loss of HSV-specific immunity
Psychological stress	Major contributor to recurrence	Elevated cortisol and catecholamines suppress cell-mediated immunity and antiviral cytokines
Ultraviolet radiation	Frequent precipitant of orolabial recurrences	UV-induced keratinocyte damage and local inflammatory changes weaken cutaneous defenses

neurons, latency-associated transcripts (LATs) are expressed and function to maintain the viral genome in a transcriptionally quiescent state while inhibiting full lytic gene expression. This molecular program permits long-term persistence of HSV without productive replication.

Reactivation occurs when the regulatory balance that enforces latency is disrupted. Under specific stimuli (Table 20.1), the suppressive influence of LATs is reduced, permitting expression of immediate-early lytic proteins followed by sequential activation of early and late genes. Viral assembly then proceeds, and newly formed virions are transported anterogradely along axons to peripheral tissues, where recurrent lesions or asymptomatic viral shedding may result.

20.3 Epidemiology

Previous studies estimate the prevalence of HSV-2 in the general population to be between 0.25% and 5%. In women with other genital infections, this prevalence rises to approximately 7%. In the United States, the prevalence of HSV-2 has declined from 21% (1988–1994) to 17% (1999–2004). Meanwhile, the seroprevalence of HSV-1 has increased from 57.7% (1988–1994) to 62% (1999–2004). The UK reports an HSV-2 incidence of 25%. In developing nations, seroprevalence rates range between 60% and 90%, influenced by risk factors such as prostitution and HIV status.

High Prevalence of HSV:

- An estimated 90–95% of adults are infected with HSV-1.
- Approximately 10–30% of adults carry HSV-2, with prevalence in those with multiple sexual partners potentially reaching 60%.
- The estimated frequency of recurrent HSV infections lies between 10% and 20%.

Although HSV-2 remains the principal cause of genital herpes, there is an increasing incidence of genital infections caused by HSV-1, particularly among young individuals. Roughly 80% of new genital herpes cases in this demographic are attributed to HSV-1, primarily linked to alterations in sexual practices and orogenital intercourse.

Serological testing in the United States indicates that 22% of pregnant women are infected with HSV-2, with 63% seropositive for HSV-1 and 13% demonstrating prior infections with both viruses. In Scandinavia, the estimated seroprevalence for HSV-2 in pregnant women is around 33%, compared to 17% in Canada. The general population prevalence of HSV-2 in isolated studies is suggested to be between 20%

and 25%, with antibody prevalence in adults estimated at 15–40% and varying from 6.3% to 8.9% in pregnant women.

In the United States, the infection rate during pregnancy ranges from 8 to 60 cases per 100,000 live births, influenced by the population studied. Reported neonatal HSV infection rates in the United States range from 1:1400 to 1:30,000 live births. Canada reports a lower incidence of 0.59 per 10,000 live births, while the UK estimates an annual rate of 1 per 60,000 live births. Data on other European regions are limited, but similar prevalence to North America is expected.

Intrauterine transmission is estimated in 4–5% of all neonatal HSV cases. Assuming an incidence of 1:5000 births with a 5% transmission rate, it can be projected that approximately one case per 100,000 births is affected by intrauterine HSV infection. The risk of intrauterine transmission is highest during the first 20 weeks of gestation, with possible outcomes including miscarriage, stillbirth, and congenital malformations. Perinatal mortality is estimated to be around 50%.

20.4 Clinical Manifestation

Primary transmission of HSV occurs by direct person-to-person contact, most commonly via exposure to active lesions or to asymptomatic viral shedding from mucosal surfaces. Fomite transmission (for example, via towels or utensils) is uncommon but possible when vesicular fluid containing high titers of infectious virions contacts susceptible mucosa or skin. Infectivity is highest during the vesicular and ulcerative phases and may continue during crusting; virus can be transmitted from areas of apparently intact mucous membrane.

After inoculation, the incubation period ranges from 3 to 20 days (mean 5–7 days). Many patients experience nonspecific prodromal symptoms that precede lesion appearance and can aid early diagnosis and treatment. Common prodromal features include mild to moderate fever, headache, and malaise beginning 24–48 h before lesions; local dysesthesias (itching, tingling, burning, or shooting pain) at the future lesion site; tender regional lymphadenopathy (for example, submandibular in orolabial infection or inguinal in genital infection); and systemic symptoms, such as myalgias and arthralgias.

Site-specific prodromes may occur: primary orolabial HSV-1 infection can present with pharyngitis, odynophagia, and tender cervical lymphadenopathy that may mimic bacterial pharyngitis; primary genital HSV-2 infection frequently produces dysuria or urethral discomfort prior to vesicle formation.

Recognition of prodromal signs permits early institution of antiviral therapy. Initiation of nucleoside analogs (for example, acyclovir and valacyclovir) at the prodromal stage—ideally within 24 h of symptom onset—reduces lesion severity, shortens healing time, and decreases viral shedding, thereby lowering transmission risk.

Symptoms of Genital Herpes Infection:

- **Mucocutaneous Manifestation:**
  - Herpes labialis, herpes facialis, herpes integumentalis (mainly caused by HSV-1).
  - Healing typically takes 10–20 days.
  - Most frequent manifestation is herpes recurrens or recidivans.
  - Gingivostomatitis and stomatitis herpetica (primarily HSV-1).
  - Genital herpes (vulvovaginitis, balanitis) is the most common sexually transmitted infection, occurring as both a primary and recurrent infection.
- **CNS Infections:**
  - Herpes encephalitis is the predominant form of necrotizing encephalitis in Central Europe, responsible for approximately 50% of cases.
  - The incidence rate is 30% post-primary infection, with recurrent herpes involved in up to 70% of cases.
  - This condition carries a high lethality rate (up to 70%), with many patients experiencing residual effects.
- **Disseminated Infections:**
  - Disseminated herpes simplex with viral spread may present as eczema herpeticatum, ocular involvement (primarily HSV-1), esophagitis, hepatitis, and involvement of other internal organs (HSV-1 and HSV-2), potentially resulting in fatal outcomes.

Herpes simplex virus (HSV) encephalitis is the most common sporadic viral encephalitis in temperate regions and constitutes a neurologic emergency. HSV-1 causes the majority of cases (HSV-2 predominates in neonates and some immunocompromised patients). The virus invades the central nervous system by retrograde axonal transport (occasionally hematogenous spread) and preferentially targets the limbic system—medial temporal lobes, insula, and orbitofrontal cortex—producing focal necrosis, edema, hemorrhage, and seizures.

Diagnosis is based on clinical suspicion with urgent MRI (T2/FLAIR hyperintensity in medial temporal regions with restricted diffusion/enhancement), CSF analysis showing lymphocytic pleocytosis and elevated protein, and CSF HSV DNA PCR for confirmation. EEG frequently demonstrates focal or periodic lateralized epileptiform discharges. CT may be normal early and should not delay further workup.

Empirical high-dose intravenous acyclovir must be initiated immediately when HSV encephalitis is suspected; treatment should not await confirmatory tests. Supportive care includes intracranial pressure management, seizure control, and critical-care support as needed. Untreated mortality approaches 70%, whereas prompt antiviral therapy reduces mortality to approximately 20% and lessens long-term neurological sequelae, such as memory loss, personality change, focal deficits, and epilepsy.

20.5 Gynecology

20.5.1 Primary Infection

Symptomatic primary genital herpes typically manifests after an incubation period of 2–20 days, most commonly between 5 and 7 days following exposure to herpes simplex virus (HSV). The initial lesions are classically composed of clusters of small, tense vesicles on the vulva, labia majora, and minora (Figs. 20.1 and 20.2), perineum, perianal skin, gluteal region, or medial aspects of the thighs. These vesicles rapidly rupture and evolve into painful, shallow ulcers that may coalesce, producing extensive mucocutaneous erosions; cervical involvement is frequently observed in females, and shallow cervical ulcerations are readily identified on speculum examination.

Prodromal symptoms are frequently reported and include intense vulvar pain and burning that often precedes lesion appearance by several hours. Dysuria is commonly experienced when ulceration involves the vestibule or urethral meatus, and a serous to purulent vaginal discharge may be observed as an expression of local inflammatory response. Tender bilateral inguinal and femoral lymphadenopathy is typical. Systemic features such as low-grade fever, cephalalgia, myalgias, and malaise are commonly reported; rare cases of viral dissemination with complications such as hepatitis or meningitis have been described.

Although the external genitalia represent the predominant sites of involvement, mucocutaneous lesions may extend to adjacent areas including the perianal skin and anal canal, perineum, inner thighs, and gluteal region. The distribution of lesions should be carefully inspected during clinical examination, and speculum assessment is advised in women to detect cervical disease.

Preexisting immunity influences the clinical course. Seropositivity for HSV-1 confers partial immune protection against severe disease during subsequent genital HSV-2 infection; affected individuals are therefore observed to experience milder initial outbreaks, shortened durations of viral shedding, and reduced lesion counts. By contrast, primary genital infections caused by HSV-1 are often more florid but are associated with lower recurrence rates, commonly reported to be less than 10% per annum. Genital HSV-2 infection, although sometimes less dramatic at presentation, is associated with higher recurrence frequencies, approximately 20–50% per year.

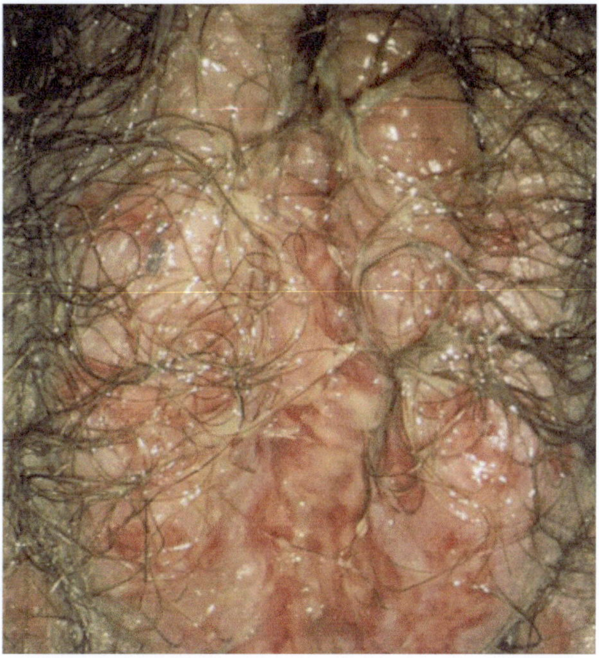

Fig. 20.1 Primary genital herpes presentation (Mylonas & Petersen 2009)

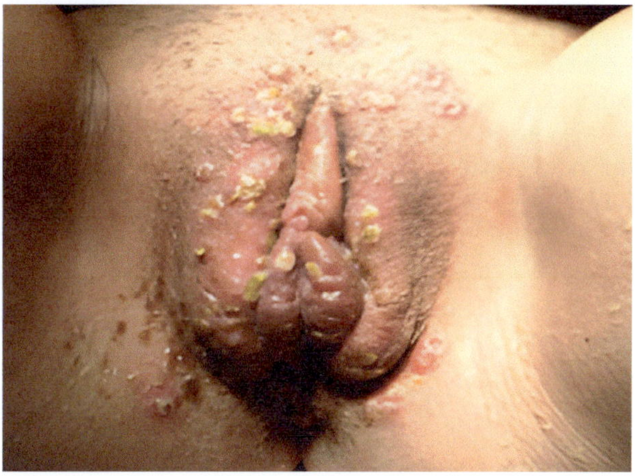

Fig. 20.2 Primary genital herpes lesion (Mylonas 2016). A bilateral inguinal lymphadenitis is noted.

20.5.2 Recurrent Infection

Recurrent HSV infection reproduces the clinical pattern of primary disease but with reduced severity, more rapid resolution, and fewer systemic manifestations (Fig. 20.3). Reactivation typically occurs at or adjacent to sites of prior involvement and is frequently heralded by a prodromal interval of localized sensory disturbance. Prodromal symptoms—classically itch, burning, paresthesia, or lancinating

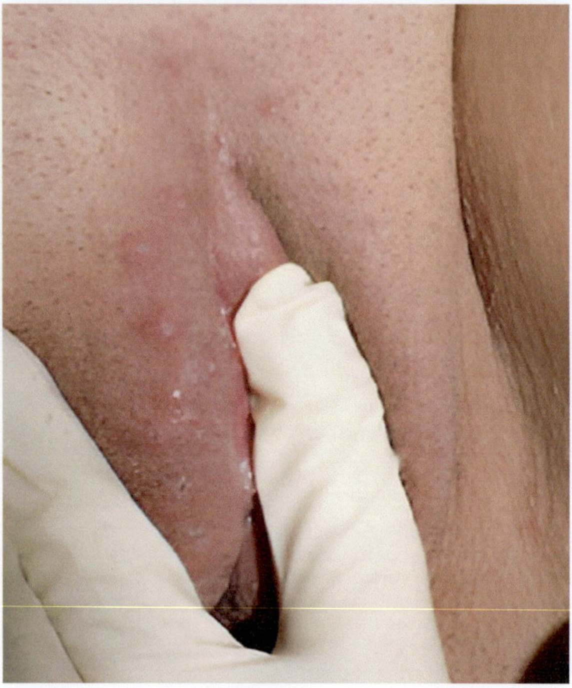

Fig. 20.3 Recurrent genital herpes presentation (Mylonas 2011, 2016)

neuralgic pain radiating from the involved sensory ganglion—usually arise within hours to 48 h before lesion appearance and provide an opportunity for early patient-initiated antiviral therapy to mitigate lesion progression and shorten symptomatic duration.

Lesions in recurrent HSV follow the same morphological sequence as primary episodes (vesiculation, ulceration, crusting, and re-epithelialization) but are generally fewer, more clustered, and smaller. Recurrent genital outbreaks typically resolve more rapidly than primary disease, most commonly within 4–7 days, and are associated with less intense pain and markedly reduced mucocutaneous destruction.

Asymptomatic viral shedding from genital or orolabial mucosa is the principal mechanism of HSV transmission. In seropositive individuals, subclinical episodes of viral replication occur intermittently and unpredictably; nucleic acid amplification testing demonstrates that viral loads during these asymptomatic intervals are sufficient to infect susceptible contacts. The frequency and duration of subclinical shedding are influenced by viral species (HSV-1 versus HSV-2), anatomic site, host immune competence, and time since primary infection. Genital HSV-2 is associated with a higher rate of asymptomatic shedding than genital HSV-1, particularly during the early years after acquisition.

The asymptomatic intervals between genital herpes outbreaks hold significant importance since HSV can periodically reactivate in latently infected cells.

Epidemiological distinctions between genital HSV-1 and HSV-2 inform prognosis and prevention. Genital HSV-1 often produces more florid primary presentations but demonstrates lower recurrence rates (commonly <10% per year), whereas genital HSV-2 is characterized by higher recurrence frequency (approximately 20–50% per year) and increased subclinical shedding (reported PCR-detectable shedding approximating 10–20% of days for HSV-2 versus 5–10% for HSV-1 in some cohorts). Reported values vary between studies and depend on surveillance intensity and population characteristics.

Approximately three-quarters of patients with genital herpes experience asymptomatic or atypical infections, regardless of the presence of symptoms.

20.6 Pregnancy

20.6.1 Primary Infections During Pregnancy

Primary infections in pregnant women are observed to present more severe disease than in nonpregnant individuals. Gingivostomatitis and vulvovaginitis herpetica have been noted to spread particularly during pregnancy, although they are rarely observed within this population. Despite low vertical transmission risk, genital herpes is regarded as the most common cause of neonatal infections, with the infected birth canal identified as the most probable transmission route. Limited data are available concerning neonatal herpes infections among immunocompromised patients. HIV-positive women have a notably higher incidence of HSV-2 infection (approximately 80%) compared to the general population, suggesting an increased risk of asymptomatic or oligosymptomatic genital viral shedding at birth.

20.6.2 Herpes Neonatorum

Herpes neonatorum refers to a severe infection in newborns caused by the herpes simplex virus (HSV). It is a critical condition requiring prompt diagnosis and treatment due to its high rates of morbidity and mortality.

Symptoms in newborns with genital herpes infection during pregnancy may include:

- Miscarriage.
- Stillbirth.
- Premature birth.

(continued)

- Herpes sepsis with aphthae, conjunctivitis, and fever.
- Generalized vesicular eruption.
- Eczema herpeticatum.
- Meningoencephalitis herpetica.
- Microcephaly.
- Seizures.
- Coma.
- Microphthalmia.
- Retinal dysplasia.
- Chorioretinitis.
- Mental disabilities.

- **Perinatal Infection:**
  - Approximately 90% of herpes neonatorum cases are attributed to perinatal transmission.
  - The primary route of transmission is through direct contact with infected maternal genital secretions during vaginal delivery.
  - The risk of viral transmission to the neonate during delivery is significant, with an estimated infection rate between 40% and 50%.
- **Neonatal Outcomes:**
  - The condition is associated with a **neonatal mortality rate of approximately 40%**, underscoring its life-threatening nature.
  - Survivors face a **morbidity rate of around 20%**, which includes potential long-term neurological complications, such as developmental delays, seizures, or cerebral palsy.
- **Recurrent Maternal HSV Infections:**
  - In cases of recurrent HSV infections in the mother, the risk of neonatal transmission is significantly lower, ranging from 1% to 5%.
  - This reduced risk is largely attributed to the presence of maternal IgG antibodies, which provide passive immunity to the newborn. These antibodies are transferred across the placenta during pregnancy and help neutralize the virus.
  - Additionally, recurrent infections typically involve lower levels of viral shedding, further decreasing the likelihood of transmission to the infant.
- **Clinical Significance:**
  - Herpes neonatorum presents a substantial public health concern due to its high rates of transmission, mortality, and morbidity.
  - Preventative measures, such as screening for genital HSV infections during pregnancy and considering cesarean delivery in mothers with active lesions, play a critical role in reducing neonatal infection risks.
  - Early antiviral therapy, typically using intravenous acyclovir, is essential for reducing viral replication, improving clinical outcomes, and preventing neurologic sequelae in affected neonates.

Neonatal herpes simplex virus infection is classified into three major clinical categories, each with distinct presentations and outcomes (Table 20.2). The

Table 20.2 Classification of neonatal HSV-infection

Feature	Mild infection (localized)	Severe CNS infection	Severe disseminated disease
Affected sites	Skin (cutis), conjunctiva/ocular tissues (oculus), oral mucosa (cavum oris)	Brain and central nervous system (CNS)	Multiple organs—liver (hepatitis), lungs (pneumonitis), coagulation system, adrenals, etc.
Prevalence (of neonates with HSV)	~45%	~30%	~25%
Key clinical features	Localized vesiculopustular eruptions without CNS or visceral involvement	Lethargy, irritability/restlessness, poor feeding, and seizures; a cutaneous rash may be present	Clinical presentation resembling neonatal sepsis with signs of multiorgan dysfunction
Untreated progression/natural history	Progression to CNS involvement and generalized dissemination is common if antiviral therapy is not administered	Rapid neurologic deterioration and increased mortality are likely without treatment	Fulminant multiorgan failure may develop rapidly in the absence of therapy
Treatment and outcome	Antiviral therapy (intravenous acyclovir when indicated) is associated with generally favorable outcomes and reduced risk of dissemination	Early intravenous acyclovir significantly reduces mortality (to approximately 6% when promptly administered)	Prompt intravenous acyclovir decreases mortality (to approximately 30%); early supportive care for organ dysfunction is required
Long-term sequelae	Recurrent cutaneous lesions may occur during childhood	Up to 50% of survivors may develop persistent neurological sequelae (developmental delay, motor deficits, epilepsy)	Survivors may exhibit organ-specific sequelae and increased long-term morbidity
Notes	Early recognition and initiation of antiviral therapy are essential to prevent progression	Rapid diagnosis and immediate initiation of acyclovir are critical to optimize neurological outcome	High index of suspicion is required; management should include empiric treatment for HSV in neonates with suspected sepsis while diagnostic workup is undertaken

"mildest form," characterized by localized involvement of the skin, eyes, and mouth (SEM disease), accounts for approximately 45% of neonatal HSV cases. Clinically, SEM disease presents with vesicular lesions on an erythematous base, often arranged in single or grouped vesicles with a linear distribution on the limbs. Ocular manifestations such as excessive lacrimation and conjunctival erythema may occur, along with localized ulcerative lesions in the oral cavity. Notably, skin lesions may be absent in up to 17% of SEM cases. If untreated, SEM disease carries a significant risk—about 50%—of progression to central nervous system (CNS) involvement or disseminated infection. However, with prompt administration of high-dose intravenous acyclovir, mortality approaches zero, and approximately 98% of treated infants achieve normal neurodevelopmental outcomes. Despite this favorable prognosis, recurrent cutaneous manifestations may occur during early childhood.

"Severe CNS infection" occurs in roughly 30% of neonatal HSV infections and presents with a spectrum of neurological symptoms, including lethargy, irritability, poor feeding, temperature instability (fever or hypothermia), seizures, tremors, and bulging fontanelle. Importantly, skin vesicles are absent in approximately one-third of cases, which can complicate diagnosis. High-dose intravenous acyclovir therapy (60 mg/kg/day) has significantly reduced mortality from about 50% in untreated infants to approximately 6%. Nevertheless, long-term neurological sequelae remain common; up to half of survivors develop impairments such as developmental delay, epilepsy, motor deficits, microcephaly, hydrocephalus, encephalomalacia, spasticity, and cognitive dysfunction. Recent studies report neurological complications in 50–76% of pediatric patients with HSV encephalitis despite adequate antiviral therapy.

The most severe form is "disseminated disease" involving multiple organs—including the liver, lungs, adrenal glands, and CNS—and accounts for about 25% of neonatal HSV infections. Clinical manifestations mimic bacterial sepsis and include temperature instability, apnea, respiratory distress, hepatomegaly, abdominal distension, necrotizing enterocolitis, disseminated intravascular coagulation, and pneumonia. Laboratory findings often demonstrate thrombocytopenia, neutropenia, coagulopathy, and elevated liver transaminases. Although high-dose intravenous acyclovir therapy reduces mortality from approximately 85% in untreated infants to 30–31%, morbidity remains substantial. Early recognition and prompt initiation of antiviral treatment are critical; delayed administration beyond 24 h after hospital admission is associated with significantly increased mortality risk.

Diagnosis of neonatal HSV infection is challenging due to nonspecific initial symptoms and the frequent absence of characteristic skin vesicles—occurring in 39% of disseminated disease and 32% of CNS disease cases. Most infections present within the first 4 weeks of life. The current standard treatment protocol involves high-dose intravenous acyclovir at 60 mg/kg/day for 14–21 days. Early empirical antiviral therapy is strongly recommended when neonatal HSV infection is suspected because delayed treatment correlates with worse outcomes.

Long-term neurodevelopmental follow-up is essential for all neonates who experience CNS involvement, as neurological deficits may emerge even if initial hospital discharge assessments are normal. This comprehensive approach ensures early identification and management of potential sequelae, optimizing developmental outcomes in affected infants.

Important Aspects of Neonatal HSV Infection

- Early recognition and the rapid initiation of acyclovir antiviral therapy are essential for managing various clinical presentations of neonatal herpes simplex virus (HSV) infections.
- Clinical outcomes vary considerably based on the severity and extent of the infection.
- Localized infections generally have a favorable prognosis with appropriate treatment; however, relapses can occur.
- Central nervous system (CNS) infections require prompt therapy to lower mortality rates, although the risk of long-term neurological complications remains significant.
- Disseminated disease is associated with a high mortality risk in the absence of treatment, highlighting the critical need for immediate therapeutic intervention.

20.7 Diagnosis

Accurate diagnosis of genital HSV infection is often challenging because classic symptoms are frequently absent or presentation may be atypical. In both nonpregnant and pregnant women, subtle clinical signs must be recognized and appropriate laboratory investigations applied to enable timely management and to reduce transmission risk.

Symptoms

- **Nonpregnant Women:** Primary infection is commonly preceded by systemic symptoms (fever, malaise, and cephalalgia), followed by localized prodromal sensations—paresthesia, pruritus, or burning—in the vulvar, perianal, or inguinal regions. Lesions are typically described as grouped, small, painful vesicles on an erythematous base that may rupture and form shallow ulcers. Up to 70% of primary infections and approximately 50% of recurrences are asymptomatic or present with atypical findings that can be mistaken for candidosis or nonspecific dermatitis.
- **Pregnant Women:** Clinical manifestations are similar to those observed in nonpregnant women but are prioritized because of the potential for neonatal transmission. Prodromal symptoms (vulvar pruritus, tingling, or lancinating pain) may be the sole presenting feature prior to vesicle emergence. Vesicular eruptions are usually small and may coalesce; subsequent rupture produces shallow ulcerations.

Laboratory Confirmation

When clinical features are equivocal or when diagnostic confirmation will alter management, the following tests are possible:

- **Viral Culture:** Live virus detection has been historically regarded as a standard method; however, culture sensitivity declines as lesions heal, and results require 48–72 h.
- **Direct Immunofluorescence (DFA):** Type-specific monoclonal antibodies are applied to lesion swabs to detect HSV antigens. Results are rapid, with moderate sensitivity.
- **Polymerase Chain Reaction (PCR):** PCR assays provide the highest sensitivity and specificity and detect HSV DNA from vesicular fluid, ulcer exudate, or crusted lesions. PCR is preferred when lesions are scant or healing.
- **Tzanck Test (Tzanck Smear):** Rapid cytologic point-of-care test for HSV/VZV. Technique: unroof fresh vesicle, scrape base, smear on slide, fix in methanol (1–2 min), stain (Giemsa/Wright/H&E). Microscopy: multinucleated giant cells, nuclear molding, chromatin margination. Performance: moderate sensitivity (~60–80%); low specificity (cannot distinguish HSV vs VZV or HSV-1 vs HSV-2). Mostly replaced by DFA/PCR but useful for immediate presumptive diagnosis in resource-limited settings.

Serologic Testing

Type-specific serology (glycoprotein G-based IgG assays) is used to differentiate prior exposure to HSV-1 versus HSV-2. Determining the serologic HSV status of pregnant women (Table 20.3) can be beneficial in certain circumstances, enhancing effective counseling and assessment of fetal infection risk. However, routine antenatal serologic screening is not recommended because of:

- **Assay Variability:** Commercial type-specific tests demonstrate inconsistent performance, particularly in low-prevalence populations.
- **Limited Clinical Impact:** There is insufficient evidence that universal screening reduces the incidence of neonatal herpes.
- **Potential Harms:** False-positive results may provoke unnecessary interventions, psychological distress, and increased healthcare costs.

Selective serologic testing may be indicated for pregnant patients who:

- Have a sexual partner with known genital herpes.
- Exhibit prodromal symptoms in the absence of visible lesions.
- Belong to higher-risk categories (recent seroconversion and multiple sexual partners).

Table 20.3 Serological parameters in herpes simplex virus (HSV) infection

	HSV serology				Genome detection		Rating
	Anti-HSV-1/2-IgG	Anti-HSV-1 IgG	Anti-HSV-2-IgG	Anti-HSV-1/2-IgM	HSV-1-PCR	HSV-2-PCR	Infection status
Negative	–	–	–	–	–	–	No infection
HSV-1	–	–	–	– or +	+	–	Primary infection (HSV-1)
	+	–	+	– or +	+	–	Primary infection (HSV-1 with HSV-2 latency)
	+	+	–	– or +	+	–	Infection or recurrence (HSV-1)
	+	+	–	–	–	–	Past infection (HSV-1)
HSV-2	–	–	–	– or +	–	+	Primary infection (HSV-2)
	+	+	–	– or +	–	+	Primary infection (HSV-2 with HSV-1 latency)
	+	–	+	– or +	–	+	Infection recurrence (HSV-2)
	+	–	+	–	–	–	Past infection (HSV-2)
Older infection (HSV 1 and 2)	+	+	+	–	–	–	Past infection (HSV 1 and 2)
Unclear findings	+	+	–	+	–	–	– Classification difficult in the absence of pathogen detection – Clinical findings
Ambiguous results	+	–	+	+	–	–	

– = negative
+ = positive
Note: A negative result for anti-HSV1/2-IgM does not exclude acute infection

20.8 Treatment

20.8.1 Gynecology

20.8.1.1 Antiviral Treatment for Genital Herpes

The objective of antiviral therapy in genital herpes is to inhibit the replication of the herpes simplex virus and relieve the symptoms of infection. Acyclovir, famciclovir, and valaciclovir are commonly employed for the oral treatment of genital herpes (Table 20.4). Medication administration is contingent upon the presentation of symptoms (Fig. 20.4).

For supportive and symptomatic management of herpes simplex infections, 0.1% zinc sulfate hydrogel can be applied locally four times daily until healing occurs.

Table 20.4 Management of herpes simplex infection. Nucleoside analogs for the treatment of HSV are not officially approved for use during pregnancy (offlabel use). However, if antiviral therapy is required, acyclovir is the preferred choice due to its extensive clinical safety data and established experience during gestation

Condition	Medication	Dosage	Duration
Herpes labialis[a]	Penciclovir cream	Apply five times daily	1–5 days
	Acyclovir cream	Apply five times daily	1–5 days
	Docosanol cream	Apply five times daily	1–5 days
	Foscarnet cream	Apply five to six times daily	1–5 days
	Valaciclovir	1000 mg orally twice daily	One day
	Valaciclovir[b]	2000 mg orally twice daily	One day
	Famciclovir	1500 mg orally twice daily	One day
Primary infection	Acyclovir	200 mg orally five times daily	7–10 days
	Acyclovir	400 mg orally three times daily	7–10 days
	Valaciclovir	1000 mg orally twice daily	7–10 days
	Famciclovir	250 mg orally three times daily	5 days
Recurrence	Acyclovir	200 mg orally five times daily	5–7 days
	Acyclovir	400 mg orally three times daily	5–7 days
	Valaciclovir	500 mg orally twice daily	5–7 days
	Famciclovir	125 mg orally twice daily	5 days
Prophylaxis	Aciclovir[c]	200 mg orally four times daily	6–12 months
	Valaciclovir	250 mg orally twice daily	6–12 months
	Valaciclovir	500 mg orally once daily	6–12 months
	Famciclovir	250 mg orally twice daily	6–12 months
	Famciclovir	125 mg orally three times daily	6–12 months
Immunosuppression	Acyclovir	400 mg orally three times daily	10 days
	Valaciclovir	1000 mg orally twice daily	10 days
	Famciclovir	500 mg orally twice daily	7 days
Immunosuppression prophylaxis	Famciclovir	250 mg orally twice daily	6–12 months
Intravenous therapy	Acyclovir	5 mg/kg body weight intravenously three times daily	7–10 days
Acyclovir resistance	Foscarnet	40 mg/kg body weight intravenously two to three times daily	7–21 days

[a] Self-medication at the first symptoms
[b] For pronounced symptoms
[c] Currently, the best therapeutic option

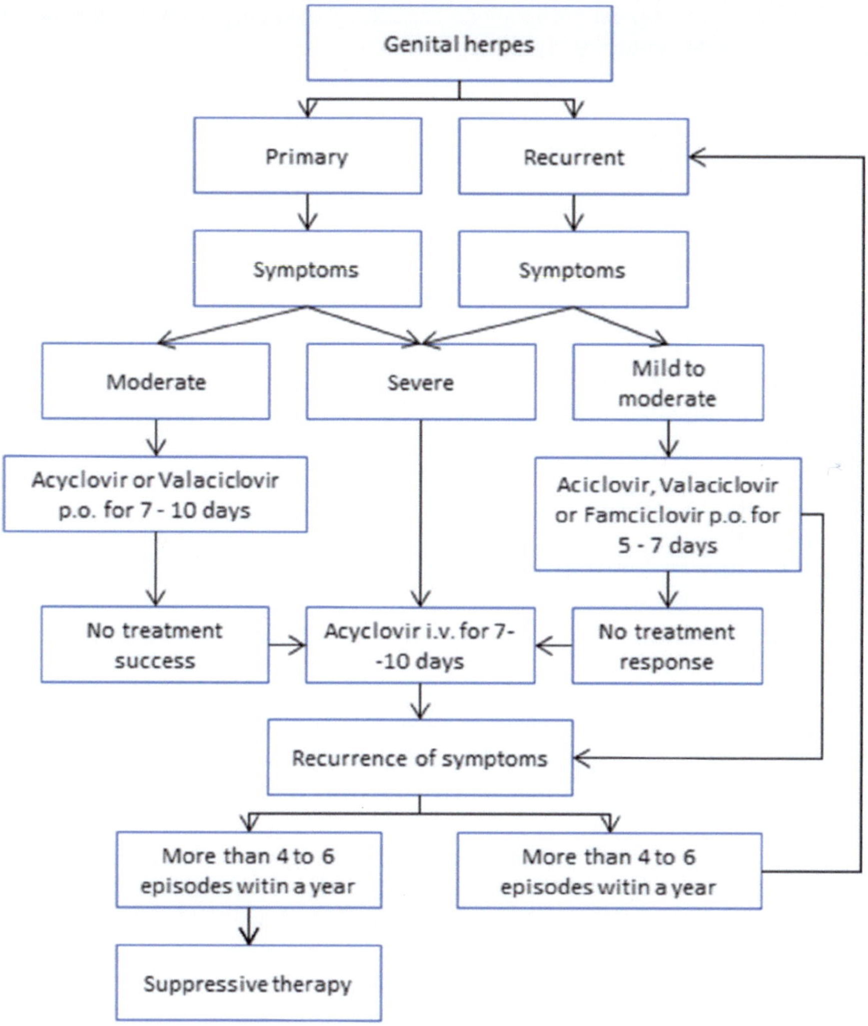

Fig. 20.4 Management algorithm for genital herpes outside of pregnancy. (Courtesy of I. Mylonas)

Tannolact® and Kamilosan® sitz baths[1] may also be beneficial, with two to three applications per day until complete resolution. During the vesicle stage, it is recommended to avoid greasy ointments and creams, opting instead for dry brushes with Clioquinol cream 2%, Clioquinol-Lotio 2%, or Pyokatanin solution 0.5%. In the

[1] Sitz baths are a form of hydrotherapy where a person sits in a shallow bath of warm water to soak the genital and anal areas. This practice can help relieve itching, irritation, and discomfort in these areas. Sitz baths are commonly used for conditions like hemorrhoids, anal fissures, and postpartum recovery, as well as for soothing symptoms associated with genital herpes symptoms.

crusting stage, oily topical preparations containing bland ingredients, such as panthenol cream at 5% concentration, may be applied.

Indications for intravenous treatment include:

- Herpes encephalitis.
- Extensive mucocutaneous herpes lesions.
- Severe symptoms.
- Extensive herpes infections.

The primary challenges in treatment often involve selecting the appropriate drug, adhering to a short treatment duration, and ensuring precise dosing. *Awareness of the bioavailability and pharmacodynamics of antiviral medications is crucial for successful treatment.* For instance, acyclovir has a half-life of approximately 3 h. Hence, a dosage of 2 × 800 mg (commonly cited) or 2 × 400 mg for suppressive therapy may prove inadequate for disease management.

20.8.1.2 Suppression Therapy

Suppression therapy for genital herpes involves long-term antiviral treatment aimed at reducing the frequency and severity of outbreaks, as well as minimizing transmission to sexual partners. This is particularly recommended for individuals with frequent recurrences (Fig. 20.4).

Indications for Suppressive HSV Therapy: Suppressive antiviral therapy is indicated for patients experiencing frequent genital herpes recurrences, commonly defined as more than four to six outbreaks per year. When fewer than six episodes have occurred, the decision to initiate continuous therapy should be individualized, weighing clinical benefit against prolonged antiviral exposure and patient preference.

Clinical Considerations: Recurrent genital herpes is associated with pain, social stigma, and psychological morbidity that can substantially reduce quality of life. A conservative "wait-and-see" strategy often delays symptomatic relief and permits ongoing asymptomatic viral shedding, with potential impact on sexual relationships and reproductive planning. In women of childbearing potential—particularly those planning pregnancy—early suppression can reduce subclinical shedding and provide clinical reassurance during conception and gestation.

Antiviral Agents for Suppressive Therapy: First-line oral agents for long-term suppression are acyclovir, valaciclovir, and famciclovir. Dosing adjustments should be made for renal impairment in accordance with standard prescribing guidelines.

- **Acyclovir:** 200 mg four times daily (alternative 400 mg orally twice daily). Extensive clinical experience supports its use; it is preferred in certain severe or complex cases.
- **Valaciclovir:** 500 mg orally once daily (alternative 250 mg twice daily). As the prodrug of acyclovir, it offers improved bioavailability permitting once-daily dosing.
- **Famciclovir:** 250 mg orally twice daily. It is well tolerated and effective for reducing clinical and subclinical recurrences.

Duration of Therapy: Suppressive therapy may be continued indefinitely in patients with persistent frequent recurrences or substantial psychosocial burden. Periodic reassessment of recurrence frequency, adverse effects, renal function, and patient preference is recommended to determine ongoing need. Long-term safety data have been reported as follows:

- **Acyclovir:** Continuous administration for up to 10 years has been reported without evidence of cumulative toxicity when dosed appropriately and monitored.
- **Valaciclovir:** Suppressive regimens have been studied for up to 1 year; tolerability was favorable and no significant long-term adverse effects were documented in the studied intervals.

Clinical Benefits of Suppressive Therapy

- **Reduction in Recurrence Frequency:** Outbreak rates are decreased by approximately 70–80%; breakthrough episodes tend to be shorter and less severe.
- **Decreased Asymptomatic Shedding and Transmission:** Daily antiviral therapy (e.g., valaciclovir) reduces subclinical shedding and lowers partner transmission risk.
- **Improved Quality of Life:** Anxiety related to prodromal symptoms and visible lesions is reduced, with consequent benefit to sexual function and interpersonal relationships.
- **Pregnancy Planning and Perinatal Safety:** Initiation of suppressive therapy at 36 weeks' gestation reduces the likelihood of active lesions at delivery and the need for cesarean delivery for herpetic lesions, thereby decreasing neonatal exposure risk.

Suppression therapy is an effective method for significantly reducing the frequency of herpes recurrences.

20.8.2 Pregnancy

Prior to initiating any treatment during pregnancy, it is essential to provide comprehensive information to the expectant mother (and her partner). In particular, patients with recurrent genital herpes should be informed about:

- The relatively low risk of transmission.
- The potential for prophylactic acyclovir administration.
- The option for cesarean delivery.

Special precautions are necessary during the first and second trimesters for patients with primary (Fig. 20.5) and recurrent (Fig. 20.6) genital herpes, to protect the unborn child from infection during childbirth. Pregnant women presenting with a first clinical episode or recurrence can be treated with either acyclovir or valaciclovir.

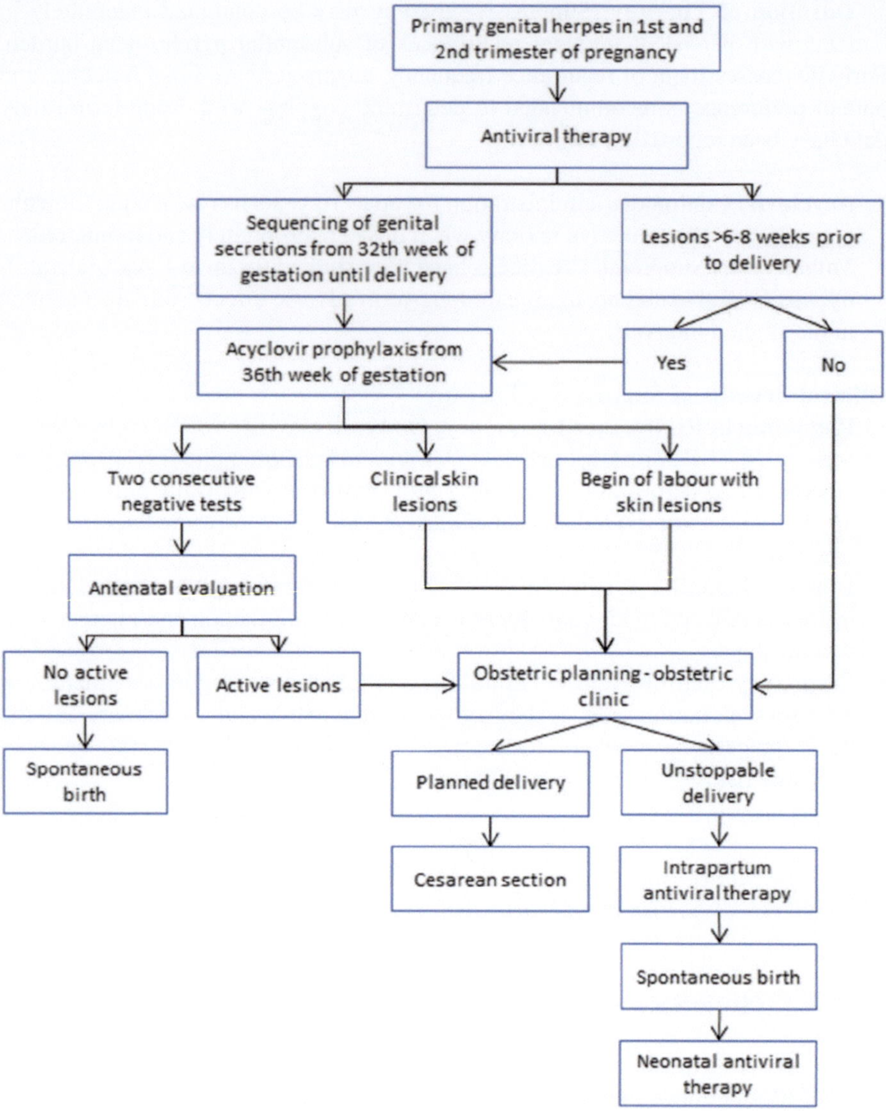

Fig. 20.5 Management algorithm for primary genital herpes during the first and second trimesters of pregnancy. (Courtesy of I. Mylonas)

As acyclovir and valaciclovir are not officially approved for use during pregnancy in most countries, it is imperative to counsel patients prior to initiating antiviral therapy. No increase in fetal malformations, premature rupture of membranes, or preterm births has been documented, though long-term outcomes remain still unclear.

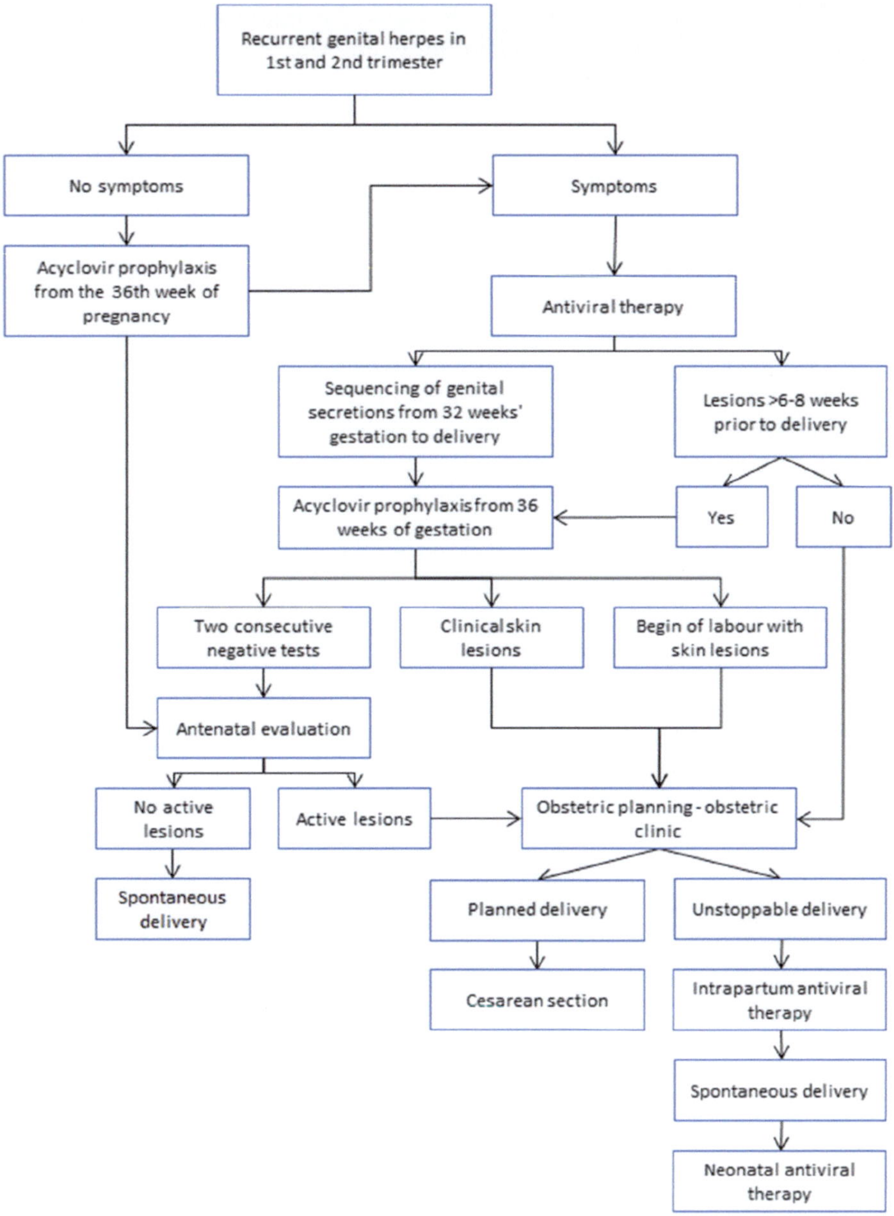

Fig. 20.6 Management algorithm for recurrent genital herpes during the first and second trimesters of pregnancy. (Courtesy of I. Mylonas)

Initiating suppressive therapy with acyclovir or valaciclovir from the 36th week of pregnancy until delivery has been shown to significantly reduce both the frequency of clinical manifestations and viral shedding at the time of birth. This approach decreases the risk of vertical transmission and helps prevent cesarean deliveries. It is advisable that all pregnant women with recurrent genital herpes or active genital HSV infections shortly before or at the time of delivery receive prophylactic acyclovir or valaciclovir in the third trimester.

Regardless of the selected medication, patients with symptomatic genital herpes in the third trimester should undergo a cesarean delivery (Fig. 20.7). In cases of labor onset, it should occur before or within 4–6 h following membrane rupture; otherwise, benefits for the infant may be compromised. Elective cesarean delivery prior to membrane rupture is recommended when active genital HSV lesions or clinical signs of recurrence are present at the onset of labor, since cesarean delivery substantially reduces intrapartum neonatal transmission. Routine prophylactic cesarean delivery is not indicated for women with a history of recurrent genital HSV who have no active lesions at term; the absolute risk of neonatal herpes in this group is low and the number of cesarean deliveries required to prevent a single neonatal case is very large. Retrospective cohort data indicate that knowledge of maternal HSV history does not increase cesarean rates among women without active lesions—cesarean rates were similar irrespective of prior HSV status or suppressive therapy—supporting avoidance of routine prophylactic cesarean delivery in asymptomatic women.

Administering 4 × 200 mg/day of acyclovir to pregnant women in the third trimester for 2–3 weeks before delivery has been shown to lead to a significant reduction in cesarean births and is beneficial for both primary and recurrent genital herpes

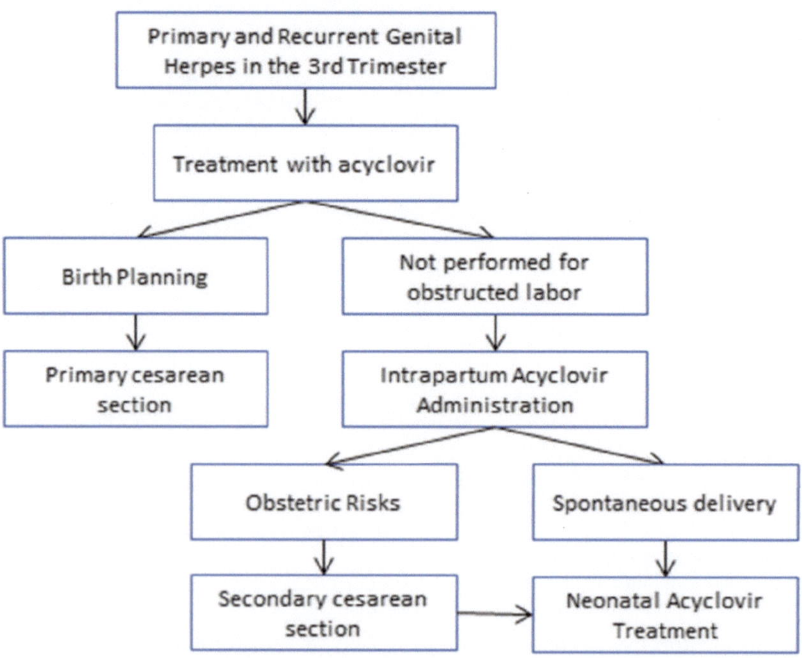

Fig. 20.7 Management algorithm for genital herpes (primary and recurrent) during the third trimester of pregnancy. (Courtesy of I. Mylonas)

infections. However, although acyclovir is generally well tolerated during pregnancy, prophylactic use warrants caution in specific fetal conditions. In cases of oligohydramnios, reduced amniotic fluid volume may concentrate drug exposure and impair renal tubular development. Similarly, fetuses with underlying renal insufficiency—whether congenital or secondary to placental insufficiency—may have diminished clearance of acyclovir, increasing the risk of nephrotoxicity and subsequent fluid–electrolyte imbalances. Therefore, when considering long-term suppressive therapy with acyclovir in pregnancy, clinicians should assess amniotic fluid indices and fetal renal function via ultrasound biometry and Doppler studies. If significant oligohydramnios or fetal renal compromise is detected, alternative strategies (such as deferment of antiviral prophylaxis until late third trimester or use of the lowest effective dose) should be discussed, and serial fetal surveillance should be intensified to ensure both maternal viral suppression and fetal well-being.

Oral and topical treatments for neonatal herpes are no longer viable options because, even with antiviral therapy, morbidity and mortality rates for disseminated neonatal herpes remain high. Additionally, these preventative measures cannot guarantee complete safety for the fetus.

20.9 Differential Diagnosis

The differential diagnosis of vesiculitis includes various conditions with similar presentations to herpes simplex infections, such as other blistering dermatoses and central nervous system infections. In men, balanitis may also exhibit similar symptoms. Herpes gestationis is a rare dermatological condition that occurs exclusively during pregnancy. Other potential differential diagnoses include contact dermatitis, lymphogranuloma venereum, molluscum contagiosum, Adamantiades-Behçet's disease, pemphigus vulgaris, syphilis, recurrent cystitis, trichomoniasis, chancroid, urethritis, varicella-zoster virus infection, and herpes zoster. Additionally, vulvitis pustulosa and vulvovaginal candidosis can present with similar symptoms, necessitating consideration during diagnosis.

20.10 Prevention

20.10.1 General

The high prevalence of asymptomatic HSV infections, which often go unrecognized, complicates the implementation of prophylactic measures. The development of a vaccine to prevent HSV-1 and HSV-2 infections would represent the most effective preventive strategy for reducing cases of herpes neonatorum. However, an effective prophylactic or therapeutic vaccine is currently unavailable.

20.10.2 Pregnancy

20.10.2.1 General

- A comprehensive medical history should be obtained from all pregnant women and their partners during the initial examination.
- Women with a history of HSV infection should be counseled to abstain from sexual intercourse (including oral sex) during relapses.
- Women with no history of HSV infection should receive detailed information about potential risks of infection. Studies have shown that condom use can reduce the risk of HSV transmission by up to 50%.
- Routine testing for serologic HSV status in pregnant women is currently not recommended (Sect. 20.5); however, in specific situations, determining serological HSV status may be useful in counseling.

20.10.2.2 Drug Prophylaxis

- All pregnant women with a history of genital herpes should receive prophylactic acyclovir (or valaciclovir) in the third trimester.
- In cases of active genital HSV infections occurring shortly before or at delivery, the administration of acyclovir (or valaciclovir) is recommended.
- Administering 200 mg of acyclovir four times daily to pregnant women in the third trimester for 2–3 weeks before delivery has been demonstrated to reduce the number of cesarean births.

Acyclovir prophylaxis has been effective for both primary and recurrent genital herpes. However, its prophylactic use may pose risks to the child under certain conditions, such as oligohydramnios or fetal renal insufficiency.

20.10.2.3 Birth Mode

Regardless of medication use, a cesarean section should be performed in all pregnant women with active genital herpes simplex virus (HSV) infections or prodromal symptoms (Figs. 20.5, 20.6, 20.7). A cesarean section conducted prior to membrane rupture reduces the risk of intrapartum transmission to the newborn.

Necessary cesarean sections should occur within 4-6 h of membrane rupture at the latest.

If initial infections happen during the first two trimesters of pregnancy, sequential virus detection in genital secretions can commence from the 32nd week of pregnancy. Pursuing vaginal delivery is possible if two consecutive pathogen tests are negative and there are no active lesions present at the time of delivery.

- Avoidance of amniotomy during labor is recommended.
- Placement of fetal scalp electrodes should be avoided because noninvasive cardiotocography (CTG) monitoring is preferred and the risk of direct fetal skin breach is eliminated.
- Operative vaginal delivery (vacuum or forceps) should be avoided when feasible because instrumentation of the fetal scalp increases the potential for viral transmission.
- Prophylactic cesarean delivery is not indicated solely for a history of recurrent genital herpes in the absence of active lesions; mode of delivery should be determined by current lesion status and standard obstetric indications.

Key Points

- HSV-2 is the primary cause of genital herpes, though HSV-1 is increasingly prevalent.
- Diagnosis is challenging due to the absence or atypical symptoms.
- The primary risk during pregnancy is the potential transmission of the virus to the fetus or newborn. HSV is a DNA virus within the Herpesviridae family, further categorized into HSV-1 and HSV-2.
- The virus remains latent in the nervous system, capable of reactivation under specific conditions.
- Primary transmission occurs through direct person-to-person contact or, on rare occasions, via contaminated objects. Highly infectious vesicles contain virus particles.
- Clinical manifestations typically arise after an incubation period of 3–20 days.
- Herpes encephalitis can result from either HSV-1 (95%) or HSV-2 (5%). Without treatment, HSV encephalitis has a mortality rate of 70%.
- Symptoms include fever, headache, nausea, and altered consciousness. Genital herpes presents with mucocutaneous symptoms, including herpes labialis, genitalis, and gingivostomatitis.
- Disseminated infections may include eczema herpeticatum, ocular involvement, and hepatitis.
- Primary infections during pregnancy are associated with an increased risk of severe disease. Herpes neonatorum has a high mortality and morbidity rate in perinatal infections.
- Diagnosis of genital HSV infections can be made clinically or via PCR diagnostics.
- Recommended treatments for HSV infections include acyclovir, famciclovir, or valaciclovir.
- Preventive strategies entail avoidance of triggers, condom use, prophylactic medications for pregnant women, and careful consideration of birth method.
- In cases of active genital HSV infections or prodromal symptoms, cesarean sections should be performed to avoid using certain delivery methods.

Mycoplasma genitalium

21

Abstract

Mycoplasma genitalium is a recently identified pathogen linked to various urogenital symptoms, particularly nongonococcal urethritis (NGU). This bacterium has a diminutive genome and lacks a cell wall, depending on host cells for survival. Prevalence varies according to different risk factors, such as sexual behaviors. In men, the infection primarily manifests as urethritis, while in women, it may lead to gynecological and obstetric complications. Detection of *Mycoplasma genitalium* is accomplished through polymerase chain reaction (PCR), although the optimal detection method remains uncertain. The efficacy of macrolide antibiotics, notably azithromycin, is declining, prompting recommendations for alternative treatments such as moxifloxacin. To date, no established prevention or screening protocols exist.

21.1 Background

Mycoplasma genitalium represents a relatively novel etiological agent of sexually transmitted infections. Following its initial identification in men with non-gonococcal urethritis (NGU) over 25 years ago, it has been implicated in urogenital infections affecting both men and women. Although the association with urethritis is well documented, the relevance of this correlation for other inflammatory diseases, particularly in women and during pregnancy, is not well understood.

***Mycoplasma genitalium* is categorized as a sexually transmitted pathogen due to its association with sexual activity, particularly among young adults.**

I. Mylonas, *Sexually Transmitted Diseases*,
https://doi.org/10.1007/978-3-031-78204-6_21

21.2 Pathogen

Mycoplasma genitalium is a member of the Mycoplasmataceae family, a group of bacteria characterized by their lack of a cell wall and dependence on host cells for survival. It is a unique organism that contains both DNA and RNA and is notable for having one of the smallest known bacterial genomes, comprising approximately 580 kb pairs. This minimal genome size reflects its highly parasitic lifestyle, where it has eliminated many biosynthetic pathways and relies heavily on host cellular processes for essential nutrients.

Unlike most bacteria, *M. genitalium* is incapable of synthesizing cholesterol, an essential component of its membrane structure. Instead, it depends entirely on the host's cellular metabolism to acquire cholesterol, as well as other lipids and nutrients necessary for membrane integrity and growth. This dependency contributes to its classification as an obligate parasite.

The organism's ability to colonize host tissues is facilitated by its specialized surface molecules, including adhesins, such as P140 and P110 proteins. These molecules play a critical role in mediating attachment to epithelial cells, particularly in the urogenital and respiratory tracts. By binding to sialylated glycoproteins or glycolipids on the host cell surfaces, *M. genitalium* establishes a tight adherence that enables persistence within the host. This attachment not only facilitates colonization but also helps the bacterium evade mucosal clearance mechanisms. Moreover, *M. genitalium* has evolved mechanisms to evade host's immune responses, including antigenic variation of its surface proteins to avoid immune recognition. This makes infections difficult to detect and treat in some cases, contributing to its role as an emerging pathogen in sexually transmitted infections.

21.3 Epidemiology

The prevalence of *Mycoplasma genitalium* varies significantly across global regions, with diverse data sets reported from studies conducted in the United States, Europe, Asia, Africa, and Latin America. In the United States, the incidence among women has been documented to range between 0.04% and 0.11%, while among men, it spans from 0.2% to 0.9%. Older studies focusing on adults aged 18–27 years estimated a prevalence of approximately 1%.

Within the EU/EEA, a study from 2021 reported prevalence rates ranging from 0.0% to 3% in both sexes. In the United Kingdom, the prevalence was found to be 1.2% in men and 1.3% in women aged 16–44 years. South Africa presented highly variable prevalence rates, ranging from 1% to 56%, with notably higher rates observed among women living with HIV. Limited data are available concerning prevalence in Latin America and Asia.

Globally, prevalence estimates suggest rates of 1–4% in men and 1–6% in women, with figures rising to as high as 38% in high-risk populations. A substantial proportion of infected individuals remain asymptomatic, with asymptomatic cases reported in 56% of men and 94% of women.

Risk factors for *M. genitalium* infection resemble those of other sexually transmitted infections (STIs) and include multiple sexual partners, early initiation of sexual activity, and coinfection with other pathogens, such as *Chlamydia trachomatis*. Despite these findings, further comprehensive epidemiological studies are necessary to gain a deeper understanding of this infection's distribution and associated risk factors globally.

Infected individuals are approximately twice as likely to contract HIV. Furthermore, the increasing antibiotic resistance, particularly against macrolides, presents significant challenges for effective treatment.

21.4 Clinical Manifestations

The most prevalent clinical manifestations of *Mycoplasma genitalium* infection in men are acute and chronic urethritis. Complications such as balanitis and prostatitis may also arise. The correlation between *Mycoplasma genitalium* infection and urethritis was established in 2001, with the infection responsible for about 15–20% of nongonococcal urethritis cases.

21.4.1 Gynecology

In women, *Mycoplasma genitalium* infection is commonly associated with vaginal discharge. The discharge characteristics can vary but are often described as yellowish-green or whitish, minimal in amount, and thin or watery in consistency. Some women may also notice a fishy odor, especially when *M. genitalium* coexists with other infections like bacterial vaginosis.

Urethritis is another symptom experienced by women infected with *M. genitalium*, often manifesting as burning or pain during urination. Cervicitis has also been reported in association with *M. genitalium* infection. Studies have shown that *M. genitalium* can be detected in 10–30% of women with clinical cervicitis. However, the precise relationship between *M. genitalium* and cervicitis remains somewhat ambiguous and requires further investigation to establish a definitive causal link.

The role of *M. genitalium* in pelvic inflammatory disease (PID) has been a subject of ongoing research. Recent studies suggest that *M. genitalium* is associated with an increased risk of PID. A systematic review and meta-analysis found that *M. genitalium* was associated with a 67% increase in the odds of PID and was detected in about one in ten clinical diagnoses of PID. This finding supports the hypothesis that *M. genitalium* infection may significantly increase the relative risk of developing PID, although the exact magnitude of this risk remains under investigation.

Regarding fertility implications, *M. genitalium* has been associated with female infertility in several studies. A meta-analysis found that women with infertility had statistically higher odds of having genital mycoplasma infections, including *M. genitalium*, compared to control groups. Another study reported that *M. genitalium* was associated with a significantly increased risk of female infertility.

Preliminary findings indicate a fivefold heightened risk of infertility related to infection in women.

Among a subset of patients with idiopathic infertility diagnosed via laparoscopy, the risk appears to be elevated ninefold. However, further epidemiological data is essential to establish a definitive link between *Mycoplasma genitalium* infection and infertility.

21.4.2 Pregnancy

The association between *Mycoplasma genitalium* infection and obstetric complications, particularly preterm delivery and premature rupture of membranes (PROM), continues to be a subject of investigation and debate within the medical community. While some studies have demonstrated potential links, the evidence remains inconclusive, with inconsistent findings across different research efforts.

Preterm Birth: A systematic review and meta-analysis indicated that women infected with *M. genitalium* may face an increased risk of preterm birth. However, conflicting evidence exists. A prospective cohort study conducted at an urban community health center found no significant association between *M. genitalium* colonization and preterm delivery.

Premature Rupture of Membranes (PROM): The association between *Mycoplasma genitalium* infection and obstetric complications, particularly preterm delivery and premature rupture of membranes (PROM), continues to be a subject of investigation and debate within the medical community. While some studies have demonstrated potential links, the evidence remains inconclusive, with inconsistent findings across different research efforts.

Preterm Birth: A systematic review and meta-analysis indicated that women infected with *M. genitalium* may face an increased risk of preterm birth. However, conflicting evidence exists. A prospective cohort study conducted at an urban community health center found no significant association between *M. genitalium* colonization and preterm delivery. In this study, the crude OR for preterm delivery among women with *M. genitalium* colonization was 1.27 (95% CI: 0.02–14.78), suggesting no meaningful difference in risk [2].

Premature Rupture of Membranes (PROM)

Limited data exist regarding the association between *M. genitalium* infection and PROM. One study reported an unadjusted odds ratio of 7.62 (95% CI: 0.40–145.86) for PROM in women infected with *M. genitalium* [1]. However, the large confidence interval underscores the uncertainty and lack of precision in this estimate, necessitating further investigation.

Other Obstetric Complications

Research has also explored associations between *M. genitalium* infection and additional adverse pregnancy outcomes, including:

Low Birthweight: A recent study conducted in Papua New Guinea observed a statistically significant association between *M. genitalium* infection and decreased birthweight. The adjusted analysis revealed a reduction of −166.9 g (95% CI: −324.2 to −9.7 g) in neonates born to infected mothers [3].

Spontaneous Abortion: Evidence regarding an association with spontaneous abortion remains inconclusive. A meta-analysis summarized data from six studies, yielding an unadjusted OR of 1.00 (95% CI: 0.53–1.89), indicating no significant relationship [1].

Perinatal Death: Findings related to perinatal death are inconsistent. A case-control study reported an unadjusted OR of 1.07 (95% CI: 0.49–2.36), while a cohort study reported an OR as high as 38.42 (95% CI: 1.45–1021.43).

The variability in these results reflects significant heterogeneity and methodological limitations [1].

> **While there have been reports of an association between *Mycoplasma genitalium* infection and obstetric complications, more scientific studies are required to establish this link definitively.**

21.5 Diagnosis

Diagnosis of *Mycoplasma genitalium* infection involves the application of molecular biological detection methods, primarily PCR. Clinical indications and typical symptoms are often unclear, thus necessitating laboratory testing. The optimal specimen type for detection has yet to be determined. Common specimens employed include vaginal swabs, cervical swabs, first-void urine, and rectal swabs. The combination of samples from different anatomical sites has demonstrated higher detection rates. For instance, combining vaginal and cervical swabs yields a detection rate of approximately 95%, while concurrent endocervical swabs with first-void urine achieve a similar detection rate. However, the establishment of uniform methodologies and standardization for detection remains to be established.

21.6 Treatment

Mycoplasma genitalium demonstrates sensitivity to macrolides, tetracyclines, and fluoroquinolones (Table 21.1). Initial treatment with tetracyclines has shown limited efficacy, whereas a single administration of azithromycin at 1g has proven more effective than higher doses of doxycycline. However, extensive use of azithromycin has prompted 15–30% resistance to the single dose. There are concerns that the single-dose therapy increases the likelihood of developing resistant strains, leading to recommendations for prolonged treatment regimens, such as 5 days of totally 1.5g azithromycin, which have demonstrated success rates of 96–100%. Emerging fluoroquinolones, such as levofloxacin, have evidenced low efficacy, while moxifloxacin is recommended for managing infections with macrolide-resistant strains, exhibiting over 95% efficacy (Fig. 21.1). Nevertheless, fluoroquinolone resistance, including to moxifloxacin, has been documented.

Treatment of sexual partners is strongly advised.

Table 21.1 Treatment options for *Mycoplasma genitalium* infection

Indication	Medication	Dosage	Duration
Standard	Azithromycin[a]	Day 1: 500 mg orally once Day 2–5: 250 mg orally once	Day 1 Day 2–5
	Josamycin[b]	500 mg orally three times daily	14 days
	Roxithromycin[b]	300 mg orally once daily	14 days
	Roxithromycin[b]	150 mg orally twice daily	14 days
First alternative	Moxifloxacin	400 mg orally once daily	14 days
Second alternative	Doxycycline[c]	100 mg orally twice daily	14 days
Case of PID	Moxifloxacin[d]	400 mg orally/intravenously once daily	14 days
Complicated cases without macrolide resistance	Doxycycline	100 mg orally twice daily	7 days
	Followed by azithromycin	Day 1: 1000 mg orally once Day 2 + 3: 500 mg orally once	Day 1–3
In complicated cases with macrolide resistance	Doxycycline	100 mg orally twice daily	7 days
	Followed by moxifloxacin	400 mg orally once daily	14 days
Complicated cases (according to Mylonas)	Doxycycline	100 mg orally twice daily	7 days
	Followed by pristinamycin[e]	1000 mg orally four times daily	10 days

[a]Azithromycin: Increasing resistance to macrolides, currently between 10% and 50% depending on the population

[b]Josamycin and roxithromycin have the most extensive experience. If Josamycin is not available, it can be obtained through international pharmacy

[c]Doxycycline alone is not sufficiently effective in about ¾ of cases, so combination therapy is preferred

[d]When treating PID, additional administration of metronidazole (500 mg three times daily) is recommended

[e]The therapy was evaluated in a study with 12 patients who did not respond to standard therapies (publication still pending). Pristinamycin is not available in every country

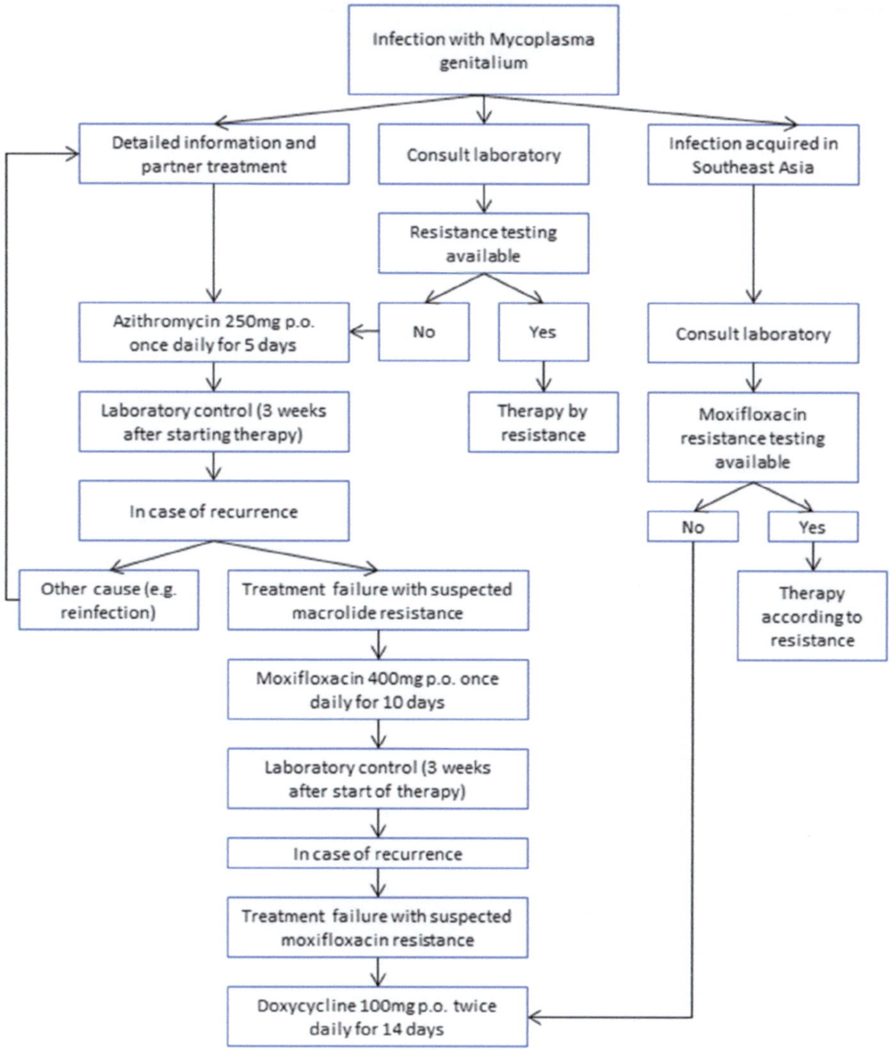

Fig. 21.1 Management protocol for Mycoplasma genitalium infection. (Courtesy of I. Mylonas)

21.7 Differential Diagnosis

Differential diagnosis for *Mycoplasma genitalium* focuses on distinguishing it from other sexually transmitted diseases (STD) presenting with similar symptoms. Key STDs to consider in this differentiation include *Chlamydia trachomatis*, *Neisseria gonorrhoeae*, and *Trichomonas vaginalis*. Nucleic acid amplification tests (NAATs) are vital in differentiating *Mycoplasma genitalium* from these other infections due to its asymptomatic presentation in certain cases.

21.8 Prevention

Currently, there is insufficient evidence to warrant the implementation of prevention or screening programs, attributed to variances in prevalence and the nascent association of *Mycoplasma genitalium* with urogenital diseases, many of which are not yet thoroughly established. Some mycoplasmas, including *Mycoplasma genitalium*, may play a role in the replication and pathogenicity of HIV, but comprehensive examination is necessary to elucidate their relationship fully. Adhesion of mycoplasmas to HIV-infected cells may enhance the excretion of the HI virus. Given that both infections are sexually transmitted, the connection may predominantly exist among high-risk individuals. Conversely, it remains plausible that HIV infection in immunocompromised individuals increases the susceptibility to *Mycoplasma genitalium*, or that *Mycoplasma genitalium* itself poses a risk factor for HIV infection and transmission.

Most published data originate from high-risk cohorts (sex workers, men who have sex with men, and STD-clinic attendees) in which co-prevalence is highest; the extent to which these associations apply to lower-risk or general populations remains uncertain.

Until higher-quality evidence is available, public-health efforts should continue to emphasize established HIV and STD prevention measures—condom use, partner notification, screening where indicated, and HIV pre-exposure prophylaxis. Testing for *M. genitalium* should be reserved for symptomatic patients or those with persistent nongonococcal urethritis or cervicitis despite standard therapy, with management guided by local diagnostic and antimicrobial-resistance resources.

Key Points

- *Mycoplasma genitalium* is a recognized pathogen linked to sexually transmitted diseases.
- Its association with nongonococcal urethritis has been established for over 25 years.
- The significance of its relationship to inflammatory diseases in women remains uncertain.
- Infection risk correlates with sexual behavior, particularly among young adults.
- This organism possesses the smallest known bacterial genome and lacks a cell wall.
- Prevalence rates show variability internationally, reaching up to 6% in women and 4% in men, with higher occurrences in at-risk groups.
- A substantial proportion of infections are asymptomatic.

(continued)

- Risk factors resemble those observed in other sexually transmitted diseases.
- *Mycoplasma genitalium* infection may double the risk of HIV exposure.
- Increasing antibiotic resistance, particularly to macrolides, poses significant treatment challenges.
- Acute and chronic urethritis are prevalent among men.
- Vaginal discharge and potential cervicitis are common in women, with unclear relationships to PID and infertility.
- Associations with obstetric complications, such as preterm birth, remain debated.
- Diagnosis primarily relies on molecular biological techniques, absent of clear clinical indications.
- Treatment options encompass macrolides, tetracyclines, and fluoroquinolones, with rising resistance noted.
- No standardized prevention or screening programs are currently established.

Sexually Transmitted Intestinal Infections

22

Abstract

Sexually transmitted intestinal infections primarily affect populations engaging in practices such as anal intercourse. Key pathogens include *Chlamydia trachomatis*, *Neisseria gonorrhoeae*, and various enteric bacteria like Shigella and Salmonella. Symptoms can range from mild proctitis to severe dysentery, characterized by abdominal pain, diarrhea, fever, and rectal bleeding. Diagnosis typically involves stool culture, serological tests, and clinical evaluations. Treatment is pathogen-specific, often consisting of antibiotics and supportive care. Preventative measures include safe sexual practices, education, and timely screening. The epidemiology of these infections highlights their higher prevalence among men who have sex with men (MSM), although they can also impact heterosexual populations. Public health initiatives aimed at increasing awareness and improving sanitation are essential to reduce gastrointestinal infections.

22.1 General

22.1.1 Background

Sexually transmitted intestinal infections are notably prevalent in certain at-risk populations. The predominant transmission routes include sexual practices such as oral–anal or genital–anal intercourse. Men who have sex with men (MSM) constitute the primary demographic affected; however, heterosexual women engaging in anal intercourse are also at risk of infection.

The spectrum of sexually transmitted intestinal infections includes a variety of diseases, including syphilis, gonorrhea, genital warts (human papillomavirus, HPV), lymphogranuloma venereum (LGV), granuloma inguinale, herpes simplex virus (HSV),

I. Mylonas, *Sexually Transmitted Diseases*,
https://doi.org/10.1007/978-3-031-78204-6_22

Table 22.1 Clinical differentiation between proctitis, proctocolitis, and enteritis

Symptom	Proctitis	Proctocolitis	Enteritis
Abdominal pain	–	+	++
Diarrhea	–	+	++
Fever	–	–	++
Loss of appetite	–	+	++
Mucus in the stool	+	+	–
Nausea	–	–	++
Palpable changes	+	+	–
Rectal bleeding	+	+	–
Vomiting	–	–	++
Weight loss	–	+	++

and *Chlamydia trachomatis*. Additionally, bacterial pathogens such as Campylobacter, Shigella, and Salmonella, along with parasitic agents like *Giardia intestinalis* and *Entamoeba histolytica*, can also be transmitted through these sexual practices.

The incubation periods for each pathogen differ significantly. In certain cases, symptomatic manifestations associated with sexually transmitted diseases (STD) may occur within days or weeks, while in others, symptoms may take months to appear.

The etiology of sexually transmitted diseases is multifactorial, involving various contributors, including unprotected anal intercourse and inadequate awareness of protective measures.

It is imperative to distinguish between proctitis, proctocolitis, and enteritis, especially in the context of sexually transmitted intestinal infections (Table 22.1):

- Proctitis: Inflammation confined to the rectum, commonly presenting with rectal bleeding, mucus in stools, and palpable changes. Abdominal pain, diarrhea, fever, loss of appetite, weight loss, nausea, and vomiting are generally absent.
- Proctocolitis: Involves both the rectum and colon, with symptoms such as rectal bleeding, abdominal pain, diarrhea, mucus in the stools, loss of appetite, weight loss, and palpable changes; fever, nausea, and vomiting are generally absent.
- Enteritis: Inflammation of the small intestine characterized by pronounced abdominal pain, diarrhea, fever, loss of appetite, weight loss, nausea, and vomiting.

Rectal bleeding, mucus in stools, and palpable changes are generally absent.

22.1.2 Clinical Manifestation

The clinical symptoms of sexually transmitted intestinal infections vary depending on the causative pathogen. Common symptoms may include abdominal discomfort, diarrhea, nausea, vomiting, fever, and fatigue. It is essential to distinguish proctitis, proctocolitis, and enteritis when assessing sexually transmitted intestinal infections (see Table 22.1). Accurate anatomic classification directs diagnostic sampling and empirical therapy.

- Proctitis: Inflammation limited to the rectum. Typical features include rectal bleeding, mucous or mucopurulent discharge, tenesmus, and local tenderness on examination. Systemic and small-bowel symptoms (significant abdominal pain, fever, anorexia, weight loss, nausea, and vomiting) are usually absent.
- Proctocolitis: Involvement of the rectum and colon. Clinical presentation combines rectal findings (bleeding, mucous discharge, and tenesmus) with lower-abdominal cramping and diarrheal symptoms; constitutional symptoms such as anorexia and weight loss may occur. High-grade fever, prominent nausea, and vomiting are less common.
- Enteritis: Inflammation of the small intestine. Presentation is dominated by diffuse or periumbilical abdominal pain, profuse watery diarrhea, fever, anorexia, weight loss, nausea, and vomiting. Rectal bleeding and prominent rectal mucous discharge are uncommon.

Perianal lesions may arise from multiple pathogens, including syphilis, herpes simplex virus (HSV), granuloma inguinale, chancroid, and condylomata acuminata.

22.1.3 Diagnosis

A thorough diagnostic evaluation is essential when anorectal infections are suspected. This systematic approach aids in accurately differentiating between various conditions, including proctitis, proctocolitis, and enteritis.

- **Proctitis** may result from infections such as gonorrhea, chlamydia, syphilis, or the herpes simplex virus (HSV).
- **Proctocolitis** may stem from pathogens like Shigella, Salmonella, Campylobacter, *E. histolytica*, or cytomegalovirus (CMV).
- **Enteritis** may be due to organisms such as Shigella, Salmonella, Campylobacter, Giardia, and CMV.

Diagnostic modalities include careful anorectal inspection, digital rectal examination, and anoscopy. These targeted examinations aid in localizing pathology and guiding specimen collection. Laboratory testing directed at specific pathogens is essential for definitive diagnosis and informed therapy; recommended tests include nucleic acid amplification tests (NAATs) on rectal swabs or stool for *Neisseria gonorrhoeae* and *Chlamydia trachomatis* (including LGV typing when indicated), stool PCR or culture for enteric pathogens (Shigella, Salmonella, and Campylobacter), antigen or PCR testing for *Entamoeba histolytica*, and HSV PCR or culture of lesions. When indicated, serologic testing (e.g., HIV and syphilis) and histopathology with biopsy may be performed. Diagnostic selection should be guided by clinical presentation, sexual history, and regional laboratory availability.

22.1.4 Therapy

The therapeutic approach should be pathogen-directed and symptom-guided.

- Antimicrobial therapy must target the identified or most likely organism (e.g., appropriate beta-lactam or third-generation cephalosporin for invasive bacterial enteritis, NAAT-guided therapy for *Neisseria gonorrhoeae*, doxycycline or azithromycin for *Chlamydia trachomatis*, targeted regimens for *Mycoplasma genitalium* guided by resistance testing, and metronidazole or tinidazole for *Entamoeba histolytica*).
- Symptom management should be provided concurrently: analgesia, antipyretics, antidiarrheals when not contraindicated, fluid and electrolyte replacement for dehydration, and topical therapies for local pain or ulceration.
- For anorectal syndromes, local measures (sitz baths, topical anesthetics, and topical or systemic anti-inflammatories) may be combined with systemic antimicrobial treatment as indicated.
- Host factors and comorbidities (pregnancy, immunosuppression, and renal or hepatic dysfunction) must inform drug selection, dosing, and duration.
- Follow-up should be arranged to confirm clinical resolution; test-of-cure (e.g., NAAT or culture) is recommended for selected pathogens (e.g., *M. genitalium*, persistent gonorrhea, or when treatment adherence or resistance is a concern).
- Sexual partners should be notified, evaluated, and treated.
- If symptoms persist or the diagnosis remains unclear, referral to infectious diseases, gastroenterology, or sexual health/STD services is recommended for further evaluation, extended diagnostics (including endoscopy/biopsy), and management.

22.1.5 Prevention

Preventive measures and early detection of sexually transmitted infections (STIs) are essential for public-health protection. Key components include:

- Public Education: Deliver clear, accessible information on transmission routes, risk factors (e.g., receptive anal intercourse, multiple partners, and inconsistent condom use), signs and symptoms, and the importance of timely testing.
- Barrier Protection: Promote consistent condom and dental-dam use for vaginal, anal, and oral sex; provide instruction on correct use.
- Routine and Targeted Screening: Implement guideline-based screening (e.g., Chlamydia and gonorrhea in sexually active young adults, HIV and syphilis screening according to risk) and offer targeted testing for high-risk groups.
- Vaccination: Ensure uptake of recommended vaccines (e.g., HPV and hepatitis B) in eligible populations.

- Access to Diagnostics and Treatment: Facilitate timely access to NAATs, point-of-care tests where validated, and evidence-based antimicrobial therapy; promote linkage to follow-up care.
- Partner Services: Perform contact notification, testing, and treatment per local public-health protocols to interrupt transmission chains.
- Harm-Reduction and Risk-Reduction Counseling: Provide behavioral interventions, safer-sex counseling, and, where appropriate, HIV pre-exposure prophylaxis (PrEP) and post-exposure prophylaxis (PEP).
- Surveillance and Reporting: Maintain robust surveillance systems and mandatory reporting where required to monitor trends and guide public-health interventions.

Early diagnosis, prompt treatment, and comprehensive prevention strategies should be prioritized to reduce individual morbidity, prevent complications, and limit onward transmission.

22.2 Frequent Sexually Transmitted Infections

22.2.1 Gonococcal Proctitis

- Primarily observed in homosexual men but may also affect women engaging in anal intercourse.
- Rectal gonorrhea can occur in women without prior anal intercourse through the transmission of infected vaginal secretions.
- Symptoms typically arise within 5–7 days post-infection, presenting as mild manifestations including constipation, anal pain, tenesmus, and purulent rectal discharge.
- Potential complications may include fistulas, abscesses, strictures, and disseminated infections.

22.2.2 Chlamydial Proctitis

- Infections caused by *Chlamydia trachomatis* and the disease lymphogranuloma venereum (LGV).
- LGV infections are associated with intense rectal discomfort, characterized by severe pain, bloody discharge, and a strong urge to defecate.
- Inguinal lymphadenopathy, similar to genital LGV, is commonly observed.
- Sigmoidoscopy may reveal extensive mucosal damage, with small rectal ulcers that could extend into the descending colon.

- Complications such as strictures and fistulas may develop, presenting a clinical picture similar to Crohn's disease or malignancies.
- Non-LGV strains of *C. trachomatis* are typically less aggressive, causing mild rectitis characterized by rectal urgency and discomfort.

22.2.3 Treponema Pallidum

- Primary anorectal ulcers caused by *Treponema pallidum* may develop 2–6 weeks following anal intercourse.
- Anorectal syphilis often remains undiagnosed until secondary or early latent stages.
- Examination may disclose anal ulcers, though asymptomatic ulcers within the anal canal and rectum should also be identified.
- Anorectal syphilis is frequently misinterpreted as anal sore, pain, constipation, rectal bleeding, or discharge.

22.3 Bacterial Intestinal Pathogens

22.3.1 *Campylobacter enteritis*

Background: *Campylobacter enteritis*, predominantly attributed to Campylobacter species, is frequently encountered in children within developing countries. The infection typically arises sporadically throughout the year, with epidemic outbreaks often following the consumption of contaminated food, particularly milk and poultry. The disease is most prevalent during the warmer months, from June to September. The predominant species are *C. jejuni* (approximately 90%) and *C. coli* (approximately 10%), with *C. lan*, *C. upsaliensis* (rare), and *C. fetus* also identified. Transmission from person to person is uncommon. The incubation period ranges from 2 to 4 days (1–7 days).

Clinical Manifestations: The clinical presentation typically includes a brief prodromal phase characterized by headache, limb discomfort, elevated fever, marked malaise, acute onset of diffuse or colicky abdominal pain, abdominal tenderness ("pseudoappendicitis"), and watery-mucous diarrhea, which may be accompanied by bloody stools, vomiting, meteorism, and occasionally delirium. The illness duration averages approximately 1 week, with relapses occurring in about 10% of patients. Possible complications comprise intestinal perforation, Guillain–Barré syndrome (rare), hemolytic uremic syndrome (rare), reactive arthritis, sepsis, systemic infections (rare), thrombotic thrombocytopenic purpura (rare), and toxic megacolon.

Pregnancy: The pathogen unlikely exerts a direct effect on the fetus. However, impaired absorption of essential nutrients and electrolyte imbalances can induce deficiency symptoms and adverse impacts on pregnancy viability.

Table 22.2 Treatment options for *Campylobacter enteritis*

Indication	Medication	Dosage	Duration
Antibiotic therapy	Azithromycin	500 mg orally/intravenously once daily	3 days
	Azithromycin	1 g orally, single dose	One day
	Ciprofloxacin	500 mg orally twice daily	3 days
	Ciprofloxacin	400 mg intravenously twice daily	3–5 days
Alternatives (older recommendations)	Erythromycin	500 mg orally/intravenously 4 times daily	7–10 days
	Clarithromycin	500 mg orally twice daily	7–10 days

Diagnosis: The diagnosis is confirmed by detecting the pathogen in stool samples during the acute phase, as well as the antigen in stool, which is detectable for approximately 2 weeks.

Treatment: Treatment is primarily symptomatic and involves the replacement of lost fluids due to diarrhea. In cases of acute infection, antimicrobial therapy is not initiated unless clinical improvement is absent despite appropriate interventions. Severe cases warrant antibiotic treatment (Table 22.2).

Differential Diagnosis: Differential diagnosis is essential to distinguish between various potential causes, including bacterial sepsis of other etiology, intestinal pathogenic *Escherichia coli*, salmonellosis, shigellosis, typhoid fever, and yersiniosis.

Prevention: *Campylobacter enteritis* is generally a self-limiting disease. It is advised to observe hygiene measures and restrict the activities and residence of suspected cases, infected persons, and carriers. Particularly for pregnant women, adherence to hygiene practices is essential, as severe disease courses can endanger the unborn child.

22.3.2 *Salmonella enteritis* (Salmonellosis)

Background: Salmonella, including *S. enteritidis*, is the causative agent of salmonellosis, a zoonotic infection that presents sporadically and epidemically worldwide. These bacteria can survive for extended periods, even months, and are not inactivated by freezing. The primary transmission route is through the ingestion of contaminated food, especially poultry, eggs, raw egg products, and ice cream. Additionally, transmission via contaminated surfaces and objects by infected individuals is possible. The incubation period typically spans hours to days, manifesting when substantial quantities of bacteria ($>10^5$) are ingested.

Clinical Manifestations: Typical signs of salmonellosis include acute onset of vomiting, diarrhea, watery stools, fever (39–40 °C), and, in certain instances, gallbladder infection. Severe cases may lead to complications such as abscesses, bacteremia, cholecystitis, endocarditis, meningitis, osteomyelitis, pleural effusions, pyelonephritis, reactive arthritis, and sepsis.

Pregnancy: The pathogen is unlikely to have a direct effect on the fetus. However, malabsorption of essential nutrients and electrolyte disturbances may induce deficiency symptoms and adverse pregnancy effects.

Table 22.3 Management of *Salmonella enteritis*

Indication	Medication	Dosage	Duration
Therapy	Ciprofloxacin	500 mg orally twice daily	5–7 days
	Co-trimoxazole	960 mg orally twice daily	5–7 days
Sepsis	Ciprofloxacin	400 mg intravenously 2–3 times daily	12–14 days
	Ceftriaxone	2 g intravenously twice daily	12–14 days
	Cefotaxime	2 g intravenously three times daily	12–14 days
Secondary prophylaxis mostly after invasive infection in HIV patients.	Ciprofloxacin	500 mg orally twice daily	6–8 months
Chronic carriers	Ciprofloxacin	500 mg orally twice daily	28 days

Diagnosis: Diagnosis depends on detecting pathogens through stool or rectal swab cultures, along with antibiogram analysis. Blood cultures usually return negative results. Serological testing, such as the Widal reaction, can be conducted starting from the tenth day of illness. Titers above 1:200 are considered conclusive, although this method is not universally reliable.

Treatment: In cases of severe illness, especially with fever and bloody stools, antibiotic therapy is indicated. Commonly prescribed antibiotics include ciprofloxacin or cotrimoxazole (Table 22.3). In immunocompromised patients, infants, young children, and the elderly, individualized therapy based on antibiogram findings should be performed. The use of antidiarrheal agents is generally ineffective, and surgical intervention for gallbladder removal may be warranted in specific cases.

Differential Diagnosis: Differential diagnoses include adenovirus infection, amoebic dysentery, *Campylobacter jejuni* infections, *Escherichia coli* infections (ETEC, EIUC), giardiasis, norovirus infection, rotavirus infection, shigellosis, and yersiniosis.

Prevention: Adherence to stringent hygiene protocols in food production is essential to prevent salmonella infections. Vigilance is also warranted against contact infections within hospitals, communal facilities, and households. The consistent implementation of hygiene measures and the establishment of protocols for infected individuals are critical.

The efficacy of therapeutic interventions targeting long-term bacterial excretors is not invariably guaranteed.

22.3.3 Shigella Dysentery (Shigellosis, Bacterial Dysentery)

Background: Shigella dysentery is primarily caused by various strains of the bacterial genus Shigella, including *Shigella dysenteriae*, *Shigella flexneri*, *Shigella boydii*, and *Shigella sonnei*. These pathogens are distributed globally but show higher prevalence in regions characterized by poor hygiene standards. The incidence is relatively low in industrialized nations. Fecal-oral transmission, typically via contaminated food—particularly dairy products—is the most frequent transmission method. Smear infections, particularly within institutions such as childcare

Table 22.4 Treatment approaches for shigellosis

Indication	Medication	Dosage	Duration
Treatment	Azithromycin	500 mg orally/intravenously once daily	3 days
	Ciprofloxacin	500 mg orally twice daily	3–5 days
	Ciprofloxacin	400 mg intravenously twice daily	3–5 days
Alternative (older recommendation)	Co-trimoxazole	960 mg orally twice daily	7–10 days
	Amoxicillin	1000 mg orally three times daily	7–10 days

facilities, also pose a significant risk. The incubation period ranges from one to 17 days, although infectious pathogens may be excreted for up to 2 months post-illness.

Clinical Manifestations: Shigella dysentery presents as an acute, febrile, and highly contagious gastrointestinal illness. Typical symptoms include mucous or bloody stools. Infection with different Shigella strains may result in tissue invasion manifested by bloody diarrhea. Disease severity can range from mild to severe, with *Shigella dysenteriae* infections potentially leading to serious complications, including encephalopathy and toxic megacolon.

Pregnancy: The pathogen is unlikely to have a direct impact on fetal development. However, malabsorption and diarrhea in pregnant women can adversely affect the fetus—a rare occurrence.

Diagnosis: The diagnosis of shigellosis is typically achieved through pathogen detection via stool or rectal swab culture. Serological examination may be conducted for *Shigella sonnei* and *Shigella flexneri* during the acute phase or through seroconversion, albeit with lower specificity and sensitivity.

Treatment: Management of shigellosis encompasses fluid and electrolyte replacement alongside antibiotic therapy, commonly consisting of macrolides or quinolones. Previously, doxycycline, sulfonamides, cotrimoxazole, and ampicillin/amoxicillin were recommended (Table 22.4). Therapy should be adapted according to antibiogram results due to rising resistance. Cotrimoxazole or ampicillin/amoxicillin are typically preferred for pediatric patients, with treatment in developing regions often utilizing ampicillin/amoxicillin, doxycycline, or cotrimoxazole based on cost-effectiveness.

Differential Diagnosis: Differential diagnoses include adenovirus infection, amoebic dysentery, *Campylobacter jejuni* and *C. coli* infections, cholera, enteropathogenic *Escherichia coli*, giardiasis, norovirus, rotavirus, and salmonellosis.

Prevention: Implementation of stringent hygiene measures is important to prevent shigellosis occurrences. Ensuring appropriate accommodations and isolation protocols is essential. Individuals suspected of having the disease or exhibiting symptoms should abstain from specific activities.

22.3.4 Yersinia

Background: The genus Yersinia comprises bacteria responsible for causing Yersinia enterocolitica and Yersinia pseudotuberculosis infections, with the latter being more commonly found in Eastern Europe and Russia. These pathogens can result in

Table 22.5 Management of *Yersinia enteritis*

Indication	Medication	Dosage	Duration
Adults	Ciprofloxacin	500 mg orally twice daily	5–7 days
	Ciprofloxacin	400 mg intravenously twice daily	5–7 days
	Co-trimoxazole	160/800 mg orally/intravenously twice daily	5–7 days
Alternative (older recommendation)	Doxycycline	100 mg orally twice daily	7–10 days
Bacteremia/sepsis	Ceftriaxone	1 g intravenously twice daily	10–14 days
	Ciprofloxacin	500 mg orally twice daily	10–14 days
	Ciprofloxacin	400 mg intravenously three times daily	10–14 days
Alternative (older recommendation)	Cefotaxime	2 g intravenously three times daily plus gentamicin initially 2 mg/kg intravenously/intramuscularly, then 1.5 mg/kg every 8 hours	10–14 days

widespread sporadic diseases, particularly in temperate climates. Epidemic outbreaks may occur due to contaminated drinking water or food sources. *Yersinia enterocolitica* resides in the intestines (and pharynx) of various warm-blooded animals and is transmitted to humans primarily through the oral ingestion of contaminated water or food. The incubation period is usually between 3 and 10 days. Yersinia infections are associated with multiple clinical manifestations, including gastrointestinal disease and reactive arthritis, which is more common post-infection than previously recognized. Characteristic findings involve preceding abdominal symptoms followed by oligoarthritis of the lower extremities. About 80% of affected patients display HLA-B27 positivity with rheumatoid factor negativity. Typically, the disease resolves spontaneously within 6 months with symptomatic treatment and antibiotic intervention.

Clinical Manifestations: Symptoms of Yersinia infections may include abdominal pain and diarrhea, which can range from watery to bloody. Additional manifestations might involve inflammation of the small intestine (enteritis), large intestine (enterocolitis), terminal ileum, and abdominal lymph nodes, sometimes resembling "pseudoappendicitis." Rarely, symptoms such as ascites, bronchitis, hepatomegaly, pharyngitis, and splenomegaly may occur, with potential complications including reactive arthritis, erythema nodosum, uveitis (particularly in HLA B27 positive patients), or severe septic conditions in immunocompromised individuals.

Pregnancy: The disease does not appear to have a direct impact on fetal development. However, it may influence maternal metabolism, potentially leading to nutrient modulation or deficiency, which could affect pregnancy outcomes.

Diagnosis: Diagnosis of a Yersinia infection is established by pathogen detection in stool samples, inflammatory exudates, or excised lymph nodes. An initial rise followed by a subsequent decline in serum antibodies may offer further diagnostic insights. Cross-reactions with Salmonella and Brucella abortus should be considered during diagnosis.

Treatment: Management of Yersinia infections is primarily supportive and symptomatic, with antibiotic treatment generally not recommended for acute infections. In cases of significant disease progression or absence of clinical improvement (Table 22.5), antibiotic therapy may be warranted, contingent upon resistance testing results. Note that antibiotics are ineffective in reactive conditions.

Differential Diagnosis: Other bacterial intestinal infections, appendicitis, and reactive arthritis of other etiology (e.g., caused by Chlamydia) should be included in the differential diagnosis.

Prevention: The implementation of hygiene measures is critical to preventing Yersinia infections. Restrictions on activities and quarantining individuals with suspected or confirmed Yersinia infections are recommended.

22.4 Viral Infections

22.4.1 Hepatitis A

Background: The hepatitis A virus (HAV) is a single-stranded, nonenveloped RNA virus that belongs to the Picornaviridae family. It has one known serotype and seven genotypes, with its distribution being widespread globally. Approximately 1.4 million new cases are reported worldwide each year. Infection is more prevalent among children living in high-prevalence regions, although these individuals typically develop immunity by adulthood. In areas with low endemicity, infections are more common in adults and can lead to serious health problems. The primary mode of transmission is fecal-oral, which accounts for the disease's higher prevalence in developing countries with inadequate hygiene and sanitation. Although rare, sexual transmission has been documented. The average incubation period is approximately 30 days.

Clinical Manifestations: Symptoms of hepatitis A can vary from mild to severe and typically manifest between 2 and 6 weeks after exposure to HAV. Not all individuals infected with HAV will exhibit symptoms, especially young children. When symptoms do occur, they often include low-grade fever, nausea, vomiting, loss of appetite, jaundice (yellowing of the skin and eyes), dark urine, abdominal pain, itching, joint pain, pale stools, and painful hepatomegaly. Symptoms generally last between 4 and 6 weeks, although, in some cases, the disease can persist for up to 6 months. Acute liver failure associated with hepatitis A is rare.

Diagnosis: Clinically, hepatitis A cannot be distinguished from other types of viral hepatitis. Diagnosis is made based on the detection of anti-HAV IgM antibodies.

Pregnancy: Pregnancy does not alter the disease's course. Vertical transmission of hepatitis A is uncommon due to the presence of anti-HAV IgG antibodies in newborns, which provide protection post-delivery. The impact of HAV infection on pregnancy varies with gestational age. There is no evidence of teratogenic effects in the first trimester, though the potential for liver damage in the fetus exists. In the third trimester, severe disease may increase the risk of placental abruption, premature rupture of membranes, and premature labor, though data on these complications are limited.

Treatment: Treatment is primarily supportive. Vaginal delivery is the preferred mode, with cesarean section indicated only for obstetric reasons. Breastfeeding is not contraindicated.

Prevention: Vaccination is the most effective preventive measure against hepatitis A. post-exposure passive immunoprophylaxis with hepatitis A immunoglobulin

(HAV-Ig) has been reported to be effective in approximately 80–90% of exposed contacts. The inactivated hepatitis A vaccine is considered safe during pregnancy and is recommended for pregnant individuals at increased risk of exposure; vaccination during gestation is advised when clinically indicated. Neonates born to mothers with acute hepatitis A should be administered HAV-Ig within 48 h of birth if maternal infection occurred within the 2 weeks before or the 1 week after delivery.

22.4.2 Hepatitis E

Background: The hepatitis E virus (HEV) is a member of the Hepeviridae family within the Orthohepevirus genus. Hepatitis E is a leading sporadic and endemic cause of hepatitis in adults in Asia and parts of Africa, with approximately 20 million infections and about 70,000 deaths annually. Genotypes 1 and 2 are predominantly found in developing nations, while genotypes 3 and 4 are more prevalent in developed countries and parts of Asia and Europe, respectively. Transmission predominantly occurs through the fecal-oral route. It is suggested that sexual transmission may also occur, especially considering the higher HEV titers found in men who have sex with men (MSM) compared to the general population. The incubation period is estimated to range from 2 to 9 weeks, with viral infectivity lasting up to 14 days post-jaundice onset. Genotypes 1 and 2 are transmitted as described, while genotypes 3 and 4 are zoonotic and transmitted through the consumption of infected pork. Vertical transmission during pregnancy is associateded with genotype 1.

Clinical Manifestations: The incubation period for hepatitis E virus (HEV) ranges from 2 to 10 weeks. In the nonpregnant population, the infection usually presents as mild to moderately severe, with a mortality rate of 0.4–4%. Clinical presentations can vary widely, from asymptomatic to anicteric, icteric, and fulminant hepatitis. HEV infections do not lead to chronic hepatitis, cirrhosis, or hepatocellular carcinoma.

Pregnancy: Infection during pregnancy can lead to fulminant liver failure, associated with a maternal mortality rate of 5–25%. Vertical transmission occurs in 33–100% of cases, with a fetal mortality rate of 33% and an 8% mortality rate in newborns. The infection may also result in various obstetric complications, including antepartum hemorrhage, premature rupture of membranes, premature labor, postpartum hemorrhage, disseminated intravascular coagulation, and intrauterine death. Newborns of mothers infected with HEV may develop mild, anicteric hepatitis and are at risk of acute liver failure, along with complications associated with premature birth.

Diagnosis: Diagnosis is based on the detection of immunoglobulin M (IgM) antibodies against HEV.

Treatment: Treatment is supportive in nature. In severe cases, delivery may be necessary to ensure the health and safety of the infant. For fulminant liver failure, liver transplantation may be considered as a treatment option.

Prevention: Currently, no vaccine or immunoglobulin is available for prevention or post-exposure prophylaxis. Vaginal delivery and breastfeeding are not contraindicated. Preventing HEV infection is critical to avoiding potentially severe consequences during pregnancy; thus, adherence to proper water hygiene and sanitation practices is essential.

22.5 Parasitic Infections

Individuals engaging in sexual activity that includes oral–anal contact are at increased risk for several parasitic infections, such as *Giardia lamblia*, *Iodamoeba butschlii*, *Dientamoeba fragilis*, *Enterobius vermicularis*, Cryptosporidium, Isospora, and Microsporidia. Among these, Giardia and *Entamoeba histolytica* are identified as the most common sexually transmitted parasitic infections, with homosexual men being the most affected demographic, although isolated cases of infection in women have been reported.

22.5.1 Amoebic Dysentery

Background: Amoebic dysentery, caused by *Entamoeba histolytica*, is a widely prevalent global infection, with prevalence rates exceeding 30% in certain tropical regions. The transmission of the parasite occurs via the fecal-oral route, through the ingestion of amoebic cysts spread via contaminated sources of food, particularly raw vegetables, or drinking water or surface water. The infection has the capacity to remain infectious for extended periods. E. histolytica undergoes two developmental stages: the cyst stage, during which cysts are excreted in the stool, and the vegetative stage, in which trophozoites develop and phagocytose erythrocytes, being subsequently termed magna forms.

Clinical Manifestations: Tissue invasion and the manifestation of typical disease symptoms occur in a limited proportion of infected individuals, approximately 10%.The clinical presentation may include various forms of enteritis, such as bloody stools accompanied by raspberry jelly-like mucus deposits, mucopurulent stools, tenesmus, and, in some cases, mild fever. Complications arising from the disease can be severe, including a fulminant course with toxic megacolon, peritonitis, intestinal perforation, or liver abscesses.

Pregnancy: Amoebic dysentery has the potential for fatal outcomes. The pathogen is unlikely to exert a direct effect on the fetus. However, impaired absorption of essential nutrients and electrolyte imbalances can induce deficiencies and adverse effects during pregnancy.

Diagnosis: Diagnosis involves a thorough travel history, microscopic detection of the pathogen, antigen detection in stool, and histological examination of colonic ulcerations. Rectosigmoidoscopy typically reveals ulcers amid intact mucosa. Serum antibody detection can also be beneficial. Various diagnostic methods, including polymerase chain reaction (PCR), can be employed to exclude nonpathogenic microorganisms in intestinal cases. Imaging techniques such as sonography, computed tomography (CT), or magnetic resonance imaging (MRI) are useful in assessing extraintestinal manifestations.

Treatment: Treatment for amoebic dysentery involves medication targeting intestinal lumen infections (asymptomatic cyst carriers), chronic intestinal infections, and acute amoebic dysentery.

Treatment Options for Amoebic Dysentery

- **Intestinal Lumen Infection (Asymptomatic Cyst Carriers):** Paromomycin 25 mg/kg/day, divided into three daily doses.
- **Intestinal Wall Amoebiasis (Chronic Intestinal Infection by Tissue Forms):** Metronidazole 750 mg three times daily for 7–10 days.
- **Acute Amoebic Dysentery:** Metronidazole 750 mg three times daily for 7–10 days.
- **Liver Abscess/Extraintestinal Manifestations:**
  1. **Metronidazole:** 750 mg three times daily for 7–10 days.
  2. **Chloroquine:** Start with 1 g/day (600 mg base) for 2 days, followed by 500 mg/day for 2–3 weeks orally.
  3. **Elimination of Intestinal Lumen Forms:** *Paromomycin* 25–35 mg/kg/day in three doses orally, or *diloxanide furoate* 500 mg three times daily for 10 days (availability varies by country).
- **Liver Abscesses:** Usually heal under conservative therapy over several months.
- **Large Abscesses with Threatened Perforation:** Aspiration performed under sonographic guidance during ongoing therapy.
- **Control:** Stool examination is recommended 2 weeks after completing medication to confirm eradication.
- **Novel Medication:** Secnidazole,[1] a novel medication administered as a 2 g granulate in a single oral dose, is typically sprinkled onto a small amount of applesauce, yogurt, or pudding and consumed immediately without chewing or mixing with liquids. It is regarded as an alternative to metronidazole but is unavailable in many countries.

Differential Diagnosis: Considering the diagnosis of amoebic dysentery requires differentiation from numerous other potential conditions, including appendicitis, Campylobacter infections, ulcerative colitis, irritable bowel syndrome, colon carcinoma, enteroinvasive *Escherichia coli* infections, hepatocellular carcinoma, hepatic echinococcosis, Crohn's disease, salmonellosis, and shigellosis.

[1] Secnidazole is FDA-approved in the United States for the treatment of amoebiasis, also in adult women and for use in females 12 years of age and older. The drug is administered as a single oral dose of 2 g, typically sprinkled onto a small amount of applesauce, yogurt, or pudding and taken immediately without chewing or mixing with liquids. Common side effects include headache, nausea, vomiting, diarrhea, and an unpleasant metallic taste. Serious side effects may include vaginal odor, white or yellowish vaginal discharge, or vaginal itching. Secnidazole should not be used during breastfeeding or suspected pregnancy and is not approved for use by anyone younger than 18 years old. It should also be avoided by individuals allergic to secnidazole or similar medications like metronidazole or tinidazole.

Prevention: Given the increasing prevalence of international travel, prioritizing hygiene measures is critical. Activity and residence restrictions, along with adherence to reporting obligations, are recommended to contain the spread of amoebic dysentery.

22.5.2 Giardiasis (Lambliasis)

Background: Giardiasis is an intestinal and/or bile duct infection caused by the noninvasive protozoan Giardia intestinalis (also known as *Giardia lamblia* or *Giardia duodenalis*, particularly in Anglo-American regions). This zoonotic parasite is widely distributed and often contaminates freshwater sources. Transmission occurs through the ingestion of viable cysts, frequently from contaminated water or food, or via fecal–oral contact. Giardia cysts resist chlorination and survive well in cold mountain streams.

Epidemiology: The incidence of giardiasis is uncertain, with estimates suggesting around 20,000 cases annually in the United States. The prevalence in the United States is approximately 4%. Waterborne outbreaks are frequent, particularly affecting children, travelers, immunocompromised individuals, and those with cystic fibrosis.

Clinical Manifestations: Symptoms of giardiasis vary widely and may include diarrhea, malaise, flatulence, foul-smelling greasy stools, abdominal cramps, nausea, loss of appetite, weight loss, vomiting, fever, hives, and constipation. Diarrhea is the most common symptom, occurring in 89% of cases, followed by malaise (84%) and flatulence (74%). The typical incubation period ranges from seven to 21 days, and some patients may remain asymptomatic. Chronic diarrhea and malabsorption are prevalent, and lactose intolerance may develop post-infection, which could be misinterpreted as a recurrent infection.

Pregnancy: Giardiasis is unlikely to directly affect the fetus. However, malabsorption and diarrhea in pregnant women can have adverse effects, although such occurrences are rare.

Diagnosis: Diagnosis is usually achieved through the microscopic examination of stool samples or duodenal aspirates. Immunoassays for Giardia antigens in stool samples offer greater sensitivity and specificity compared to microscopy. Laboratory tests, including serum albumin and vitamin B12 levels, help exclude malabsorption as a cause.

Treatment: Treatment may involve nonpharmacological measures, such as avoiding dairy products, in addition to drug therapies, including metronidazole, tinidazole, and albendazole, depending on severity and patient age (Table 22.6). Paromomycin is considered safe during pregnancy. However, albendazole and paromomycin exhibit lower efficacy compared to other medications. A stool examination is recommended 2 weeks following treatment, with additional treatment

Table 22.6 Management strategies for giardiasis

Indication	Medication	Dosage	Duration
Adults	Metronidazole	500 mg orally three times daily	7 days
	Metronidazole	1 g orally twice daily	5 days
	Tinidazole[a]	2 g orally once daily	4 days
Alternatives	Albendazole	400 mg orally daily	5–7 days
	Paromomycin	25–35 mg/kg in 3 single doses	7 days
Pregnancy	Metronidazole[b]	500 mg orally three times daily	7 days
	Paromomycin	25–35 mg/kg in 3 single doses	7 days

[a]The availability of tinidazole should be verified
[b]Metronidazole should be avoided during the first trimester, according to local authority approval

warranted in the event of recurrence. Secnidazole[2], a novel medication administered as a 2 g granulate in a single oral dose, is typically sprinkled onto a small amount of applesauce, yogurt, or pudding and consumed immediately without chewing or mixing with liquids. It is not available in many countries.

Differential Diagnosis: A differential diagnosis is necessary to determine the underlying cause of diarrhea. Other infectious and noninfectious causes of malabsorption should also be considered.

Prevention: Individuals traveling to endemic areas should be advised to boil drinking water or utilize water purification tablets, as chlorination may not be effective. Chronic giardiasis in developing countries can be associated with stunted growth and developmental issues in children.

22.6 Other Pathogens

Evidence suggests that sexual transmission of Cryptosporidium, Isospora belli, and Microsporidia may occur more frequently among HIV-infected homosexual men, although evidence for such transmission remains limited. These protozoa predominantly infect the small intestine, leading to nonspecific, watery diarrhea, abdominal cramps, and flatulence. Diagnosis can be challenging. In immunocompetent patients experiencing self-limiting diarrhea, treatment for Cryptosporidium or Isospora infections is typically unnecessary. In HIV-infected patients, management should prioritize symptom relief, with a focus on ensuring adequate fluid intake and electrolyte replacement, either orally or intravenously. Although various antibiotics, such as paromomycin and azithromycin, are employed, chronic infections and

[2]Secnidazole is FDA-approved in the United States for the treatment of giardiasis in adult women and for use in females 12 years of age and older. The drug is administered as a single oral dose of 2 g, typically sprinkled onto a small amount of applesauce, yogurt, or pudding and taken immediately without chewing or mixing with liquids. Common side effects include headache, nausea, vomiting, diarrhea, and an unpleasant metallic taste. Serious side effects may include vaginal odor, white or yellowish vaginal discharge, or vaginal itching. Secnidazole should not be used during breastfeeding or suspected pregnancy and is not approved for use by anyone younger than 18 years old. It should also be avoided by individuals allergic to secnidazole or similar medications like metronidazole or tinidazole.

relapses remain common. The most efficacious treatment currently available involves highly active antiretroviral therapy.

Other Potential Sexually Transmitted Intestinal Pathogens

- **Cryptosporidium parvum**
  - **Transmission and Epidemiology**: This microorganism is primarily transmitted via the fecal–oral route and is frequently observed in immunocompromised individuals, such as those with HIV/AIDS or undergoing immunosuppressive therapy. Contaminated water and food sources are common vectors for transmission, making outbreaks more likely in areas with poor sanitation.
  - **Clinical Features**: The primary symptom is watery diarrhea, which can be severe and persistent in immunocompromised patients. Malabsorption may also occur, leading to nutritional deficiencies. The condition can be self-limiting in immunocompetent individuals but tends to be chronic in those with weakened immune systems.
  - **Diagnosis**: Diagnosis involves testing stool samples; however, if initial results are negative, further diagnostic evaluations like small bowel aspiration or biopsies may be necessary. Diagnostic methods include microscopic examination using modified acid-fast staining techniques, immunofluorescence assays, enzyme-linked immunosorbent assay (ELISA) methods, and polymerase chain reaction (PCR) for detecting Cryptosporidium DNA.
  - **Treatment**: Nitazoxanide is recommended for immunocompetent patients aged ≥1 year. Supportive care, including adequate fluid and electrolyte replacement, is critical to manage dehydration resulting from diarrhea. Immunocompromised individuals may require additional supportive measures and close monitoring.
- **Cyclospora cayetanensis**
  - **Transmission and Epidemiology**: Cyclospora is also transmitted via the fecal–oral route, often through contaminated water or food, particularly fresh produce such as berries or leafy greens. It is commonly associated with travel to tropical or subtropical regions where the parasite is endemic.
  - **Clinical Features**: Symptoms include prolonged watery diarrhea, which may be accompanied by malabsorption, fatigue, abdominal cramping, and weight loss. The infection can persist for weeks if left untreated.
  - **Diagnosis**: Stool sample analysis is the primary diagnostic method. If stool tests are inconclusive, small bowel aspiration or biopsies may be required. Microscopic examination using modified acid-fast staining is the standard diagnostic procedure.
  - **Treatment**: The antibiotic combination of trimethoprim–sulfamethoxazole is the treatment of choice. Supportive care, including hydration and electrolyte replacement, is essential to manage symptoms and prevent complications.
- ***Isospora belli***
  - **Transmission and Epidemiology**: *Isospora belli* infections occur via fecal–oral transmission and are more frequently seen in immunocompromised

individuals, particularly those with HIV/AIDS. Poor hygiene and environmental contamination contribute to its spread.
  - **Clinical Features**: This parasite causes watery diarrhea accompanied by malabsorption, leading to potential dehydration and nutritional deficiencies. Chronic or recurrent infections are common in immunocompromised patients.
  - **Diagnosis**: Stool sample examination is the initial diagnostic step; however, negative results may necessitate small bowel aspiration or biopsies for further evaluation. Diagnostic techniques include microscopic examination with modified acid-fast staining and PCR for detecting Isospora DNA.
  - **Treatment**: Trimethoprim–sulfamethoxazole is the first-line treatment. Supportive care, including fluid and electrolyte replacement, plays a vital role in managing symptoms and preventing complications.
- **Microsporidia**
  - **Transmission and Epidemiology**: Microsporidial infections are transmitted via the fecal–oral route and are predominantly observed in immunocompromised individuals. Common sources of infection include contaminated water, food, or direct contact with infected animals or humans.
  - **Clinical Features**: Symptoms include watery diarrhea and malabsorption, which can lead to significant weight loss and dehydration in severe cases. In immunocompromised patients, microsporidiosis can cause chronic gastrointestinal symptoms.
  - **Diagnosis**: Stool sample analysis is the initial diagnostic tool. If stool tests are inconclusive, small bowel aspiration or colon biopsy may be needed for further evaluation. Diagnostic methods include microscopic examination using special staining techniques (e.g., chromotrope-based stains) and PCR for identifying microsporidial species.
  - **Treatment**: Albendazole is commonly used for treating microsporidiosis caused by *Enterocytozoon bieneusi* or *Encephalitozoon intestinalis*. Fumagillin[3] may also be effective but is not widely approved for use. Supportive care, including hydration therapy and nutritional support, is essential for symptom management, particularly in immunocompromised patients.
- ***Balantidium coli***
  - **Transmission and Epidemiology**: Transmission occurs via the fecal–oral route, primarily through ingestion of contaminated water or food. *Balantidium coli* infections are more common in regions with poor sanitation and hygiene practices. Zoonotic transmission from infected pigs can also occur.
  - **Clinical Features**: Clinical manifestations include bloody diarrhea and dysentery-like symptoms, such as abdominal pain and cramping. Severe cases may lead to complications, such as intestinal perforation or secondary bacterial infections if left untreated.

[3] Fumagillin, which is sometimes used for microsporidiosis caused by *Enterocytozoon bieneusi* and *Encephalitozoon intestinalis*, has not been universally approved for use in clinical practice.

- **Diagnosis**: Diagnosis relies on stool sample analysis through microscopic examination to identify the characteristic trophozoites or cysts of *Balantidium coli*.
- **Treatment**: Tetracycline is the preferred treatment option, with metronidazole serving as an alternative in cases where tetracycline is contraindicated. Supportive care, including fluid replacement therapy, is crucial to manage dehydration and maintain electrolyte balance.

Key Points

- Sexually transmitted intestinal infections predominantly affect at-risk populations, especially men who have sex with men (MSM) and heterosexual women practicing anal intercourse.
- Routes of transmission include oral-anal and genital-anal sexual practices.
- Common infections include syphilis, gonorrhea, HPV, lymphogranuloma venereum (LGV), granuloma inguinale, herpes simplex virus (HSV), Chlamydia trachomatis, and various bacterial pathogens (e.g., Campylobacter, Shigella, Salmonella) as well as parasites (e.g., Giardia intestinalis, Entamoeba histolytica).
- Distinctions among proctitis, proctocolitis, and enteritis are clinically significant.
- Clinical symptoms associated with sexually transmitted intestinal infections vary according to the causative pathogen, with common manifestations including abdominal discomfort, diarrhea, nausea, vomiting, fever, and fatigue.
- Conditions include proctitis (gonorrhea, chlamydia, syphilis, HSV), proctocolitis (Shigella, Salmonella, Campylobacter, E. histolytica, CMV), and enteritis (Shigella, Salmonella, Campylobacter, Giardia, CMV).
- Additional methods include anorectal examination, digital rectal examination, and anoscopy, with laboratory tests remaining critical for definitive diagnosis.
- Therapy is determined by the specific infectious microorganism involved.
- Accurate distinction among conditions related to sexually transmitted intestinal infections is critical for effective diagnosis and treatment planning.
- Inclusive understanding of symptomatology, transmission pathways, and prevention strategies should be promoted across the healthcare community to enhance the clinical and public health response to these infections.

Trichomoniasis

23

Abstract

Trichomoniasis is a sexually transmitted infection caused by the protozoan parasite *Trichomonas vaginalis*. This disease constitutes the most common sexually transmitted infection globally, with an estimated 174 million new cases reported annually. In females, the pathogen can manifest with symptoms, including colpitis and the production of a malodorous vaginal discharge. Conversely, males frequently remain asymptomatic. Symptoms typically develop between 5 and 28 days post-infection, although asymptomatic cases may also occur. In pregnant women, *T. vaginalis* infection can lead to premature birth, premature rupture of membranes, and low birth weight. Diagnosis is generally achieved through microscopic examination. Treatment with metronidazole has proven effective, and the use of condoms can serve as an important preventive measure. Coinfection with HIV increases the transmission risk for both diseases.

23.1 Background

The protozoan parasite Trichomonas vaginalis was initially described in 1836 by Alfred Donne in a preliminary communication presented to the Paris Academy of Sciences. For an extended duration, trichomonads were regarded as a prevalent but clinically irrelevant element of the normal vaginal flora. In the year 1916, the Kiel-based gynecologist Hoehne introduced the term "trichomonas colpitis."

In humans, multiple trichomonas species are organ-specific, colonizing distinct anatomical sites. *Trichomonas tenax* inhabits the gingiva, *Trichomonas hominis* resides in the intestine, while *T. vaginalis* targets the genital tract.

I. Mylonas, *Sexually Transmitted Diseases*,
https://doi.org/10.1007/978-3-031-78204-6_23

23.2 Pathogen

Trichomonas vaginalis is a unicellular, pear-shaped pathogen belonging to the flagellate family, capable of motility through the action of its flagella. The organism features four short flagella and one long flagellum, along with an undulating membrane and axial rod, measuring up to 25 μm in length. The reproduction of trichomonads occurs through simple longitudinal division, utilizing an anaerobic metabolic pathway. Unlike many other parasites, *T. vaginalis* possesses a direct life cycle, necessitating no intermediate hosts or distinct developmental stages.

As an obligate pathogen, *T. vaginalis* reproduces solely within the vaginal and urethral mucosa. The protozoa are sensitive to desiccation, low temperatures, and light, thereby requiring direct and intimate contact for transmission.

Trichomonas vaginalis is transmitted predominantly by sexual contact, affecting the genital tract and lower urinary tract; in males, extension to the prostate and seminal vesicles may occur. Alternative fomitic transmission routes (for example, bath towels, hand towels, toilet seats, or swimming-pool water) have been proposed but are generally regarded as improbable.

23.3 Epidemiology

Trichomoniasis represents the most widely distributed sexually transmitted infection globally, with approximately 174 million cases reported annually.

Data on the incidence and prevalence of the disease remain fragmented. According to the World Health Organization (WHO), there were 10.6 million new cases in Western Europe, 13.1 million in Eastern Europe and Central Asia, and 8.2 million in the United States as of 1999. Key points regarding the prevalence of trichomoniasis include:

- The disease occurs more frequently in women than in men, reporting a ratio of 16 infected women for every 10 infected men.
- A prevalence of 3.1% was observed among 4000 women examined in the United States.
- Notably, the prevalence of infection escalates with age, peaking in women over 40, where it exceeds 11%.
- Certain ethnic groups exhibit higher prevalence rates. In the United States, for instance, the prevalence among non-Hispanic women of color stands at 13.3%, compared to 1.3% in non-Hispanic white women.
- Among a study of 14–17-year-old girls, predominantly of color, a prevalence of 6.0% was recorded in the United States, with approximately 1% experiencing recurrent infections.
- Moreover, the prevalence of trichomonas infection in pregnant women appears to be elevated due to hormonal changes favoring trichomonad proliferation. However, data vary significantly across regions. Projections from the WHO in the 1990s suggested prevalence rates of 2.1% in Brazil, 8% in Nicaragua, and 41.4% in South Africa.

- In many countries, prevalence data remain unavailable. In Western nations, it is estimated that approximately 1% of symptomatic women of childbearing age are infected, with the highest infection rates occurring in women aged 19–35.

23.4 Clinical Manifestation

23.4.1 Gynecology

Typically, the male partner exhibits no symptoms with infection manifesting as a minimal parasitic load in 50–90% of cases. Severe cases may present as urethritis, featuring mucous-milky discharge, which can progress to painful prostatitis, epididymitis, and potential infertility.

In females, *T. vaginalis* infection often presents with a foul-smelling genital discharge, accompanied by sensations of burning and itching in the vagina (Table 23.1). Severe erosive inflammation may develop in the cervical region, in addition to potential affliction of the urethra, paraurethral glands, and urinary bladder. Symptoms may be exacerbated by concurrent infections, such as bacterial vaginosis or gonococcal infections, with an increase in anaerobic bacterial flora frequently noted.

A distinguishing feature of *T. vaginalis* infection is the presence of yellow-greenish genital discharge observable upon clinical examination, which can coincide with bacterial infections in 5–50% of cases. The variability in the frequency of symptoms is indicative of the varying severity of the infection and the individual physiological responses of the patient.

Initial symptoms typically arise between five and 28 days post-infection. Nonetheless, untreated infections may persist for months or years, with symptoms potentially appearing at any time and fluctuating over time within the same

Table 23.1 Key clinical features of trichomoniasis

Clinical feature	Description	Prevalence
Pruritus and dysuria	Intense pruritus of the vulva or urethra; burning on micturition; men may report dysuria or pain associated with ejaculation	Very common
Frothy, malodorous discharge	Yellow-green, frothy vaginal or urethral discharge often associated with a fishy odor	Characteristic
Strawberry cervix	Punctate petechial hemorrhages on the cervical epithelium, best seen on speculum examination or colposcopy	~30%
Vesicles (blisters)	Small, fluid-filled vesicles on the vaginal mucosa; may be transient	~33%
Vaginal mucosal emphysema	Subepithelial gas within the vaginal wall producing crepitus on palpation; uncommon	Rare
Concurrent bacterial vaginosis	Mixed infection with bacterial vaginosis organisms identified by microscopy or culture; may alter discharge characteristics	Up to 15%

individual. Approximately 70–85% of those infected remain asymptomatic, with one-third of asymptomatic women developing symptoms within 9 months.

Clinical manifestations include:

- Pruritus and local irritation
- Local erythema
- Dysuria or painful ejaculation
- Increased quantity of foul-smelling, yellowish-greenish discharge
- Dyspareunia
- Sensation of friction within the vagina

Trichomoniasis is a parasitic infection that can manifest with a variety of symptoms, including itching and local irritation. It can also lead to local erythema, a burning sensation during urination (dysuria) or ejaculation (in males), and an increased, foamy discharge from the vagina or urethra. This discharge is often yellowish-green and has a foul smell. In symptomatic infections, up to one-third of cases may exhibit small blisters (Fig. 23.1). The predominant symptoms consist of irritation and bleeding of the vaginal epithelium in the posterior fornix region. Colposcopic examination of the cervix may reveal small bleedings (petechiae), indicative of granular colpitis—also referred to as maculitis granularis or “strawberry cervix.”

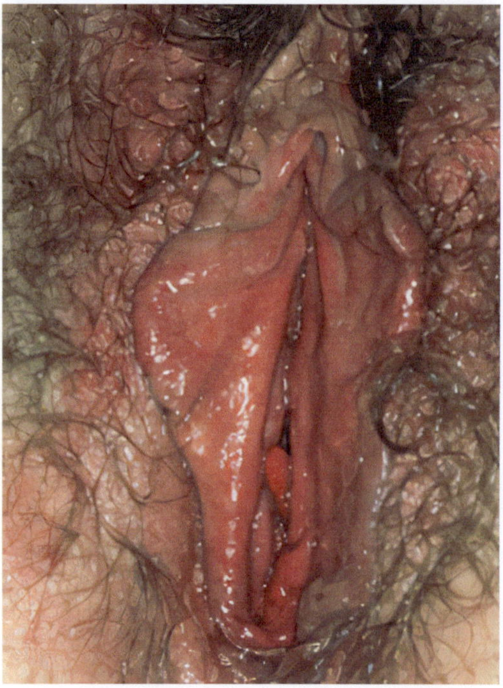

Fig. 23.1 Clinical presentation of trichomoniasis, indicating a markedly erythematous vulva (Weissenbacher 2013)

Additionally, vaginal mucosal emphysema has been documented as a rare complication associated with vaginitis caused by *Trichomonas vaginalis*. The discharge is frequently accompanied by an unpleasant odor. Coexisting bacterial vaginosis is observed more commonly with a *T. vaginalis* infection, with a prevalence of up to 15%.

23.4.2 Pregnancy

Pregnant women infected with *T. vaginalis* face an increased risk of complications adversely influencing pregnancy, including:

- Premature birth
- Premature rupture of membranes
- Low birth weight

The risk of preterm birth is increased by approximately 27–42% in pregnant women with *Trichomonas vaginalis* infection. Multiple cohort and meta-analytic studies have demonstrated a consistent association between maternal trichomoniasis and earlier delivery, with effect estimates clustered within this range after adjustment for measured confounders.

The risk of pre-labor rupture of membranes (PROM) is also elevated, with reported relative risks or odds ratios ranging from approximately 1.41–1.87. This association suggests that infection may contribute to weakening of fetal membranes or the inflammatory processes that precipitate membrane rupture.

Low birth weight (LBW) and small-for-gestational-age (SGA) infants are more frequently observed among pregnancies complicated by trichomoniasis; some studies report up to a two-fold increase in LBW risk. These findings indicate an adverse impact on fetal growth and/or gestational duration that may be mediated by infection-related inflammation or altered placental function.

Importantly, the reported associations have persisted after statistical adjustment for common confounders, including tobacco use and coexisting genital infections, supporting an independent relationship between *T. vaginalis* and these adverse outcomes. Nevertheless, residual confounding cannot be entirely excluded.

No robust evidence currently supports a causal link between maternal *T. vaginalis* infection and miscarriage or confirmed intrauterine infection. Although isolated case reports have described intrauterine detection of the organism in the context of pregnancy loss or delivery, high-quality epidemiological data demonstrating an association with early pregnancy loss are lacking.

The presence of a trichomonas infection during pregnancy is a risk factor for premature birth, low fetal birth weight, and low birth weight in premature babies.

No evidence currently substantiates transmission of *T. vaginalis* to the fetus. However, the pathogen can be transmitted from an infected mother to the newborn during birth, potentially resulting in urethritis and vaginitis. It is hypothesized that up to 5% (and in some older studies, up to 17%) of female newborns may experience vaginal colonization with trichomonads if the mother was infected and untreated at the time of birth. Clinical symptoms generally appear approximately 1 week after birth, presenting as redness and swelling of the vulva.

Prevalence of trichomonas vaginitis correlates with the degree of estrogenization of the vagina. Due to maternal hormonal influences, newborn girls may experience genital changes shortly after birth, facilitating pathogen transmission during delivery and the development of associated symptoms. Trichomoniasis is practically absent during the hormonal resting phase in young girls.

Although prepubescent children are almost never infected with trichomonas, infants may get vaginitis as a result of exposure after birth. Sexual assault must therefore be investigated as a possible cause of vaginal trichomonas infection in minors.

23.5 Diagnosis

Clinical observation frequently identifies initial indications of a trichomonas infection. In females, the acute phase is characterized by increased, foamy vaginal or urethral discharge, often yellowish-green in color and occasionally odorous. Diagnosing trichomoniasis in males presents greater challenges due to lower pathogen levels and less pronounced inflammatory responses.

Under direct wet mount microscopic examination, motile trichomonads can be identified during the acute stage (Fig. 23.2). Trichomonads are easily distinguishable from leukocytes, fungal spore cells, and epithelial cells. In most cases, wet mount microscopy is sufficient for diagnosis, as these protozoa are readily identifiable due to their distinctive morphology and irregular motility. The sensitivity of microscopic examination is estimated to range from 66% to 88%. However, a negative microscopic result does not definitively exclude infection.

In some instances, utilizing a 0.5% methylene blue solution when examining native preparations from vaginal secretions may enhance the visibility of bacteria, assisting in differentiating trichomonads from the stained background. Giemsa staining may also facilitate the detection of trichomoniasis, resulting in the plasma of trichomonads appearing blue while their nuclei, flagella, and axial rod present as red.

Staining preparations for trichomonad diagnosis is generally ineffective, as the pathogens typically exhibit only weak staining or quickly perish.

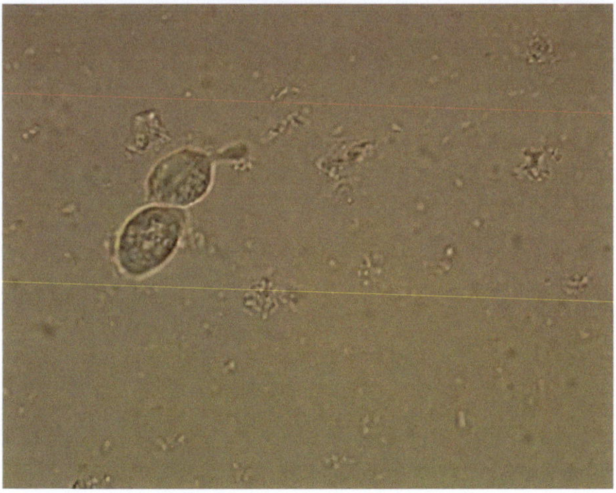

Fig. 23.2 Trichomonas vaginalis (Mylonas 2013, 2016)

Table 23.2 Diagnostic methods for detection of *Trichomonas vaginalis*

Test	Sensitivity (%)	Specificity (%)	Advantages	Disadvantages
Wet mount microscopy	62–88	>99	– Fast results – Cost-effective – High specificity	– Lower sensitivity depending on experience – Depending on the quality of the sample
Culture	95	100	– High sensitivity and specificity – Possibility for further analysis	– Organism can die quickly if the wrong medium or transport delay occurs – Duration approx. 3–7 days – Not available in most clinical laboratories
PCR/NAAT	95	98	– Fast results compared to culture	– Most expensive option – Not available in many clinical laboratories

The most reliable diagnostic method for a trichomonas infection currently remains pathogen cultivation (Table 23.2). However, this requires special media and rapid transport of samples, presenting organizational challenges in everyday practice. An alternative is utilizing DNA detection via polymerase chain reaction (PCR). Recent years have seen the approval of several tests by the US FDA for detecting *T. vaginalis* in vaginal, cervical, or urine samples from women, including the APTIMA *T. vaginalis* assay (Hologic Gen-Probe, San Diego, CA) and the BD ProbeTec TV Qx.

Immunochromatographic flow dipstick tests are also available for point-of-care diagnostics, having a sensitivity of 82–95% and a specificity of 97%. Although not typically diagnosed via cervical cytology (Papanicolaou test), it may be detected incidentally.

Following a positive diagnosis of trichomoniasis, comprehensive diagnostics must be conducted to rule out other sexually transmitted diseases (STD), including gonococcal infection, chlamydial infection, syphilis, HIV, and hepatitis B and C, along with bacterial vaginosis and candidosis.

23.6 Treatment

Trichomonads are susceptible to nitroimidazole drugs due to their anaerobic energy metabolism, resulting in cure rates ranging from 90% to 95% (Table 23.3). The effective treatment is derived from hydroxymetabolites produced in the liver; however, certain studies indicate a potential efficacy of localized treatment.

Metronidazole may be administered as a single 2-g oral dose or 500 mg twice daily for 7 days. Evidence indicates that the twice-daily regimen may provide greater efficacy than a single oral dose. For patients coinfected with HIV, twice-daily dosing demonstrates superior effectiveness compared to single-dose treatment, making it the preferred option in these cases. Alcohol consumption during metronidazole treatment is contraindicated due to the potential for an antabuse-like reaction.

Administration of treatment during pregnancy can be performed safely from the second trimester using nitroimidazole derivatives. In cases requiring treatment during the first trimester, clotrimazole may be utilized, offering symptom relief but achieving a cure in only 20% of instances.

Table 23.3 Treatment options for trichomoniasis. Metronidazole is not approved in most countries for use during the first trimester of pregnancy

Therapy	Medication	Dosage	Duration
Systemic therapy	Metronidazole	500 mg orally twice daily	7 days
	Metronidazole	250 mg orally three times daily	7 days
	Metronidazole	2 g orally	Single dose
	Tinidazole[a]	2 g orally	Single dose
	Tinidazole[a]	400 mg orally twice daily	5 days
Treatment failure	Metronidazole	500 mg orally twice daily	7 days
	Metronidazole	2 g orally once daily	5 days
	Tinidazole[a]	2 g orally once daily	5 days
Pregnancy	Metronidazole	1–2 vaginal ovules of 500 mg daily	10 days
	Clotrimazole	100 mg intravaginally	7 days
	Metronidazole	500 mg orally twice daily[b]	10 days
	Metronidazole	500 mg orally three times daily[c]	7 days

[a] The availability of tinidazole should be verified

[b] In some countries, metronidazole is available in 500 mg and 400 mg tablet formulations. Adherence to the 500 mg dosage should be ensured

[c] Consideration should be given to increasing the dosage based on the overall constitution of the pregnant woman, particularly in cases of high distribution volume, such as obesity

- In the first trimester, clotrimazole 100 mg is given intravaginally for seven days.
- In the second and third trimesters, metronidazole 500 mg is administered orally twice daily for 10 days or three times daily for 7 days.

All pregnant women, regardless of HIV status, should undergo retesting for cure within 3 months following the initial infection.

Given the common association between vaginitis and urethral infection, systemic treatment is warranted. Local treatment with metronidazole should be reserved for exceptional cases.

Treatment failure should initially be attributed to nonadherence or partner-mediated reinfection. When treatment failure is suspected, a second therapeutic course should be administered (Fig. 23.3).

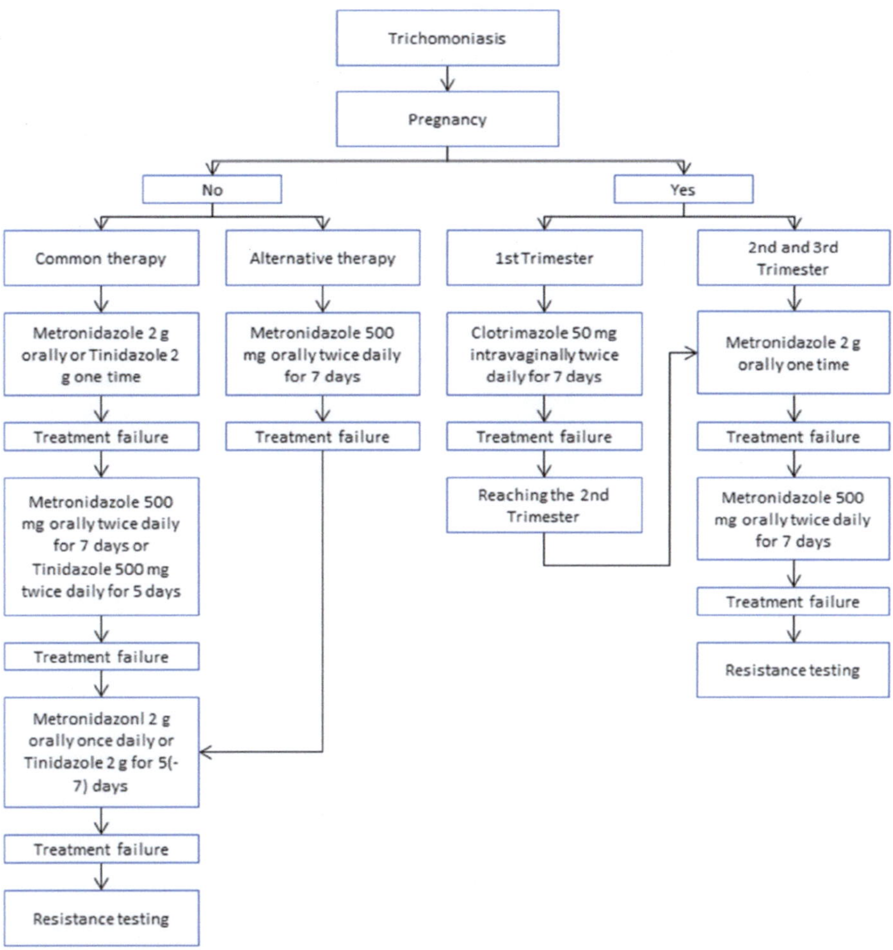

Fig. 23.3 Treatment algorithm for trichomoniasis (courtesy of I. Mylonas)

Metronidazole resistance among *Trichomonas vaginalis* clinical isolates has been reported to be increasing, with an estimated prevalence of approximately 5% and exhibiting variable degrees of reduced susceptibility. For certain resistant infections, a high-dose metronidazole regimen (2 g once daily for 3–5 days) has been shown to be effective. The CDC recommends metronidazole 2 g once daily for 7 days for resistant infections, while advising that administration of more than a single 2 g dose should be avoided because of an associated increased risk of preterm birth.

Tinidazole has been reported to be active against up to 60% of metronidazole-resistant *T. vaginalis* isolates. Availability of tinidazole has, however, been reduced in multiple countries following discontinuation of production by some pharmaceutical manufacturers for economic reasons.

For patients exhibiting a confirmed allergy to metronidazole, desensitization should be performed prior to treatment initiation.

Breastfeeding and Metronidazole: Recommendations and Pharmacokinetic Considerations

Metronidazole is excreted into human milk at concentrations approximating maternal plasma levels, with reported milk-to-plasma ratios near 0.9 for the parent compound and 0.76 for the major active metabolite. Peak milk concentrations have been measured at approximately 15.5 mg/L for metronidazole and 5.7 mg/L for hydroxymetronidazole, yielding an estimated infant exposure of 10–15% of the maternal weight-adjusted dose. Such exposure was considered clinically relevant and warrants careful assessment of risk versus benefit when lactation is to be continued.

Neonates and young infants demonstrate markedly prolonged elimination of metronidazole relative to adults because of immature hepatic metabolic pathways and renal clearance. In full-term neonates, the elimination half-life has been reported between 22.5 and 109 h, with preterm infants typically exhibiting half-lives at the upper end of this range. These pharmacokinetic characteristics increase the potential for drug accumulation and consequent exposure when breastfeeding is continued during maternal therapy.

Manufacturer guidance has recommended that breastfeeding be suspended for the duration of metronidazole therapy and for 48–72 h after the final dose to allow for sufficient drug clearance from the infant's circulation. This conservative approach is intended to minimize infant exposure, particularly in neonates, preterm infants, or when prolonged or repeated maternal dosing is required. In contrast, published expert reviews and population studies have reported minimal adverse events in breastfed infants after standard short-course maternal treatment (for example, 400 mg three times daily for 7 days), and some authorities therefore consider brief courses compatible with continued breastfeeding provided that the infant is closely monitored for gastrointestinal disturbance, oral candidiasis, and adequate weight gain.

Clinical recommendations should be individualized: when metronidazole is deemed essential during lactation, the benefit of maternal therapy must be weighed against the risk of infant exposure. If therapy is prolonged, involves preterm or neonatal infants, or repeated dosing is anticipated, temporary suspension of breastfeeding for up to 72 h after the final dose is prudent to reduce the risk of accumulation. For short courses in term infants, continuation of breastfeeding may be permitted with vigilant clinical monitoring and documentation of infant well-being.

23.7 Differential Diagnosis

The differential diagnosis of trichomoniasis encompasses various conditions (Table 23.4) with overlapping symptoms, including bacterial vaginosis, candidosis, gonorrhea, chlamydial infection, genital herpes, and infections caused by Ureaplasma and *Mycoplasma genitalium*, as well as human papillomavirus (HPV). These conditions can also present with discharge, itching, or genital pain.

Table 23.4 Differential diagnoses for trichomoniasis

	Pathogen	Symptoms	Differences to trichomoniasis
Bacterial vaginosis	Overgrowth of bacteria such as *Gardnerella vaginalis*	Fishy odor, gray discharge, itching or burning	Absence of foamy discharge; vaginal pH often increased
Vulvovaginal candidosis	Candida species	Itching, redness, white "curd-like" discharge	Absence of foamy and foul-smelling discharge
Gonorrhea	*Neisseria gonorrhoeae*	Pain during urination, purulent discharge	Purulent instead of foamy discharge; may be asymptomatic
Chlamydia	*Chlamydia trachomatis*	Mild to no symptoms, pain during urination, discharge	Often less pronounced symptoms than with trichomoniasis
Genital herpes	Herpes simplex virus (HSV) type 1 and 2	Painful blisters or ulcers in the genital area	Presence of blisters, not mainly discharge
Mycoplasma infections	*Ureaplasma urealyticum*, *Mycoplasma genitalium*	Similar to chlamydia: pain during urination, discharge	More difficult to diagnose; often similar treatment to chlamydia
Human papillomavirus (HPV)	Human papillomavirus	Warts in the genital area; sometimes asymptomatic	Presence of warts instead of discharge or itching

23.8 Prevention

The utilization of condoms serve as a preventative measure against trichomonas infection. It is critical that infected partners also undergo treatment to avert relapses. Given the absence of immunity post-infection, reinfection with trichomonads is a possibility at any time.

Trichomonas infections frequently co-occur with other STDs and yeast infections. In HIV-positive women, trichomonas infections are detected approximately twice as frequently as in HIV-negative counterparts. Furthermore, a vaginal infection with trichomonads can augment the risk of acquiring HIV. Research conducted in Africa has shown that the HIV transmission rate is doubled in the presence of a trichomonas infection. The significant prevalence rates of trichomonads in specific communities, particularly in Africa and the United States, indicate their substantial role in the dissemination of HIV.

A trichomonas infection increases the risk of acquiring HIV and promotes the transmission of the virus in individuals who are already infected with HIV.

Key Points

- *Trichomonas vaginalis* is an obligate pathogen that proliferates within the mucous membranes of the vagina and urethra. The pathogen is incapable of surviving in low humidity, cold temperatures, or low light, necessitating direct contact for infection.
- It is a unicellular, pear-shaped protozoan equipped with flagella, reaching a maximum size of 25 μm. This organism is characterized by its anaerobic metabolism.
- Primary transmission occurs via sexual contact, although the possibility of transmission through contaminated objects, such as towels and toilets, cannot be excluded.
- Approximately 174 million cases of trichomoniasis are reported globally each year, making it the most prevalent sexually transmitted disease.
- The infection is often asymptomatic, but can cause a variety of symptoms, including vaginitis, foul-smelling vaginal discharge, itching, and burning. The severity and duration of symptoms may vary over time in a given individual, and complications, including infertility, are possible.
- Pregnant women have an increased risk of preterm delivery, premature rupture of membranes, and low birth weight. While the likelihood of direct fetal transmission remains unproven, neonatal infection is a possible outcome.

- Diagnosis primarily relies on microscopic examination of native preparations, cultures, or polymerase chain reaction (PCR) techniques.
- Considering concomitant infections is essential in the diagnosis of sexually transmitted diseases.
- Treatment initiation involves nitroimidazoles, starting in the second trimester of pregnancy (e.g., metronidazole).
- Adhering to prescribed treatment regimens and ensuring partner treatment are critical in preventing reinfection.
- Utilizing condoms is strongly recommended as a protective measure against infection.
- There exists a correlation between trichomoniasis and an increased risk of HIV infection.

Part V

Sexually Transmitted Diseases Through Close Skin Contact

Monkeypox (mpox)

24

Abstract

Monkeypox is a zoonotic disease caused by the orthopoxvirus. The condition typically presents with fever and a rash and can be transmitted both person to person and animal to person. The incubation period is estimated to range from 7 to 21 days. Given the global spread of the disease, the World Health Organization (WHO) has issued an alert. Diagnosis is primarily based on polymerase chain reaction (PCR) testing. Clinically, monkeypox manifests as skin lesions, which commonly appear on the face and extremities and progress to pustules and crusts. Treatment is symptom oriented, with antiviral options available for severe cases. Infected individuals should be isolated, and vaccination is recommended for at-risk groups as a preventive measure. Special caution should be exercised during pregnancy and breastfeeding regarding medication and vaccine selection. Implementing educational measures and hygiene protocols is crucial to prevent disease transmission.

24.1 Background

Monkeypox (mpox) is a viral disease caused by the monkeypox virus, displaying symptoms similar to those of smallpox, although generally milder. The disease can be transmitted from person to person and, although rare, from animal to person. The natural reservoir of the virus remains unidentified, although various small mammals, including squirrels and monkeys, have been found to be susceptible. The incubation period for monkeypox is estimated to be between 5 and 21 days. Viremia correlates with the signs and symptoms of monkeypox infection, progressing through distinct phases, from exposure to the eventual emergence of skin and mucous membrane lesions.

I. Mylonas, *Sexually Transmitted Diseases*,
https://doi.org/10.1007/978-3-031-78204-6_24

24.2 Pathogen

The monkeypox virus (MPXV) is a zoonotic Orthopoxvirus within the family Poxviridae. The virus is enveloped and brick-shaped, containing a linear double-stranded DNA genome of approximately 197 kilobase pairs; virion dimensions are typically 200–250 nm. MPXV is antigenically and genomically related to other orthopoxviruses, including variola (smallpox), cowpox, and vaccinia viruses.

MPXV is classified into two principal clades with differing geographic distributions and clinical severity:

- Clade I (Formerly "Congo Basin"): associated with higher virulence and greater human-to-human transmissibility; historical case fatality ratios in unvaccinated populations have approached 10%.
- Clade II (Formerly "West African"): associated with lower virulence and case fatality ratios typically under 1%. Clade II is subdivided (IIa and IIb); recent international transmission has been driven predominantly by Clade IIb.

Wild mammals—principally rodents (for example, rope squirrels and Gambian pouched rats) and various nonhuman primates—act as reservoirs. Human infection is typically acquired through direct contact with infected animals (blood, bodily fluids, or lesion material) or by consumption of undercooked infected meat.

Human transmission occurs via:

- Large respiratory droplets during prolonged close face-to-face contact.
- Direct contact with active skin or mucosal lesions and indirect contact via contaminated fomites (for example, bedding or clothing).
- Possible Sexual Transmission: viral DNA has been detected in semen, rectal swabs, and genital lesions.

Epidemiologic clusters among men who have sex with men have implicated intimate contact as an important driver of recent spread, although the precise efficiency of sexual transmission remains under investigation.

On August 14, 2024, the World Health Organization designated the multi-country monkeypox outbreak as a Public Health Emergency of International Concern. Notable features of this outbreak include:

- Wide geographic dissemination across Europe, the Americas, and parts of Africa without clear travel links
- Predominance of Clade IIb, frequently associated with atypical clinical presentations, such as localized genital lesions and prolonged courses in some immunocompromised individuals.
- Continued circulation of Clade I in Central African regions, with higher morbidity and mortality observed historically where that clade persists.

24.3 Epidemiology

The World Health Organization has declared the global spread of mpox a Public Health Emergency of International Concern; laboratory-confirmed infections have been reported in 95 non-endemic countries. Human-to-human transmission occurs via large respiratory droplets and by contact with lesion exudate or contaminated fomites, and recent outbreaks have demonstrated efficient spread through prolonged close physical contact, including intimate sexual contact.

In Africa, the epicenter has remained the Democratic Republic of the Congo (DRC). By mid-August 2024, the DRC had recorded more than 17,000 suspected and confirmed cases and over 500 deaths, yielding an overall case-fatality ratio of approximately 3%, representing the highest burden observed in any single country during this outbreak. Neighboring countries reporting imported or autochthonous transmission have included Burundi, Kenya, Rwanda, Uganda, and Côte d'Ivoire. Public health responses have focused on enhanced surveillance, targeted vaccination of high-risk groups with third-generation smallpox/orthopox vaccines, and rigorous contact tracing to limit further spread.

The disease primarily affects males, with a notably higher prevalence among men who have sex with men (MSM). Individuals living with HIV are particularly susceptible to severe outcomes.

24.4 Clinical Manifestation

24.4.1 Gynecology

Monkeypox presents with a variety of clinical symptoms that can be categorized into prodromal and rash phases. The disease exhibits similarities to smallpox but is generally less severe.

24.4.1.1 Prodromal Phase

The prodromal phase typically begins 1–2 weeks after exposure and lasts for 2–10 days. Symptoms during this phase may include:

- **Fever:** This is one of the earliest symptoms, often accompanied by chills.
- **Severe Headaches:** Patients frequently report intense headaches, which may be debilitating.
- **Lymphadenopathy:** Unlike many viral infections where lymph nodes may remain normal, monkeypox often leads to significant swelling of lymph nodes, especially in the cervical and axillary regions. This lymphadenopathy can precede or coincide with the rash.

- **Muscle Pain (Myalgia):** Generalized muscle aches may accompany fever and weakness.
- **Back Pain:** Many patients experience discomfort or pain in the back.
- **Fatigue and Malaise:** A profound feeling of tiredness and general unwellness is common during this phase.

24.4.1.2 Rash Phase

The rash phase typically occurs 1–3 days after the onset of fever and can last 2–4 weeks. This phase involves several distinct stages:

- **Initial Lesion Formation:** The rash often starts as flat macules or spots, which may initially appear on the face and extremities before spreading to other body parts.
- **Progression to Papules:** The macules evolve into raised papules, which are firm and palpable. This stage is characterized by redness and inflammation around the lesions.
- **Vesicle Development:** The papules then progress to vesicles, which are fluid-filled blisters. These vesicles can be quite itchy or painful.
- **Formation of Pustules:** As the disease progresses, the vesicles turn into pustules, which contain thick, yellowish fluid. The pustules are typically umbilicated (having a central depression) and often resemble those seen in smallpox.
- **Crusting:** Eventually, the pustules dry up and form crusts or scabs, which subsequently fall off. This process marks the transition toward healing.

24.4.1.3 Distribution of Lesions

The rash can appear on various surfaces of the body, including:

- **Face:** Lesions commonly involve the face, including the forehead, cheeks, and nasal region.
- **Extremities:** The rash frequently spreads to the arms and legs, including the palms of the hands and soles of the feet.
- **Genital Area:** It can also compromise the genital region, with lesions manifesting on or around the genitals and the anus.
- **Oral Mucosa:** Some individuals may develop lesions in the mouth, throat, and other mucosal surfaces, which may complicate eating and swallowing.

24.4.1.4 Additional Symptoms and Complications

Monkeypox can lead to extracutaneous complications that affect other organ systems, including:

- **Pneumonia:** Respiratory complications may arise, particularly in individuals with weakened immune systems.
- **Ophthalmological Issues:** Inflammation or infection of the eyes (conjunctivitis or keratitis) may occur, potentially leading to vision impairment.

- **Encephalitis:** Although rare, inflammation of the brain can occur, presenting with neurological symptoms such as confusion, seizures, or altered consciousness.
- **Secondary Soft Tissue Infections:** Bacterial superinfections can develop in the skin lesions leading to additional complications.

24.4.1.5 Differences from Other Conditions

The rash associated with monkeypox is distinctive, permitting differentiation from other similar conditions:

- **Varicella (Chickenpox):** Unlike chickenpox, where lesions appear at different stages of development, monkeypox lesions usually progress simultaneously, presenting a more uniform appearance.
- **Smallpox:** While the rashes of smallpox and monkeypox are similar in appearance, monkeypox is distinguished by the presence of prominent submandibular or cervical lymphadenopathy, which is less common in smallpox.

24.4.1.6 Severity Assessment

The severity of monkeypox infection is often gauged by the number of skin manifestations:

- An infection is considered mild if it presents with approximately ten lesions.
- Moderate-to-severe infections are typically characterized by more than 100 lesions or the involvement of critical areas such as the eyes or genitals.

Health care providers often assess the overall condition of the patient, including systemic symptoms, lesion extensiveness, the presence of complications, and individual health factors to determine the necessary level of care and treatment.

Overall, monkeypox poses a significant health challenge, and understanding its clinical manifestations is crucial for diagnosis, treatment, and monitoring of affected individuals.

24.4.2 Pregnancy

Data related to monkeypox during pregnancy is limited. However, severity of infection in pregnant women has been observed to vary, with adverse pregnancy outcomes noted in cases of moderate-to-severe infection. In a study involving 122 patients in the Democratic Republic of Congo, four pregnant women contracted monkeypox. One woman gave birth to a healthy infant, while two experienced miscarriages during the early weeks of pregnancy, and one woman died. The newborn exhibited cutaneous lesions and other signs of monkeypox infection, suggesting vertical transmission of the virus.

24.5 Diagnosis

- Monkeypox should be suspected in patients, including pregnant women, who have traveled to monkeypox endemic regions within the past 21 days and present with unexplained skin rashes or genital ulcers.
- Nonspecific symptoms such as fever, headache, myalgia, fatigue, and lymphadenopathy warrant further diagnostic evaluation, particularly in individuals returning from affected areas.
- A history of close contact with infected persons or sexual activity during travel to endemic regions further supports the suspicion of monkeypox.
- The preferred diagnostic method for monkeypox is the detection of viral DNA using polymerase chain reaction (PCR). Samples should ideally be collected directly from skin lesions, including vesicles, pustules, or crusts.
- In cases where direct sampling is not feasible, a skin biopsy may also be considered.
- Serological methods, including antigen and antibody detection, are generally of limited diagnostic utility due to their inability to distinguish between orthopoxviruses.

24.6 Treatment

24.6.1 General

Monkeypox treatment primarily focuses on supportive care to alleviate symptoms and prevent complications. There is no specific antiviral treatment for the monkeypox virus. In cases of severe illness, antiviral medications such as cidofovir or brincidofovir may be considered, although their efficacy is limited. Other potential treatments, while still in experimental stages, may include immunomodulators such as interferons and antibiotics for secondary bacterial infections. Smallpox vaccines exhibit approximately 85% cross-reactivity against monkeypox, playing a vital role in the prevention of the disease, particularly for individuals at increased risk.

Timely diagnosis, isolation of infected individuals, and implementation of appropriate hygiene measures are critical to containing monkeypox virus transmission and preventing further infections.

24.6.2 Pregnancy

Treatment options for monkeypox during pregnancy remain highly limited, as no specific antiviral therapy has been approved for this condition. The management of monkeypox in pregnant individuals primarily focuses on symptom alleviation, supportive care, and the prevention of complications. Supportive care measures may include adequate hydration, nutritional support, and antipyretics to manage fever. Analgesics may be administered to relieve pain, while secondary bacterial infections resulting from skin lesions should be addressed with appropriate antibiotics.

Although there is no targeted treatment specifically for monkeypox, some antiviral agents or vaccinations have been used under compassionate-use protocols or in severe cases. However, their safety and efficacy during pregnancy remain uncertain, as data on their use in pregnant individuals is limited.

Brincidofovir: This medication is recommended at a dosage of 600 mg orally twice daily over a course of 2 weeks, with caution advised due to potential side effects, including the risk of QT prolongation. An electrocardiogram (ECG) should be performed prior to use in pregnant individuals, as torsade de pointes (TdP) poses a risk, which can manifest asymptomatically or have fatal consequences. Notably, women are at a greater risk than men due to longer QT intervals. Caution is also warranted when considering combination therapy with erythromycin, as both drugs can prolong the QT interval.

Vaccinia Immunoglobulin-Intravenous (VIGIV): VIGIV can be given intravenously at a dose of 6000 units/kg, with the infusion rate tailored according to the patient's weight. Caution is essential for patients who are pregnant or have diabetes mellitus, as VIGIV contains maltose, which may produce falsely elevated blood glucose levels. Additionally, the risk of venous thromboembolism must be considered, especially in pregnant women, with infusion rates adjusted accordingly. For patients with a history of venous thromboembolism (VTE), the infusion rate should not exceed 12,000 units/kg. Pregnant women with additional VTE risk factors may require concurrent administration of low-molecular-weight heparin (LMWH). Care should be taken with patients who have allergies, as VIGIV can cause life-threatening hypersensitivity reactions.

Vaccines: The MVA-BN vaccine is recommended for prophylaxis, offering an inactivated vaccine with 85% cross-protective immunity against monkeypox. To date, more than 300 pregnant women have safely received this vaccine. Conversely, the live vaccine ACAM2000 poses a risk of fetal vaccinia, making the MVA-BN vaccine the preferred option for pregnant healthcare workers and other individuals at high risk.

Labor and Delivery: If vaginal and anorectal lesions are present, or if the vaginal and rectal MPXV PCR tests are positive, a cesarean section should be performed. It is critical that isolation measures be *enacted immediately*. Extended antibiotic therapy with cefazolin and azithromycin is recommended, with preoperative skin antisepsis using povidone-iodine considered safer than chlorhexidine–alcohol. Nonadhesive surgical drapes should be utilized for extensive abdominal lesions. Furthermore, it is advised to conduct placental histology and MPXV PCR tests on amniotic fluid, cord blood, placenta, and vaginal and rectal swabs. Regarding postpartum care, it is essential to provide appropriate attention to the newborn. The use of LMWH for postpartum thrombosis prophylaxis in monkeypox is not contraindicated, and consent should be obtained for MPXV PCR testing of expressed breast milk.

Breastfeeding should begin as soon as possible following delivery; however, it should be postponed until the mother's rash has crusted over. If the mother chooses to breastfeed before this point, stringent precautions must be taken.

In routine gynecological practice, patients with suspected monkeypox infection should be referred or transferred to facilities equipped with the necessary expertise and isolation capabilities.

24.7 Differential Diagnosis

The differential diagnosis for maculopapular rashes includes measles, rubella, cytomegalovirus, toxoplasmosis infections, secondary syphilis, atopic pregnancy dermatosis, and itchy urticarial papules and plaques during pregnancy. Vesiculopustular rashes may arise from varicella zoster, gestational pemphigoid, or hand-foot-and-mouth disease. Anogenital ulcers could indicate herpes simplex or lymphogranuloma venereum.

24.8 Prevention

Preventing and controlling mpox depends on two fundamental strategies: increasing public awareness and providing comprehensive training for healthcare workers to prevent infection and interrupt transmission. Avoiding close contact with infected individuals and contaminated materials is crucial to reducing the spread of the virus. To address concerns related to racism and stigmatization, the World Health Organization (WHO) officially recommended renaming the disease from "monkeypox" to "mpox" on November 28, 2022.

Key Points

- The monkeypox virus (MPXV) is classified in the genus Orthopoxvirus and is a zoonotic virus related to variola, cowpox, and vaccinia; it is transmitted via respiratory droplets, skin contact, and contaminated objects.
- The virus can be transmitted both person-to-person and from animals to humans. The natural reservoirs of the virus remain unidentified. The incubation period ranges from 5 to 21 days, with gradual symptom development.
- MPXV can be detected in semen; however, the potential for sexual transmission has yet to be definitively established.
- The WHO has classified monkeypox outbreaks as an international public health emergency.
- Symptoms include fever, headache, lymphadenopathy, muscle pain, back pain, and weakness.

(continued)

- The rash typically lasts for 2–4 weeks and may appear as plaques, pustules, or scabs. Lesions can occur on various body parts, including the palms, soles, groin, and genital area, along with anal swelling and dysuria.
- The most definitive diagnosis is achieved through PCR testing on samples from skin lesions.
- Treatment is primarily supportive, with no specific antiviral therapy currently available.
- Smallpox vaccines with cross-reactivity are crucial for prevention.
- Isolation measures for monkeypox patients are essential.
- Treatment options during pregnancy are limited; cesarean delivery and isolation measures should be considered in cases of monkeypox in pregnant individuals.
- Public education and training of healthcare staff in infection control are critical. Avoidance of direct contact with infected individuals and contaminated materials is imperative.

Molluscum Contagiosum

25

Abstract

Molluscum contagiosum is a viral dermatological condition typically transmitted through direct skin contact. It presents as painless, skin-colored lesions. This disease is caused by the molluscum contagiosum virus (MCV), part of the poxvirus family. Although it most commonly affects children and young adults who are sexually active, it may also impact individuals across all age groups. The presence of numerous lesions often indicates an underlying immunocompromised state, such as in cases of HIV. Vertical transmission of the virus from mother to child during delivery is also possible. Diagnosis is primarily clinical, with no standardized therapeutic protocols currently available. Nevertheless, various treatment options exist, while many cases resolve spontaneously. In the absence of specific recommendations, the primary preventive strategy is to avoid direct skin contact with lesions.

25.1 Background

Molluscum contagiosum is caused by the molluscum contagiosum virus (MCV) and can be transmitted both sexually and nonsexually. The average duration of a solitary lesion is approximately 2 months. However, due to the potential for rapid spread through autoinoculation (such as scratching or trauma), the duration of infection may average around 8 months, with some cases extending to 12 months or longer.

Molluscum contagiosum is considered a benign, self-limiting disease.

I. Mylonas, *Sexually Transmitted Diseases*,
https://doi.org/10.1007/978-3-031-78204-6_25

25.2 Pathogen

The molluscum contagiosum virus (MCV) belongs to the poxvirus family and is phylogenetically distinct from other poxviruses, exhibiting unique biological properties. Viral replication occurs exclusively within human epidermal cells. MCV has three genotypes, with genotype 1 being the most prevalent. The primary transmission route is via direct skin-to-skin contact, though rare cases have been documented involving fomite transmission.

25.3 Epidemiology

Molluscum contagiosum is hypothesized to be more prevalent in tropical climates; however, comprehensive epidemiological data remain limited. Individuals may often refrain from seeking medical evaluation due to the asymptomatic nature of the disease, thus complicating efforts to ascertain accurate data on incidence and prevalence.

It is estimated that men are affected approximately twice as frequently as women. Children, sexually active adults, and immunocompromised individuals are particularly vulnerable to infection. The virus typically spreads through direct contact, with infrequent instances of transmission via contaminated objects or environments (e.g., swimming pools, bath towels). Comprehensive data regarding contagion rates, epidemiology, and transmission efficiency are currently lacking.

Vertical transmission during childbirth has been documented; however, relevant epidemiological information remains unavailable.

25.4 Clinical Manifestation

25.4.1 Gynecology

Clinically, the most common presentation involves the emergence of skin-colored, painless lesions, ranging from 2 to 5 mm in diameter, characterized by a superficially waxy appearance. These lesions typically cluster, with some displaying a depression at the apex (Fig. 25.1). The lesion count usually does not exceed 20; however, immunocompetent individuals may present with more than 100 lesions, particularly those with HIV. Trauma or mechanical disruption can lead to the formation of a creamy, grayish-white exudate.

Lesions are commonly localized to the anogenital region and lower abdomen in sexually transmitted cases. Molluscum contagiosum can also occur on other extremities, including the palms, soles, face, and trunk, suggesting nonsexual transmission

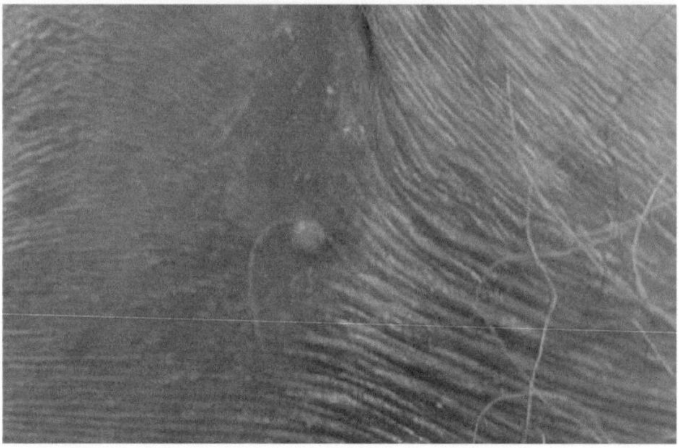

Fig. 25.1 Isolated skin lesion of molluscum contagiosum (Mylonas 2016)

in these regions. The disease may affect individuals of any age, although it predominantly presents in children and young adults. Genotype 2 of MCV has been identified in specimens of vaginal lesions. Traumatic autoinoculation during itching may result in lesions arranged in a linear manner, known as the pseudo-Koebner phenomenon. The surrounding area may also demonstrate an associated molluscum dermatitis. The development of pustules within molluscum contagiosum lesions signals an inflammatory response, often indicating the initiation of host immune activity and subsequent infection resolution.

25.4.2 Pregnancy

Given that MCV primarily replicates within the epidermis, systemic spread and consequent fetal infection during pregnancy is unlikely. Nonetheless, the virus can be transmitted to the newborn during vaginal delivery, which may result in the clinical manifestation of molluscum contagiosum. It is advisable to prevent direct contact between lesions and the newborn, for instance, by covering existing lesions. Caesarean delivery is not warranted to prevent transmission.

To date, only a limited number of congenital molluscum contagiosum cases have been documented, with lesions appearing at various postnatal intervals, ranging from 1 week to 3 months. In each reported case, maternal infection with MCV was confirmed, suggesting the possibility of congenital transmission. The morphological characteristics of lesions in infants resemble those observed in adult cases.

25.5 Diagnosis

Diagnosis is predominantly clinical. However, histological confirmation (identification of inclusion bodies) or virion detection via electron microscopy may be employed in cases of uncertainty. Indirect detection of the virus using polymerase chain reaction (PCR) or antibody assays employing enzyme-linked immunosorbent assay (ELISA) is theoretically feasible, although these methods are not routinely utilized due to a lack of standardization.

25.6 Treatment

Currently, no specific antiviral therapy exists for molluscum contagiosum. Surgical or surface-destructive interventions may be warranted in certain cases, including trichloroacetic acid applications, laser therapy, electrocoagulation, or cryotherapy (Table 25.1). Curettage or liquid nitrogen application can be performed 40–60 min

Table 25.1 Treatment strategies for molluscum contagiosum. The availability of medications should be verified before subscribing

Measure	Method/medication	Application
Surgical measures	Curettage	Curettage under local anesthesia
	Cryotherapy	Cryospray (liquid nitrogen) for 10–20 s for each lesion; repeat in 1 week if necessary
	Laser therapy	Laser therapy (585 nm) under local or general anesthesia; repeat in 1 week if necessary
Physical measures	Electrocoagulation	Electrocoagulation under local or general anesthesia; repeat if necessary
	Photodynamic therapy	Application of "photosensitizer" with light (short wavelength)
Destructive medicinal measures	Trichloroacetic acid 80–100%	Sparing application on lesions; repeat in 2 weeks if necessary
Nondestructive measures	Cantharidin 0.9%	Sparing application on each lesion, wash off after 4 h; repeat in 3–4 weeks if necessary
	Podophyllotoxin 0.3–0.5% Solution; 0.15% cream	Twice daily for 3 days, followed by a 4-day break; repeat after 1 week. Treatment duration: 4 weeks
	Salicylic acid gel 12%	1–2 times per week for 4 weeks
	Benzoyl peroxide 10%	Twice daily for 4 weeks
	Vitamin a 0.5% cream	Twice daily on each lesion for 4 weeks
Immunomodulators	Imiquimod 5% cream	Apply overnight (8 h), wash off in the morning, 3–5 times per week until clinical cure or up to 16 weeks
	Cimetidine	40 mg/kg/day divided into 2–3 doses per day, for 2 months
Antiviral agents	Cidofovir cream 1–3%	Apply 3% cidofovir cream on individual lesions once daily, 5 days per week for 8 weeks. Occlusion for 12 h
	Cidofovir intravenously	3–5 mg/kg intravenously per week, weekly for 1–2 weeks followed by infusions every other week. Four to nine infusions until clinical cure

Note: The availability of medications should be verified before subscribing

after administering a topical anesthetic cream, such as EMLA cream (lidocaine/prilocaine) or a 4% lidocaine cream, provided it has been applied under occlusion. Caution is advised with EMLA cream due to potential systemic side effects, especially in pediatric populations. While curettage is a highly effective procedure in adults, it can be exceedingly painful without appropriate anesthesia.

The efficacy of therapeutic modalities exhibits considerable variation, with certain treatments—such as cidofovir—having been predominantly investigated in HIV-positive patients.

A significant proportion of MCV infections resolve on their own, indicating that extensive interventions may not be required in many cases.

25.7 Differential Diagnosis

In the differential diagnosis of molluscum contagiosum, consideration must be given to other dermatological conditions with similar clinical presentations (Table 25.2).

Table 25.2 Important differential diagnostic considerations in molluscum contagiosum

Differential diagnosis	Description	Notes (distinguishing features)
Scabies	Infestation by the mite Sarcoptes scabiei, producing intensely pruritic papules, excoriations, and characteristic burrows in interdigital webs, wrists, and flexural sites	No central umbilication; nocturnal pruritus is pronounced and burrows may be visualized; diagnosis is confirmed by identification of mites, eggs, or fecal pellets on skin scrapings
Lichen planus	A T-cell-mediated inflammatory dermatosis characterized by polygonal, flat-topped, violaceous papules that frequently involve flexor surfaces and mucous membranes	Wickham's striae and polygonal morphology are typical; lesions lack the central dimple/core of molluscum and histology shows a lichenoid lymphocytic infiltrate rather than intracytoplasmic inclusion bodies
Milia	Small keratin-filled epidermal cysts presenting as firm, white to yellowish papules, most commonly on the face and periorbital region in infants and adults	Lesions are 1–2 mm, firm and non-umbilicated; no spontaneous central discharge is produced on pressure; histology demonstrates a keratin-filled cyst lined by stratified squamous epithelium
Molluscum pendulum (skin tag)	Acrochordons: soft, pedunculated fibroepithelial polyps occurring in skin folds (neck, axillae, and groin), varying from skin-colored to hyperpigmented	Pedunculated, soft, and fleshy morphology distinguishes them; central umbilication is absent and histology lacks molluscum (Henderson-Patterson) bodies

(continued)

Table 25.2 (continued)

Differential diagnosis	Description	Notes (distinguishing features)
Genital warts (HPV)	Papillomatous, exophytic, or flat-topped lesions caused by human papillomavirus on the vulva, penis, perineum, or perianal region; lesions may be solitary or clustered	Rough, verrucous, or flat surfaces are typical; central umbilication is absent; acetowhitening with 5% acetic acid supports HPV; and histology shows koilocytosis rather than molluscum inclusion bodies
Verrucae (common warts)	Firm, hyperkeratotic papules or nodules with a papillomatous surface, commonly affecting the hands and digits; caused by cutaneous HPV types	Hyperkeratosis and black punctate hemorrhages are characteristic; central umbilication is absent; and histology lacks intracytoplasmic molluscum bodies

25.8 Prevention

Currently, no formal, evidence-based international guidelines exist for the prevention of molluscum contagiosum (MCV). Preventive measures are therefore based on fundamental principles of barrier protection and hygiene intended to interrupt skin-to-skin and fomite transmission.

- Avoid Direct Skin Contact: Direct touching, scratching, or picking of visible lesions should be avoided. Individuals with active lesions should be advised to refrain from close-contact sports or activities (for example, wrestling or gymnastics) until lesions have resolved or have been appropriately treated.
- Minimize Fomite Transmission: Personal items (towels, razors, clothing, bath sponges, washcloths, and sports equipment) should not be shared. Clothing, towels, and bedding used by infected persons should be laundered in hot water with detergent and dried on a high-heat cycle.
- Promote Hand Hygiene: Thorough handwashing with soap and warm water should be performed after contact with affected skin; alcohol-based hand rubs may be used when washing facilities are unavailable.
- Cover Lesions: Individual lesions should be covered with a waterproof adhesive dressing or clothing during outbreaks to reduce direct and indirect transmission risk; dressings should be changed daily and disposed of safely.
- Disinfect Shared Surfaces: Surfaces and objects that contact skin (for example, gym mats, shower floors, and bath seats) should be cleaned with detergent and then disinfected using a standard household disinfectant.
- Patient and Caregiver Education: Patients and caregivers should be informed that MCV is usually self-limited in immunocompetent persons but remains contagious until lesions resolve or are treated. The importance of avoiding sharing personal items and maintaining good skin care to prevent autoinoculation and onward transmission should be emphasized.

Key Points

- Molluscum contagiosum: Caused by the molluscum contagiosum virus (MCV), presenting as a viral skin disease predominately transmitted via skin contact.
- The condition manifests as painless, skin-colored lesions.
- It is commonly found in children and young, sexually active adults; a multitude of lesions may indicate an impaired immune response.
- Diagnosis is typically clinical; in ambiguous cases, histological confirmation or virion detection may be performed.
- Spontaneous resolution frequently occurs, although surgical or surface-destructive interventions may be indicated, including trichloroacetic acid tamponade or laser therapy.
- Treatment success rates vary, with cidofovir available as an option for patients who are HIV-positive and exhibit severe symptoms.
- There are no established prevention recommendations, and direct skin contact with lesions should be avoided.

Nonvenereal Treponematoses

26

Abstract

Nonvenereal treponematoses, encompassing framboesia, endemic syphilis, and pinta, are bacterial infections predominantly found in developing countries and are caused by Treponema spp. These illnesses are primarily transmitted through direct skin contact, with transmission through infected objects occurring less frequently. The clinical manifestations of these infections vary and may progress from initial skin lesions to severe, late-stage bone and skin damage. Diagnosis is typically clinical, supported by serologic tests that share similarities with, but lack specificity for, syphilis. Treatment is primarily conducted with penicillin, whereas azithromycin is utilized as an alternative option. Preventive strategies encompass the treatment of all close contacts to mitigate the transmission of disease.

26.1 Background

Nonvenereal treponematoses consist of framboesia, endemic syphilis, and pinta, which mainly affect developing nations. The pathogens involved share similarities with those causing syphilis but differ in their epidemiological patterns and clinical presentations. Transmission predominantly occurs through direct contact; however, endemic syphilis may also involve transmission via infected objects. Evidence supporting blood or blood product transmission remains scarce, although transplacental transmission from pregnant women to their unborn children is theoretically possible. The predominant mode of dissemination appears to be close physical contact, encompassing sexual intercourse.

I. Mylonas, *Sexually Transmitted Diseases*,
https://doi.org/10.1007/978-3-031-78204-6_26

26.2 Pathogens

The genus Treponema comprises four bacterial species recognized as human pathogens. These bacteria are challenging to culture and are morphologically and immunologically indistinguishable. Research primarily relies on a limited number of clinical isolates. Genome sequencing of *T. pallidum* has revealed genetic loci that permit the differentiation of these organisms:

- *Treponema pallidum* subsp. *pallidum*: Syphilis (lues venereum)
- *Treponema pallidum* subsp. *endemicum*: Nonvenereal endemic syphilis (bejel)
- *Treponema pallidum* subsp. *pertenue*: Yaws
- *Treponema carateum*: Pinta

26.3 Epidemiology

Endemic treponematoses manifest in developing countries, exhibiting variable geographical distributions. However, they tend to be rare above or below the 30th geographical parallel. Framboesia is distributed worldwide, while endemic syphilis predominantly occurs in the arid regions of North Africa and the Arabian Peninsula. Pinta has been reported in the Caribbean Islands, Central, and South America. Limited access to sanitary facilities correlates with elevated infection rates.

Despite nearing eradication in the 1970s, the incidence of these diseases has resurged, with estimates indicating that over 2.5 million individuals are currently affected.

26.4 Clinical Manifestations

26.4.1 Gynecology

These infections are classified as chronic bacterial diseases that are transmitted through direct contact with infectious materials. They progress through well-defined clinical stages, from early localized manifestations to later disseminated forms (Table 26.1). The initial lesions emerge at the inoculation site following an incubation period ranging from 9 to 90 days, with an average duration of 21 days. Primary lesions in yaws and pinta typically heal spontaneously without intervention, although recurrences may occur in the secondary stage for up to 5 years, with recurrence frequency diminishing over time.

Recurrent secondary manifestations of early endemic treponematoses mainly feature dermatological symptoms; however, a substantial proportion of affected

Table 26.1 Features of nonvenereal treponematoses

Feature	Yaws (*Treponema pallidum* subsp. pertenue)	Endemic syphilis—Bejel (*Treponema pallidum* subsp. endemicum)	Pinta (*Treponema carateum*)
Primary lesion	"Mother yaw": papillomatous or ulcerative sore on exposed skin (face, limbs); often moist and highly infectious	Painless mucosal ulcer in the oropharynx or a small papule on the face or trunk; lesions are typically non-genital	Small, scaly, pink papules on exposed skin (classically lower limbs)
Secondary features	Multiple moist papillomas and papuloulcerative lesions; regional lymphadenopathy common	Mucosal patches and condyloma-lata-like lesions in intertriginous sites; regional lymphadenopathy may be present	Coalescing plaques with centrifugal spread; pruritus is uncommon
Tertiary manifestations	Chronic destructive lesions of bone and cartilage (e.g., periostitis, bowing of long bones, gummatous nodules)	Gummatous destruction of bone and nasal cartilage leading to sabre-shins and facial disfigurement in advanced disease	Irreversible pigmentary alteration (hypo- and hyperpigmented macules); no systemic or destructive visceral disease
Microbiology/ serology	Caused by *T. pallidum* subsp. pertenue; serologic tests (treponemal and non-treponemal) are usually positive but cannot distinguish subspecies	Caused by *T. pallidum* subsp. endemicum; serology mirrors venereal syphilis (treponemal and non-treponemal positivity)	Caused by *T. carateum*; serology may be variable and less consistently positive than in yaws or bejel
Key epidemiology	Endemic in warm, humid, rural areas of West and Central Africa, Southeast Asia, and Pacific islands; predominantly affects children <15 years	Occurs in arid and semi-arid regions (Sahel, parts of the Middle East, Afghanistan); primarily a childhood, non-sexual disease	Focal rural distribution in Latin America; affects school-age children; transmission by direct skin-to-skin contact
Transmission	Direct skin-to-skin contact with infectious lesions; predominantly non-sexual in children	Non-sexual transmission through close contact, often via shared utensils or household contact in dry climates	Direct skin-to-skin contact; confined to skin without systemic spread
Public health notes	WHO endemic disease elimination initiatives (mass azithromycin campaigns) have reduced prevalence in many areas	Requires community-level control measures; improvement in sanitation and access to care reduces transmission	Control focuses on early detection and treatment to prevent pigmentary sequelae

individuals may develop osteitis or bony lesions. Late-stage infections impact a minority of untreated patients with yaws and endemic syphilis, presenting destructive manifestations that commonly include ulcerative or hyperkeratotic cutaneous lesions and complications associated with bone and joint health.

26.4.1.1 Yaws

Yaws, caused by *T. pallidum* subsp. *pertenue*, is the most prevalent endemic treponematosis. The primary transmission route is via direct contact, wherein infectious exudate is transferred from lesions to uninfected individuals. The disease predominantly affects children aged 2–15 years.

Initial manifestations are usually pruritic, leading to potential self-infection, and may be accompanied by mild regional lymphadenopathy. Secondary-stage lesions primarily affect the skin, bones, and cartilage, often healing without treatment and without scarring. However, approximately 10% of untreated patients may later develop changes characterized by hyperkeratotic plaques, destructive bony lesions, or periodontal disease. Gangosis refers to these disfiguring chronic outcomes that result in the destruction of bone, cartilage, and soft tissue within the oral and nasal cavities. Serologic tests for syphilis may remain reactive for years, even following appropriate therapy.

26.4.1.2 Endemic Syphilis (Bejel)

Endemic syphilis, caused by *T. pallidum* subsp. *endemicum*, predominantly occurs in arid regions within rural communities. Its highest prevalence is noted in North Africa, Southwest Asia, and the Eastern Mediterranean. Similar to framboesia, endemic syphilis primarily affects children, with most cases reported in individuals aged 2–15 years.

Secondary manifestations often include cutaneous rashes, mucosal lesions, and involvement of bone and cartilage. Complications such as gingival lesions or chronic ulcerative eruptions are common. In contrast to these earlier lesions, late-stage manifestations exhibit a more destructive tendency, with the potential to result in deforming bony and cartilaginous facial lesions termed gangrene.

26.4.1.3 Pinta

Pinta, attributable to *T. carateum*, is a nonvenereal treponematosis endemic to the New World, principally occurring in several South American countries and the Caribbean.

Transmission occurs through direct contact with lesions, with untreated efflorescences persisting for extended periods. The initial pinta lesion typically presents as a nodule or a reddish, thickened skin area, which progressively enlarges and transforms into a darkly pigmented lesion. Additional pigmented skin changes may develop later in the disease course Interstingly, no other known disabilities or complications have been associated with pinta.

26.4.2 Pregnancy

In contrast to syphilis, evidence of transmission via blood or blood products remains scant, although such transmission is theoretically feasible. Additionally, the possibility of transplacental transmission from pregnant women to their unborn children exists. However, no documented cases of such occurrences have been reported.

26.5 Diagnosis

The diagnosis of individual cases of endemic treponematoses is predominantly dependent on clinical assessments supplemented by serologic testing for confirmation alongside syphilis serologic tests. Although not widely utilized, visualization of characteristic treponemes using dark-field microscopy on lesion exudates can provide immediate and highly specific diagnoses. Immunofluorescent antibody staining for treponemes is also available in select facilities and allows specific identification of infections. However, resources for dark-field or immunofluorescence microscopy are rare in regions where endemic treponematoses are prevalent.

Currently, no serological tests have been specifically developed for the diagnosis of endemic treponematoses. Due to the indistinguishable humoral antibody response between these diseases and syphilis, serologic testing for syphilis remains vital in confirming clinically suspected infections. Serologic tests for syphilis (and endemic treponematoses) are classified into nontreponemal and treponemal categories. Most false-positive serologic results for syphilis manifest at dilutions of 1:4 or less. Accordingly, in many resource-limited settings with high prevalence of such infections, nontreponemal test titers exceeding 1:4 are interpreted as indicative of active infections, guiding management decisions for both endemic treponematoses and syphilis.

Following effective treatment, patients typically experience a twofold or greater decrease in serologic test titers, although many may retain test reactivity post-treatment. A twofold or greater increase in serologic titer may be indicative of reinfection or relapse.

26.6 Treatment

Penicillin remains the first-line treatment for endemic treponematoses and continues to be widely utilized. The World Health Organization (WHO) recommends administering a single intramuscular dose of benzathine penicillin G (600,000 IU for children under 10 years of age and 1.2 million IU for individuals aged 10 years and older) for each endemic treponematosis.

Azithromycin, at a dosage of 30 mg/kg (up to a maximum of 2.0 g) as a single oral dose, may also be employed for the treatment of early framboesia. Azithromycin proves to be an effective alternative for patients with penicillin allergy.

26.7 Differential Diagnosis

The differential diagnosis of nonvenereal treponematoses such as yaws (*T. pallidum* subsp. *pertenue*), endemic syphilis (*T. pallidum* subsp. *endemicum*), and pinta (*T. carateum*) is critical due to their clinical similarities to other dermatological and systemic conditions. Early stages often present with skin lesions that may mimic tropical diseases, including leprosy, cutaneous leishmaniasis, and fungal infections (e.g., chromoblastomycosis). In later stages, bone abnormalities may be confused with osteomyelitis or chronic multifocal osteitis. Given the clinical overlap, including ulcerative skin lesions, pain, and systemic symptoms, definitive diagnosis necessitates advanced serological testing, dark-field microscopy, or molecular techniques such as polymerase chain reaction (PCR) to identify the specific Treponema species.

26.8 Prevention

To avert the development of infection in exposed individuals, it is recommended that all household members and close personal contacts receive treatment. Although reduced azithromycin susceptibility has been noted in *T. pallidum* subsp. *pallidum*, similar resistance has not been confirmed in endemic treponematoses. Although studies are lacking, extrapolation from experiences with venereal syphilis suggests that doxycycline administered over 14 days may also yield effective outcomes.

Therapeutic response may be assessed based on the resolution of early lesions or, in cases of late infections, inhibition of progressive disease. Serologic response to therapy may manifest as a twofold or greater decrease in nontreponemal test results for syphilis (e.g., rapid plasma reagin [RPR] or Venereal Disease Research Laboratory [VDRL]). After treatment, titers may continue to indicate seropositivity for prolonged durations.

Key Points

- Nonvenereal treponematoses include framboesia, endemic syphilis, and pinta, which are prevalent primarily in developing countries.
- Transmission mainly occurs through direct contact, and potentially through infected objects in the case of endemic syphilis, with significant differences from syphilis in epidemiology and clinical presentations.
- The genus *Treponema* consists of four bacterial species recognized as human pathogens, which are challenging to culture and differentiate.

(continued)

- These species are: *Treponema pallidum* subsp. *pallidum*, *Treponema pallidum* subsp. *endemicum*, *Treponema pallidum* subsp. *pertenue*, and *Treponema carateum*.
- The geographic distribution of endemic treponematoses varies, and they are predominantly rare in areas above or below 30° latitude.
- The incidence of these diseases has been rising since the 1970s, with over 2.5 million affected individuals currently estimated worldwide.
- Infections progress through well-defined clinical stages, transitioning from an early localized form to a later disseminated form.
- Framboesia, caused by *T. pallidum* subsp. *pertenue*, is primarily observed in children and may lead to serious skin and bone lesions.
- Endemic syphilis, caused by *T. pallidum* subsp. *endemicum*, is most common in arid regions and frequently results in gingival lesions.
- Pinta, caused by *T. carateum*, is confined to the New World and typically presents with cutaneous manifestations.
- Diagnosis predominantly relies on clinical findings, with serologic tests assisting in confirming cases, including syphilis tests, which may lack specificity.
- Specific diagnostic methods such as dark-field microscopy or immunofluorescence staining exist but are infrequently available in endemic regions.
- Penicillin is the treatment of choice, as per WHO guidelines, while azithromycin serves as an alternative for those allergic to penicillin.
- To prevent disease transmission, treatment of all household members and close contacts is strongly advised.
- Assessment of therapeutic response relies on the resolution of lesions and a decrease in serologic titers, although serologic positivity may persist long after successful treatment.

Pubic Lice (Phthirus pubis) 27

Abstract

Phthirus pubis, commonly known as pubic lice, are parasitic insects that predominantly infest the pubic hair region. They are transmitted through close physical contact, especially during sexual intercourse. The ova measure approximately 1.0–1.6 mm in diameter, with each louse capable of laying up to five eggs daily. Common symptoms include intense itching and scratching, particularly at night. Additionally, pubic lice can cause blue-red spots (maculae coeruleae) and may lead to secondary bacterial infections. Diagnosis is based on the identification of lice, nits, and associated skin changes. Various medications are utilized in treatment regimens; however, pregnant women should avoid using pyrethrum solutions. Maintaining good personal hygiene and avoiding close contact with affected individuals are recommended as preventive measures. While intimate shaving may decrease the risk of infestation, it cannot guarantee complete prevention.

27.1 Background

Lice are flattened, wingless insects, measuring approximately 1.5–4.5 mm in size. Notable features include robust legs and distinctive mouthparts. The principal types of human lice are:

- Head louse (*Pediculus humanus capitis*)
- Clothes louse (*Pediculus humanus corporis*)
- Pubic louse (*Phthirus pubis*)

Pubic lice primarily inhabit the pubic hair, with transmission occurring through close contact with infected individuals, particularly during sexual activity.

I. Mylonas, *Sexually Transmitted Diseases*,
https://doi.org/10.1007/978-3-031-78204-6_27

There is a prevailing assumption that the prevalence of head lice and pubic lice in Central Europe may be underestimated. Head lice infestations pose significant challenges for children due to the discomfort and distress they cause.

27.2 Pathogen

The pubic louse (*Phthirus pubis*) is distinct from both the head louse and the clothes louse. It is a small, oval to shield-shaped parasite measuring approximately 1.0–1.6 mm in length (Fig. 27.1). The life span of female lice is about 1 month, during which they can lay up to five eggs (nits) daily, adhering them to hair using a specialized adhesive. Larvae develop into adult lice over two additional stages, with the complete developmental cycle lasting approximately 3–4 weeks.

Pubic lice require human body temperature and are exclusively adapted to humans as hosts, meaning that animals do not transmit them to humans.

Transmission predominantly occurs through close physical contact, such as during sexual activity, though direct transmission may also occur through the sharing of mattresses, laundry, or bedding.

Both male and female lice depend on frequent blood meals, allowing them to maintain close contact with their host. Pubic lice can feed on blood up to ten times daily.

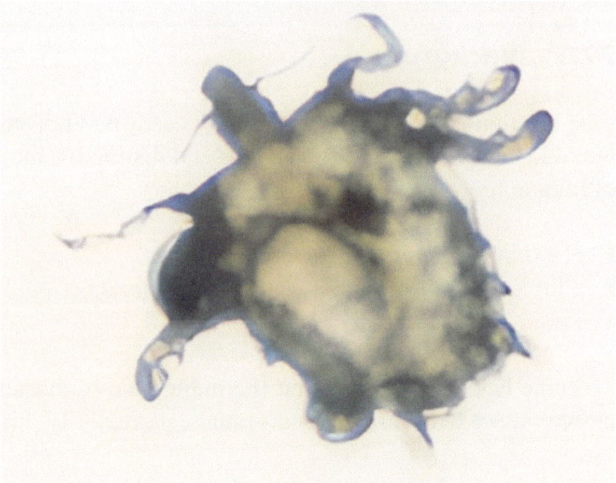

Fig. 27.1 Pubic louse observed under microscopy (Mendling 2006)

27.3 Epidemiology

In developed countries, pubic lice (*Pthirus pubis*) primarily cause medical concerns related to the direct effects of infestation. These include intense pruritus, erythematous papules, and secondary skin changes resulting from scratching. Diagnosis is typically confirmed by visual identification of live lice or nits, often aided by dermoscopy or microscopy. Although pubic lice most commonly infest the pubic area, they can also colonize other areas of coarse body hair, such as the axillae, chest, beard, eyebrows, and eyelashes. Transmission occurs predominantly through close physical or sexual contact but can also result from exposure to contaminated bedding, towels, or clothing. Importantly, pubic lice infestation may serve as a marker for other sexually transmitted infections (STIs), thereby warranting a comprehensive evaluation for coexisting infections.

Unlike body lice (*Pediculus humanus humanus*), which are established vectors of serious infectious diseases such as epidemic typhus (*Rickettsia prowazekii*), trench fever (*Bartonella quintana*), and relapsing fever (*Borrelia recurrentis*), pubic lice have not been definitively implicated in disease transmission. However, molecular studies have identified DNA from potential pathogens—including *Bartonella quintana* and Acinetobacter species—in pubic lice specimens, suggesting a possible but unconfirmed vectorial role that requires further investigation. Currently, the main health burden associated with pubic lice remains the discomfort and psychosocial impact of infestation as well as the risk of secondary bacterial infections due to excoriation.

Pubic lice (*Pthirus pubis*) are obligate human ectoparasites primarily transmitted through sexual contact, with infestations historically affecting 0.3–4.6% of adults worldwide and prevalence estimates around 2% in adults. The highest rates are seen among sexually active individuals aged 15–45, with men who have sex with men (MSM) and sex workers at increased risk. Infestations are also associated with other sexually transmitted infections and can occur in crowded or low-hygiene environments.

The incidence of pubic lice infestations in developed countries has declined in recent years, likely reflecting increased pubic hair removal practices, which reduce available habitat for lice. Nevertheless, pubic lice continue to represent a public health concern, particularly among sexually active adults and in populations with close personal contact.

Pubic lice are relatively common, particularly in areas exhibiting poor hygiene standards.

27.4 Clinical Manifestation

27.4.1 Gynecology

Pubic lice primarily infest the hairy regions of the pubic and perianal areas. In rare instances, they may also appear in the abdominal and axillary regions. Extremely rare cases may involve the eyelashes, eyebrows, beard, and nipple hair.

The predominant symptomology includes pronounced itching, leading to scratching lesions in the pubic region or other affected areas. The nocturnal itching is often exacerbated due to warmth and a personally lower itching threshold. Characteristic bluish-red spots may develop on the mons pubis, with diameters ranging from a few millimeters to 1 cm (maculae coeruleae).

Scratching can result in bacterial infections; untreated cases may lead to dry, hyperpigmented skin with thick crusting and scaling, potentially resulting in permanent scarring. Lice are capable of carrying and transmitting *Staphylococcus aureus* and Group A *Streptococcus pyogenes*.

Itching in the pubic area, particularly at night, should be considered a potential indicator of a pubic lice infestation.

27.4.2 Pregnancy

While pubic lice can cause discomfort and itching, they typically do not pose a significant risk to the unborn child or the mother. Treatment during pregnancy can be complicated, as many conventional products contain chemical components whose safety for the fetus is uncertain. Additionally, the psychological impact of an infestation during pregnancy can be particularly distressing. Pregnant women should implement preventive measures similar to those recommended for the general population, including regular personal hygiene, avoiding close contact with infected individuals, and ensuring the use of clean bedding and clothing.

Prompt treatment of pubic lice is crucial to prevent further spread of the infestation.

27.5 Diagnosis

Diagnosis is primarily based on clinical presentation. Specific symptoms, such as evening itching in the pubic area, serve as important indicators for a comprehensive examination.

Characteristic Findings

- **Detection of Pubic Lice:** Lice can typically be seen without magnification, although using a magnifying glass or microscope may enhance visibility. They are commonly located at the base of hair shafts.
- **Detection of Nits:** Nits are found 2-3 mm above the hair root, firmly fixed with a water-resistant adhesive and positioned at a distinct angle, making them identifiable during inspection.
- **Presence of Blood Crusts and Fecal Pellets:** Blood crusts and fecal matter from lice may be found among the pubic hairs during examination.
- **Scratch Marks in the Pubic Hair Region:** Scratching can lead to skin lesions that may subsequently become infected. Slate-blue spots (maculae coeruleae) may also be observed on the mons pubis, often accompanying itching.
- **Occasional Eczematous Changes:** In some cases, eczematous lesions may be observed as a result of lice bites.

27.6 Treatment

In cases of mild infestation, mechanical removal of nits using specialized combs can be effective. For more severe infestations, shaving the pubic hair is advisable to eliminate both nits and adult lice.

A variety of pharmacological treatments are available (Table 27.1). While pyrethrum solution is safe for use during pregnancy, breastfeeding, and in neonatal care,

Table 27.1 Treatment options for pubic lice. Note: Verify medication availability before prescribing. Nits can be removed with vinegar water and by extracting with tweezers or a comb. Follow-up after one week is advised, with repeat treatment if needed. Examine and treat contacts and partners to prevent reinfestation. Maintain strict hygiene for body and laundry

Indication	Medication	Dosage	Duration
Recommendation	Permethrin 5% cream	Once for 8–12 h	Day 1 and 8
	Allethrin and piperonyl butoxide	Once for 10 min	Day 1 and 8
	Pyrethrum extract	Once for 30 min	Day 1 and 8
Alternative	Ivermectin	0.2 mg/kg orally once	Day 1 and 8
	Phenothrin 0.2% lotion	Once for 2 h	Day 1
	Malathion 0.5% lotion	Once for 12 h	Day 1
Pregnancy	Pyrethrum extract	Once for 30 min	Day 1 and 8

other treatment options are contraindicated in these instances. Given the resistance of nits to many topical treatments, it is advisable to repeat the treatment one week later to address any freshly emerging lice.

In cases of secondary bacterial infections, local disinfectants or antibiotic ointments may be employed. For secondary eczema, topical glucocorticoids may also be considered.

It is advisable to provide treatment for others who may have been exposed to the infestation.

27.7 Differential Diagnosis

Differential diagnoses for pubic lice may include scabies, pediculosis (head lice and clothes lice), contact dermatitis, urticaria, various parasitic skin diseases, dermatitis, allergic reactions, and bacterial infections.

27.8 Prevention

Preventing pubic lice (*Pthirus pubis*) infestations requires a multifaceted approach combining personal hygiene, behavioral precautions, and timely treatment. Although the prevalence of pubic lice in developed countries has declined—largely due to changes in grooming habits such as increased pubic hair removal—these measures do not provide absolute protection.

- Personal Hygiene: Regular cleansing of the body, clothing, and bedding may reduce infestation risk but is not fully protective, as pubic lice are primarily transmitted through close physical or sexual contact rather than poor hygiene alone.
- Grooming Practices: The widespread adoption of pubic hair removal methods (e.g., shaving and waxing) has contributed to a notable decrease in pubic lice infestations. However, lice can still colonize other coarse body hair areas, including the axillae, chest, beard, and eyelashes; thus, hair removal does not guarantee complete prevention.
- Avoidance of Shared Personal Items: Avoid sharing towels, bedding, clothing, and grooming tools such as combs or brushes to minimize indirect transmission risk, although this route is less common.
- Sexual Health Practices: Limiting the number of sexual partners and notifying partners promptly if infestation is diagnosed are critical steps. Given the frequent association of pubic lice with other STD, comprehensive STD screening is recommended following diagnosis.

- Prompt Treatment and Partner Notification: Early detection and treatment with recommended topical pediculicides (such as permethrin or pyrethrins) are essential. Simultaneous treatment of all sexual partners and close contacts is necessary to prevent reinfestation.

Additional preventive strategies involve the routine laundering of garments, bed linens, and towels at elevated temperatures, as well as the avoidance of close physical interactions with individuals who are infected.

Key Points

- Pubic lice infestation is caused by the presence of *Phthirus pubis* in the pubic hair.
- Transmission primarily occurs through close contact, particularly during sexual intercourse.
- The prevalence of lice infestations is notable among children and in conditions of poor hygiene.
- The lice are small, oval to shield-shaped, measuring approximately 1.0–1.6 mm. Females can lay up to five eggs daily, with the development to adulthood taking approximately 3–4 weeks. Transmission is exclusively through close physical contact.
- The prevalence of pubic lice in Central Europe is especially marked in contexts of inadequate hygiene standards.
- Clothing lice can serve as carriers of various pathogens.
- The main symptom experienced is pruritus (itching) in the pubic and perianal areas, as well as in other hairy regions.
- Associated symptoms may include bluish-red spots (maculae coeruleae), scratches, and secondary bacterial infections.
- Diagnostic findings in the pubic area include the presence of lice, nits, blood crusts, fecal pellets, and scratch marks.
- For mild infestations, mechanical removal of nits is advised In the event of a moderate to severe infestation, shaving is recommended.
- Various active ingredients are available for pharmacological treatment.
- A second course of treatment should be administered one week post-initial treatment if nits prove resistant.
- Careful personal hygiene is essential for the prevention of lice infestations.
- Intimate shaving may serve as a preventive measure, though it does not provide complete protection.
- Regular washing of clothing, bed linens, and towels at high temperatures, along with minimizing contact with infected individuals, is recommended.

Scabies

28

Abstract

Scabies, also referred to as mange, is an infestation caused by the mite *Sarcoptes scabiei hominis*. Transmission occurs primarily through physical and sexual contact. Female mites burrow into the dermis to lay eggs, resulting in severe pruritus, particularly at night and in predilection sites such as the interdigital spaces. Diagnosis is established based on characteristic cutaneous manifestations and the identification of mites, their eggs, or feces, typically via visual or microscopic examination. First-line treatment employs topical antiscabiosa such as permethrin, with ivermectin as a systemic alternative. Prevention strategies focus on minimizing close contact with infested individuals, emphasizing hygiene practices and the treatment of contacts to impede further spread. While scabies is prevalent globally, it remains relatively uncommon in developed countries.

28.1 Background

Scabies is an intensely pruritic dermatosis caused by the obligate human ectoparasite *Sarcoptes scabiei* var. *hominis*. Although the term "scabies" itself was first recorded in the sixteenth century, descriptions of the disease date back to ancient civilizations, including Hippocratic texts that detail characteristic itching and burrow lesions. Historically, scabies has surged during periods of overcrowding, social upheaval, and famine—conditions that facilitate prolonged skin-to-skin contact and impede effective hygiene.

Transmission requires direct and prolonged skin-to-skin contact, making household and institutional outbreaks common. While nonsexual close contact suffices, scabies is also recognized as a sexually transmitted infestation, particularly among young adults, where intimate contact promotes rapid mite transfer. Fomite transmission—via bedding, clothing, or furniture—is less efficient but can occur in settings with heavy infestation or "crusted" (Norwegian) scabies.

I. Mylonas, *Sexually Transmitted Diseases*,
https://doi.org/10.1007/978-3-031-78204-6_28

28.2 Pathogen

Following mating on the skin surface, male scabies mites (*Sarcoptes scabiei hominis*) (Fig. 28.1) perish, while females burrow into the epidermis to lay eggs. Respiration occurs via diffusion through the cutaneous surface, thus deeper skin layers remain unaffected. As the female can vacate the initial burrow to create new tunnels in the skin, the number of burrows is not directly correlated with the number of mites present. A single female mite can survive up to 60 days, laying two to four eggs that hatch into larvae within 2–7 days. These larvae subsequently burrow into the epidermis, undergoing several developmental stages to become adult mites.

Outside the human host, scabies mites exhibit limited survival capability. Transmission occurs almost exclusively through direct person-to-person contact. Consequently, adult scabies is often transmitted during sexual encounters, categorizing it as a sexually transmitted infection.

The transmission rate increases with prolonged and intense physical contact. Higher mite burdens, poor personal hygiene, and immunosuppression in the host also contribute to transmission. Transmission via contaminated clothing or bedding is uncommon; for example, the risk of acquiring scabies from sleeping on infested bedding is estimated to be less than 1 in 200.

In contrast to the classic scabies mite, *Sarcoptes scabiei* var. *norvegica* (crusted scabies) is highly contagious and capable of airborne transmission via mite-containing skin particles. Other common mites, such as house dust mites and *Demodex follicularis*, are largely harmless.

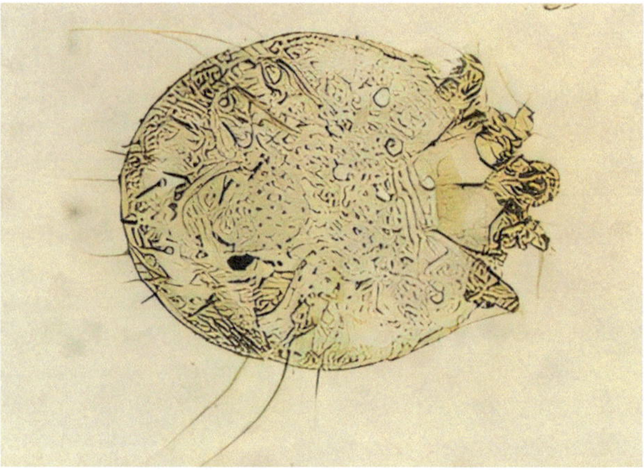

Fig. 28.1 Detection of Sarcoptes scabiei hominis via light microscopy (Mendling 2006)

28.3 Epidemiology

Scabies remains a highly prevalent and often neglected parasitic skin disease, with epidemiological patterns shaped by geography, age, seasonality, and social determinants.

Global Burden
Worldwide, scabies affects over 200 million people at any given time, with annual incidence estimates ranging from 150 to 300 million new cases. It accounts for approximately 0.21% of the global burden of disease measured by disability-adjusted life years (DALYs), ranking among the top 50 causes of non-fatal disease burden globally. The burden is particularly high in tropical and resource-poor settings, where secondary complications such as pyoderma, glomerulonephritis, and rheumatic heart disease further increase morbidity.

Regional Prevalence
In Oceania, including northern Australia and Pacific islands, prevalence can reach 35–50% in some Indigenous and remote communities. This high prevalence is largely driven by overcrowding and limited access to healthcare. In sub-Saharan Africa, prevalence rates commonly range from 10% to over 30%, particularly in rural or nomadic populations; however, data are often extrapolated due to limited surveillance. Southeast and South Asia report prevalence between 5% and 15%, frequently linked to monsoonal overcrowding and seasonal migration. In Latin America and the Caribbean, urban slums and informal settlements experience prevalence rates up to 10–20%, with national averages around 2–5%. In Europe and North America, general population prevalence remains low at 0.5–2%, although institutional outbreaks in care facilities, prisons, and shelters can exceed 10%.

Age and Sex Distribution
Children aged 5–14 years bear the highest incidence of scabies worldwide, reflecting transmission in school and household settings. Outbreaks among young adults in congregate environments such as dormitories and military barracks underscore the potential for rapid spread. Sex distribution is generally balanced; however, some studies report slightly higher rates among females, possibly related to caregiving roles.

Seasonality
In temperate climates, scabies incidence peaks during autumn and winter months, correlating with increased indoor crowding. In tropical regions, seasonality is less pronounced but may intensify during wet seasons due to crowding.

Outbreak Dynamics and Control
Institutional outbreaks can result in attack rates exceeding 80% if not promptly recognized and managed. Mass drug administration (MDA) with oral ivermectin has demonstrated up to a 90% reduction in scabies prevalence within 12 months in

hyperendemic communities, illustrating the effectiveness of community-wide interventions. Challenges to control include diagnostic limitations, treatment failures, and reinfection from untreated contacts.

Public Health Implications
Scabies is a significant public health challenge beyond its dermatological impact. Effective control strategies require integrated approaches that combine pharmacotherapy, community-based interventions, enhanced diagnostics, and improvements in living conditions to reduce transmission and associated complications.

28.4 Clinical Manifestations

28.4.1 Gynecology

Clinical manifestations typically include pruritic nodules and distinct skin changes such as exanthema, mite burrows, and secondary excoriations. Symptom severity may vary (Table 28.1).

Predilection sites frequently involve the interdigital spaces of the hands (Fig. 28.2), the volar surfaces of the wrists, the anogenital area, the vulva, the anterior axillary fold, the elbows, the umbilicus, or the medial aspect of the feet. In infants, involvement of the face, scalp, and palms of the hands and feet may be observed. In older individuals, the scalp may also be affected.

The initial lesion of scabies typically presents as a palpable, often curved or comma-shaped burrow on the skin. These burrows range in length from a few

Table 28.1 Various forms of scabies

Form	High-risk group	Clinical manifestations
Classical scabies (scabies vulgaris)	Infants, children, sexually active adults, MSM	– Intense itching, especially at night – Inflammatory papules on fingers, wrists, elbows, armpits, buttocks, genital area, breasts – Lesions spare face, head, neck – Secondary lesions: eczema, excoriation, impetigo
Scabies of the scalp	Infants, children, institutionalized older adults, AIDS patients	– Atypical encrusted papular lesions – Affects scalp, face, palms of hands, soles of feet
Encrusted scabies (scabies norvegica, scabies crustosa)	Institutionalized older adults, homeless people, immunocompromised individuals	– Psoriasiform lesions – Affects scalp, face, neck, hands, feet, with nail involvement – Eczematization and often impetigo
Nodular scabies	Sexually active adults, MSM, HIV-positive individuals	– Purple itchy nodules on genitals, groin, armpits – Hypersensitivity reaction to mite antigens

MSM Men who have sex with men

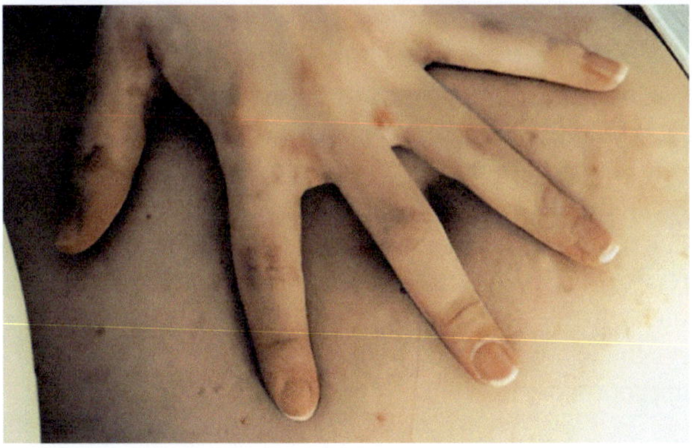

Fig. 28.2 Scabies infestation in a patient at 20 weeks' gestation involving the hands and trunk (Friese et al. 2003)

millimeters up to one centimeter. At the distal end of the burrow lies the mite, which may sometimes be visible as a small dark spot known as the mite mound. This structure represents the site where the female *Sarcoptes scabiei* mite tunnels into the stratum corneum to deposit eggs.

The intense pruritus associated with scabies arises from a hypersensitivity reaction to mite antigens, feces, and eggs, leading to significant inflammation and eczematous changes. This pruritus is characteristically more severe at night, which is thought to be related to increased mite activity and reduced distractions during sleep.

The resulting skin manifestations are diverse and can include papulovesicular lesions, inflammatory pruritic papules, crusted plaques, and excoriations caused by persistent scratching. Collectively, these lesions are referred to as scabies exanthema and may extend well beyond the primary sites of mite infestation due to the generalized hypersensitivity response. The widespread eczema and scratch-induced skin damage can predispose patients to secondary bacterial infections, further complicating the clinical picture.

Overall, the combination of the distinctive burrow lesion, nocturnal pruritus, and polymorphic rash forms the hallmark of scabies infestation, guiding clinical diagnosis and management.

Symptoms vary in severity, with immunocompromised patients (e.g., those with HIV infection) exhibiting more pronounced clinical manifestations.

Treatment may give rise to skin irritation, persistent pruritus, and papular eruptions (Fig. 28.2). These effects can mimic treatment failure. However, if skin symptoms persist for longer than 2–3 weeks, the possibility of reinfestation should be evaluated.

28.4.2 Pregnancy

Scabies does not appear to present with increased severity during pregnancy compared to nonpregnant women. There is no evident primary risk to the fetus.

Scabies in pregnancy manifests with clinical severity and symptomatology similar to that in non-pregnant women, and there is no evidence of increased mite burden or more extensive skin involvement. Maternal infestation does not pose a direct teratogenic risk or adverse effect on fetal development. Standard treatment regimens, including topical permethrin 5% cream, remain safe and effective throughout pregnancy, with no demonstrated increase in maternal or fetal complications when appropriately applied.

28.5 Diagnosis

A clinical history indicating the presence of highly pruritic skin lesions predominantly occurring at night, conjunction with the identification of close contacts, suggests the possibility of scabies in differential diagnoses. Definitive evidence of infestation includes the identification of mites, their eggs, or fecal remnants. In cases of suspected infestation, characteristic skin eruptions should be sought at the typical predilection sites. These lesions may be obscured by secondary scabietic eczema.

As mites typically reside at the end of a burrow, they may be extricated tangentially. Mites are often discernible to the naked eye as dark specks. Extracted materials can subsequently be analyzed under a light microscope (Fig. 28.1).

Diagnosis relies on clinical assessment, though biopsy may be beneficial in rare instances. The most salient diagnostic criterion is the identification of burrows through dermatoscope or magnifying glass. Confirmation is typically achieved through the detection of fecal globules, with the less common detection of the mite itself.

28.6 Treatment

Numerous antiscabietic agents are now licensed for clinical use (Table 28.2), but "permethrin 5% cream" remains the cornerstone of therapy for all patient populations (Fig. 28.3)—including infants over 2 months of age, children, adults, and pregnant or lactating women. Lindane preparations are either tightly restricted by prescription or have been withdrawn entirely in many regions (for example, the European Union) due to concerns about neurotoxicity.

Permethrin cream should be applied in a thin, even layer to "all skin surfaces below the mandible," extending from the neck down to the toes, paying special attention to skin folds. After an "8 to 12-h" contact period, the cream is rinsed off with warm water. In patients with suspected or confirmed "scalp involvement" (more common in infants and the elderly), permethrin may be carefully applied to

Table 28.2 Management approaches for scabies

Indication	Medication	Application	Duration
Recommendations	Permethrin 5% cream	Apply once, leave on skin for 8–12 h	Day 1 and day 8; repeat after 14 days if needed
	Ivermectin	0.2 mg/kg orally, single dose	Day 1 and day 8
Alternatives	Benzyl benzoate 25%	Apply once, leave on skin for 12 h	Days 1–3; repeat after 7 days if needed
	Benzyl benzoate 10%	Apply once, leave on skin for 12 h	Days 1–3; repeat after 7 days if needed
	Crotamiton 10% cream/lotion	Apply once, leave on skin for 24 h	3–5 consecutive days; repeat after 7 days if needed
	Ivermectin 1% lotion	Apply once, leave on skin for 12 h	Day 1 and day 8
	Sulfur cream/ointment/lotion 6–33%	Apply once, leave on skin for 12 h	Days 1–4; repeat after 1 week if needed
Others	Malathion 0.5%a	Apply once, leave on skin for 12 h	Day 1
	Lindane 0.3%b	Apply once, leave on skin for 12 h	Days 1–3
Eczematous skin	Methylprednisolone/hydrocortisone	Apply locally 1–2 times daily	2–3 days
Severe inflammation	Disinfectants	Apply locally once or twice daily	5–7 days
	Systemic antibiotic therapy	As prescribed	7–10 days
Pregnancy	Permethrin 5% cream	Apply once, leave on skin for 8–12 h	Day 1 and day 8; repeat after 14 days if needed
Pregnancy-alternative	Benzyl benzoate 25%c	Apply once, leave on skin for 12 h	Days 1–3; repeat after 7 days if needed
	Crotamiton 10% cream/lotion	Apply once, leave on skin for 24 h	3–5 days; repeat after 7 days if needed

[a]Malathion 0.5%: This medication is unavailable in several countries but can be obtained through international pharmacies if needed

[b]Lindane 0.3%: Lindane has been withdrawn from the market in many countries, including all European Union member states. Use may be considered only via international pharmacies when no alternatives are available

[c]Benzyl benzoate 25%: In North America, benzyl benzoate is contraindicated due to its association with "gasping syndrome," a serious and potentially fatal condition in premature infants and neonates. Clinical manifestations include metabolic acidosis, seizures, respiratory distress, and gasping respirations. The syndrome results from accumulation of benzyl alcohol caused by immature hepatic and renal clearance in newborns

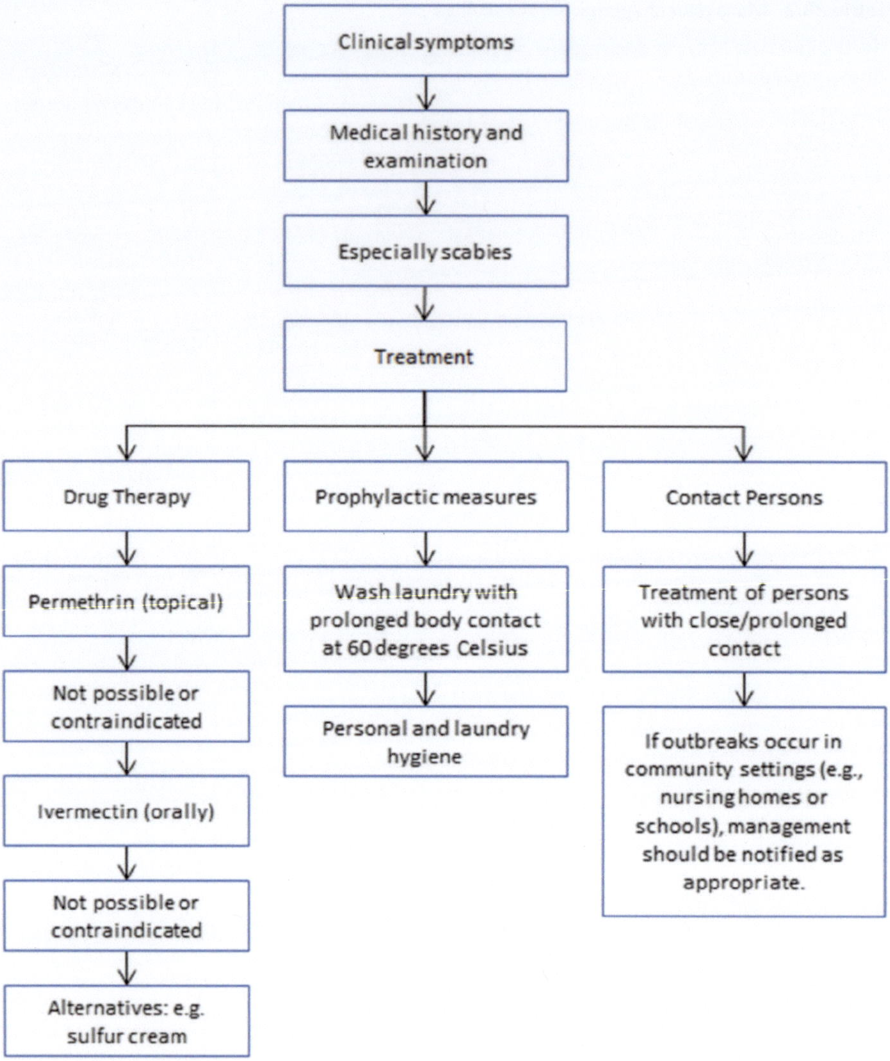

Fig. 28.3 Management protocol for scabies infestation. (Courtesy of I. Mylonas)

the hair-bearing scalp—avoiding contact with the "eyes and mouth"—using the same contact time. If live mites or new lesions are evident at follow-up (typically 2 weeks after initial treatment), a "second application" should be administered 10–14 days after the first.

Oral "ivermectin"—dosed at "200 μg/kg in a single dose, repeated after 7–14 days"—serves as an effective systemic option, particularly in outbreaks or in cases of crusted scabies. However, ivermectin is not approved for scabies treatment in all countries and should be used with caution in children weighing less than 15 kg, pregnant women, and individuals with underlying neurologic disorders.

Topical alternatives—including "benzyl benzoate," "crotamiton," "sulfur preparations," and "malathion"—remain useful in settings where permethrin or ivermectin are unavailable, contraindicated, or poorly tolerated. When selecting any antiscabietic regimen, simultaneous treatment of household and close contacts, laundering of linens and clothing, and environmental decontamination are essential to prevent reinfestation.

During treatment, daily laundering of clothing and bedding is advised. Contacts exhibiting skin symptoms should be treated concurrently for a duration of 3 days, while those without symptoms require treatment for just 1 day. For eczematous lesions, the short-term use of topical glucocorticoids is recommended following the conclusion of antiparasitic therapy.

28.7 Differential Diagnosis

Conditions that may mimic scabies include:

- **Allergic Reactions**: Allergic dermatoses may exhibit symptoms similar to scabies.
- **Other Parasitic Infections**: Parasitic conditions such as pediculosis, pseudoscabies (resulting from zoonotic mite transmission), and *Sarcoptes scabiei* var. *norvegica* (crusted scabies) may yield analogous presentations.
- **Dermatitis**: Various dermatitis conditions, including bullous pemphigoid and impetigo, may cause rashes and pruritus akin to scabies.
- **Eczema**: Several forms of eczema manifest with rashes and severe pruritus, which can be confused with scabies (e.g., contact dermatitis, pruritic eczema, atopic dermatitis).
- **Psoriasis**: Psoriasis may produce symptoms resembling those of scabies, such as erythematous, scaly plaques.
- **Urticaria**: Urticaria may overlap with scabies in terms of pruritic skin reactions.
- **Other Infectious Diseases**: Conditions such as pustular candidosis, eosinophilic folliculitis, framboesia, herpes simplex infection, and pyoderma may be considered.
- **Other Diseases**: Injuries, poisons, insect stings, insect bites, and Langerhans cell histiocytosis should be differentiated from scabies.

28.8 Prevention

The prevention of scabies is contingent upon the avoidance of direct skin contact with infested individuals. It is imperative to note that infection can occur even in the absence of awareness regarding one's own infestation. The probability of transmission is directly proportional to the duration and intensity of physical contact, with the overall transmission risk remaining relatively low; for instance, transmission does not typically occur through brief interactions such as handshakes.

In instances of close contact with an infected person, a clinical examination should be performed, irrespective of the presence of characteristic symptoms. Treatment and necessary adjunct measures (Table 28.2) should be meticulously adhered to, to prevent further dissemination of the infestation.

Additional preventive measures for scabies include:

- **Hygiene measures**:
  - Thorough cleaning and disinfection of linens, bedding, and clothing used in the days preceding treatment (Table 28.3).
  - Intensive vacuuming and sanitation of living environments.
- **Management of contacts**:
  - Identification and treatment of close contacts to disrupt the transmission chain.
  - In communal living settings, isolation of affected individuals may be mandated until treatment efficacy is confirmed.
  - Caregivers maintaining close contact with infected individuals should also receive concurrent treatment.

Table 28.3 Necessary accompanying measures for scabies

Overview	Measures
General	– The typical lifespan of mites under ambient conditions (i.e., a temperature of 21°C and a relative humidity of 40–80%) is approximately 2–3 days.
	– Under colder conditions or with higher humidity, survival for several weeks may be possible
	– Below 20 °C, the movement and reproduction of the mites are halted
	– At temperatures above 50 °C, mites are eliminated within 10 min
Dealing with scabies	– Isolation of individuals with scabies in communal facilities or accommodations is necessary. Individuals can be accommodated in either individual rooms or shared spaces for multiple affected persons
	– Isolation must continue until treatment is effective, which is usually 10–24 h after the start of topical therapy or ivermectin
	– Identification of all persons who had close physical contact with the infected individuals
	– Comprehensive monitoring and, if necessary, treatment of all exposed persons in care and community facilities, regardless of symptom presence
	– Minimizing the number of caregivers per affected person
	– Use of protective clothing and disposable gloves for close physical contact with affected individuals
	– Daily change of body clothing, underwear, bed linen, blankets, and towels until no live mites are present on the affected person
	– Cooperation between the health authorities and the facility management

(continued)

Table 28.3 (continued)

Overview	Measures
Carrying out disinfection	– Wash all textiles at 60 °C if possible and then dry them (in a dryer at over 50 °C for at least 10 min)
	– Dry cleaning is recommended for delicate garments
	– Alternatively, pack dry items airtight and store at room temperature for at least 3 days, or near a radiator for 48 h
	– Items such as slippers or soft toys can be treated by freezing them in a plastic bag for at least 24 h
	– Thorough and repeated vacuuming is recommended for mattresses, upholstered furniture, and carpets
	– Contaminated, dry objects can be wrapped in thick foil and stored for 3 days at room temperature in a separate room if necessary
	– Mattresses can also be sterilized in special disinfection systems that operate at 90 °C for 5 min
	– It is not necessary to treat rooms with chemical agents
Additional measures for scabies crustosa	– Isolation of infected individuals for 14 days in individual accommodation. If multiple people are affected, they can be housed together in separate rooms
	– Following this isolation period, a mandatory subsequent disinfection procedure is required for highly contagious scabies crustosa

- **Behavioral recommendations**:
  - Avoidance of close skin contact and communal activities until treatment efficacy has been confirmed.
  - Avoidance of scratching to mitigate the risk of secondary infections.
- **Monitoring and follow-up**:
  - Post-treatment follow-up examinations to ascertain treatment effectiveness.
  - If symptoms persist, reevaluation and potential retreatment may be warranted.

While personal hygiene may influence the progression of the disease, it cannot entirely prevent infestation.

Key Points

- Scabies is induced by the scabies mite (*Sarcoptes scabiei hominis*) and is predominantly transmitted through physical and sexual contact.
- The condition is widespread globally but relatively infrequent in developed nations.
- Scabies has been recognized as an itchy dermatosis since ancient times.
- Transmission primarily occurs through intimate physical interaction and sexual intercourse.
- Scabies presents significant epidemiological challenges, especially in developing regions, largely attributed to inadequate hygiene and socioeconomic conditions.
- Current estimates suggest that scabies impacts several hundred million individuals globally, with heightened prevalence noted in low-income areas characterized by poor hygiene.
- Clinical symptoms encompass pruritic nodules, cutaneous changes in favored regions, and intense pruritus, particularly nocturnally.
- Diagnosis is established through clinical history along with the visual or microscopic identification of mites, their eggs, or fecal remains.
- Treatment options include topical antiscabiosis such as permethrin as the primary choice, with ivermectin as a systemic alternative.
- Preventive measures focus on avoiding contact with affected individuals, regularly changing clothing, and treating close contacts.

Part VI

Sexually Transmitted Diseases With Systemic Impact

Cytomegaly (CMV) 29

Abstract

Cytomegaly is a prevalent viral infection that can lead to serious consequences for pregnant women and their newborns. Approximately 1–4% of women experience primary infection during pregnancy, with the potential for transmission to the fetus. The transmission rate increases with gestational age; however, the severity of the disease is inversely related to the duration of pregnancy. Around 15–20% of infected infants may develop sequelae, including hearing loss, intellectual disabilities, and developmental delays. Preventive measures, such as limiting contact with young children and practicing frequent hand hygiene, can help mitigate the risk of infection. Routine screening for CMV during pregnancy is not typically recommended. Currently, no specific antiviral therapy exists for CMV, although treatments, such as hyperimmunoglobulin and valaciclovir, are under investigation. Further research is essential to substantiate their efficacy and safety.

29.1 Background

The significance of cytomegaly, also referred to as cytomegalic inclusion body disease, has garnered increased attention in recent years. The infection is attributed to the cytomegalovirus (CMV), a member of the herpesvirus group. While CMV infrequently causes mononucleosis in immunocompetent individuals, individuals with acquired or congenital immunodeficiency—including those undergoing organ transplantation, living with HIV, or diagnosed with malignancies—are particularly vulnerable.

I. Mylonas, *Sexually Transmitted Diseases*,
https://doi.org/10.1007/978-3-031-78204-6_29

Cytomegalovirus (CMV) generally does not evoke significant symptoms in individuals with healthy immune systems; however, it can trigger severe complications in immunocompromised individuals, including pneumonia, retinitis, and encephalitis.

During pregnancy, the virus can be transmitted to the fetus, possibly resulting in serious conditions, including congenital malformations and long-term complications. Globally, approximately 0.2–2.3% of newborns are infected with CMV. The risk of congenital disease at birth, with the potential for late sequelae, strongly correlates with primary maternal infection, characterized by the detection of IgG seroconversion and elevated IgM antibody titers. Recurrent infections are indicated by the presence of IgG antibodies prior to conception, alongside congenital infection in the newborn. In contrast to other pathogens, such as rubella virus or *Toxoplasma gondii*, both primary and recurrent maternal infections can lead to fetal infection. Nevertheless, fetal damage due to recurrent maternal infection is relatively uncommon.

Cytomegalovirus (CMV) is the predominant cause of congenital infection related to disease at birth and long-term infantile impairments.

Transmission occurs primarily through direct contact with infectious secretions and inhalation of infectious droplets. Infection is usually initiated through contact with bodily secretions containing the virus, with potential routes including saliva, urine, feces, or breast milk. Sexual transmission may also occur via infected cervical and vaginal secretions or semen. Parenteral transmission typically transpires through blood transfusions or organ transplant procedures, where the virus may exist latently within monocytes.

29.2 Pathogen

Cytomegalovirus (CMV) possesses double-stranded (ds) DNA and is a member of the herpesvirus group. It features the largest genome among herpesviruses, with structural similarities to herpes simplex virus (HSV) type 1. The term "cytomegalovirus" is derived from the enlargement of infected cells, which typically exhibit large eosinophilic inclusions in the nucleus. Upon infection with CMV, the virus persists throughout the individual's lifetime; virus isolates share up to 80% sequence homology, signifying no distinct serotypes.

The incubation period for CMV infection is highly variable, spanning from 20 to 60 days, although cases extending to 100 days have been documented. The precise pathogenesis of CMV infection remains largely elusive. CMV has the capacity to infect various cell types, with replication occurring through either lysis of the host cell or latent persistence until reactivation.

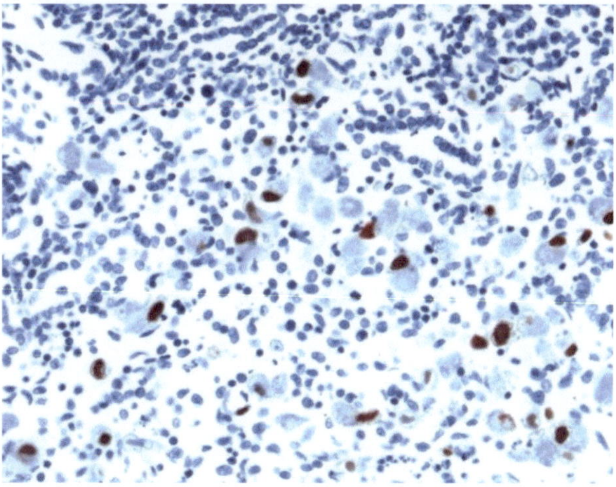

Fig. 29.1 Cytomegalovirus placentitis with immunohistochemical detection of CMV inclusions (Kost et al. 2007)

In instances of primary maternal infection, intrauterine infection is believed to arise from maternal viremia affecting the endothelial cells in placental vessels and/or chorionic fibroblasts (transplacental) (Fig. 29.1). When the chorion is infected, the virus may disseminate to the fetus via amniotic fluid. However, alternative transmission routes remain incompletely understood, as fetal infection can occur in cases of recurrent maternal infection despite low maternal viremia and the presence of IgG antibodies.

Perinatal transmission typically occurs during passage through the birth canal, with maternal secretions serving as the infectious source. Early postnatal transmission is primarily facilitated through breastfeeding, although child-to-child transmission can also occur, particularly in communal settings.

29.3 Epidemiology

29.3.1 Degree of Infection

The prevalence of cytomegalovirus (CMV) infection exhibits considerable variation across global populations, influenced by several critical factors:

- **Socioeconomic Status**: A lower socioeconomic status and restricted access to healthcare are correlated with elevated rates of CMV infection. Research indicates that CMV seroprevalence and congenital CMV infection rates are more pronounced in low- to middle-income countries (LMICs) compared to high-income countries (HICs).
- **Geographical Location**: Differences in environmental conditions and public health practices contribute to the variance in prevalence rates between regions. For instance, the World Health Organization (WHO) Eastern Mediterranean region demonstrates higher CMV seroprevalence rates relative to the WHO European region.
- **Ethnicity**: Susceptibility to and transmission of CMV can be affected by cultural habits and genetic predispositions. Cultural practices in childcare and sexual behaviors exhibit significant variation among different ethnic groups.

- **Birth and Infant Care Practices**: Childbirth and neonatal care practices influence transmission and prevalence. For example, breastfeeding and maternal contact in neonatal care can elevate the risk of CMV transmission.
- **Sexual Behavior**: The sexual transmission of CMV is impacted by factors such as the age of first intercourse and the frequency of sexual activities, affecting the spread of infection.

Globally, CMV infection rates range from 30% to 90%, reflecting these diverse factors. The highest seroprevalence rates are frequently observed in developing countries and among populations with limited healthcare access. This underscores the necessity for targeted public health strategies to mitigate CMV transmission, particularly among vulnerable groups such as pregnant women and individuals with compromised immune systems.

29.3.2 Pregnancy

29.3.2.1 Primary Infection

The prevalence of cytomegalovirus (CMV) infection varies significantly based on socioeconomic factors, with higher rates of congenital CMV observed in infants of color compared to Hispanic and non-Hispanic white infants. CMV seropositivity rates are approximately 40–50% among women from middle and high socioeconomic backgrounds and range from 60% to over 80% in those from lower socioeconomic strata. The age-adjusted seroprevalence of CMV has remained consistent from 1988–1994 to 1999–2004. Global estimates place the seroprevalence among women of childbearing age at approximately 86%, with the highest rates in the WHO Eastern Mediterranean Region (92%) and the Americas (79%), and the lowest in the WHO European Region (70%).

Annually, approximately 1–4% of seronegative pregnant women acquire a primary CMV infection. In the United States, this rate averages 1%, while some low-prevalence countries report rates of 0.2–0.3%. Long-term fetal impairment occurs in around 50% of clinically abnormal newborns and in approximately 15% of

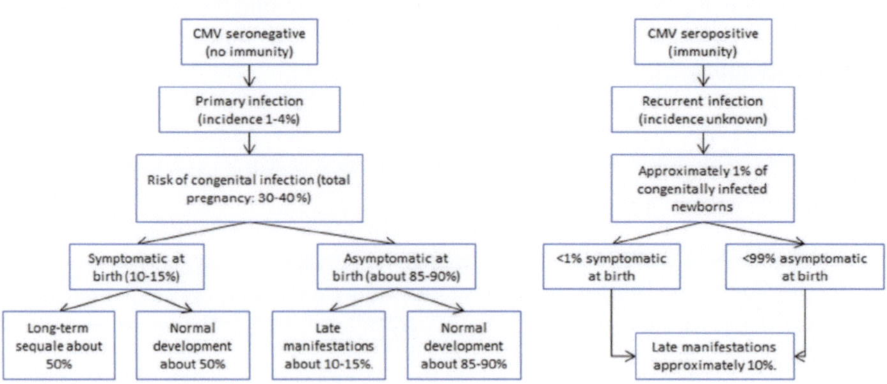

Fig. 29.2 Consequences of cytomegalovirus infection. (Courtesy of I. Mylonas)

asymptomatic children. The rate of intrauterine infection is about 40% for primary maternal infections and approximately 1% for recurrent infections (Fig. 29.2).

Mothers from lower social classes exhibit the highest risk of delivering congenitally infected children. Young adults (ages 14–20 years) typically acquire primary CMV infection through sexual intercourse, while pregnant women from middle and upper socioeconomic classes often contract their first infection at ages 20–30 years, primarily through contact with virus-excreting infants and toddlers.

Primary CMV infections during pregnancy are generally not more severe than those encountered in nonpregnant women, with over 90% of cases remaining asymptomatic or presenting with nonspecific symptoms. There is no established increased rate of miscarriage or intrauterine fetal death (IUFD), although the incidence of preterm birth is elevated. During primary infection, the potential for CMV transmission to the fetus exists throughout pregnancy during the maternal viremic phase.

Primary maternal infection at conception and during early pregnancy presents the highest risk for fetal infection and associated damage.

29.3.2.2 Recurrent Infections

Recurrent infections, resulting from either reactivation of endogenous CMV or reinfection with a different strain, are almost universally asymptomatic. These infections predominantly occur in CMV-seropositive pregnant women during the second and third trimesters. However they might result in a spontaneous abortion (Fig. 29.2). A 5-year follow-up study found late sequelae in 8% of congenitally CMV-infected children who appeared asymptomatic at birth, with observed complications including unilateral hearing loss (5%), chorioretinitis (2%), and microcephaly (2%).

The incidence of congenital infection in neonates born to seropositive pregnant women is approximately 1%. Congenital damage, either at birth or subsequently, is uncommon, affecting fewer than 1% of these cases.

29.4 Clinical Manifestations

29.4.1 Gynecology

Following infection, the viremic phase ensues after CMV enters the body through mucous membranes of the respiratory and genital tracts, leading to local replication. The initial infection is often unnoticed during childhood. Even among adolescents, most infections remain asymptomatic or present with nonspecific symptoms such as malaise, fatigue, fever, and lymphadenopathy. Rarely, mononucleosis-like illness, pneumonia, hepatitis, meningoencephalitis, hemolytic anemia, colitis, esophagopharyngitis, retinitis, myocarditis, and even Guillain–Barré syndrome may manifest (Table 29.1).

Table 29.1 Symptoms associated with cytomegalovirus infection

Symptoms		Comments
General	CMV mononucleosis	– CMV mononucleosis and EBV mononucleosis present with a similar clinical picture
		– The clinical manifestation of a primary CMV infection in an immunocompetent patient
		– It is relatively uncommon, occurring at any age, including in older patients following blood transfusions and in young adults following sexual contact
		– The patient may present with a gradual increase in body temperature (up to 40 °C), accompanied by fatigue, discomfort in the extremities, pharyngitis, and enlargement of the cervical lymph nodes
		– Rare complications include pneumonia, pleurisy, myocarditis, arthritis, and encephalitis
		– The disease typically resolves within 2–6 weeks, although residual fatigue may persist for several months
Eyes	CMV retinitis	– The eye is painless and not reddened
		– Visual disturbances, including blurred vision and flashes of light
		– Visual field defects
		– Visual acuity is diminished, and vision is blurred and hazy (also known as "misty vision")
Respiratory symptoms	CMV pneumonia	– Dyspnea
		– A dry, irritating cough is also a common symptom
		– Radiological evidence of interstitial infiltrates throughout the lungs was observed
Gastrointestinal symptoms	CMV esophagitis	– Presents as difficulty swallowing
		– Additionally, the patient reported a sensation of retrosternal burning
		– Additionally, ulcerations may be observed
		– Submucosal bleeding
	CMV enterocolitis	– Characterized by fever
		– Patients may experience weight loss
		– Diarrhea may be observed
		– Cramps are also a potential symptom

(continued)

Table 29.1 (continued)

Symptoms		Comments
Neurological symptoms	CMV encephalitis	– Diffuse central nervous system (CNS) symptoms
		– Apathy
		– Decreased motivation
		– Additionally, the patient presented with cephalalgia
		– Additionally, there is a notable slowing of psychomotor function
		– Epileptic seizures
		– Additionally, memory and concentration disorders may manifest
	CMV polyradiculitis	– Urinary retention
		– Difficulty with defecation
		– Saddle anesthesia
		– Additionally, there may be motor deficits
		– Sensory disturbances
		– Additionally, the patient's partner may experience erectile dysfunction.
		– Rapid onset of disorders affecting the emptying of the legs and bladder
	Mononeuritis multiplex	– Sensory disturbances
		– The majority of cases present with a predominantly unilateral paresis
		– Isolated paresis of the arm or leg
		– The symptoms exhibited a rapid progression
		– The onset of symptoms typically occurs within a single day

In immunocompetent individuals, reactivated CMV infections are almost always asymptomatic. In contrast, in immunocompromised individuals, both primary and recurrent infections can manifest with severe and potentially life-threatening clinical courses.

29.4.2 Pregnancy

While cytomegalovirus can be transmitted sexually, the majority of maternal CMV infections arise from close contact with young children—either in the household or in childcare settings—where asymptomatic viral shedding in saliva and urine is common. Occupational exposures among daycare workers and pediatric healthcare personnel similarly increase risk. In the United States, modeling studies estimate that every 2 years between 31,000 and 168,000 CMV-susceptible pregnant women acquire infection from an infected child.

Approximately 90% of maternal primary infections are asymptomatic or present with nonspecific symptoms such as low-grade fever, malaise, or mild lymphadenopathy, making clinical recognition difficult. Although definitive data on CMV-associated miscarriage and intrauterine fetal demise are lacking, there is clear evidence of an elevated risk of preterm delivery in women with primary CMV infection.

Once maternal viremia occurs, transplacental transmission to the fetus can take place at any point during the remainder of the pregnancy. The likelihood of fetal infection correlates with gestational timing of maternal seroconversion—highest in first-trimester infections—and with maternal viral load. Continuous placental exposure to virus during maternal viremia underlies the risk of congenital infection, which may lead to a spectrum of neonatal sequelae ranging from asymptomatic seroconversion to severe multisystem disease.

Primary maternal infection at conception and early pregnancy poses the highest risk of fetal infection and congenital damage.

In instances of primary maternal infection, intrauterine infection is likely attributed to maternal viremia. If the chorion becomes infected, the virus may disseminate to the fetus via amniotic fluid. However, other transmission routes remain feasible (e.g., direct infection from reactivated focal infections in the endometrium, fallopian tubes, or spermatozoa, as well as ascending infection from the vagina prior to and especially after the rupture of membranes). Fetal infection can occur despite low viremia and the presence of maternal IgG antibodies, even in cases of recurrent maternal infection. Neonates infected prenatally with CMV shed the virus in urine and the pharynx at birth, with urinary viral shedding often persisting for several

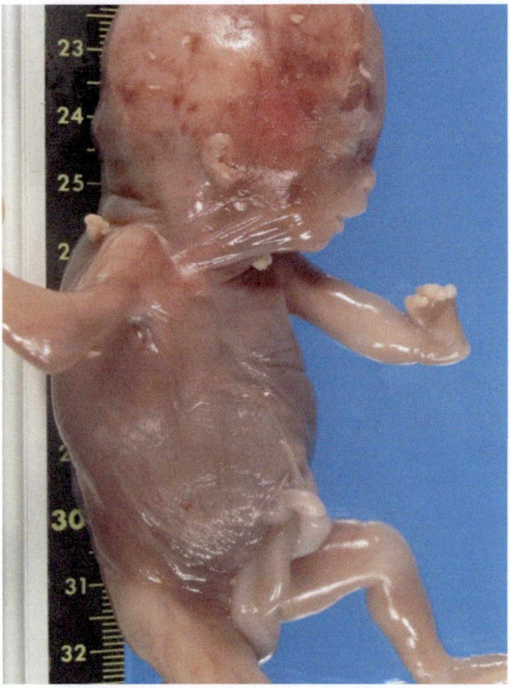

Fig. 29.3 Spontaneous abortion at 16 weeks of gestation due to fetal cytomegalovirus infection (Kost et al. 2007)

years. Primary maternal infection during the first to early third trimester carries the highest risk for fetal damage (Fig. 29.3).

Primary maternal infection during the first to early third trimester of pregnancy carries the highest risk for congenital defects and long-term complications. Recurrent infections may result in fetal infection but seldom lead to congenital anomalies. However, in approximately 5–8% of cases, long-term damage, particularly in the form of auditory impairment, is anticipated.

29.4.3 Concerns Regarding CMV Infection and Pregnancy

- **Risk of Fetal Transmission**: Primary CMV infection during pregnancy poses the greatest risk of fetal transmission, estimated at approximately 30%. Periconceptional primary CMV infection (acquired around the time of conception) presents a lower risk, ranging from 5–16%, with the likelihood diminishing over time.
- **Maternal–Fetal Transmission Rates**: Data from 17 studies indicate variable maternal-fetal transmission rates: 5.5% for infection during the "periconceptional period" (defined as the 3 months preceding the last menstrual period), 21% during the "periconceptional period" (ranging from 4 weeks before to 6 weeks after the last menstrual period), 36.5% in the first trimester, 40.3% in the second trimester, and 66% in the third trimester.
- **CMV Reactivation**: The potential for CMV reactivation is a significant concern, indicating that "zero risk" of intrauterine transmission is never achievable, regardless of the time elapsed since the primary CMV infection.
- **Transmission Throughout Pregnancy**: CMV can be transmitted at any point during gestation, creating a continuous risk for the fetus.
- **Neurological Sequelae**: The risk of severe neurological sequelae is greater when primary infection occurs in the first trimester. Conversely, fetal infection occurring later in pregnancy is unlikely to result in significant neurological impairments.

29.4.4 Neonatology

Perinatal CMV infection most commonly occurs when a neonate is exposed to virus-laden secretions during passage through the birth canal. Early postnatal infection is predominantly acquired via breast milk from CMV seropositive mothers. Following exposure, the incubation period ranges from 4 to 12 weeks, after which CMV may be shed in the infant's saliva and urine.

Among infants infected in utero, approximately 10% are symptomatic at birth. Roughly half of these—about 5% of all congenitally infected neonates—exhibit the classic triad of congenital CMV disease (jaundice, petechiae, and

Table 29.2 Symptoms of congenital CMV infection

Category	Symptoms
Asymptomatic CMV infection	No overt abnormalities
	Normal hearing
Asymptomatic CMV infection with hearing loss	No overt abnormalities except: Sensorineural hearing loss (≥21 dB)
Mildly symptomatic CMV disease	Isolated signs may include
	– Mild hepatomegaly
	– Low platelet count
	– Elevated liver enzymes
Moderately to severely symptomatic CMV disease	Symptoms may include
	– Abnormal cerebrospinal fluid (CSF) values
	– Chorioretinitis
	– Hepatitis (elevated transaminases or bilirubin)
	– Hepatomegaly and splenomegaly
	– Intrauterine growth restriction
	– Presence of CMV DNA in the cerebrospinal fluid
	– Sensorineural hearing loss
	– Thrombocytopenia and petechiae
	– Central nervous system involvement, including microcephaly and radiological abnormalities

Table 29.3 Clinical manifestations in newborns with symptomatic congenital CMV infection

	Clinical finding	Frequency among survivors (%)
General	Prematurity (<38 weeks' gestation)	30–50
	Low birth weight (SGA or LBW)	40–60
	Petechiae/cutaneous rash	30–50
Hematologic	Thrombocytopenia	30–50
Hepatobiliary	Hepatomegaly and/or splenomegaly	40–60
	Jaundice/clinical icterus	30–50
Respiratory	Pneumonitis/pneumonia	20–40
Central nervous system	Microcephaly	30–50
	Intracranial calcifications	30–50
	Neurological abnormalities	30–90
	Lethargy/poor feeding/weak suck	30–50
	Seizures/convulsions	20–40
Sensory	Sensorineural hearing loss	40–58
	Chorioretinitis/posterior segment disease	20–30

hepatosplenomegaly) or other manifestations, such as microcephaly, intracranial calcifications, or chorioretinitis (Table 29.2). In this symptomatic subgroup, 12–30% will go on to develop severe late sequelae, including sensorineural hearing loss, visual impairment, intellectual disability, and other neurological deficits (Table 29.3).

Even infants who appear asymptomatic at birth are at risk: 8–15% will manifest delayed complications—most commonly hearing loss—during the first 2–3 years of life (Table 29.4). By contrast, term neonates acquiring CMV perinatally or postnatally seldom display overt acute illness or long-term sequelae. Symptomatic early postnatal disease—characterized by a sepsis-like syndrome with thrombocytopenia,

Table 29.4 Late manifestations in infants with congenital CMV infection regardless of initial symptoms

Type of late manifestation	Frequency of symptomatic children at birth (%)	Frequency at birth of asymptomatic children (%)
Hearing loss (up to 6 months)	40–58	8–15
Bilateral hearing loss	30–50	5–10
Speech disorders	30–70	5–10
Chorioretinitis (with/without optic atrophy)	20–30	1–2
Visual disturbances	20–30	1–2
IQ < 70	30–70	5–10
Microcephaly (with convulsions and paresis)	30–90	8–15

CMV cytomegalovirus, *IQ* intelligence quotient

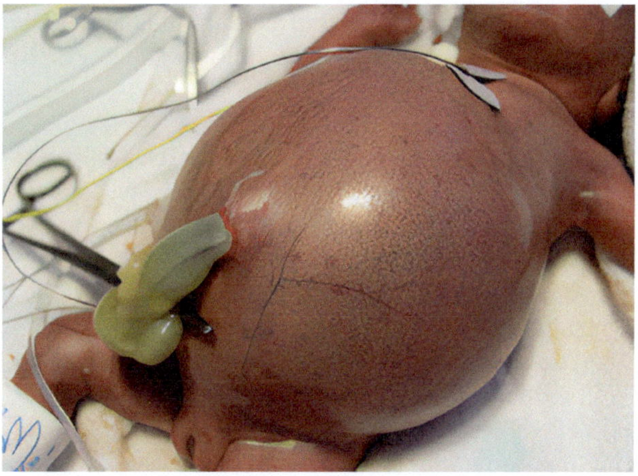

Fig. 29.4 Clinical presentation of a premature infant with prepartum-acquired cytomegalovirus infection and maternal preconception seropositivity (Wintergerst et al. 2006)

hepatosplenomegaly, and respiratory compromise—is rare and occurs almost exclusively in very low-birth-weight, preterm infants (Fig. 29.4), reflecting infection transmitted via breast milk. Continuous audiological monitoring and neurodevelopmental assessment are therefore recommended for all infants with confirmed congenital CMV infection, regardless of initial symptom status.

29.4.5 Concerns in Neonates with Symptomatic CMV Infection

- **Premature Mortality**: A significant concern is the elevated mortality rate within the first three months of life, affecting 5–10% of symptomatic newborns. This highlights the severe ramifications of intrauterine CMV infection and underscores the importance of early diagnosis and timely intervention.
- **Neurological Complications**: Neurological issues are common among affected children. Microcephaly, characterized by abnormally small head size and

associated brain malformations, occurs in 35–50% of cases, often correlating with delayed cognitive development and intellectual impairments. Furthermore, approximately 20-40% of these children may experience seizures or epilepsy, necessitating ongoing medication and close monitoring.

- **Chorioretinitis**: This eye condition affects 20–30% of newborns and can lead to partial or complete blindness if not promptly diagnosed and treated.
- **Developmental Delays**: Up to 70% of children with congenital CMV infection exhibit developmental delays in areas such as motor skills, language, and cognition. These impairments may become evident or worsen over time, necessitating regular monitoring and early intervention.
- **Sensorineural Hearing Loss (SNHL)**: Among the most common and severe complications, SNHL affects 25–50% of symptomatic infants. Alarmingly, this hearing loss worsens in approximately half of these cases within the first 2 years of life, potentially leading to progressive hearing loss or deafness. Early screening and appropriate use of hearing aids are essential to support language and cognitive development and to mitigate long-term detrimental effects.

29.4.6 Concerns for Newborns with Asymptomatic CMV Infection

- **Sensorineural Hearing Loss (SNHL)**: A primary concern is the potential development of SNHL. Approximately 10% of asymptomatic newborns are diagnosed with hearing loss at birth. In contrast, the risk in infants with symptomatic congenital CMV infection is significantly higher, ranging from 30% to 50%. These statistics highlight the need for diligent monitoring of hearing development, even in asymptomatic newborns.
- **Neurodevelopmental Monitoring**: While initial studies suggest that the cognitive and motor skills of asymptomatic CMV-infected newborns may be comparable to those of healthy controls, reports indicate that neurological problems may manifest later in life. Continuous neurodevelopmental assessments are critical for identifying and addressing any delayed symptoms or complications.
- **Chorioretinitis**: This inflammation of the choroid and retina occurs in approximately 2% of asymptomatic newborns. Despite its relatively low incidence, chorioretinitis requires vigilant monitoring, as it can result in visual impairment or blindness if not promptly detected and treated.
- **Long-Term Developmental Outcomes**: Generally, normal development by 12 months of age correlates with a higher likelihood of maintaining normal development in the long term. However, the emergence of developmental abnormalities after the second year of life is atypical and should prompt detailed investigation.
- **Vestibular Dysfunction**: Recent findings suggest potential vestibular dysfunction, or impaired balance, in asymptomatic CMV-infected children. This issue

may adversely affect motor development and necessitates increased attention. Effective measures include raising awareness of vestibular dysfunction, conducting targeted testing, and referring children for early physiotherapy when necessary. These steps can aid in identifying and managing potential motor development delays or impairments promptly.

Overall, it is imperative to closely monitor asymptomatic newborns with congenital CMV infection and to intervene at the first sign of developmental abnormalities. Early detection and treatment of potential complications are essential for minimizing long-term consequences for affected children.

29.5 Diagnosis

29.5.1 Laboratory Diagnosis

Antibody determinations are performed to clarify immune status or to establish the presence of an acute or recurrent infection. Both virus and antibody detection are employed in prenatal and pediatric diagnostics. The virus can be detected in various biological specimens, including urine, saliva, throat secretions, cervical secretions, amniotic fluid, fetal blood, ascites, chorionic villi, tissue biopsies, and breast milk. Possible diagnostic methods include:

- **Isolation in Cell Culture**: Traditional cell culture involves isolating CMV from clinical specimens using cell culture techniques. While it can be effective, it often takes considerable time, typically up to 16 days, to yield results [2].
- **Early Antigen Detection Following Rapid Cultivation**: Early antigen fluorescent foci (DEAFF) is a method used to quickly detect CMV in fibroblasts cultured from clinical specimens. This technique uses a pool of monoclonal antibodies against CMV early antigens and can provide results within 24 hours, making it significantly faster than traditional cell culture methods.
- **Direct Detection of pp65 Antigen in Blood**: The CMV pp65 antigenemia assay involves direct erythrocyte lysis followed by indirect immunofluorescence staining. This method allows for the rapid detection of CMV antigens in blood samples.
- **Nucleic Acid Detection via Real-Time PCR**: This method involves the extraction and amplification of CMV DNA using real-time polymerase chain reaction (PCR). It is highly sensitive and specific, allowing for the detection and quantification of CMV DNA in plasma. This method is used to determine the need for antiviral therapy, diagnose active CMV disease, and monitor the response to treatment.

29.5.2 Diagnosis During Pregnancy

Primary CMV infection is often undiagnosed due to its typically uncharacteristic symptoms or subclinical presentation. However, in pregnant individuals, laboratory tests for CMV are increasingly performed as a rule-out diagnosis when symptoms are present.

Prenatal diagnosis is routinely performed in both asymptomatic and symptomatic pregnant individuals with abnormal serologic findings (particularly borderline to positive IgM results) or abnormal ultrasound findings while having unremarkable CMV serology.

Serologic differentiation between primary and recurrent infections during pregnancy is essential due to the increased risk of fetal harm associated with primary infection compared to recurrent infection (Table 29.5). The following considerations are important:

- **Negative IgG Result**: If the IgG result is negative, the pregnant individual should be advised on methods to reduce the risk of infection.
- **Positive IgG and Negative IgM Results**: If the IgG result is positive and the IgM result is negative, it is unlikely that the infant will be congenitally affected, and reassurance can be provided to the pregnant patient.
- **Positive IgG and IgM Results**: If both IgG and IgM results are positive, further testing is required to differentiate between primary and reactivated infection. Should these results be abnormal, prenatal diagnosis must be conducted to rule out fetal infection (Fig. 29.5).

Table 29.5 CMV serology in pregnancy (primary testing)

CMV IgG	CMV IgM	IgG avidity	Rating
-	–	–	– No infection
-	+	–	– Questionable infection – False-positive CMV IgM possible – Repeat the test in 10–14 days
+	+	High	– Before 16 weeks' gestation: CMV latency, CMV recurrence – After 16 weeks' gestation: CMV primary infection possible (periconceptional or early pregnancy)
+	–	High	– Before 16 weeks' gestation: CMV latency – After 16 weeks' gestation: CMV latency, CMV primary infection possible (periconceptional or early pregnancy)
+	+/–	Intermediate	– No statement possible, possibly retesting (in 14 days)
+	+	Low	– CMV primary infection, additional examination may be necessary, clarification of a possible fetal infection

Positive viral detection from urine or cervical smears has limited utility as a diagnostic tool for differentiating between primary and recurrent maternal infections.

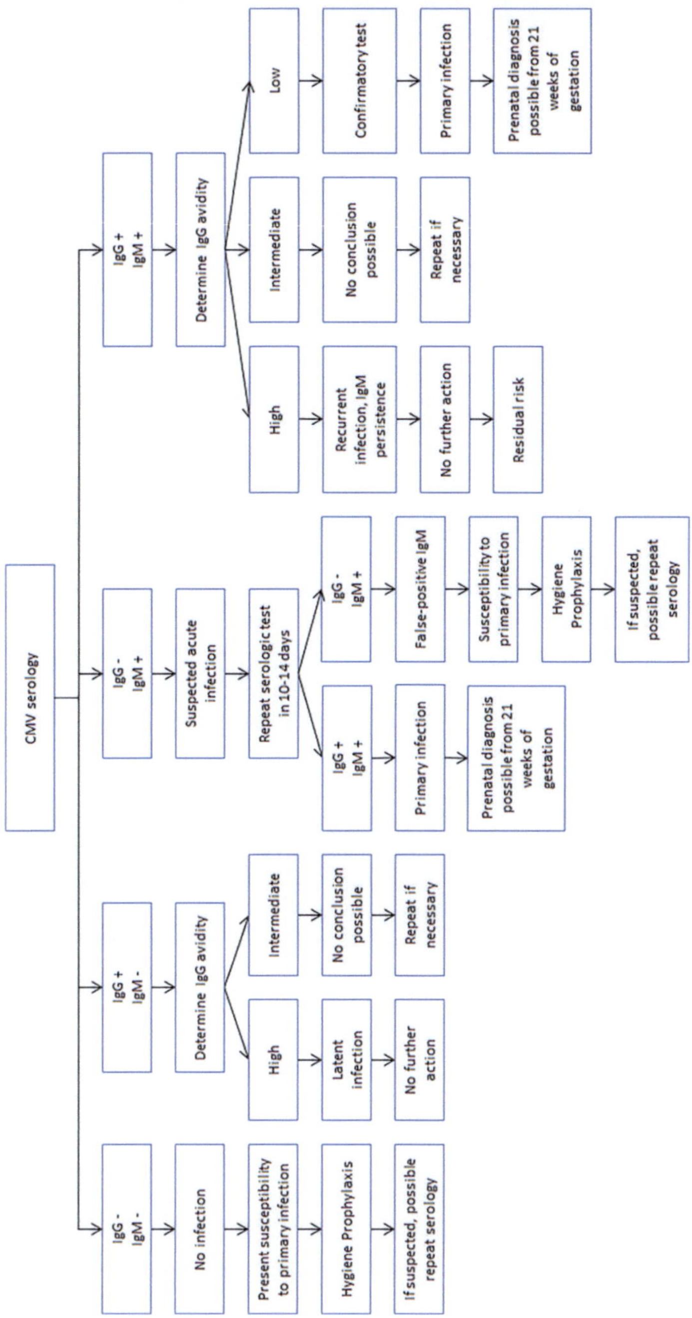

Fig. 29.5 Cytomegalovirus serology for diagnostic purposes during pregnancy. (Courtesy of I. Mylonas)

29.5.3 Prenatal Diagnosis

Chorionic villi and amniotic fluid are both viable fetal specimens for evaluation during early pregnancy (11–19 weeks of gestation), while fetal EDTA blood and amniotic fluid are utilized in late pregnancy (≥22 weeks of gestation). The overall sensitivity of prenatal diagnosis is approximately 80%, while specificity reaches 100% when amniocentesis is performed before 21 weeks gestation and after a 7-week interval following the diagnosis of maternal infection.

29.5.3.1 Fetal (In Utero) Testing

Timely and appropriately timed molecular testing of fetal specimens is essential for accurate prenatal diagnosis of congenital CMV infection:

- Enhanced Sensitivity: Diagnostic sensitivity increases markedly when fetal sampling occurs at least 6 weeks after confirmed maternal primary infection, allowing sufficient time for viral replication and shedding into amniotic fluid.
- Amniocentesis Timing: Performing amniocentesis between 18 and 21 weeks' gestation—and only after a minimum 6-week interval from maternal seroconversion—yields PCR sensitivity of 85–95% and specificity approaching 100%. False-negative PCRs under these conditions are exceedingly rare, and subsequent positive conversions have not been linked to significant neonatal sequelae.
- Recommendation for Prenatal Testing: Targeted prenatal CMV testing is advised for all women with documented primary infection, especially when seroconversion occurs before 20 weeks' gestation.
- Optimal Diagnostic Strategy: A dual approach combining high-resolution fetal ultrasound (for detection of ventriculomegaly, calcifications, growth restriction, and fluid collections) with amniotic fluid PCR provides the most comprehensive assessment of fetal infection and potential disease burden.
- Interpreting Positive Results: A positive CMV PCR confirms in utero infection but does not correlate reliably with the severity or spectrum of fetal organ involvement; therefore, positive findings should prompt serial imaging and multidisciplinary counseling rather than definitive prognostication.
- Role of Quantitative PCR: While quantitative viral load in amniotic fluid or fetal blood is investigational, current evidence does not support its use as a standalone predictor of clinical outcome or disease severity.

However, abnormal ultrasound findings paired with a positive CMV IgM antibody result are critical for making informed decisions about the continuation or termination of pregnancy (Figs. 29.6 and 29.7).

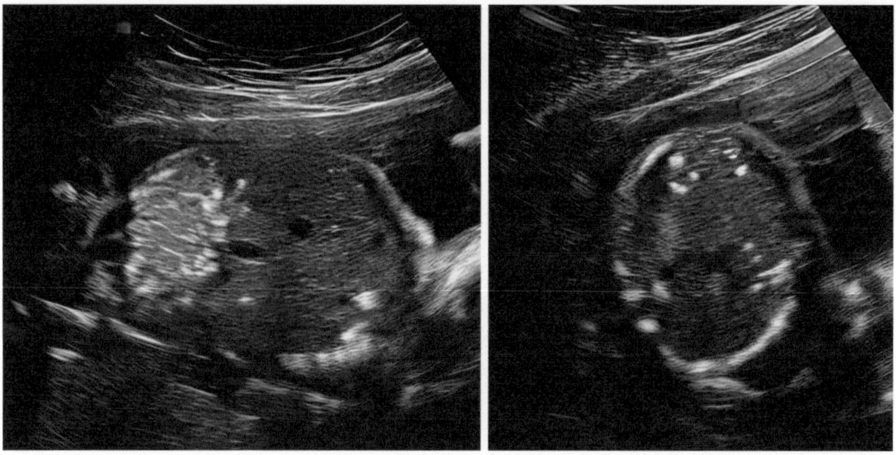

Fig. 29.6 Characteristic hyperechogenic bowel and hepatic calcifications observed in fetal cytomegalovirus infection (Kagan et al. 2011)

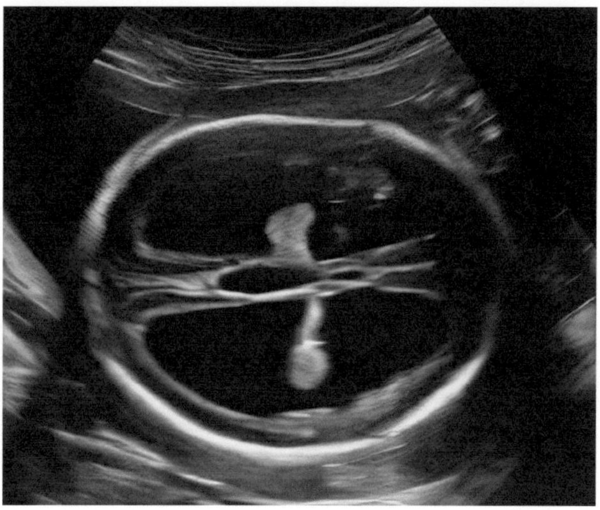

Fig. 29.7 Ventriculomegaly with echogenic rim in fetal cytomegalovirus infection (Kagan et al. 2011)

29.5.3.2 Ultrasound

Ultrasound findings can yield crucial insights into potential congenital CMV infection, facilitating early diagnosis and management. Key ultrasound findings associated with congenital CMV infection include, but are not limited to (alphabetical):

- **Abdominal Calcifications**: Abnormal calcium deposits within the abdomen may indicate underlying pathology associated with CMV infection.
- **Amniotic Fluid Abnormalities**: Oligohydramnios (reduced amniotic fluid) and polyhydramnios (excessive amniotic fluid) can signify complications in fetal health, necessitating further investigation.

- **Ascites**: The accumulation of fluid in the peritoneal cavity may indicate intrauterine infection, including CMV.
- **Cerebral Ventriculomegaly**: Enlargement of the brain's ventricular system may suggest increased intracranial pressure or underlying abnormalities resulting from CMV infection.
- **Hepatomegaly**: Ultrasound may reveal an enlarged liver, which could indicate fetal infection or other hepatic conditions.
- **Hydrops Fetalis**: This severe condition is characterized by the accumulation of fluid in multiple fetal compartments (e.g., skin, abdomen, and around the heart and lungs). Hydrops fetalis poses a high risk of morbidity and mortality.
- **Hyperechogenic Bowel**: Increased echogenicity observed in the fetal bowel may suggest several conditions, including CMV infection.
- **Intracranial Calcifications**: Calcium deposits in the fetal brain serve as a hallmark sign of congenital CMV infection and may correlate with neurological impairment and developmental delays.
- **Intrauterine Growth Restriction (IUGR)**: Delayed or restricted fetal growth can result from congenital infections, including CMV, warranting close monitoring and potential intervention.
- **Microcephaly**: A condition where the fetal head circumference is significantly smaller than expected, often associated with developmental issues and neurological damage due to CMV.
- **Pleural or Pericardial Effusion**: The presence of fluid in pleural (around the lungs) or pericardial (around the heart) cavities may indicate widespread infection and inflammation.
- **Pseudomeconium Ileus**: The appearance of meconium-like material within the bowel, noted on ultrasound, may suggest intestinal obstruction or other gastrointestinal abnormalities.

The presence of these ultrasound signs cannot always be regarded as predictors of the extent of fetal damage. While the sensitivity of fetal ultrasound remains challenging to assess, it is likely around 30-50% for identifying symptomatic congenitally infected infants.

29.5.4 Pediatric Diagnostics

In neonates born to mothers with documented CMV infection during pregnancy, as well as in infants with clinical signs suggestive of CMV—regardless of maternal serostatus—comprehensive virological testing within the first 14 days of life is essential to confirm congenital infection. Such testing should include viral culture or PCR of urine, saliva, or throat swabs, supplemented by CMV-specific serology.

Detection of CMV DNA or replication in these specimens before day 14 provides definitive evidence of in utero transmission, whereas IgM serology alone may miss up to one-third of symptomatic infants, particularly when maternal infection occurs late in gestation.

By contrast, maternal and neonatal IgG titers at birth largely reflect passive antibody transfer and cannot distinguish congenital from perinatal or postnatal acquisition. If virological assays are delayed beyond 3–4 weeks of age, distinguishing congenital infection from postnatal acquisition becomes untenable in otherwise asymptomatic infants. In that scenario, persistent CMV-specific IgG beyond 8–10 weeks of age—measured by enzyme immunoassay or immunofluorescence—is required to document established infection.

All infants with confirmed CMV infection warrant long-term follow-up, with particular attention to neurodevelopmental milestones, auditory function, and growth. Universal or targeted newborn hearing screening should be performed soon after diagnosis, given the high risk of delayed-onset sensorineural hearing loss in congenitally infected children. In infants receiving antiviral therapy—most commonly intravenous ganciclovir or oral valganciclovir—quantitative PCR of CMV DNA in peripheral blood leukocytes can guide treatment response and inform duration of therapy. Regular monitoring of hematological and renal parameters is also indicated to detect potential drug toxicity.

29.6 Treatment

Multiple antiviral agents with distinct mechanisms of action are currently available for the treatment of cytomegalovirus infections, allowing for targeted and resistance-adaptive therapeutic strategies (Table 29.6).

First-Line Therapy

- **Ganciclovir**, an acyclic nucleoside analog (DHPG = dihydroxypropoxymethylguanine), and its orally bioavailable prodrug **Valganciclovir** constitute the cornerstone of CMV therapy. Ganciclovir penetrates the cerebrospinal fluid and inhibits viral DNA polymerase following intracellular phosphorylation by the viral UL97 kinase. Intravenous administration is preferred in cases of severe CMV disease, whereas Valganciclovir is typically used for mild infections or maintenance therapy.
- **Letermovir** represents a significant prophylactic alternative, particularly in hematopoietic stem cell transplant recipients. As a terminase complex inhibitor, Letermovir exhibits a unique mechanism of action without cross-resistance to other CMV antivirals and does not induce myelosuppression. Randomized controlled trials have demonstrated non-inferiority of Letermovir compared to Valganciclovir for prophylaxis in high-risk kidney transplant patients.

Table 29.6 Management strategies for cytomegalovirus infection. IV = intravenously

Condition	Strategy type	Medication	Dosage	Duration
Congenital infection	First-line	Ganciclovir	5 mg/kg IV twice daily	3–6 weeks (extend if needed)
	Alternative	Valganciclovir	16 mg/kg orally twice daily	6 weeks to 6 months
	Second-line	Foscarnet	60 mg/kg IV every 8 h	3 weeks
	Alternative	Cidofovir	5 mg/kg IV every 7 days	2–3 doses
Transplant recipients	Prophylaxis	Letermovir	480 mg orally once daily	Up to 100 days post-transplant
	Prophylaxis	Valganciclovir	900 mg orally once daily	3–6 months
	Pre-emptive Therapy	Ganciclovir/ valganciclovir	5 mg/kg IV twice daily/900 mg orally twice daily	Until viral clearance plus 1–2 weeks
Resistant CMV infection	Second-line	Foscarnet	60 mg/kg IV every 8–12 h	Until viral clearance
	Alternative	Cidofovir	5 mg/kg IV every 7–14 days	2–3 doses
	Alternative	Maribavir	400 mg orally twice daily	Until viral clearance
Adjunct therapy	Adjunct	CMV Hyperimmune Globulin	100 mg/kg IV every 2 weeks (typical dosing range: 50–150 mg/kg)	Variable; often for severe or refractory cases
	Investigational	Adoptive T-cell therapy	Ex vivo expanded CMV-specific T cells	Refractory or resistant cases
Uveitis, retinitis	First-line	Ganciclovir/ valganciclovir	5 mg/kg IV twice daily/900 mg orally twice daily	3–6 weeks (extend if needed)/6 weeks to 6 months
	Second-line	Foscarnet	60 mg/kg IV every 8–12 h	3 weeks
	Alternative	Cidofovir	5 mg/kg IV every 7–14 days	2–3 doses
CMV pneumonia	First-line	Ganciclovir/ valganciclovir	5 mg/kg IV twice daily/900 mg orally twice daily	2–3 weeks; extend if needed
	Adjunct	CMV Hyperimmune Globulin	100 mg/kg IV every 2 weeks (typical dosing range: 50–150 mg/kg)	Severe or life-threatening cases

(continued)

Table 29.6 (continued)

Condition	Strategy type	Medication	Dosage	Duration
Suppression/ maintenance		Valganciclovir	900 mg orally once daily	After initial therapy
		Ganciclovir	5 mg/kg IV once daily	After initial therapy

Notes:
- Adoptive T-cell Therapy: Experimental; involves infusion of CMV-specific T cells expanded ex vivo
- Cidofovir: Given weekly or biweekly depending on indication, with probenecid and hydration to reduce toxicity
- CMV Hyperimmune Globulin: Typical dose ranges from 50 to 150 mg/kg every 2 weeks; dosing individualized per protocol
- Foscarnet: Reserved for resistant cases due to nephrotoxicity risk; dosing interval varies by clinical protocol
- Ganciclovir: IV dosing commonly at 5 mg/kg twice daily for induction; maintenance dosing may be once daily
- Letermovir: Recommended for primary prophylaxis in allogeneic hematopoietic stem cell transplant (HSCT) recipients and is being studied in solid organ transplant (SOT) patients
- Maribavir: Oral agent for resistant CMV infections; recent approval expands options in refractory cases
- Valganciclovir: Oral prodrug of ganciclovir; dosing adjusted by weight and renal function

Second-Line Therapy in Case of Resistance

Resistance to Ganciclovir, primarily due to mutations in the UL97 kinase or UL54 DNA polymerase genes, necessitates alternative treatments:

- **Foscarnet**, a pyrophosphate analog, directly inhibits viral DNA polymerase and remains effective against UL97 mutant strains. The standard dosing regimen is 90 mg/kg intravenously every 12 h. However, nephrotoxicity and electrolyte disturbances limit its clinical use.
- **Maribavir**, a benzimidazole riboside, inhibits UL97 kinase through an alternative mechanism and shows efficacy against ganciclovir-resistant CMV strains. Phase III clinical trials have demonstrated superior efficacy and improved tolerability of Maribavir compared with investigator-selected therapies in refractory or resistant CMV infections.
- **Cidofovir**, a nucleotide analog, is reserved for multidrug-resistant CMV strains but is associated with significant nephrotoxicity. Its administration requires concomitant intravenous hydration and probenecid to mitigate renal toxicity. In a cohort study, nephrotoxicity occurred in over one-third of patients, and a quarter developed uveitis.

Adjuvant Immunotherapy

- **CMV hyperimmune globulin (CMV-HIG)** is frequently administered alongside antiviral agents in immunocompromised patients. CMV-HIG contains high titers (≥100 U/mL) of CMV-specific antibodies that neutralize the virus by binding to surface antigens. Meta-analyses provide moderate evidence supporting its benefit in preventing severe CMV disease among solid organ transplant recipients. Notably, some studies have reported that standard intravenous immunoglobulin (IVIG) preparations may exhibit higher CMV-neutralizing activity than specific CMV-HIG products, highlighting the role of the IgG3 subclass in CMV neutralization.

- **Adoptive T-Cell Therapy Against CMV:** Adoptive T-cell therapy (ATCT) represents a promising immunotherapeutic approach for the treatment and prevention of cytomegalovirus (CMV) reactivations in severely immunocompromised patients. By the targeted infusion of CMV-specific T lymphocytes, durable antiviral immune surveillance can be established, thereby circumventing antiviral resistance and the toxicities associated with conventional antiviral agents.

Therapy During Pregnancy

Antiviral treatment during pregnancy requires careful consideration due to potential teratogenicity:

- **Ganciclovir is not recommended for pregnant women with acute primary CMV infection** because the teratogenic risk outweighs unproven maternal benefit; controlled safety data are lacking.
- **Valaciclovir** at high doses (8 g daily) has shown promising results in reducing maternofetal transmission in confirmed maternal primary infection. A randomized controlled trial demonstrated a 71% reduction in fetal infection rates (11% versus 30% in placebo). Current guidelines recommend antiviral therapy during pregnancy only within clinical trial settings (see Sect. 29.8.5.).
- **Intrauterine ganciclovir therapy** for fetuses with confirmed CMV infection remains controversial due to unpredictable developmental risks and absence of long-term safety data. Experimental approaches involving fetal valaciclovir after amniocentesis-confirmed infection are reserved for high-risk cases and require multidisciplinary expertise.
- **Cytomegalovirus hyperimmune globulin (CMV-HIG)** is an intravenous preparation of pooled human immunoglobulin enriched with high titers of CMV-specific antibodies, primarily used as adjunctive therapy or prophylaxis in high-risk populations such as seronegative solid organ transplant recipients of seropositive donors and hematopoietic stem cell transplant patients. In these groups, CMV-HIG reduces peak viral loads and the incidence or severity of CMV disease when combined with antiviral agents like ganciclovir or valganciclovir. It may also be considered in select pregnant women with primary CMV infection, although routine use outside clinical trials is not widely recommended due to limited evidence. The therapeutic effect of CMV-HIG is mediated through neutralization of circulating virions by binding to viral surface antigens, thereby preventing cellular entry and by enhancing immune clearance mechanisms, such as antibody-dependent cellular cytotoxicity and opsonization.

Currently, treatment with ganciclovir is not recommended for pregnant women with acute primary CMV infection, and intrauterine therapy with ganciclovir presents difficulties in fetuses infected with CMV.

29.7 Differential Diagnosis

In nonpregnant individuals, the differential diagnosis of suspected CMV infection includes other viral infections (e.g., Epstein–Barr virus, hepatitis viruses, HIV), bacterial infections (e.g., mononucleosis, sepsis), autoimmune diseases, and malignancies. In pregnant women, considerations for differential diagnoses extend to other viral infections (e.g., rubella, varicella, parvovirus B19, herpes simplex virus), toxoplasmosis, listeriosis, syphilis, and other etiologies of fetal abnormalities, including chromosomal abnormalities, malformations, or growth retardation.

Accurate laboratory diagnosis is important to distinguish CMV infection from other conditions and to initiate appropriate treatment when indicated.

29.8 Prevention

Exposure prophylaxis for CMV remains complex due to its multiple transmission routes and the often asymptomatic nature of the infection. Although CMV screening during pregnancy has been recommended, the practicality and effectiveness of such screening continue to be debated (Table 29.7).

29.8.1 Recommendations for Seronegative Women

- **Informed Awareness**: Seronegative women should be educated regarding primary sources of CMV infection, including sexual intercourse, close contact with young children (particularly those in daycare), and occupational exposure to

Table 29.7 Preventive hygiene measures against CMV transmission

Category	Recommendations/Guidelines
Hand hygiene	– Wash hands thoroughly with warm water and soap
Personal care	– Ensure proper hygiene during diaper changes and when assisting with toileting
	– Maintain cleanliness while feeding
	– Wipe away runny noses, tears, or saliva promptly
	– Handle saliva-contaminated objects (toys, pacifiers, etc.) with care
Avoid shared items	– Do not share eating and drinking vessels
	– Avoid sharing toothbrushes, washcloths, or towels
Personal contact	– Refrain from mouth-to-mouth kisses
	– Avoid touching your mouth, nose, or eyes with unwashed hands
Day care centers	– Clean toys frequently with water, soap, and a brush or disinfect them regularly
	– Wear disposable gloves when changing diapers
	– Pregnant seronegative caregivers should not care for small children (see legal requirements)

children who shed the virus. They should be made aware of the infection risks and advised on preventive behaviors.

29.8.2 Intravenous Immunoglobulin (IVIG) for Passive Immunization

- **Available Products**: Various intravenous immunoglobulin (IVIG) products are available for passive immunization and are primarily used prophylactically in CMV-seronegative individuals prior to blood transfusions and organ transplants. Additionally, these products may be used therapeutically in conjunction with ganciclovir for immunocompromised patients, particularly for premature infants exhibiting CMV symptoms.
- **Consideration for Pregnant Women**: The administration of IVIG to seronegative pregnant women, particularly those with occupational CMV exposure, is under consideration. However, the efficacy of this approach during pregnancy remains inconclusively determined and is the subject of ongoing clinical trials.

Exposure prophylaxis remains challenging due to the transmission characteristics of cytomegalovirus (CMV). However, it is essential to educate seronegative women about the risks of infection and preventive behaviors.

29.8.3 Preventive Measures for CMV Infection in Contact with Infants

Preventive measures for CMV infection are particularly important for pregnant women who have close contact with children in settings such as daycare centers or nursing homes. A variety of measures are recommended (Table 29.7). These simple hygiene practices can reduce the risk of primary CMV infection in pregnant women by 50-85%.

29.8.4 Hyperimmunoglobulin (HIG) as a Preventive Measure Against CMV Infection During Pregnancy

Hyperimmunoglobulin (HIG) is being considered as a preventive approach to reduce the risk of congenital CMV infection during pregnancy. Initial positive results regarding CMV suppression by HIG were observed over 20 years ago in *kidney transplant patients*. Since then, its use in transplantation medicine has been officially approved under clearly defined situations and continues to be successfully employed.

29.8.4.1 Study Results on HIG Efficacy During Pregnancy

- **Variable Efficacy**: The efficacy of HIG during pregnancy varies widely across studies. One randomized controlled trial (RCT) suggested that passive immunization with a CMV-specific hyperimmunoglobulin formulation might reduce the risk of congenital transmission, although the results were not statistically significant. Conversely, an earlier nonrandomized study demonstrated a more pronounced effect of HIG.
- **Associated Risks**: The aforementioned RCT also noted an increased incidence of fetal growth retardation and preterm delivery associated with HIG use.

29.8.4.2 Safety and Outcomes

- **Primary CMV Infection**: HIG administration in pregnant women with primary CMV infection has been shown to be safe and effective. While HIG may not significantly reduce the rate of infection, it appears to be safe and may confer beneficial effects on symptomatic outcomes for infected fetuses.
- **Fetal Outcomes**: For fetuses without ultrasound abnormalities prior to HIG administration, the risk of long-term adverse outcomes remains low. Therefore, HIG is considered a reasonable therapeutic option for fetuses infected with CMV.

In conclusion, while HIG shows promise as a preventive measure against congenital CMV infection, its efficacy varies and associated risks must be carefully weighed. Despite some studies indicating benefits, further research is required to establish standardized guidelines for its use during pregnancy.

29.8.5 Valaciclovir as a Preventive Option for CMV Infection in Pregnancy

29.8.5.1 Potential Benefits

- **Reduction of Primary CMV Infection**: Valaciclovir may lower the incidence of primary CMV infection in seronegative pregnant women, thereby reducing the likelihood of congenital CMV infection in the fetus.
- **Minimizing Risk of Reactivation or Reinfection**: In seropositive pregnant women at heightened risk of CMV reactivation or reinfection, valaciclovir may help lessen the risk of vertical transmission to the fetus.
- **Prophylaxis Against Severe Outcomes**: Prophylactic use of valaciclovir could potentially prevent severe consequences of congenital CMV infection, including hearing loss, neurological damage, and growth retardation in the fetus.

29.8.5.2 Unresolved Questions and Concerns

- **Regulatory Data**: Although acyclovir and valaciclovir are approved for treating and preventing HSV and VZV infections in nonpregnant patients, they lack approval for use during pregnancy to prevent HSV, VZV and CMV infection. Although studies indicate that acyclovir usage during pregnancy is not associated with an increased rate of birth defects, potential benefits must be carefully weighed against potential risks, particularly in cases of maternal toxicity.
- **Pharmacodynamics**: Valaciclovir, with a half-life of approximately 3–4.5 h after oral administration, is rapidly converted to acyclovir by enzymes in the small intestine and liver. Both drugs are primarily excreted through the kidneys, with about 90% excreted unchanged in the urine. Impaired renal function can lead to drug accumulation, raising concerns regarding toxicity.
- **Dosage**: Effective CMV prophylaxis necessitates high dosing of valaciclovir, with recommended doses reaching up to 8 g/day—four to eight times higher than doses utilized for the treatment of herpes simplex (1 g/day) or in transplant patients (2 g/day). To reduce renal stress, a dosing regimen of 2 g four times daily is advised. Extended high-dose treatment appears to increase the risk of toxicity.
- **Side Effects**: High doses of valaciclovir may lead to side effects, including neurological issues and altered kidney function. Instances of kidney failure have also been reported in pregnant women, underscoring the need for vigilant monitoring.
- **Duration of Treatment**: The treatment duration for CMV prophylaxis varies from weeks to months, potentially heightening toxicity risks, especially at elevated doses.
- **Efficacy**: The prophylactic efficacy of valaciclovir against CMV infection remains uncertain. While some studies suggest favorable outcomes, such as reduced CMV transmission to newborns, these studies often lack randomization or control, limiting the reliability of their findings.
- **Use of Valaciclovir**: Valaciclovir, a prodrug of acyclovir, inhibits herpes virus replication by binding to viral DNA and obstructing DNA polymerase. While the precise mechanism of valaciclovir against CMV is not fully understood, acyclovir evidences resistance or minimal effect at higher doses. Valaciclovir is generally reserved for exceptional instances of CMV prophylaxis in transplant patients, given that valganciclovir is more specifically targeted against CMV.

Currently, the routine application of valaciclovir for CMV prophylaxis during pregnancy raises several concerns. However, in certain high-risk situations, prophylaxis may be considered on an individual basis. Additional studies are needed to accurately assess the risks and benefits involved.

29.8.5.3 International Recommendations on Valaciclovir Prophylaxis for Primary CMV Infection During Pregnancy

Overview

Most professional societies in Europe and North America do not recommend routine use of valaciclovir for prophylaxis against primary cytomegalovirus (CMV) infection during pregnancy (Table 29.8). Instead, some organizations—though not the majority—advocate its use only within research protocols or after individualized risk-benefit assessment.

Professional Society Recommendations

- **Restrictive Recommendations (Specialized Centers or Clinical Studies Only):**
  - Germany (AWMF S2k, DGGG/BVF): Oral valaciclovir therapy is not recommended outside research protocols; emphasis placed on prevention and diagnostics.
  - United Kingdom (RCOG): Valaciclovir use for primary CMV infection before 12 weeks of gestation is limited to specialized research centers; no routine recommendation outside controlled studies (Evidence level C).
  - USA (ACOG, SMFM): Valaciclovir should only be used within controlled clinical trials; no off-label recommendation for routine care.
- **Conditional Recommendations (Individual Risk-Benefit Assessment):**
  - Canada (SOGC): Valaciclovir at 8 g/day may be considered until PCR negativity or for up to 6 weeks in documented primary infection as a case-by-case decision (evidence level B based on RCT data).
  - Experimental or Limited Programs:
  - France (CNGOF): No formal therapeutic recommendation; antiviral use limited to pilot and research programs (evidence level C).
  - Italy (SIGO): Valaciclovir treatment only in selected cases or study settings, not as standard therapy.
  - Switzerland (SGGG): Off-label valaciclovir at 8 g/day may be considered after careful individualized assessment 4–6 weeks post-diagnosis (evidence level C).
- **No Recommendation:**
  - The majority of societies restrict valaciclovir use to controlled studies or, more commonly, do not recommend general antiviral prophylaxis.
  - European Union (ISUOG/EFC, EMA): Focus on hygiene and screening guidelines; no broad antiviral prophylaxis or Grade A recommendation for valaciclovir. Early treatment recommended for primary infection by EFC but no widespread valaciclovir use recommended by ISUOG.

Table 29.8 Valaciclovir recommendations for primary CMV infection during pregnancy

Country/ region	Institution (type)	Valaciclovir recommendation for primary CMV infection in pregnancy	Dosage and duration	Evidence grade
Argentina	SADOG (Professional Society)	No antiviral therapy; prevention and hygiene counseling; valaciclovir only in study protocols	–	D (research context)
	Ministerio de Salud de la Nación (State)	No antiviral therapy in official guidelines	–	D (no recommendation)
Australia/ New Zealand	RANZCOG (Professional Society)	No routine screening; focus on education and hygiene	–	D (hygiene measures preferred)
	Department of Health Australia (State)	Local protocols without national coordination	–	D (no national guidelines)
Belgium	BVGOG (Professional Society)	Serology if suspected; antiviral therapy not routinely recommended	–	D (local protocols)
	FÖD Volksgesundheit (State)	Optional CMV screening; valaciclovir generally not recommended		C (local protocols)
Brazil	FEBRASGO (Professional Society)	Individualized approach; therapy only in exceptional cases	–	D (regional differences)
	Ministério da Saúde (State)	No nationwide guideline; regional protocols vary	–	D (no standardization)
Bulgaria	Bulgarian Society of Obstetrics and Gynecology	Education and prevention; valaciclovir only in clinical studies	–	D (research context)
	Ministry of Health Bulgaria (State)	No national CMV guidelines; no therapy recommendation	–	D (no recommendation)
Canada	SOGC (Professional Society)	Valaciclovir may be considered for documented primary infection	8 g/day (2 g × 4), until PCR negativity or 6 weeks	B (RCT, grade B)
	Health Canada (State)	No national recommendation; provincial guidelines apply	–	D (uneven implementation)

(continued)

Table 29.8 (continued)

Country/ region	Institution (type)	Valaciclovir recommendation for primary CMV infection in pregnancy	Dosage and duration	Evidence grade
China	CMA (Professional Society)	Preconception screening; no antiviral therapy during pregnancy	–	D (developmental phase)
	NHC (State)	Treatment guidelines in development; no recommendation	–	D (no recommendation)
Egypt	Egyptian Society of Obstetrics and Gynecology	No standardized CMV screening; focus on education	–	D (prevention focus)
	Ministry of Health and Population (State)	No CMV therapy recommendations; prevention prioritized	–	D (no recommendation)
France	CNGOF (Professional Society)	Early antiviral therapy recommended for primary infection	8 g/day (2 g × 4), until PCR result (4–6 weeks)	C
	Ministère de la Santé (State)	Pilot antiviral therapy programs planned for 2025–2026	8 g/day during pilot; 6 weeks	B (pilot programs planned)
Germany	AWMF S2k-Guideline CMV (Consensus)	Consider valaciclovir for primary infection <14 weeks gestation	8 g/day (2 g × 4), until 20 weeks gestation (max 6 weeks)	B
	DGGG/BVF (Professional Society)	Same as AWMF plus serology monitoring every 4 weeks until 16 weeks if seronegative	8 g/day (2 g × 4), until 20 weeks gestation (max 6 weeks)	B (Professional Society Consensus)
	BMG (State)	No general recommendation; individual decisions	–	D
Greece	HSOG (Professional Society)	No routine screening; valaciclovir only in study context	–	D (research context)
	Ministry of Health Greece (State)	Guidelines in preparation; no antiviral therapy recommended	–	D (developmental phase)

(continued)

Table 29.8 (continued)

Country/ region	Institution (type)	Valaciclovir recommendation for primary CMV infection in pregnancy	Dosage and duration	Evidence grade
India	FOGSI (Professional Society)	No routine screening; risk counseling and hygiene emphasized	–	D (prevention focus)
	ICMR (State)	Guidelines under development; no antiviral therapy recommended	–	D
Israel	ISOG (Professional Society)	Recommendation limited to study context; no routine use	–	C (early RCTs)
	Ministry of Health Israel (State)	Diagnostic costs covered; no antiviral therapy recommended	–	D (prevention focus)
Italy	SIGO (Professional Society)	Risk-based screening; valaciclovir only in studies or specific cases	8 g/day (2 g × 4), until PCR result (4–6 weeks)	D
	SSN (State)	No standard treatment; reimbursement only in special cases	8 g/day (2 g × 4), until PCR result (4–6 weeks) until negative PCR	D
Japan	JSOG (Professional Society)	Valaciclovir only within clinical studies; no routine recommendation	–	D
	MHLW (State)	First practice guidelines expected in 2024, limited to study context	–	C
Mexico	AMEG (Professional Society)	Risk-based serology and hygiene education only; no antiviral therapy	–	D (prevention focus)
	Secretaría de Salud (State)	National guideline pending; no routine CMV therapy	–	D

(continued)

Table 29.8 (continued)

Country/ region	Institution (type)	Valaciclovir recommendation for primary CMV infection in pregnancy	Dosage and duration	Evidence grade
Netherlands	NVOG (Professional Society)	Risk-based approach; valaciclovir not recommended	–	D
	RIVM (State)	Opportunistic testing for high-risk pregnancies only	–	D
Norway	NGF (Professional Society)	Risk-based screening; no routine therapy recommended	–	D (pilot phase)
	Folkehelseinstituttet (State)	No official position on antiviral therapy	–	D
Austria	OEGGG (Professional Society)	Individual decision-making advised	–	D
	BMSGPK (State)	Screening not included in mother-child pass program	–	D
Poland	Polish Society of Gynecologists and Obstetricians	Risk-based screening; no routine antiviral therapy recommended	–	D
	Ministry of Health Poland (State)	No specific recommendations for CMV therapy during pregnancy	–	D
Portugal	SPGO (Professional Society)	Hygiene education and risk avoidance counseling only; no antiviral therapy recommended	–	D
	DGS (State)	No universal screening established	–	D
Romania	Romanian Society of Obstetrics and Gynecology	Focus on screening and counseling; valaciclovir not recommended	–	D
	Ministry of Health Romania (State)	No universal CMV screening or antiviral therapy recommended	–	D

(continued)

Table 29.8 (continued)

Country/ region	Institution (type)	Valacidovir recommendation for primary CMV infection in pregnancy	Dosage and duration	Evidence grade
Russia	Russian Society of Obstetricians and Gynecologists	Recommendation only within research settings; no routine use	–	D
	Ministry of Health, Russian Federation (State)	National guidelines focus on prevention; antiviral therapy not planned	–	D
Sweden	SFOG (Professional Society)	Evaluation ongoing; no standard valaciclovir recommendation yet	–	D
	Socialstyrelsen (State)	Regional protocols without uniform therapy recommendations	–	D
Switzerland	SGGG (Professional Society)	Off-label valaciclovir use allowed after individual risk-benefit assessment for primary infection	8 g/day (2 g × 4), for 4–6 weeks post diagnosis	C
	BAG (State)	No binding guidelines; physician makes case-by-case decisions	–	D
Spain	SEGO (Professional Society)	Risk-based screening; emphasis on hygiene and education only	–	D
	Ministerio de Sanidad (State)	No universal strategy; regional programs exist	–	D
Thailand	Thai College of Obstetricians and Gynecologists	Preventive measures and education only; no routine antiviral therapy recommended	–	D
	Ministry of Public Health (State)	National CMV guidelines under development; antiviral therapy currently not recommended	–	D

(continued)

Table 29.8 (continued)

Country/ region	Institution (type)	Valaciclovir recommendation for primary CMV infection in pregnancy	Dosage and duration	Evidence grade
United Kingdom	RCOG (Professional Society)	Yes, for primary infection <12 weeks gestation in specialized centers with risk-benefit assessment recommended	8 g/day (2 g × 4), until 21 weeks gestation or 4 weeks post start	B
	NHS (State)	No general recommendation; local protocols vary widely	–	D
USA	ACOG (Professional Society)	Valaciclovir use restricted to controlled clinical trials; no off-label recommendation	–	D
	SMFM (Professional Society)	Therapy only within research protocols	–	D
	CDC (State)	No universal screening or antiviral therapy outside studies due to insufficient evidence	–	D
European Union	EFC/ISUOG (Professional Societies)	Early treatment recommended for primary infection by EFC but no widespread valaciclovir use recommended by ISUOG; emphasis on hygiene and screening guidelines	8 g/day (2 g every 6 h), until 20 weeks gestation, max 8 weeks duration	B

- **Public Health Authorities: Most Governmental Health Agencies Do Not Recommend Routine Valaciclovir Therapy During Pregnancy.**
  - Canada (Health Canada): No national policy; provincial guidelines vary.
  - Germany (BMG): No systematic evaluation; decisions made on a case-by-case basis.
  - Italy (SSN): No widespread reimbursement for valaciclovir in pregnancy.
  - Switzerland (BAG): No binding guidelines; clinical judgment on individual cases.
  - UK (NHS): No national routine recommendation; local protocols vary.
  - USA (CDC): No universal screening or antiviral therapy outside studies.

The international evidence demonstrates a cautious approach toward routine valaciclovir prophylaxis for primary CMV infection during pregnancy. Only Switzerland and Canada recommend conditional therapy based on individual risk-benefit assessment. The majority of professional societies and governmental authorities limit the use of valaciclovir to controlled clinical trials or entirely refrain from issuing general antiviral prophylaxis recommendations.

Key Points

- The significance of cytomegaly has recently increased, with cytomegalovirus (CMV) identified as the causative agent. It possesses double-stranded DNA and is classified within the herpes virus group.
- CMV is the most common cause of intrauterine viral infection, impacting approximately 0.5–2.3% of all newborns.
- Pregnant women typically become infected through interactions with children in home or professional settings.
- Approximately 1–4% of women (IgG negative) acquire primary CMV infection during pregnancy, and about one-third of these women transmit the infection to their unborn child.
- The transmission rate increases with gestational age (greatest in the third trimester); however, the severity of the disease inversely correlates with gestational age, with the child most significantly affected if maternal infection occurs in the first trimester.
- Overall, around 15–20% of infected infants develop secondary symptoms.
- Complications in infants with congenital CMV infection include jaundice, petechiae, thrombocytopenia, hepatosplenomegaly, growth retardation, microcephaly, intracranial calcifications, nonimmune hydrops, premature births, and subsequent issues such as hearing loss, intellectual disability, psychomotor delays, chorioretinitis, optic atrophy, seizures, expressive language delays, and learning disabilities. The long-term mortality rate for severely affected infants is approximately 5%.
- Preventive measures are advisable for pregnant women, including avoiding close contact with children, frequent handwashing, and glove use, which may influence behavior and effectively reduce CMV infections during pregnancy.
- Routine CMV screening during pregnancy is not currently recommended in most countries until appropriate fetal interventions have been validated to reduce neonatal morbidity due to maternal CMV infection.

(continued)

- Maternal diagnosis of primary CMV infection is confirmed by serum IgM, and fetal diagnosis is established by detecting the virus in amniotic fluid via polymerase chain reaction (PCR).
- The presence or absence of fetal abnormalities on ultrasound can assist in counseling, but ultrasound is not sensitive and fails to adequately predict whether an infant will be affected (symptomatic), particularly when maternal serology information is lacking.
- There is no *in utero* therapy for CMV. Hyperimmunoglobulin has been shown in randomized controlled trials to be ineffective in preventing vertical transmission of CMV; however, it may provide benefits in certain cases. Valaciclovir has demonstrated positive effects in small studies, but concerns regarding dosage, duration, and side effects persist. Further studies are required to evaluate these aspects comprehensively.

Hepatitis B and D

30

Abstract

Hepatitis B is transmitted primarily through blood transfusions, contaminated needles, sexual contact, and vertical transmission from mother to child. The prevalence of the virus varies globally, with higher rates observed in Africa, Asia, and South America. Only a small percentage of those infected exhibit symptoms, with many remaining asymptomatic. Acute hepatitis B can progress to a chronic form, which is associated with cirrhosis and hepatocellular carcinoma. Coinfection with hepatitis D virus (HDV) often results in more severe disease. Diagnosis is made through serologic and molecular biological tests. Pregnant women should be screened for hepatitis B virus (HBV) to prevent transmission to newborns. While acute hepatitis B is typically managed symptomatically, chronic cases may require treatment with interferon-alpha or nucleoside/nucleotide analogs. Antiviral therapy during pregnancy presents challenges. Vaccination is recommended for newborns of HBV-positive mothers to confer protection against both HBV and HDV. Generally, prevention efforts should focus on screening, vaccination, and avoidance of risk factors.

30.1 Background

Hepatitis B, caused by the hepatitis B virus (HBV), is the most prevalent form of hepatitis worldwide, affecting approximately 300–350 million people chronically. The prospect of vertical transmission raises significant concerns, though this risk can generally be controlled in developed countries through vaccination.

Hepatitis D, resulting from infection with the hepatitis delta virus (HDV), was first identified in 1973 when a new antigen (D) was detected in the hepatocytes of patients with severe hepatitis B. Initially thought to be a variant of the HBV core protein, further research in the 1980s established it as an independent pathogen.

I. Mylonas, *Sexually Transmitted Diseases*,
https://doi.org/10.1007/978-3-031-78204-6_30

Basic Classification of HBV Infection

- **Acute Hepatitis B**: Newly acquired infection that is often asymptomatic and self-limiting.
- **Persistent Hepatitis B**: Infection lasting longer than 6 months, characterized by intermittent or prolonged asymptomatic periods.
  - **Highly Viremic HBsAg Carrier Status**: Chronic HBV infection without evidence of liver cell damage, typically resulting from vertical transmission or early infection. Transition to chronic hepatitis B is possible at any time.
  - **Low-Viremic HBsAg Carrier Status**: Persistent HBV infection without signs of liver cell damage, with potential for reactivation at any stage.
- **Chronic Hepatitis B**: Persistent infection demonstrating evidence of liver cell damage.

30.2 Pathogens

30.2.1 Hepatitis B

The virion, referred to as the Dane particle in honor of its discoverer in 1970, is the only known hepatotropic virus composed of double-stranded DNA. Due to its intermediate RNA stage and pronounced replication mechanisms, mutations can occur in various regions of the HBV genome, leading to a significant variability. HBV is characterized by its complex structure, high viral concentrations in the bloodstream, and environmental stability. Mutations in regions that encode for the envelope antigen (HBsAg) and the core protein (HBeAg) are particularly important for both vertical transmission and neonatal disease outcomes.

The immune response following acute or chronic hepatitis B infections is essential; its effectiveness depends on numerous factors, some of which remain unidentified, and it may be delayed by weeks, months, or even years. If the immune response is delayed, the virus is free to replicate, resulting in significant viremia. Once the immune response is initiated, the viral load in the bloodstream diminishes.

While hepatic inflammation may be mild, the disease course can be marked by episodes of heightened activity, advancing toward cirrhosis. During the infection, liver cells are not directly harmed by the virus itself (lack of cytopathic effect), but rather by the host's immune response. The more effective the elimination of the virus, the greater the consequent cellular destruction.

30.2.2 Hepatitis D

The hepatitis D virus (HDV) is a spherical, enveloped RNA virus measuring approximately 36 nm in diameter. It is currently classified within the Kolmioviridae family.

This reclassification is relatively recent, as HDV was formerly considered the sole member of the genus Deltavirus. The Kolmioviridae family is part of the realm Ribozyviria, and it is the sole member of the Deltaviridae family. The genome encodes a singular protein, HD-Ag, which exists in both small (24 kDa) and large (27 kDa) forms. The incubation period for coinfection with HBV, is estimated at 4-8 weeks, while superinfection may take 50–180 days to manifest.

While replication of the HDV genome can occur independently of HBV infection, HBV envelope proteins are essential for the morphogenesis, release, and infectivity of HDV. The viral envelope comprises around 95% HBsAg. HDV is transmitted similarly to HBV, with percutaneous inoculation being the predominant infection route. However, HDV is less frequently transmitted through sexual contact compared to HBV.

HDV exhibits a cytopathic effect; coinfection with HDV typically results in more significant liver damage than HBV infection alone. Notably, hepatitis B-infected cells exhibit marked necrotic progression in vitro following HDV transfection, without immune response involvement.

30.3 Epidemiology

30.3.1 Hepatitis B

30.3.1.1 Global and Regional Prevalence of Chronic HBV Infection

- An estimated 300–350 million individuals worldwide are living with chronic HBV infection, with a global prevalence rate of approximately 3.6% for hepatitis B surface antigen (HBsAg). The highest rates over 8.8% are found in Africa and 5.3% in the Western Pacific.
- **United States**
  - **Prevalence**: Chronic HBV infections account for approximately 0.3–0.4% of the population.
  - **Trend**: Since 1982, acute hepatitis B cases have decreased by about 90%, from 9.6 to 1.0 cases per 100,000 population by 2018.
  - **High-Risk Groups**: Increased prevalence is noted among intravenous drug users (between 3.5% and 20%) and migrants from high-endemic regions.
- **Europe**
  - **Reported Cases**: The European Centre for Disease Prevention and Control (ECDC) recorded 16,187 hepatitis B cases in the EU and European Economic Area in 2021.
  - **Case Classification**: Of these, 15,380 were registered, resulting in an overall rate of 4.7 cases per 100,000 population. The classification comprised 7% as acute, 43% as chronic, and 43% as "unknown," with 7% not distinctly classified.
  - **Demographics**: The highest incidence of both acute and chronic infections was observed in the 35–44 age group, with a sex ratio of 1.4 men to 1 woman.
  - **Trend**: There has been a steady decline in reported acute cases, likely due to the effectiveness of national vaccination programs.

- **Asia**
  - **Prevalence**: With a prevalence rate of 5.3%, Asia remains a region of significant HBV endemicity.
  - **Vaccination Programs**: Comprehensive vaccination efforts have considerably reduced new infection rates in certain countries, exemplified by Taiwan.
- **Africa**
  - **Prevalence**: Africa holds the highest global prevalence of HBsAg at 8.8%.
  - **High-Impact Countries**: Countries such as South Africa, Kenya, Nigeria, and Congo demonstrate particularly high prevalence.

30.3.1.2 Primary Routes of HBV Transmission

- **Parenteral transmission**
  - **Blood Transfusions**: Contaminated blood transfusions can facilitate HBV transmission.
  - **Needlestick Injuries**: Healthcare workers face risk from accidental needlestick injuries.
  - **Contaminated Syringes or Cannulas**: Sharing needles among drug users substantially increases infection risk.
- **Contact with mucous membranes**
  - **Sexual Intercourse**: HBV can be transmitted through mucosal contact during sexual activity.
- **Perinatal transmission**
  - **Newborns of HBeAg and/or HBsAg Positive Mothers**: The perinatal transmission rate ranges from 70% to 90% for newborns born to HBeAg and/or HBsAg-positive mothers.
  - The likelihood of vertical transmission correlates directly with maternal viremia. Intrauterine diaplacental transmission is rare but can occur, particularly in late pregnancy, without negatively influencing the course of pregnancy.
  - Perinatal and early postnatal infections pose substantial risks due to the high viral concentration in the vaginal secretions of infected mothers, detectable in approximately 35% of amniotic fluid, around 50% of umbilical cord blood, and more than 70% of breast milk.
- **Reservoir for HBV**
  - **Chronically Infected Persons**: The primary reservoir for HBV comprises chronically infected individuals (HBsAg-positive) who often exhibit minimal or no symptoms, playing a significant role in ongoing transmission.

Currently, unprotected sexual intercourse is considered the most significant mode of Hepatitis B virus (HBV) transmission.

30.3.2 Hepatitis D

30.3.2.1 Global Overview

It is estimated that 15–20 million individuals worldwide are infected with HDV, primarily in regions with high hepatitis B prevalence, such as parts of Africa, Asia, and South America. Due to the interrelationship between HBV and HDV, areas with a high HBV prevalence are often associated with increased rates of HDV.

30.3.2.2 Regional Prevalence

- **Asia**: High HBV prevalence results in elevated HDV rates.
- **Africa, Asia, and South America**: Similar patterns emerge due to high HBV prevalence.
- **Southern and Eastern Europe**: Hepatitis D is prevalent in these regions, mirroring the distribution of HBV.
- **Middle East, Africa, and South America**: An increase in HDV prevalence in these regions parallels the spread of HBV.

30.3.2.3 Relationship to HBV Prevalence

- The prevalence of HDV is closely associated with the rate of chronic hepatitis B infection:
  - **Low HBV Carrier Rate**: In countries with low HBV carrier rates, HDV infections primarily occur in high-risk groups such as drug users, hemophiliacs, homosexuals, and individuals from endemic areas.
  - **Moderate to High HBV Prevalence**: In regions where chronic hepatitis B infection is moderate to high, the prevalence of HDV coinfection may reach up to 20%. Among patients with HBV-related liver disease, the detection rate of HDV ranges from 30% to 60%.

30.3.2.4 Impact of HBV Vaccination

- The relationship between HBV and HDV prevalence is particularly evident in Southern Europe, where the incidence of anti-HDV antibodies significantly decreased from 40% to nearly 10% following the introduction of HBV vaccination and improvements in socioeconomic conditions in the 1980s.
- HDV prevalence remains closely linked to HBV distribution. Public health initiatives, including HBV vaccination and targeted education, are essential for effectively managing and reducing HDV infections in high-risk regions and populations.

With the implementation of HBV vaccination programs, hepatitis D prevalence has declined. However, precise epidemiologic data remain unavailable.

30.4 Clinical Manifestations

30.4.1 Gynecology

30.4.1.1 Hepatitis B

30.4.1.1.1 Acute HBV Infection

Acute hepatitis B virus (HBV) infection is frequently oligosymptomatic or asymptomatic. After an incubation period of approximately 6–25 weeks, a prodromal phase typically ensues and is characterized by nonspecific systemic symptoms, including malaise, anorexia, nausea, vomiting, low-grade fever, and arthralgia. The prodrome is followed in many patients by an icteric phase of variable duration (commonly 2–6 weeks), during which hepatobiliary and systemic manifestations are observed. Characteristic features that may be present during the icteric phase include:

- Icterus (jaundice), caused by hyperbilirubinemia due to impaired hepatic conjugation and excretion
- Hepatomegaly, reflecting hepatic inflammation and cellular swelling
- Splenomegaly, indicative of reticuloendothelial activation and portal pressure changes
- Lymphadenopathy, representing immune activation and viral antigen presentation
- Dark urine (bilirubinuria) and pale, acholic stools, resulting from increased conjugated bilirubin excretion in the urine and reduced bile pigment delivery to the intestine

Laboratory findings during the acute phase are commonly characterized by elevated serum aminotransferases (ALT and AST, often markedly increased), elevated total and direct bilirubin, and variable changes in alkaline phosphatase and gamma-glutamyl transferase. Serologic markers diagnostic of acute HBV infection include hepatitis B surface antigen (HBsAg) and hepatitis B core IgM antibody (anti-HBc IgM); hepatitis B e antigen (HBeAg) may be present and generally correlates with high viral replication. Clinical course is usually self-limited in immunocompetent adults; however, fulminant hepatic failure may develop rarely. Supportive management is indicated for most patients, and antiviral therapy is reserved for those with severe or protracted disease, significant hepatic decompensation, or high risk for progression as determined by current guideline criteria. Follow-up with serial liver function tests and HBV serology is recommended to document viral clearance or progression to chronicity.

Occasional complications, including pancreatitis or alterations in hematopoiesis, may arise. In rare instances, an acute hepatitis B infection can progress to a fulminant course.

30.4.1.1.2 Chronic HBV Infection

Chronic hepatitis B virus (HBV) infection is associated with significant long-term morbidity and mortality, including hepatic fibrosis, cirrhosis, hepatic decompensation, and hepatocellular carcinoma (HCC). The natural history after acute infection varies according to host age, immune status, and viral factors. Approximately 90% of immunocompetent adults with acute HBV infection recover spontaneously and develop protective immunity, whereas roughly 5–10% progress to chronic infection; the risk of chronicity is markedly higher in neonates and young children.

Clinical and Virologic Phenotypes of Chronic HBV Infection

- Asymptomatic HBV Carrier (Inactive HBsAg Carrier): HBsAg persists for >6 months, but HBV DNA levels are low or undetectable and alanine aminotransferase (ALT) is normal. Hepatic necroinflammation is minimal and the short-term prognosis is favorable, although the risk of reactivation persists, particularly with immunosuppression.
- Chronic Persistent Hepatitis: Low-grade hepatic inflammation is present with persistent HBsAg positivity and minimally elevated or fluctuating ALT. Progression to advanced fibrosis is slow and the overall prognosis is relatively good compared with more active disease.
- Chronic Active Hepatitis (Immune-Active Phase): Ongoing hepatic necroinflammation is accompanied by persistently or intermittently elevated ALT and higher HBV DNA levels. This phenotype confers a higher risk of progressive fibrosis and cirrhosis; historically, the risk of progression to cirrhosis and related complications has been estimated to be substantial (figures vary between cohorts), and untreated active disease is associated with increased long-term morbidity.

Complications and Long-Term Outcomes

- Cirrhosis: Progressive hepatic fibrosis may culminate in cirrhosis, with subsequent complications such as portal hypertension, ascites, variceal hemorrhage, and hepatic encephalopathy. The annual incidence of progression from chronic hepatitis B to cirrhosis is variable and is influenced by viral load, duration of infection, age at infection, alcohol use, metabolic comorbidities, and coinfection (e.g., hepatitis D virus). When cirrhosis is established, the risk of hepatic decompensation and HCC is increased.
- Hepatocellular Carcinoma (HCC): Chronic HBV infection is a major etiologic factor for HCC, both in the presence and absence of cirrhosis. Cumulative risk estimates vary by population, duration of infection, and presence of cofactors; in patients with cirrhosis, the 10–15-year incidence of HCC has been reported in some series to approximate 15% but varies widely. Regular HCC surveillance with abdominal ultrasound ± serum alpha-fetoprotein (AFP) every 6 months is recommended for at-risk individuals in accordance with guideline recommendations.

Management Implications

- Patients with chronic HBV infection should be stratified for antiviral therapy based on HBV DNA level, ALT, degree of fibrosis, age, and comorbidities. Nucleos(t)ide analogs with high genetic barrier to resistance (e.g., entecavir, tenofovir disoproxil fumarate, and tenofovir alafenamide) are preferred for long-term viral suppression. Antiviral therapy has been shown to reduce the risks of cirrhosis, hepatic decompensation, and HCC but does not eliminate them entirely.
- Periodic monitoring of liver enzymes, HBV DNA, HBsAg status, and noninvasive assessment of fibrosis (transient elastography and serum fibrosis biomarkers) is required to detect disease activity, guide treatment decisions, and identify progression.
- Vaccination of susceptible contacts and implementation of preventive measures are essential to reduce transmission.

While a significant proportion of acute HBV infections resolve spontaneously with lasting immunity, a subset may progress to chronic infection, associated with serious long-term complications, particularly if acquired at a younger age.

30.4.1.1.3 Age-Related Progression

The probability of progression from acute to chronic hepatitis B virus (HBV) infection is highly dependent on the age at initial exposure.

- Adults: When HBV infection is acquired in adulthood, chronicity develops in approximately 5–10% of cases. Chronic infection acquired in adulthood is associated with an increased long-term risk of cirrhosis and hepatocellular carcinoma (HCC), which may manifest after decades (commonly 20–30 years) of persistent hepatic inflammation and hepatocyte regeneration.
- Infants (Older Infants and Young Children): Infection occurring during infancy and early childhood carries an intermediate risk of chronicity, with approximately 20–30% of infected infants progressing to chronic HBV infection.
- Neonates (Perinatally Acquired Infection): When infection is acquired in the perinatal period, the risk of progression to chronic infection is highest, reaching up to 85–90% in the absence of post-exposure prophylaxis (hepatitis B immunoglobulin and timely vaccination). Perinatally acquired chronic infection confers a high lifetime risk of cirrhosis and HCC unless viral replication is controlled.

Infectivity persists as long as HBsAg, HBeAg, or HBV DNA remains detectable in serum. Co-infection with HDV is also possible and should be ruled out in cases of HBV infection.

30.4.1.2 Hepatitis D

30.4.1.2.1 Coinfection with HBV and HDV

Simultaneous infection with HBV and HDV results in hepatitis clinically indistinguishable from hepatitis B alone. In over 90% of instances, both pathogens are cleared following the acute phase of co-infection; however, co-infection may lead to acute hepatitis that is more severe than hepatitis B alone.

- **Acute Phase**: A biphasic pattern of transaminases reflects liver damage by both viruses or the immune response. Clinical symptoms generally resolve within 3–12 weeks.
- **Chronic Transition**: Approximately 5% of cases progress to a chronic course.
- **Severe Disease**: Co-infection can lead to fulminant hepatitis, particularly in individuals with a history of drug use.

30.4.1.2.2 HDV Superinfection in HBV Carriers

Superinfection of hepatitis B virus (HBV) carriers with hepatitis D virus (HDV) often precipitates a severe and frequently fulminant form of hepatitis. The interplay between these two viruses results in a more aggressive disease course and poorer outcomes than HBV infection alone.

- Chronic Progression: Up to 90% of HBV carriers who acquire HDV develop chronic hepatitis D, a rate substantially higher than the chronicity observed in acute HBV infection alone. Once established, chronic hepatitis D tends to progress more rapidly to advanced liver disease.
- Mechanism of Increased Severity: HDV is a defective virus that relies on the HBV surface antigen (HBsAg) for assembly and secretion of new virions. In an HBV-infected host, abundant HBsAg production provides the essential helper function for HDV replication. This viral synergy amplifies liver injury through direct cytopathic effects of HDV and heightened immune-mediated damage.
- High Mortality in Fulminant Cases: When HDV superinfection triggers fulminant hepatitis, mortality rates exceed 30%. This dramatic outcome reflects massive hepatocyte necrosis, profound coagulopathy, and rapid hepatic decompensation.
- Accelerated Cirrhosis Development: HDV superinfection accelerates fibrogenesis, with cirrhosis occurring in as many as 70–80% of patients within 5–10 years—significantly faster than the 20–30% progression rate seen in chronic HBV monoinfection over the same period.
- Spontaneous Clearance: Spontaneous HDV clearance is rare but most often observed in asymptomatic HBsAg carriers who mount an effective immune response. In these individuals, HDV may be eradicated before establishing chronic infection, although they remain at risk for reactivation if HBV replication intensifies.

30.4.1.2.3 Other Forms of HDV Infection

Other Forms of HDV Infection

In addition to the well-characterized scenarios of acute HBV/HDV coinfection and HDV superinfection in chronic HBV carriers, a rare but clinically important presentation involves HBV superinfection in the setting of clinically latent HDV infection. This pattern is most often encountered in transplantation medicine and other immunocompromised states. In these patients, HDV can persist at low levels without causing overt liver injury. However, if HBV replication is reactivated—either by deliberate withdrawal of antiviral prophylaxis after transplantation, immunosuppressive therapy adjustments, or through true HBV superinfection—the sudden surge in HBV surface antigen provides the essential helper function for HDV. The resulting boost in HDV replication can then precipitate fulminant liver inflammation and injury.

Notably, reinfection with other hepatotropic viruses does not carry the same risk. For instance, HCV reinfection in an HDV-infected host does not induce significant hepatic damage, even when HDV replication continues unchecked. Only an increase in HBV antigen expression—through HBV reactivation or new HBV superinfection—triggers the pathogenic cascade that leads to clinically apparent hepatitis in these patients. This underscores the unique dependency of HDV on HBV for virion assembly and highlights the critical need for vigilant HBV monitoring in immunosuppressed individuals with latent HDV carriage.

30.4.1.3 Summary

- **Coinfection with HBV and HDV**: This combination leads to acute hepatitis, which may be more severe than HBV alone, but is typically resolved after the acute phase in over 90% of cases. Approximately 5% transition to chronic infection, and severe forms such as fulminant hepatitis are more likely, particularly among drug users.
- **HDV Superinfection in HBV Carriers**: This situation often results in severe hepatitis, with 70–90% of cases progressing to chronic hepatitis D. This form is more aggressive than chronic hepatitis B without HDV, showing higher rates of liver cirrhosis and mortality.
- **HBV Superinfection in Latent HDV**: In transplantation contexts, this scenario is uncommon and primarily significant, as superinfection can result in hepatic damage.

30.4.2 Pregnancy

30.4.2.1 Hepatitis B

It can be assumed that neither acute nor chronic hepatitis B adversely affects an existing pregnancy. Fulminant courses leading to liver failure have been reported only in rare instances. However, a significant percentage of HBV-infected women (up to 95% when HBeAg positive) can transmit the infection intrauterine or perinatally to the child unless the newborn receives postpartum vaccination, which includes both active and passive immunization.

If the mother is an HBsAg carrier, the risk of transmitting hepatitis B virus (HBV) to her infant is approximately 40%, but this risk increases to 90% if she is also HBeAg positive. The presence of HBeAg reflects high-level viral replication and correlates strongly with infectivity. In addition, a detectable maternal HBV DNA load further escalates the likelihood of perinatal transmission: every ten-fold increase in viral DNA roughly doubles the transmission risk.

30.4.2.2 Hepatitis D

Hepatitis D Virus in Pregnancy

Hepatitis D virus (HDV) infection complicating hepatitis B virus (HBV)-infected pregnancies is uncommon, and the precise prevalence of HDV among pregnant women remains undetermined due to limited epidemiological data. When HDV does occur alongside HBV in pregnancy, it represents a distinct clinical scenario that carries a higher risk of maternal morbidity and mortality compared to HBV monoinfection. Consequently, obstetric care providers should include HDV screening (anti-HDV and, if positive, HDV RNA testing) in HBV-infected pregnant patients, particularly in regions with known HDV endemicity.

Vertical transmission of HDV is rarely documented but has been reported in isolated cases; when it occurs, infants are at high risk of developing chronic hepatitis D, mirroring the natural history of HDV superinfection in adults, which is characterized by accelerated progression to cirrhosis and hepatic decompensation. Although HBV infection during the postpartum period and through breastfeeding may influence viral kinetics, current evidence suggests that the risk of HDV transmission via breast milk is negligible if standard HBV immunoprophylaxis protocols are followed.

Prevention of HDV in infancy hinges on established HBV immunization strategies. Active immunization with recombinant HBV vaccine, combined with passive prophylaxis using hepatitis B immune globulin at birth, not only prevents HBV transmission but also indirectly blocks HDV infection by eliminating the necessary HBV surface antigen "helper" function. Completion of the HBV vaccine series in infancy effectively abolishes the risk of both HBV and HDV acquisition in early life. Continuous post-vaccination serologic testing at 9–12 months ensures immune protection and identifies nonresponders who may require additional vaccination.

Newborns vaccinated against HBV can be safely breastfed, and there is no necessity for isolation or separation of the mother and infant following birth.

30.5 Diagnosis

30.5.1 Hepatitis B

Available serologic and molecular biological tests enable reliable detection and characterization of both acute and chronic forms of hepatitis B (Table 30.1). HBV infection should be considered in the differential diagnosis of jaundice during pregnancy.

Following infection, the hepatitis B surface antigen (HBsAg) generally becomes detectable within 2 to 8 weeks. In chronic forms, persistence of HBsAg after 4–6 months indicates ongoing viral replication. Characteristic serologic antigen-antibody patterns facilitate clear conclusions regarding the course, infectivity, and viral replication of hepatitis B infections. In the case of HBsAg detection, it is important to determine anti-HDV antibodies to diagnose acute hepatitis D.

30.5.2 Hepatitis D

Acute or past HDV infection is diagnosed by detecting anti-HDV antibodies through enzyme-linked immunosorbent assay (ELISA). Persistent HDV infection is identified by the presence of HDV RNA, with quantitative detection available in specialized laboratories, which is crucial for therapeutic monitoring. Acute and chronic infections can be distinguished by the presence of IgM antibodies; however, this detection lacks specificity and should ideally be replaced by HDV RNA determination. Chronic HDV infection is defined by the persistence of HDV RNA for at least 6 months.

Diagnostic clarification is essential, given that the mortality rate for superinfection with hepatitis D is approximately ten times higher than that for HBV infection alone.

HDV antibodes are often not included in the primary diagnosis of acute hepatitis. In acute infections, hepatitis B markers are prioritized, as anti-HDV antibodies generally become detectable only at the conclusion of the acute phase. However, delta antigen and HDV RNA can be identified shortly after the onset of clinical symptoms. As the disease progresses, HDV markers, particularly HD-Ag, HDV RNA, and anti-HDV IgM, gradually decline.

Both viral infections persist in superinfected HBV carriers. During the transition to chronic phase, anti-HDV antibodies (IgG and IgM) maintain persistently high titers, while HD-Ag and HDV RNA remain detectable.

HDV diagnostics should be recommended for newly diagnosed HBV infections, especially in cases where HDV testing has not been previously conducted. In cases of clinical deterioration and exacerbation of chronic hepatitis B, HDV superinfection should be considered.

Table 30.1 Evaluation of diagnostic methods for hepatitis B virus (HBV) infection

HBs antigen	Anti-HBc-AK	Anti-HBs-AK	Assessment	
–	–	–	No evidence of HBV infection	– Hepatitis B infection in the incubation period (2–6 months) – Further diagnostics (if a fresh infection is suspected): controls: HBs-Ag, anti-HBc, anti-HBc-IgM, anti-HBs, if necessary HBV-DNA-PCR – 5–10% of HBV infections remain HBs-Ag-negative!
+	–	–	Onset of (clinical) HBV infection	– Time window of this constellation: a few weeks (then the formation of anti-HBc takes place) – Assume infectivity – The anti-HBc-IgM often becomes positive earlier – Further diagnosis: anti-HBc-IgM; HBV-DNA-PCR
+	+	–	Acute, infectious hepatitis B	– HbS antigen >6 months: transition to a chronic course – Anti-HBc-IgM almost always positive – Further diagnosis: anti-HBc-IgM; HBV-DNA-PCR
			Chronic hepatitis B	– Persistence of the HbS antigen >6 months – CAVE: later seroconversions possible – If HBV DNA persists for >8 weeks: chronic course – Anti-HBc-IgM often negative – Further diagnosis: HBs-Ag, anti-HBc, anti-HBc-IgM, anti-HBs, if necessary HBV-DNA-PCR
–	+	+	HBV infection contracted	– No infectivity – Immunity is dependent on the anti-HBs antibody
–	–	+	Vaccination	– Immunity is dependent on the anti-HBs antibody
			HBV infection contracted	– Mostly anti-HBc positive (rarely isolated anti-HBs) – No infectivity – Immunity depends on the level of the anti-HBs antibody
–	+	–	HBV infection contracted	– No infectivity – Questionable immunity
			Low-level HBs antigen carriers	– Chronic course with below the detection limit – Mostly inconspicuous progression – Further diagnosis: HBs-Ag, anti-HBc, anti-HBc-IgM, anti-HBs, if necessary HBV-DNA-PCR

HBs-Ag hepatitis B surface antigen, *anti-HBc* hepatitis B core antibody, *Anti-HBc-IgM* immunoglobulin M antibody to hepatitis B core antigen, *Anti-HBs* hepatitis B surface antibody, *HBV DNA-PCR* hepatitis B virus DNA polymerase chain reaction

30.6 Treatment

30.6.1 Hepatitis B

30.6.1.1 Acute Form

Acute hepatitis B is characterized by a sudden onset of symptoms, including fever, malaise, anorexia, and jaundice. In immunocompetent adults, spontaneous virologic clearance occurs in 95–99% of cases, so specific antiviral therapy is generally not indicated. Management focuses on supportive care such as rest, hydration, nutritional support, and avoidance of hepatotoxic medications.

Antiviral therapy is reserved for cases of fulminant or protracted acute hepatitis B, which present with signs of hepatic synthetic failure, encephalopathy, rapid clinical deterioration, or in patients with high-risk comorbidities. Hepatic synthetic failure is indicated by markedly elevated transaminases (ALT, AST often >1000 IU/L) and coagulopathy, reflected by an international normalized ratio (INR) >1.5 or Quick value <50%. Encephalopathy may manifest as new-onset confusion, asterixis, or rising bilirubin levels above 10 mg/dL, often accompanied by progressive jaundice or worsening ascites. High-risk comorbidities include underlying chronic liver disease such as cirrhosis or fatty liver and states of immunosuppression like chemotherapy or HIV infection.

In cases of fulminant acute hepatitis B, nucleos(t)ide analogs with high potency and strong genetic resistance barriers are preferred. Tenofovir disoproxil fumarate (TDF) and entecavir are the recommended agents due to their rapid viral suppression and favorable safety profiles (Table 30.2). Therapy should begin promptly once fulminant features are identified and continue until HBsAg clearance or transition to chronic management if HBsAg persists beyond 6 months.

Close monitoring is essential during treatment, including daily assessment of liver enzymes, coagulation parameters (INR/Quick value), bilirubin levels, and neurological status. Renal function requires frequent evaluation when patients are receiving tenofovir. Immediate referral to a transplant center is critical if there is rapidly rising INR despite treatment, worsening encephalopathy, or refractory coagulopathy.

30.6.1.2 Chronic Hepatitis B

Chronic hepatitis B is diagnosed when hepatitis B surface antigen (HBsAg) persists for more than 6 months. Antiviral therapy is indicated when HBV DNA exceeds 2000 IU/mL in conjunction with one or more of the following: elevated serum aminotransferases, histologic evidence of at least minimal inflammation or mild fibrosis, or high-grade fibrosis, cirrhosis, or detectable HBV DNA by PCR regardless of enzyme levels. Treatment decisions should be individualized on the basis of virologic, biochemical, and histologic parameters.

First-Line Therapy: Pegylated interferon-α (Peg-IFN-α) is recommended as a first-line option for treatment-naive adults with compensated liver disease, irrespective of hepatitis B e antigen (HBeAg) status. The therapeutic course is administered

Table 30.2 Oral nucleos(t)ide analogs for chronic HBV

Agent (generic)	Potency/resistance barrier	Typical adult dose (oral)	Key points
Entecavir	High/High	0.5 mg once daily (1 mg if prior lamivudine exposure)	Check renal function; adjust dose for reduced creatinine clearance
Tenofovir DF (TDF)	High/High	300 mg once daily	Monitor renal function and serum phosphate; assess bone density if at risk
Tenofovir AF (TAF)	High/High	25 mg once daily	Lower renal and bone toxicity vs TDF; preferred in renal impairment when available
Lamivudine	Moderate/Low	100 mg once daily	Rapid resistance (YMDD); generally avoided as monotherapy
Telbivudine	Moderate–High/ Moderate	600 mg once daily	Risk of myopathy/ neuropathy; check CK with muscle symptoms
Adefovir dipivoxil	Low–Moderate/ Moderate	10 mg once daily	Nephrotoxicity possible; monitor renal function and phosphate; adjust dose for renal impairment

for 48 weeks. Advantages of Peg-IFN-α include a finite duration of therapy, the potential for sustained off-therapy virologic response, and the possibility of HBsAg seroclearance. The agent is administered by injection and is associated with systemic effects such as influenza-like symptoms and neuropsychiatric adverse events, including depression; therefore, it is contraindicated in patients with decompensated cirrhosis and in those with autoimmune disease.

Oral Nucleos(t)ide Analogs: When interferon-based therapy is contraindicated, poorly tolerated, or unsuccessful in achieving adequate viral suppression, long-term oral nucleos(t)ide analog therapy is advised (Table 30.2). Selection of an oral agent should be guided by the stage of liver disease, prior antiviral exposure and resistance profile, and renal function; adherence and the emergence of resistance must be monitored during therapy.

Treatment goals are focused primarily on sustained suppression of HBV DNA to undetectable levels. Secondary objectives include normalization of alanine aminotransferase (ALT), HBeAg seroconversion where applicable, and prevention of progression to cirrhosis and hepatocellular carcinoma (HCC). Monitoring is recommended at regular intervals: HBV DNA quantification and liver enzyme testing every 3–6 months, HBsAg quantitation at least annually, and HCC surveillance with abdominal ultrasound, with or without alpha-fetoprotein (AFP), every 6 months in patients at high risk.

In patients with cirrhosis, whether compensated or decompensated, antiviral therapy should be initiated irrespective of ALT or HBV DNA levels, and agents with a high barrier to resistance (entecavir or tenofovir) are preferred. In patients with renal impairment, tenofovir alafenamide is favored over TDF when available, and dose adjustments for entecavir and adefovir should be implemented according to creatinine clearance.

30.6.1.3 Pregnancy

Tenofovir disoproxil fumarate (TDF) and tenofovir alafenamide (TAF) are now established as first-line treatments during pregnancy. Both agents have demonstrated safety, with no increased risk of congenital anomalies. TAF has received approval based on recent clinical data showing birth defect rates comparable to those in the general population. Furthermore, studies confirm that tenofovir can be safely initiated in the first trimester, effectively achieving full viral suppression and preventing mother-to-child transmission.

The **2024 WHO guidelines** recommend:

- All HBsAg-positive pregnant women with HBV DNA >200,000 IU/mL should start TDF or TAF early, ideally before the second trimester.
- In settings without viral load testing, universal TDF prophylaxis is advised for all HBsAg-positive pregnant women.
- Women planning multiple pregnancies may continue treatment between pregnancies. For example, Canadian guidelines suggest immediate treatment for women planning pregnancy within 1–2 years, especially if over 30 with high viral loads. Initiating tenofovir (TDF or TAF) before conception maximizes viral suppression, reducing mother-to-child transmission risk and preventing hepatic disease progression, especially in women over 30 with longer infection duration. This approach leverages tenofovir's established safety profile in early pregnancy, avoids delays in viral control, and simplifies antenatal management by minimizing medication changes during gestation.

Lamivudine vs. Tenofovir: While lamivudine is effective, tenofovir (TDF/TAF) is preferred due to stronger antiviral effects and higher resistance barrier. Safety profiles are similar, but tenofovir offers superior viral suppression and is the recommended agent.

Interferon-α: Interferon-α is contraindicated during pregnancy due to teratogenicity but may be used postpartum if needed. Oral antivirals remain preferred for ongoing management.

30.6.1.4 Postpartum Period

Current evidence and guidelines, including those from the World Health Organization (WHO), affirm the safety of breastfeeding among HBsAg-positive mothers under appropriate conditions:

- Breastfeeding is considered safe when infants have received appropriate immunoprophylaxis, comprising hepatitis B immune globulin (HBIG) and the hepatitis B vaccine administered promptly after birth.
- Mothers may continue antiviral therapy during breastfeeding, especially with nucleos(t)ide analogs such as tenofovir disoproxil fumarate (TDF) and lamivudine, without contraindication.
- Although small quantities of antiviral agents are excreted into breast milk, no adverse effects have been documented in nursing infants.

Recent pharmacokinetic studies demonstrate that concentrations of tenofovir in breast milk are substantially lower than maternal serum levels and are unlikely to exert any biological effect on the infant. A prospective study following infants breastfed by mothers on TDF therapy for up to 96 weeks revealed no abnormal clinical signs or symptoms attributable to drug exposure.

Postpartum Management and Breastfeeding Support
- Antiviral therapy should be continued postpartum, particularly in mothers with high HBV viral loads, to reduce the risk of hepatic flares and maintain viral suppression.
- Breastfeeding should be actively supported while mothers continue tenofovir or tenofovir alafenamide (TAF) therapy, given the established safety profile.
- Infants must receive HBIG and the first dose of hepatitis B vaccine within 12 h of birth to maximize prophylactic efficacy against vertical transmission.
- Infants should undergo clinical monitoring and serologic testing for HBV infection and immunity status between 9 and 12 months of age to confirm effective immunoprophylaxis and absence of infection.

30.6.2 Hepatitis D

Causal treatment for HDV infection remains challenging and is generally associated with the successful treatment of chronic hepatitis B. The efficacy of newer therapeutic interventions for HDV infection remains to be determined.

While treatment with nucleoside analogons to reduce the high viral load in hepatitis B is theoretically feasible, it is unlikely to impact HDV RNA levels.

30.7 Differential Diagnosis

The differential diagnosis of hepatitis B includes other viral hepatitis forms such as hepatitis A, C, and E, along with nonviral causes like alcoholic hepatitis, drug-induced hepatitis, autoimmune hepatitis, and nonalcoholic fatty liver disease (NASH). Additionally, other liver diseases, including cirrhosis, liver tumors, and liver failure, as well as systemic diseases with liver involvement like Wilson's disease, hemochromatosis, and alpha-1-antitrypsin deficiency, should be considered. Clinical symptoms, laboratory values, serologic markers, imaging studies, and, if necessary, liver biopsy play critical roles in identifying the underlying cause of hepatic injury.

30.8 Prevention

30.8.1 Hepatitis B

30.8.1.1 Primary Prevention: Objective—Prevention of New Infection Through Immunization and Behavioral Measures

Vaccination: Recombinant inactivated HBsAg vaccines are administered at 0, 1, and 6 months; an accelerated 0, 1, 2-month series with a 12-month booster may be employed for urgent situations. Vaccination is recommended for newborns, infants (often included in hexavalent formulations), persons with occupational or medical exposure, dialysis and transplant recipients, individuals with HIV, HCV, or diabetes mellitus, and travelers to areas with HBsAg prevalence >2%. Anti-HBs titers are to be measured 1–2 months after completion of the primary series in at-risk persons; if concentrations <10 IU/L are found, additional vaccine doses or a booster are indicated.

Behavioral Precautions: Standard precautions are to be applied to prevent parenteral transmission: disposable gloves, eye protection, appropriate protective clothing, and safe sharps handling and disposal. Sexual transmission risk is to be reduced by consistent condom use and by avoidance of unprotected intercourse with partners of unknown serostatus. Sharing of potentially blood-contaminated items (e.g., razors and toothbrushes) is to be avoided. Blood and plasma donations are screened for HBV DNA. Patients are to be counseled regarding infection risks associated with tattoos, piercings, and traditional practices, and providers performing such procedures should be verified to adhere to hygienic standards.

30.8.1.2 Secondary Prevention: Objective—Early Detection and Interruption of Transmission Routes

Screening: Diagnostic testing for HBsAg, anti-HBs, and anti-HBc is recommended in relevant circumstances (e.g., after percutaneous exposure). Targeted screening is advised for healthcare and emergency personnel, dialysis patients, pregnant women during prenatal care, and persons with known HIV or HCV infection.

Post-exposure Prophylaxis (PEP): After needlestick injury or exposure to infectious blood, unvaccinated persons should be given the hepatitis B vaccine series (0, 1, and 6 months) and immediate passive immunization with HBIG; additional HBIG or a 4-week vaccine dose may be administered according to exposure risk and serology. Partially vaccinated persons should have the series completed and may receive a single HBIG dose depending on exposure and serologic status. For fully vaccinated persons, anti-HBs titers are to be measured; if <10 IU/L, a booster dose should be considered and further management individualized. PEP decisions are to be guided by risk assessment including the source's HBsAg status.

30.8.1.3 Tertiary Prevention: Objective—Prevention of Complications in Chronic Infection

Management of Chronically HBsAg-Positive Patients: Chronic HBsAg-positive patients are monitored regularly with liver enzymes (ALT and AST), serum bilirubin, and HBV DNA quantification; treatment indications are determined by viral replication, transaminase elevations, and fibrosis stage. Antiviral therapy (e.g., tenofovir disoproxil fumarate, tenofovir alafenamide, or entecavir) is initiated when indicated. Hepatocellular carcinoma surveillance is performed with hepatic ultrasound, with or without alpha-fetoprotein, at 6-month intervals in patients with advanced fibrosis, cirrhosis, or other risk factors.

Education and Lifestyle Interventions: Patients are counseled to abstain from alcohol or to substantially reduce intake. Household contacts and close contacts are to be screened for immune status and vaccinated if susceptible; post-exposure or pre-exposure prophylaxis is to be provided when indicated. Psychosocial support is offered to optimize adherence to therapy.

The effectiveness of hepatitis B prevention is ensured by consistent vaccination aligned to individual risk profiles, strict hygiene practices in healthcare and community settings, timely risk-based post-exposure prophylaxis, and structured chronic disease monitoring with antiviral intervention when warranted.

30.8.1.4 Recommended Standard Hepatitis B Vaccinations for Infants, Children, and Adolescents

Vaccination: The objective of hepatitis B vaccination from infancy through adolescence is to prevent acute HBV infection and long-term complications such as cirrhosis and hepatocellular carcinoma. Recombinant HBsAg vaccines are used for primary immunization (Table 30.3). Vaccination is routinely initiated in infancy, either as a monovalent vaccine or within combination (e.g., hexavalent) formulations, and is usually administered on a 0–1–6-month schedule. Accelerated schedules are employed when exposure risk is elevated. The standard adult schedule is 0, 1, and 6 months; accelerated schedules are available when rapid protection is required. Higher antigen doses or additional doses are recommended for hemodialysis and immunocompromised patients to improve seroconversion.

Table 30.3 Monovalent preparations: dosage, schedules, and boosters

Preparation	Dose	Standard schedule	Accelerated schedule	Booster/remarks
Engerix® B	20 µg	0, 1, 6 months	0, 1, 2 months; booster at 12 months	Booster every 5–10 years if at risk; standard vaccine with high seroprotection; suitable for pregnant women and immunosuppressed
HBVAXPRO® Paed.	10 µg	0, 1, 6 months	0, 1, 2 months; booster at 12 months	Booster every 5–10 years if at risk; licensed for children; good immunogenicity in childhood; multiple dosage forms available
HBVAXPRO®	5/10/40 µg	0, 1, 6 months	0, 1, 2 months; booster at 12 months	Booster every 5–10 years if at risk; doses adjusted for children/adults; higher dose for high-risk adults (dialysis/immunosuppression); protection against liver cancer
Sci B Vac®	10 µg + PreS	0, 1, 6 months	0, 1, 2 months; booster at 12 months	Booster every 5–10 years based on risk; contains PreS1/PreS2 antigens; effective for non-responders; broader immune coverage
Fendrix®	20 µg (adult)	0, 1, 2, 6 months	—	Especially for high-risk patients (dialysis/renal insufficiency); booster every 5–10 years; high antibody persistence; four-dose schedule recommended
Heplisav-B®	20 µg (adult)	0, 1 months	—	Booster every 5 years if at risk; CpG adjuvant; two-dose schedule with rapid protection; adults only; usually no routine booster needed
Twinrix® (HAV+HBV)	20 µg (HBV)	0, 1, 6 months	0, 7, 21–30 days; booster at 12 months	Recommended only for high-risk individuals; combined hepatitis A+B vaccine; mainly for travelers; booster only if risk persists

Revaccinations: Catch-up vaccination is provided for older children and adolescents who remain susceptible. Post-vaccination anti-HBs testing is recommended 1–3 months after completion of the primary series for persons at increased risk; an anti-HBs concentration ≥10 IU/L denotes protective immunity. Individuals with anti-HBs <10 IU/L should receive revaccination according to national protocols (repeat a full primary series or additional doses as specified) and undergo repeat serologic testing to confirm seroconversion. Routine booster doses are not indicated for immunocompetent adults who achieved protective titers; periodic monitoring and booster administration are advised for hemodialysis patients, transplant recipients, other immunosuppressed persons, and similar high-risk groups.

Contraindications: These are limited to acute severe febrile illness and documented allergy to vaccine components. Vaccination should be recorded in official immunization records, and guardians or adolescents should be educated regarding benefits and follow-up. Combination vaccines that include hepatitis B also confer protection against diphtheria, tetanus, pertussis, poliomyelitis, *Haemophilus influenzae* type b, and in some formulations, pneumococcus. Accelerated schedules with an additional early dose (third or fourth month) are utilized for short-term travel or other high-risk situations.

30.8.1.5 Legal Regulations and Recommendations Outside Pregnancy

Screening for hepatitis B in adults is targeted to persons with epidemiologic or clinical risk factors rather than performed universally. Indications include healthcare workers with blood-exposure risk, chronic hemodialysis patients, people who inject drugs, sexual or household contacts of HBsAg-positive individuals, persons from high-endemic regions, people living with HIV, candidates for immunosuppression or transplantation, pregnant women, and those with unexplained transaminase elevation. A serologic panel (HBsAg, anti-HBs, and anti-HBc) is performed when indicated; HBV DNA and HBeAg/anti-HBe testing are reserved for viremia and disease-activity assessment. Screening intervals and assays are to be determined by national guidance and local infection-control policies, and results must be documented to inform vaccination, counseling, or treatment.

Mandatory reporting for hepatitis B is required to support surveillance, contact tracing, and prevention. Clinicians and laboratories must notify confirmed or suspected cases to public health authorities within legally prescribed timeframes, providing essential data such as patient identifiers, key clinical findings, laboratory results (HBsAg, HBV DNA if available), vaccination status, and exposure history. Reporting enables identification of contacts for testing, post-exposure prophylaxis, or vaccination and informs outbreak response. Data protection and confidentiality must be maintained, and local statutory requirements (e.g., national infection notification laws) should be followed for specific reporting procedures and timelines.

30.8.1.6 Legal Regulations and Recommendations During Pregnancy

Screening: In many jurisdictions, antenatal HBsAg screening is routine and is performed at the first prenatal visit (Table 30.4); repeat testing in the third trimester is advised when ongoing exposure risk or local guidance indicates. Positive results must be reported to public-health authorities and communicated immediately to obstetric and neonatal teams to arrange maternal antiviral therapy if indicated and to ensure neonatal hepatitis B immunoglobulin and timely vaccination. Maternal status, counseling, and planned peripartum measures must be documented while maintaining consent and data-protection requirements.

Vaccination During Pregnancy: Vaccination during pregnancy is not routinely recommended in most countries (Table 30.4). Women lacking prior immunity, who exhibit high-risk behaviors or have documented exposure, are to be offered vaccination. The same recombinant HBsAg vaccines and schedules as used in nonpregnant adults are to be employed; initiation is preferred in the second or third trimester for safety considerations. In select jurisdictions (e.g., Canada and Australia), vaccination may be offered during pregnancy after clinical risk assessment. Routine antenatal vaccination without identified risk is not advised.

Table 30.4 Legal regulations and recommendations during pregnancy for hepatitis B

Country	Screening timing	Vaccination during pregnancy	Newborn management
Australia	Universal early pregnancy	Not routine; risk-based vaccination	HBIG + vaccine within 12 h; vaccines at 2, 4, 6 months
Canada	Universal early pregnancy	Not routine; offered if high risk	HBIG + vaccine within 12 h; vaccines at 1, 2, 6, 12 months
China	Universal early pregnancy	Not routine	HBIG + vaccine within 12 h; vaccines at 1, 2, 7 months
France	Universal first trimester	Not routine	HBIG + vaccine within 12 h; vaccines at 1, 6, 12 months
Germany	Mandatory first trimester; third trimester	Not routine	HBIG + vaccine within 12 h; vaccines at 1, 2, 6 months
India	Risk-based; moving toward universal	Not routine	HBIG + vaccine within 24 h; vaccines per national schedule (6, 10, 14 weeks + booster)
Italy	Universal first trimester	Not routine	HBIG + vaccine within 12 h; vaccines at 1, 6, 12 months
Japan	Universal early pregnancy	Not routine	HBIG + vaccine within 12 h; vaccines at 1, 6 months
Switzerland	First trimester; repeat if risk	Not routine	HBIG + vaccine within 12 h; vaccines at 1, 2, 12 months
UK	Universal 8–12 weeks gestation	Not routine	HBIG + vaccine within 24 h if high risk; vaccines at 1, 2, 12 months
USA	Universal early pregnancy	Not routine	HBIG + vaccine within 12 h; vaccines at 1, 6 months

Reporting Obligations During Pregnancy: Maternal HBsAg positivity must be reported promptly to public-health authorities per legal timelines. Reports should include identifiers, test result, gestational age, and brief exposure/clinical history and be communicated to obstetric, neonatal, and infectious-disease teams to ensure timely maternal antiviral therapy (if indicated) and newborn post-exposure prophylaxis. Confidentiality must be maintained and notification, counseling, and planned interventions documented in the maternal record.

30.8.1.7 Newborns of HBsAg-Positive Mothers

- Passive-active immunoprophylaxis with hepatitis B immune globulin (HBIG) plus the first dose of hepatitis B vaccine is considered standard care in most countries (Table 30.5). Continuation of the vaccine series is to follow national immunization schedules, commonly at 1 and 6 months or as part of combination vaccines. Several active and passive immunization products are currently available (Table 30.5).

Table 30.5 Active and passive immunization in newborns born to mothers with hepatitis B (Note: Current national guidelines and product specifics must be observed)

Immunization type	Examples	Active class	Ingredient/dose/schedule and mechanism
Passive immunization	Hepatitis B immunoglobulin (HBIG)	Human immunoglobulin (anti-HBs IgG)	Usually 30–100 IU/kg IM (commonly 1 mL = 200 IU); single dose within 12 h postpartum. Provides immediate protection via passive antibody transfer
	Médihép HBIG®	Human immunoglobulin (anti-HBs IgG)	Single IM injection of 0.5–1 mL (100–200 IU); immediate passive immunity through specific antibody transfer
	Bayhep Hepatitis B Immunoglobulin	Human immunoglobulin (anti-HBs IgG)	Single IM dose of 0.5–1 mL; passive immunity by direct antibody transfer
	CSL Behring HBIG	Human immunoglobulin (>200 IU/mL)	Single dose IM at usual dose per body weight providing immediate protection via anti-HBs antibodies

(continued)

Table 30.5 (contiuned)

Immunization type	Examples	Active class	Ingredient/dose/schedule and mechanism
Active immunization	Engerix B Paediatric	Recombinant HBsAg produced in *Saccharomyces cerevisiae* yeast	Dose: 10 μg/0.5 mL; schedule: 0, 1, 6 months or alternatively 0, 1, 2, and 12 months. Induces active immunity with long-lasting anti-HBs antibody production
	HBVAXPRO® Paediatric	Recombinant HBsAg produced in *Saccharomyces cerevisiae* yeast	Dose: 5 μg/0.5 mL; schedule same as above. Induces active antibody formation
	Sci B Vac® Paediatric	Recombinant HBsAg plus PreS1/PreS2 antigens	Dose: 5 μg/0.5 mL; schedule: 0, 1, 6 months. Enhanced antigen presentation via PreS antigens improves immunogenicity
	Twinrix® Paediatric (HAV+HBV)	Recombinant HBsAg (10 μg) plus HAV antigen	Dose: 0.5 mL; schedule: 0, 1, and 6 months from age 1 year onward. Simultaneous induction of immunity against HAV and HBV via combined antigen administration
	Hexavalent vaccines	Includes HBsAg plus DTaP IPV Hib components	Schedule typically at months 2, 4, and 11 or 2, 3, 4, and 11 for preterm infants. Provides combined protection inducing multiple specific immune responses simultaneously

- Maternal HBV DNA quantification is to be performed; antiviral therapy (most commonly tenofovir) is initiated in pregnancy when viral load exceeds defined thresholds (typically ≥200,000 IU/mL), generally beginning in the late second trimester to reduce vertical transmission risk. Country-specific postpartum protocols for continuation of the infant series are to be applied.
- All infants born to HBsAg-positive mothers are to receive HBIG plus hepatitis B vaccine. If maternal HBsAg status is discovered after delivery, HBIG

administration may be provided up to 7 days postpartum. Premature infants are to be vaccinated with schedule adjustments based on gestational age and birth weight.

- Anti-HBs titers are to be measured 4–8 weeks after completion of the primary series; if levels <10 IU/L are detected, a booster dose is to be given and serology repeated.

Vaccination against hepatitis B during pregnancy can safely occur with recombinant vaccines, posing no risk to the mother or the child.

All newborns of HBsAg-positive mothers should receive concomitant immunoprophylaxis with hepatitis B immunoglobulin and the hepatitis B vaccine (10 μg within 12 h, followed by doses at 1 and 6 months postpartum) immediately after delivery and within 12 h of birth (Table 30.2).

- If the mother is subsequently found to be HBsAg-positive, hepatitis B immunoglobulin can be administered to the newborn within 7 days of birth. Premature infants can also receive vaccination.
- After active and passive immunization, breastfeeding can proceed. There is no necessity for maternal and infant separation after birth.
- These preventive measures can reduce infection rates by 85–95%, depending on HBeAg/anti-HBe status and replication level.

The transmission of the hepatitis B virus from mothers who are positive for both HBeAg and HBV-DNA to their newborns is highly probable. Therefore, the consideration of cesarean delivery, combined with simultaneous passive and active immunoprophylaxis, is being explored as an improved preventive strategy, especially in cases where the viral load is extremely high.

Tenofovir disoproxil fumarate (TDF) and tenofovir alafenamide (TAF) are now established as first-line treatments during pregnancy. Both agents have demonstrated safety, with no increased risk of congenital anomalies.

30.8.2 Hepatitis D

Exposure prophylaxis mirrors that of hepatitis B. HBsAg carriers should receive detailed counseling about appropriate precautions when traveling to endemic areas.

Though perinatal transmission to the infant is rare. However, timely postnatal hepatitis B vaccination is crucial as it protects against both hepatitis B and perinatal transmission of hepatitis D. Prevention measures should be applied regardless of the mother's HBV status if there is any suspicion of hepatitis D.

Active immunization against HBV provides protection against hepatitis D. Consequently, pre-exposure and post-exposure active immunizations should be administered concurrently.

Key Points

- The hepatitis B virus (HBV) is the causative agent of hepatitis B and is primarily transmitted via blood transfusions, contaminated needles, sexual contact, and vertical transmission from mother to child. The hepatitis D virus (HDV) can only infect individuals with HBV or can be transmitted concurrently with HBV.
- It is estimated that 300–350 million people worldwide live with chronic HBV infection, with the highest prevalence observed in Africa (8.8%) and the Western Pacific (5.3%).
- The rate of vertical transmission is contingent on the mother's viremia, while intrauterine prenatal diaplacental transmission is rare.
- Clinical manifestations of hepatitis B can be both acute and chronic. Acute cases are often asymptomatic but may progress to chronic infection, which increases the risks of cirrhosis and hepatocellular carcinoma.
- Coinfection of HBV with HDV can lead to severe disease progression. Diagnosis is based on the detection of anti-HDV antibodies and the quantification of HDV RNA.
- Serologic and molecular biological tests are employed to diagnose hepatitis B, and screening during pregnancy is critical to prevent transmission to the newborn.
- Treatment of hepatitis B incorporates symptomatic measures for acute cases and interferon-alpha and nucleoside/nucleotide analogons in chronic cases. Tenofovir disoproxil fumarate (TDF) and tenofovir alafenamide (TAF) are now established as first-line treatments during pregnancy. Both agents have demonstrated safety, with no increased risk of congenital anomalies.
- Preventive measures encompass screening programs, vaccination, and avoidance of risk factors to decrease the incidence of hepatitis B. Vaccination against HBV also protects against HDV.

Hepatitis C

31

Abstract

Hepatitis C is a significant disease caused by the hepatitis C virus (HCV), which can persist chronically and affects approximately 170 million individuals worldwide. The primary modes of transmission include contact with infected blood and blood products. Acute infections may be asymptomatic, resulting in a frequent lack of diagnosis. Chronic HCV infection can cause liver damage and cirrhosis. The virus is characterized by a diverse range of genotypes, necessitating genotype-specific treatments that include novel antiviral agents. While a cure is achievable, there is currently no vaccine available, underscoring the importance of prevention. Universal screening during pregnancy is not routinely recommended in many countries due to the low prevalence of HCV and a minimal vertical transmission rate.

31.1 Background

Hepatitis C represents the most prevalent infectious disease transmitted parenterally through blood or blood products. Globally, approximately 170 million persons (around 3% of the population) are chronically infected with HCV.

Definition of Hepatitis C

- **Active hepatitis C**
  - HCV infection contracted within the preceding six months, which may be accompanied by elevated aminotransferase activity and potential reductions in liver function.

I. Mylonas, *Sexually Transmitted Diseases*,
https://doi.org/10.1007/978-3-031-78204-6_31

- **Chronic hepatitis C**
  - Characterized as a persistent liver infection lasting six months or longer, as evidenced by the continuous presence of HCV RNA.
  - This condition may lead to a spectrum of clinical, biochemical, and histological effects, including extrahepatic manifestations.

Due to the pronounced tendency for chronicity, the often-subclinical nature of the disease, and the limited efficacy of antiviral treatments, early diagnosis and ongoing monitoring are critical.

31.2 Pathogen

Hepatitis C virus (HCV) is an enveloped, positive-sense RNA virus belonging to the "Flaviviridae" family. Virions are spherical, with diameters ranging from approximately 40 to 60 nm, and consist of a lipid envelope studded with two viral glycoproteins, E1 and E2. Beneath this envelope lies the icosahedral nucleocapsid, which packages the viral genome and is detectable in patient serum during active infection. HCV exhibits extensive genetic diversity: to date, "eight major genotypes" (numbered 1–8) have been conclusively characterized, along with numerous subtypes (e.g., 1a and 1b) and a high degree of quasi-species variation within each infected individual. This heterogeneity has important implications for transmission patterns, disease progression, and treatment response.

The extensive genetic variability of HCV, manifesting as multiple genotypes, subtypes, and intra-host quasispecies, significantly impacts clinical management. Specific genotypes exhibit differing geographic distributions and show variable responses to direct-acting antiviral regimens. For example, genotype 1 historically required longer and more complex treatment courses compared with genotype 2 or 3, although current pangenotypic regimens have largely mitigated these differences. Continuous surveillance of emerging variants remains critical to ensure sustained efficacy of antiviral therapies.

31.3 Epidemiology

According to estimates from the World Health Organization (WHO), approximately 58 million individuals globally were chronically infected with HCV as of 2019. The regions of the Eastern Mediterranean and Europe are notably affected, with around 12 million infections recorded.

- **Global prevalence:** In recent years, the global prevalence of HCV has experienced a decline. In 2019, approximately 1.5 million new HCV infections were reported alongside 290,000 HCV-related deaths worldwide.

- **High-prevalence regions:**
  - **Asia:** Exhibits considerable HCV prevalence, often correlated with high rates of hepatitis B.
  - **Latin America:** Reports an overall HCV prevalence of 1.5%, with elevated rates observed in countries such as Mexico and Brazil.
- **Regional prevalence:**
  - **Europe:** The estimated prevalence of HCV antibodies stands at 1.1%, classifying Europe as a low-prevalence region. However, significant variability exists among European countries.
  - **Latin America:** The overall HCV prevalence is estimated at 1.5%, particularly in countries like Mexico and Brazil.
  - **Africa:** Antibody prevalence may reach as high as 5.3%.
- **High-risk groups:**
  - **Hemophiliacs:** Display a prevalence of HCV infection up to 90%.
  - **Intravenous Drug Users:** Prevalence ranges from 50% to 90%.
  - **Dialysis Patients:** Prevalence ranges from 5% to 30%.

The global and regional prevalence of HCV exhibits substantial variability, with the most considerable burdens identified in specific WHO regions and among high-risk populations. While Europe generally shows lower prevalence, important differences exist between individual countries. High-risk demographics, such as hemophiliacs, intravenous drug users, and dialysis patients, continue to demonstrate elevated rates of infection.

The most prevalent modes of HCV transmission encompass:
- Parenteral transmission through blood and blood products.
- Needlestick injuries and the use of contaminated needles.
- Sexual contact.

Intravenous drug use is recognized as a *significant risk factor* for the acquisition of HCV infection. Despite the implementation of relevant prevention strategies, the risk of HCV infection among drug users remains elevated. HCV transmission may also occur through household contact with blood-contaminated objects, with an estimated risk of transmission ranging from 1% to 5%. Therefore, HCV screening is recommended for individuals with close contact to an HCV-infected person (e.g., family members).

HCV can also be transmitted sexually, as the virus has been identified in both semen and vaginal secretions. Hence, sexual intercourse is acknowledged as a crucial transmission route. However, the risk of infection within stable partnerships is extremely low, estimated at less than 1% per year. The risk of transmission increases with the number of sexual partners and specific sexual practices. Additionally, there exists a statistical correlation with positive syphilis, HBV, or HIV serology.

A total of 18 distinct HCV genotypes have been recognized, further classified into subtypes and strains. Genotypes 1–6 are the most prevalent, with genotype distribution showing considerable variability between nations and regions. For example, HCV genotype 1 accounts for approximately 60% of HCV infections in the United States, genotype 2 for over 50% of infections in China, genotype 3 for over 76% of HCV infections in India, and genotype 5 being the predominant genotype in South Africa.

Approximately 25–30% of individuals infected with HIV and up to 10% of those infected with HBV are also positive for HCV. Therefore, testing for HCV co-infection should be considered reasonable.

31.4 Clinical Manifestations

31.4.1 Gynecology

Hepatitis C virus infection may present as acute hepatitis, although symptomatic cases are uncommon. When symptoms occur, they typically develop after an incubation period and include jaundice, fatigue, nausea, and malaise. However, the majority of acute HCV infections remain asymptomatic or subclinical, contributing to delayed diagnosis and underrecognition.

Spontaneous viral clearance occurs in only 15–50% of cases, resulting in chronic infection in 50–85% of individuals. Chronic hepatitis C often remains clinically silent or presents with nonspecific complaints such as mild fatigue. Notably, up to 40% of patients with chronic HCV may have normal liver enzyme levels, complicating diagnosis if based solely on biochemical markers or clinical symptoms.

Progression to Chronic Disease and Associated Complications
Over 80% of patients with acute HCV infection progress to chronic hepatitis C, which may subsequently lead to progressive hepatic fibrosis and cirrhosis. Chronic HCV infection markedly increases the risk of hepatocellular carcinoma (HCC), a leading cause of liver-related morbidity and mortality.
During the acute phase, rare but serious complications have been reported, including:

- Acute pancreatitis
- Hematologic abnormalities such as aplastic anemia and agranulocytosis

Chronic hepatitis C is also linked to multiple extrahepatic manifestations, including:

- Mixed cryoglobulinemia, characterized by immune complex-mediated vasculitis with potential renal involvement
- Membranoproliferative glomerulonephritis, due to deposition of circulating immune complexes in glomeruli

- Sjögren's syndrome, an autoimmune exocrinopathy causing xerostomia and keratoconjunctivitis sicca
- Autoimmune thyroiditis (Hashimoto's thyroiditis), reported occasionally in HCV-infected patients
- Additional associations include autoimmune hepatitis, porphyria cutanea tarda, lichen planus, and periarteritis nodosa

Co-infection with Hepatitis B Virus (HBV)
HBV/HCV co-infection affects approximately one-third of HCV-infected patients, especially in regions with high endemicity for both viruses. This co-infection is associated with:

- An increased risk of accelerated progression to cirrhosis
- A substantially higher incidence of hepatocellular carcinoma compared to monoinfection

In patients with established cirrhosis, interferon-based therapies have demonstrated up to a sixfold reduction in HCC risk; however, this benefit is observed predominantly in those without HBV coinfection. The presence of HBV complicates clinical management and prognosis, highlighting the necessity for comprehensive viral screening and individualized treatment strategies.

> **Hepatitis C is a liver disease attributed to HCV that, if left untreated, can lead to severe complications including cirrhosis and liver cancer.**

31.4.2 Pregnancy

Horizontal and Vertical Transmission of Hepatitis C Virus (HCV)

- **Horizontal Transmission:** Intrafamilial horizontal transmission of HCV within households and sexual transmission are both rare events. The risk of sexual transmission between monogamous partners is very low; however, it is increased among individuals with multiple sexual partners, concurrent sexually transmitted infections, or HIV co-infection.
- **Viral Dynamics During Pregnancy:** Pregnancy induces a state of relative immunosuppression characterized by altered T-cell-mediated immunity and a shift toward Th2 immune responses. Consequently, HCV viral load typically rises during pregnancy, especially in the third trimester. In contrast, serum transaminase levels (ALT and AST) usually decline due to reduced immune-mediated hepatocyte injury. After delivery, immune function normalizes, and both viral load and transaminase levels return to pre-pregnancy baselines. Importantly, pregnancy does not significantly affect the clinical course of chronic hepatitis C infection.

- **Vertical (Perinatal) Transmission of HCV:** Current evidence indicates that mother-to-child transmission of HCV occurs more frequently than previously estimated. The overall perinatal transmission rate among HCV mono-infected mothers is approximately 7.2% (95% CI: 5.6–8.9%), exceeding prior estimates of 1–6%. This rate increases to about 12.1% (95% CI: 8.6–16.8%) in mothers co-infected with HIV.
- Prerequisites for Transmission:
  - Detectable maternal viremia (HCV RNA) is essential for vertical transmission to occur.
  - Although no definitive viral load threshold has been established, higher maternal HCV RNA levels (>1,000,000 IU/mL) correlate with increased transmission risk.
  - Rare cases exist of infant infection despite undetectable maternal HCV RNA; these cases remain exceptional.

The risk of perinatal infection of HCV from mother to child is about 1–6%.

Mode of Delivery and Transmission Risk

Extensive studies have demonstrated no significant difference in HCV vertical transmission rates between cesarean section and vaginal delivery. A meta-analysis encompassing eight international studies with 641 HCV-positive, HIV-negative mothers found no statistically significant reduction in transmission associated with cesarean delivery. Accordingly, many guidelines advise against cesarean section solely for the indication of maternal HCV infection.

No recommendation can presently be made regarding a prophylactic cesarean delivery for women infected with HCV.

Influence of Maternal HIV Co-infection

Maternal HIV co-infection substantially increases the risk of perinatal HCV transmission, with some studies reporting up to a 36-fold increase in odds. However, access to effective highly active antiretroviral therapy (HAART) during pregnancy significantly mitigates this risk, reducing transmission rates to levels comparable to those observed in HCV mono-infected mothers when HIV viral suppression is achieved.

Special Considerations in Multiple Births

In twin pregnancies complicated by vertical HCV transmission, infection more frequently affects the second-born twin or the twin with the higher birth weight. Proposed mechanisms include placental abruption or partial placental insufficiency affecting the second-born infant. Cesarean delivery does not appear to reduce transmission risk to either twin in these cases.

Infant Screening and Diagnosis

- **Diagnostic Challenges:** A diagnostic window exists wherein HCV RNA may be intermittently detectable or undetectable during the early postnatal period. Sensitivity of HCV PCR testing is approximately 22% during the first months due to low or intermittent viremia. Sensitivity improves to 70–85% after 1 month of age.
- **Recommended Screening Schedule:** HCV RNA testing at 6 months of age is optimal for reliable diagnosis. For infants born to mothers positive for anti-HCV antibodies but negative for HCV RNA, anti-HCV antibody testing at 15 months is recommended to confirm clearance of maternal antibodies and exclude infection.
- **Spontaneous Clearance:** Recent data indicate spontaneous resolution of HCV infection in up to 65.9% of perinatally infected infants, with only 3.9% remaining chronically infected by 5 years of age.

At present, cord blood testing is not considered to be a reliable indicator of fetal or infant infection, and therefore, it is not recommended as a diagnostic tool.

31.5 Diagnosis

The “indirect detection of HCV infection” is primarily performed by identifying “virus-specific antibodies in serum.” This is most commonly achieved through “enzyme-linked immunosorbent assay (ELISA)” screening tests. When ELISA results are positive or indeterminate, “confirmatory testing with immunoblotting techniques,”” such as the recombinant immunoblot assay (RIBA), is employed to verify seropositivity (see Table 31.1).

It is critical to note that the mere “presence of HCV antibodies does not differentiate between acute, chronic, or resolved infection,” nor does it predict immunity. Therefore, “quantitative detection of HCV RNA” via nucleic acid amplification tests is essential in various clinical contexts:

- In “acute hepatitis C cases where antibodies may not yet be detectable (seronegative window period).
- “Perinatal infection diagnosis.
- To assess “infectivity in asymptomatic anti-HCV-positive carriers.”
- To guide initiation, monitoring, and efficacy evaluation of antiviral therapy.
- To determine the “viral genotype,” which is critical for tailoring treatment regimens (Table 31.2).

Due to typically “low levels of free virus in serum,” “direct detection of HCV antigens” is not a feasible or reliable diagnostic approach. Instead, advanced

Table 31.1 Evaluation of diagnostic methods for hepatitis C virus (HCV) infection

Test	Material	Rating
HCV ELISA	Serum	– Sensitive search test
		– Antibody formation starts after 4–6 weeks at the earliest (usually 2–6 months!)
		– Positive results should be checked with a specific method (e.g., immunoblot) due to possible false positive results
		– Causes of false-positive findings include paraproteinemia, autoantibodies, and EBV infections
		– Cannot distinguish between acute, chronic (infectious), or cured (no longer infectious) disease
HCV immunoblot	Serum	– Confirmation test
		– Interpretation of band pattern allows for differential diagnosis between disease and non-specific reaction
		– If a specific band is detected, the result is questionable and control is recommended
		– If more than one specific band is detected, the result is positive
		– Cannot distinguish between acute, chronic (infectious), or cured (no longer infectious) disease
HCV PCR	EDTA blood	– Indications include antibody-positive patients, differential diagnosis of acute or cured hepatitis, fresh infection before the appearance of antibodies, diagnosis/progression of a chronic infection without antibody detection, and unclear serological findings
		– Currently the only available method to detect activity and infectivity of hepatitis C disease

ELISA enzyme-linked immunosorbent assay, *PCR* polymerase chain reaction

Table 31.2 Serological results in HCV testing

HCV RNA/ antigen	HCV antibodies (IgG + IgM)	Infection status
–	–	No infection
+	–	Acute infection
+	?	Acute infection
+	+	Acute or chronic infection
–	+	Cured (spontaneously or at least 6 months after the end of therapy)

antibody assays utilizing various "recombinant viral proteins" allow for "high sensitivity and specificity." Earlier generations of these tests were prone to false positives related to "cross-reactivity with sera from patients with hypergammaglobulinemia, paraproteinemia, or autoimmune hepatitis," but such occurrences are now rare owing to improved assay design and specificity. This progress has facilitated notably "earlier detection of acute HCV infections."

Breastfeeding and the Potential Risk of HCV Transmission

The possibility of "HCV transmission through breast milk" remains a relevant clinical question, especially given concerns about vertical transmission. At present, there is "no compelling evidence that HCV is transmitted via breastfeeding." However, data remain limited and somewhat inconsistent, stemming from variable results of HCV RNA detection in breast milk samples.

In clinical practice, if a mother's "anti-HCV antibody status is unknown or uncertain," it is recommended to perform "HCV RNA testing on maternal serum prior to initiating breastfeeding." In cases where HCV RNA is detectable, individualized counseling regarding the "potential but low risk of transmission" may be warranted, and discussions surrounding the possibility of weaning should be undertaken collaboratively with the mother and her healthcare providers.

Despite these uncertainties, current international guidelines generally "encourage breastfeeding in HCV-infected mothers," considering the well-established benefits of breastfeeding and the lack of definitive evidence of transmission through breast milk.

In cases of HCV infection, breastfeeding may not need to be discouraged, provided there is no inflammation or injury to the nipple. However, women co-infected with HIV and HCV, as well as individuals with a history of drug abuse, should refrain from breastfeeding.

31.6 Treatment

31.6.1 Acute Hepatitis C Virus Infection: Natural History and Treatment Evolution

Acute hepatitis C virus (HCV) infection may either **resolve spontaneously** or progress to **chronic infection**. Spontaneous viral clearance occurs in approximately **10–50% of cases**, with variability influenced by factors including symptom presence, host gender, genetic determinants of both the virus and the host immune response, and possibly ethnicity. Infection persisting beyond **6 months** is classified as **chronic HCV infection**.

Historically, treatment of HCV relied on the use of **pegylated interferon-α (PEG-interferon-α)** to stimulate the host immune response and suppress viral replication. Two formulations have been commonly used:

- **PEG-interferon-α 2a** administered at **180 µg subcutaneously once weekly** for 24 weeks
- **PEG-interferon-α 2b** dosed at **1.5 µg/kg subcutaneously once weekly** for similar durations

These interferon-based regimens were often combined with **ribavirin** to enhance antiviral efficacy. Response rates in acute HCV infection during the interferon era ranged between **85% and 98%**, with **sustained virologic response (SVR)**—defined as undetectable HCV RNA by PCR 24 weeks after treatment completion (SVR24)—indicating virological cure. It is important to note that the term SVR5 in your text is likely a typographical error; the accepted endpoint in interferon-based therapy was SVR24.

Acute HCV infection itself is *not typically associated with increased mortality*, but the risk of chronicity presents significant long-term morbidities including cirrhosis, hepatocellular carcinoma, and liver failure.

31.6.2 Advances in Direct-Acting Antiviral (DAA) Therapy

Therapeutic approaches to HCV have been revolutionized in recent years by the advent of **direct-acting antivirals (DAAs)**, which directly inhibit viral enzymes essential for replication. These agents have rendered most interferon-based treatments obsolete due to substantially higher efficacy, improved safety profiles, and shorter treatment durations. Currently, **over 95%** of chronic hepatitis C cases can achieve cure with **interferon-free DAA regimens**.
DAA therapy is now individualized based on:

- Viral genotype
- Stage of liver disease (fibrosis/cirrhosis)
- Baseline viral load
- Other patient-specific characteristics such as prior treatment history and comorbidities

Commonly used DAAs include **sofosbuvir, ledipasvir, velpatasvir, glecaprevir, pibrentasvir, elbasvir, grazoprevir**, and the adjunctive **ribavirin** in select cases. Treatment durations typically range from **8 to 24 weeks**, adapted to regimen, genotype, and disease severity (refer to Table 31.3 for detailed regimen and duration guidance).

Given the continuous advancements in diagnostic techniques and therapeutic options for hepatitis C, consultation with or referral to a hepatology or infectious disease specialist is strongly recommended to ensure optimal patient management.

Table 31.3 Treatment options for chronic hepatitis C

Genotype	Medication	Duration
Genotype 1	Elbasvir 50 mg/grazoprevir 100 mg (combination) orally once daily ± ribavirin 500–600 mg orally twice daily	12–16 weeks
	Glecaprevir 300 mg/pibrentasvir 120 mg (combination) orally once daily	8–16 weeks
	Ledipasvir 90 mg/sofosbuvir 400 mg (combination) orally once daily	8–24 weeks
	Paritaprevir 150 mg/ritonavir 100 mg/ombitasvir 25 mg (combination) orally once daily + dasabuvir 250 mg orally twice daily + ribavirin 500 to 600 mg orally twice daily	12–24 weeks
	Sofosbuvir 400 mg orally once daily + simeprevir 150 mg orally once daily ± ribavirin 500 to 600 mg orally twice daily	12–24 weeks
	Sofosbuvir 400 mg orally once daily + daclatasvir 60 mg orally once daily ± ribavirin 500 to 600 mg orally twice daily	12–24 weeks
	Velpatasvir 100 mg/sofosbuvir 400 mg (combination) orally once daily	12 weeks
Genotype 2	Glecaprevir 300 mg/pibrentasvir 120 mg (combination) orally once daily	8–16 weeks
	Sofosbuvir 400 mg orally once daily + daclatasvir 60 mg orally once daily	12–24 weeks
	Sofosbuvir 400 mg/velpatasvir 100 mg (combination) orally once daily	12 weeks
Genotype 3	Glecaprevir 300 mg/pibrentasvir 120 mg (combination) orally once daily	8–16 weeks
	Sofosbuvir 400 mg orally once daily + daclatasvir 60 mg orally once daily ± ribavirin 500 to 600 mg orally twice daily	12–24 weeks
	Sofosbuvir 400 mg/velpatasvir 100 mg (combination) orally once daily	12 weeks
Genotype 4	Elbasvir 50 mg/grazoprevir 100 mg (combination) orally once daily	12 weeks
	Glecaprevir 300 mg/pibrentasvir 120 mg (combination) orally once daily	8–16 weeks
	Ledipasvir 90 mg/sofosbuvir 400 mg (combination) orally once daily	12 weeks
	Paritaprevir 150 mg/ritonavir 100 mg/ombitasvir 25 mg (combination) orally once daily	12 weeks
	Velpatasvir 100 mg/sofosbuvir 400 mg (combination) orally once daily	12 weeks
Genotype 5 and 6	Glecaprevir 300 mg/pibrentasvir 120 mg (combination) orally once daily	8–16 weeks
	Ledipasvir 90 mg/sofosbuvir 400 mg (combination) orally once daily	12 weeks
	Velpatasvir 100 mg/sofosbuvir 400 mg (combination) orally once daily	12 weeks

31.6.3 Key Considerations in Hepatitis C Virus (HCV) Treatment

Treatment Selection and Duration

The selection of an antiviral regimen and its duration should be individualized based on several critical clinical factors (see Fig. 31.1):

- **Cirrhosis Status:** Patients with **compensated cirrhosis** usually tolerate standard DAA regimens administered over 8–12 weeks. Those with **decompensated cirrhosis** often require modified treatment approaches, including the addition of ribavirin and extended therapy duration. Management should be conducted by hepatology specialists due to increased complexity and risk.
- **Prior Treatment History:** Individuals with previous DAA treatment failure may necessitate more potent regimens, longer durations, or combinations targeting resistant viral strains to achieve viral eradication. Salvage therapies, such as triple combination regimens, are considered in these cases.
- **Resistance-Associated Substitutions (RAS):** Presence of RAS can diminish susceptibility to specific DAAs, particularly NS5A inhibitors. Resistance testing is advisable in select scenarios—such as treatment-experienced patients or those infected with genotype 1a—guiding regimen choice and duration. Extended treatment or ribavirin addition may be required to overcome resistance.
- **Comorbidities:** Coexisting conditions including HIV coinfection, chronic kidney disease, and immunosuppression influence regimen selection and monitoring strategies. For instance, some DAAs require dose adjustments or avoidance in severe renal impairment, whereas others are safe across a broad spectrum of comorbidities.

Treatment Duration

- Most contemporary DAA regimens provide high cure rates with **8–12 weeks** of therapy, even among patients with compensated cirrhosis or prior treatment history.

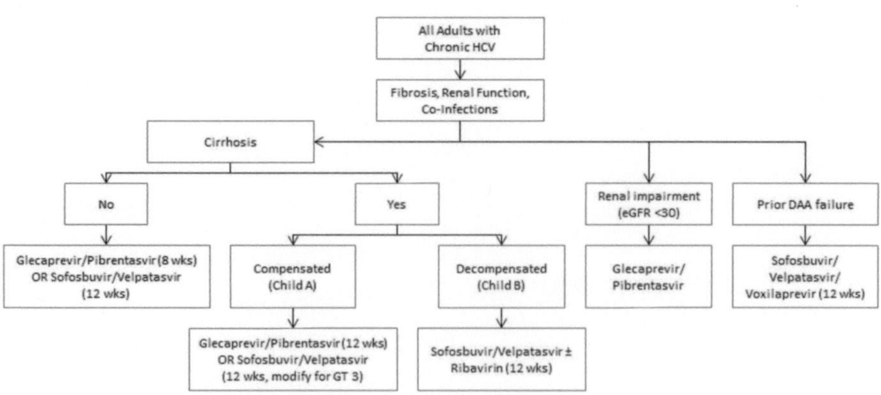

Fig. 31.1 Treatment decision algorithm for chronic hepatitis C

- **Treatment extension to 16–24 weeks** is reserved for complex clinical situations such as decompensated liver disease, significant RAS presence, or multiple prior treatment failures.

Ribavirin Use

- Ribavirin is no longer routinely recommended due to its adverse effect profile, particularly hemolytic anemia, but remains a valuable adjunct in selected contexts:
  - Patients with **decompensated cirrhosis**, where it enhances antiviral efficacy.
  - Certain **treatment-experienced individuals** harboring resistant viral variants may benefit from ribavirin addition to improve sustained virologic response rates.

Efficacy and Monitoring

- Direct-acting antivirals achieve **sustained virologic response (SVR) rates exceeding 95%**, equating to a functional cure of chronic HCV infection.
- SVR is defined as **undetectable HCV RNA 12 weeks after completion of therapy (SVR12)**, a robust predictor of long-term viral suppression.
- Routine monitoring includes:
  - Quantitative HCV RNA at baseline and 12 weeks post-treatment completion.
  - Additional on-treatment viral load assessments when clinically indicated.
  - Safety labs including liver function tests and hematologic profiles (especially if ribavirin is used). Renal function should be monitored in susceptible individuals.

Special Populations

- **Liver Transplant Recipients:** DAAs are highly effective in treating recurrent HCV posttransplantation. Attention to potential **drug–drug interactions with immunosuppressive agents** (e.g., tacrolimus and cyclosporine) is essential, necessitating close therapeutic drug monitoring.
- **HIV/HCV Coinfection:** Similar SVR rates (>95%) are achieved compared to HCV monoinfection. Coordination with antiretroviral therapy (ART) is critical to avoid clinically significant drug interactions and preserve HIV viral suppression.
- **Renal Impairment:** Regimens such as **glecaprevir/pibrentasvir** and **elbasvir/grazoprevir** are safe and effective in patients with severe renal impairment or on dialysis. Sofosbuvir-containing regimens require caution due to renal clearance of the drug and its metabolites; specialist consultation is advised for patients with eGFR <30 mL/min/1.73 m^2.

Future Directions in HCV Therapy

- **Shortened Regimens:** Emerging clinical trials are investigating ultra-short DAA courses (4–6 weeks), primarily for selected patients with low baseline viral loads and absence of advanced fibrosis or prior treatment failure.

- **Novel Antiviral Combinations:** Development of new agents aims to overcome resistant HCV variants and improve outcomes in difficult-to-treat populations, including patients with multidrug resistance or complex comorbidities.
- **Global Access Expansion:** Efforts continue to reduce costs and increase availability of DAAs worldwide, focusing on low- and middle-income countries where hepatitis C prevalence remains high but therapeutic access is limited.

31.6.4 Treatment Decision Algorithm: Chronic Hepatitis C

31.6.4.1 Step 1: Confirm Diagnosis and Complete Pre-treatment Assessment

- Confirm active infection with quantitative HCV RNA.
- Stage fibrosis by transient elastography (FibroScan), biopsy if indicated, or FIB-4/APRI.
- Screen for Coinfections: HIV, HBV (HBsAg, anti-HBc total; test HDV when HBsAg positive).
- Assess renal function (serum creatinine, eGFR, with attention to eGFR <30 mL/min/1.73 m^2).
- Other Baseline Tests: Liver function tests, INR, CBC (if ribavirin anticipated), pregnancy test, and hepatitis serologies.
- Review concomitant medications carefully for drug–drug interactions (antiretrovirals, immunosuppressants, statins, anticonvulsants, etc.).

31.6.4.2 Step 2: First-Line Regimens (Treatment-Naïve, Compensated Liver Disease). Preferred Pangenotypic Options

- **Glecaprevir 300 mg/Pibrentasvir 120 mg** (fixed-dose combination, three tablets once daily with food). Recommended Duration: 8 weeks for treatment-naïve patients without cirrhosis; 12 weeks for compensated cirrhosis or patients with prior treatment exposure.
- **Sofosbuvir 400 mg/Velpatasvir 100 mg** (fixed-dose combination, one tablet once daily). Recommended Duration: 12 weeks for all genotypes. In genotype 3 with cirrhosis or adverse predictors, consider 16 weeks of treatment or add ribavirin 500–600 mg orally twice daily for 12 weeks.

31.6.4.3 Step 3: Alternative Regimens (When Pangenotypics Unavailable or Contraindicated)

- **Ledipasvir 90 mg/Sofosbuvir 400 mg** (one tablet once daily). Duration: 12 weeks for genotypes 1, 4, 5, and 6; may shorten to 8 weeks in non-cirrhotic genotype 1 with low viral load.
- **Elbasvir 50 mg/Grazoprevir 100 mg** (one tablet once daily). Duration: 12 weeks for genotypes 1 and 4. Resistance testing is recommended for genotype 1a where available.

- **Paritaprevir 150 mg/Ritonavir 100 mg/Ombitasvir 25 mg** (once daily) plus **Dasabuvir 250 mg** (twice daily) with or without **ribavirin 500–600 mg** twice daily. Duration: 12–24 weeks. Legacy regimen for genotype 1 only.
- **Sofosbuvir 400 mg plus Daclatasvir 60 mg** (both once daily) with or without **ribavirin 500–600 mg** twice daily. Duration: 12–24 weeks. Useful in resource-limited settings, particularly for genotypes 2 and 3.

31.6.4.4 Step 4: Management of Special Populations

- **Renal Impairment (eGFR <30 mL/min/1.73 m² or dialysis):** Glecaprevir/Pibrentasvir is preferred. Sofosbuvir-containing regimens should generally be avoided or used only with specialist guidance.
- **Genotype 3 with Compensated Cirrhosis:** Either sofosbuvir/velpatasvir for 16 weeks or sofosbuvir/velpatasvir plus ribavirin 500–600 mg twice daily for 12 weeks (based on resistance profile and tolerability).
- **Decompensated Cirrhosis (Child-Pugh B–C):** Sofosbuvir/velpatasvir for 12 weeks with or without ribavirin 500–600 mg twice daily under hepatology supervision. Protease inhibitors (such as glecaprevir, grazoprevir, and voxilaprevir) are contraindicated. Patients should be evaluated for liver transplantation and managed for cirrhosis complications.
- **Prior DAA Treatment Failure:** Sofosbuvir 400 mg/velpatasvir 100 mg/voxilaprevir 100 mg (fixed-dose combination, one tablet daily with food) for 12 weeks across all genotypes.
- **Pregnancy:** DAAs are generally not recommended during pregnancy. Initiate treatment postpartum unless a specialist deems therapy essential during gestation.

31.6.4.5 Step 5: Treatment Monitoring and Endpoints

- **Primary Endpoint:** Sustained virologic response at 12 weeks post-treatment (SVR12), defined as undetectable HCV RNA.
- **Viral Monitoring:** HCV RNA at baseline and again 12 weeks after treatment completion. Additional on-treatment testing as clinically indicated.
- **Safety Monitoring:** Liver function tests, renal function as appropriate, and CBC if ribavirin is prescribed. Monitor for drug–drug interactions at each follow-up.
- **Post-SVR Management:** Patients with advanced fibrosis (F3–F4) or prior hepatocellular carcinoma require lifelong HCC surveillance with ultrasound (± AFP) every 6 months. Counsel all cured patients regarding alcohol abstinence, reinfection risks, and harm-reduction strategies.

31.6.5 Current Perspectives on Treatment of Acute HCV

Most cases of acute hepatitis C resolve spontaneously without treatment; hence, immediate antiviral therapy is not universally required. However, treatment may be indicated in certain clinical scenarios, including:

- Post-exposure prophylaxis, for example, after needlestick injuries in healthcare workers to accelerate viral clearance and reduce transmission risk.

- Patients with symptomatic or severe disease, where prompt viral eradication may improve clinical outcomes and reduce disease-related symptoms.

Despite the excellent outcomes with DAAs for chronic hepatitis C, there is limited evidence and experience regarding their use in acute HCV infection, and formal recommendations vary. Use of DAAs in acute infection is emerging but requires further supporting data.

31.6.6 Treatment Considerations During Pregnancy

All antiviral agents approved for HCV, including DAAs and ribavirin, are contraindicated during pregnancy due to insufficient safety data and potential teratogenicity (especially ribavirin). Similarly, pegylated interferon-based regimens are contraindicated in pregnancy. Therefore, for pregnant individuals with acute or chronic HCV infection, deferral of antiviral therapy until after delivery is generally advised unless benefits outweigh risks and specialist consultation is obtained.

No safe treatment options for hepatitis C are currently established during breastfeeding. The administration of ribavirin and interferon-alpha in the postpartum period is contraindicated due to their teratogenic potential and adverse side effect profiles. Furthermore, direct-acting antivirals (DAAs) are not recommended during lactation because of insufficient safety data. If maternal HCV treatment is considered essential during this period, breastfeeding cessation is advised prior to initiating therapy.

At present, no pharmacologic agents have received approval for the treatment of chronic hepatitis C during pregnancy. Antiviral therapy is generally deferred until the postpartum period owing to insufficient data regarding fetal safety and potential teratogenicity. During gestation, clinical management prioritizes close monitoring of maternal and fetal well-being, including serial quantitative assessments of maternal HCV RNA levels to evaluate viral activity.

31.7 Differential Diagnosis

If hepatitis C is suspected, alternative etiologies of hepatic injury should be excluded or differentiated. Differential diagnoses include viral hepatitides (hepatitis A, B, and E), alcoholic liver disease (alcoholic steatohepatitis), drug- or toxin-induced liver injury (hepatotoxicity), autoimmune hepatitis, primary biliary cholangitis, primary sclerosing cholangitis, nonalcoholic fatty liver disease, and other infectious causes such as Epstein–Barr virus (EBV) and cytomegalovirus (CMV).

31.8 Prevention

Despite extensive research, no effective vaccine against hepatitis C virus (HCV) has been developed and no HCV-specific immunoglobulin preparations are available. Consequently, prevention is principally predicated on exposure prophylaxis.

Primary Preventive Measures

- Avoidance of Blood Exposure: Contact with blood and blood products should be minimized to prevent transmission. Risks should be assessed and mitigated in clinical and nonclinical settings.
- Screening of Blood and Organ Donors: All blood and solid-organ donations should be screened for HCV to prevent transfusion- and transplant-associated transmission.
- General Hygiene Prophylaxis: Rigorous hygiene protocols should be implemented, including routine disinfection of surfaces and instruments potentially contaminated with blood or bodily fluids.
- Avoidance of Sharing Items Potentially Contaminated with Blood: Personal articles that may be contaminated with blood should not be shared; examples include razors, nail scissors, syringes, and toothbrushes. The sharing of dishes and cutlery is not considered a significant route of transmission.

Additional Considerations

- Standard precautions should be applied universally in healthcare environments, with appropriate use of personal protective equipment (PPE) and safe injection practices.
- Occupational exposures should be managed according to established postexposure protocols, including immediate wound care and timely reporting.
- Harm-reduction strategies (for example, needle and syringe programs and opioid substitution therapy) should be employed for people who inject drugs to reduce HCV transmission risk.

Given the low prevalence of HCV infection in many developed countries (less than 0.5%), the minimal vertical transmission rate (between 1% and 6%), and the effectiveness of preventive measures, universal screening for HCV infection during pregnancy is currently not recommended.

Key Points

- Hepatitis C is the most prevalent disease transmitted through blood and blood products globally.
- There are both acute and chronic forms of hepatitis C.
- The hepatitis C virus (HCV) belongs to the Flaviviridae family and comprises various genotypes.
- The prevalence of HCV infection varies by region and country.
- The main transmission routes are parenteral (through blood and blood products) and sexual.
- Risk groups for HCV infection include intravenous drug users, hemophiliacs, and dialysis patients.
- Acute hepatitis C is often asymptomatic, whereas chronic hepatitis C can lead to liver damage and extrahepatic manifestations.
- Vertical transmission of HCV from mother to child is rare but possible.
- Hepatitis C is diagnosed by detecting HCV antibodies and HCV RNA in the blood.
- Treatment for hepatitis C has significantly improved with the advent of novel antiviral drugs (DAAs).
- No specific drug treatments for hepatitis C have been approved during pregnancy or breastfeeding.
- There is currently no effective vaccine for hepatitis C.
- Exposure prophylaxis and hygiene measures are vital for preventing HCV transmission.
- Universal screening for HCV infection during pregnancy is not currently recommended.

HIV Infection and AIDS

32

Abstract

Infection with the human immunodeficiency virus (HIV) culminates in acquired immunodeficiency syndrome (AIDS). This global pandemic has approximately 35 million individuals infected, significantly affecting sub-Saharan Africa. Acute HIV infection typically presents with symptoms resembling mononucleosis, followed by a latency period during which opportunistic infections may arise. In the AIDS stage (stage C), severe infections and malignancies occur. Diagnosis is established through the detection of antibodies, antigens, and reverse transcriptase polymerase chain reaction (RT-PCR). The primary objective of therapy is to achieve complete suppression of HIV replication, which is accomplished through a combination of various classes of antiviral drugs. Pregnant women are provided with specific recommendations to minimize mother-to-child transmission of the virus. HIV screening during pregnancy has been implemented in many developed countries. Since no effective HIV vaccine is currently available, exposure prophylaxis remains a critical intervention.

32.1 Introduction

The definition of acquired immunodeficiency syndrome (AIDS) emerged from epidemiologic and clinical studies conducted in 1981. These studies revealed that high-risk groups, including homosexual men, intravenous drug users, and recipients of blood transfusions or blood products, were particularly vulnerable to the disease. The pathogen was isolated in 1983, subsequently identified as an RNA retrovirus known as the human immunodeficiency virus (HIV). The later identification of HIV-2 was attributed to its milder, more protracted course and lower transmission rates via sexual or perinatal routes.

I. Mylonas, *Sexually Transmitted Diseases*,
https://doi.org/10.1007/978-3-031-78204-6_32

The significance of HIV in gynecology and obstetrics is profound, as infection can have extensive implications for a woman's reproductive health. HIV-positive women necessitate specialized medical care and education to prevent complications during pregnancy, childbirth, and for the fetus. With advancements in treatment options, the rate of fetomaternal transmission of HIV in the Western world has decreased from approximately 15–20% without treatment to less than 2%. Nevertheless, HIV infection is associated with an increased risk of pregnancy complications, including preterm labor, premature delivery, and fetal growth restriction. As such, regular checkups and close collaboration among gynecologists, obstetricians, and HIV specialists are paramount.

Currently, HIV infection is not regarded as a contraindication for pregnancy.

32.2 Pathogen

HIV is categorized as a retrovirus within the lentivirus family and contains its genetic material as diploid single-stranded RNA (ssRNA). Lentiviruses are characterized by persistent viremia and prolonged clinically asymptomatic latency periods. HIV is classified into two main types: HIV-1 and HIV-2. Isolates of HIV-1 can be further divided into groups M and O, with the majority belonging to group M, which comprises ten distinct subtypes (A–J). These subtypes display variability in the viral genome and geographic distribution. Subtype B of HIV-1 predominates in Western Europe and North America, while all major HIV-1 subtypes and HIV-2 (subtypes A–E) are prevalent in Africa. HIV-2 infections are infrequent in Western Europe. Generally, HIV-2 exhibits lower pathogenicity and a significantly reduced risk of mother-to-child transmission.

The target cells for HIV include all human cells expressing the CD4 receptor. HIV may be transmitted in both cell-bound and cell-free forms, primarily affecting immune system cells such as:

- CD4-positive T lymphocytes (T helper cells)
- Cells of the monocyte–macrophage system (e.g., dendritic cells, dermal Langerhans cells, brain microglia, intestinal antigen-presenting cells)

Moreover, cells that exhibit passive CD4 receptors during their development and maturation can also become infected, such as:

- Bone marrow stem cells
- Thymic T cells
- CD8-positive cytotoxic T cells

Additionally, cells that possess only HIV coreceptors (e.g., neuronal and epithelial cells) may also be susceptible to infection.

A HIV infection ultimately leads to the acquired immune deficiency syndrome (AIDS). Integration of proviral HIV DNA into the host cell genome induces latent infection. The persistence of HIV within lymphoid tissues results in a gradual but progressive depletion of immunocompetent cells. As the disease advances, an abnormal increase in activation-induced lymphocyte apoptosis occurs, contributing to a global dysfunction of effector cells, ultimately manifesting clinically as AIDS. The terminal stage of the disease is characterized by extensive destruction of lymphatic organ architecture, resulting in a deficiency of competent immunoregulatory effector cells, which predisposes the organism to infections by opportunistic pathogens, autoimmune disorders, and malignancies.

32.3 Epidemiology

The spread of HIV has caused a global pandemic over recent decades. According to UNAIDS estimates, approximately 35 million individuals are currently living with HIV, while over 25 million have died from AIDS. The most pronounced impact of the disease is observed in southern Africa, where around 22.5 million (76%) of the HIV-infected population resides. In certain areas of southern Africa, the HIV infection rate among pregnant women exceeds 30%, with only a small fraction (approximately 9%) having access to medical care.

32.3.1 Global Perspective

- The epidemiology, prevalence, and incidence of HIV reveal considerable variation across different regions worldwide
  - **Prevalence:** UNAIDS reports that approximately 39 million individuals globally are living with HIV, which includes 37.5 million adults and 1.5 million children under 15 years of age. The global prevalence of HIV among pregnant women is approximately 1.4%.
  - **Incidence:** The global incidence rate of HIV among pregnant women is estimated to be around 0.7 per 100 person-years.

32.3.2 Regional HIV Prevalence Statistics

- **Africa:**
  - Sub-Saharan Africa remains the most affected region globally, accounting for nearly two-thirds of all individuals living with HIV worldwide.
  - South Africa has one of the highest HIV prevalence rates globally, with approximately 7.7 million people living with HIV in 2020.

  - East African countries, such as Kenya and Uganda, have made considerable progress in reducing HIV prevalence, with Kenya's rate declining from 7.2% in 2007 to 4.9% in 2020.
- **Asia:**
  - While the overall prevalence of HIV in Asia is lower than in Africa, certain Southeast Asian countries report higher infection rates. For instance, Thailand is estimated to have 440,000 individuals living with HIV as of 2020.
  - India ranks third in the global HIV epidemic, with approximately 2.5 million individuals living with the virus in 2020.
  - In Cambodia, targeted prevention strategies have significantly decreased HIV prevalence from 1.7% in 2014 to 0.3% in 2020.
- **Europe:**
  - Eastern Europe and Central Asia have experienced rising HIV prevalence in recent years, with about 1.7 million individuals living with HIV in the region by 2020.
  - In Western Europe, the HIV epidemic is predominantly concentrated among key populations, including men who have sex with men (MSM) and people who inject drugs.
  - Countries such as Spain and Italy have successfully implemented HIV prevention and treatment programs, resulting in the reduction of new infections and improved outcomes for individuals living with HIV.
- **North America:**
  - The United States faces ongoing challenges related to the HIV epidemic, with approximately 1.2 million individuals living with HIV as of 2020.
  - Canada has witnessed a decline in new HIV infections due to enhanced testing and treatment accessibility, which has contributed to better health outcomes for individuals living with HIV.
  - In Mexico, initiatives aimed at increasing HIV awareness and improving access to care have achieved success in reducing new infections and enhancing treatment adherence rates.

32.3.3 Epidemiology, Prevalence, and Incidence of HIV During Pregnancy

- **Global perspective:**
  - **Prevalence:** According to UNAIDS, the prevalence of HIV among pregnant women globally is approximately 1.4%.
  - **Incidence:** The global incidence rate of HIV among pregnant women is estimated to be around 0.7 per 100 person-years.
- **Regional breakdown:**
  - **Africa:** The prevalence of HIV among pregnant women in Africa varies from 1.4% to 30.9% across different countries, with Nigeria reporting an overall pooled prevalence of 7.22% among pregnant women.

- **Asia:** In Asia, the prevalence of HIV among pregnant women generally ranges from 0.1% to 1.4% across various countries.
- **Europe:** The prevalence of HIV among pregnant women in Europe is relatively low, ranging from 0.1% to 1.1%.
- **United States:** In the United States, the prevalence of HIV among pregnant women is approximately 0.4%.

32.3.4 Factors Influencing HIV Prevalence and Incidence

- **Age:** Younger women, particularly those under 25, are at an elevated risk for HIV infection.
- **Geographic Location:** Significant disparities exist in HIV prevalence and incidence across regions, with Africa being the most affected.
- **Behavioral Factors:** Risky behaviors such as unprotected sexual intercourse and having multiple sexual partners facilitate the spread of HIV.
- **Access to Healthcare:** Availability of antiretroviral therapy (ART) and other healthcare services has profound implications for HIV prevalence and incidence.

32.3.5 Trends and Progress

- **Decline in HIV Prevalence:** There has been a notable decline in HIV prevalence among pregnant women globally, especially in locales with robust healthcare systems and effective prevention programs.
- **Increased Access to ART:** Enhanced access to antiretroviral therapy has resulted in a significant reduction in mother-to-child transmission of HIV, with some countries achieving transmission rates as low as 0.9%.

The epidemiology, prevalence, and incidence of HIV during pregnancy exhibit considerable variability across different regions worldwide. Comprehending these trends and influencing factors is nessesary for formulating effective prevention and treatment strategies necessary to address the ongoing HIV epidemic.

32.4 Clinical Manifestations

32.4.1 Gynecology

Following an incubation period of 16–25 days, individuals may experience a clinical picture resembling mononucleosis. The illness typically lasts from several days to a few weeks, generally not exceeding 14 days.

- **Important symptoms in individuals with potential HIV exposure:**
  – Maculopapular rash, predominantly affecting the trunk (in 40–80% of cases)
  – Aseptic meningitis (in some cases)
  – Mucocutaneous ulcerations of the oral mucosa, gingiva, palate, esophagus, and anus
- **Other symptoms:**
  – Fever and malaise (70–90%)
  – Exanthema (40–80%)
  – Headache (32–70%)
  – Lymphadenopathy (40–70%)
  – Pharyngitis (50–70%)
  – Myalgia and arthralgia (50–70%)
  – Nausea, vomiting, and diarrhea (30–60%)
  – Aseptic meningitis (24%)
  – Oral and genital ulcers (5–20%)
  – Thrombocytopenia and leukopenia (40–45%)

The acute phase is succeeded by a *latency period*, typically lasting 8–10 years. During this time, opportunistic infections, such as candidosis, may arise due to compromised cellular immune defenses (stage B), although these infections do not qualify as AIDS-defining conditions (stage C).

32.4.2 Staging of HIV Infection

The classification of HIV infection is based on the 1993 CDC (Centers for Disease Control and Prevention) classification system, which considers the lowest recorded CD4 cell count (Table 32.1). This classification encompasses three clinical stages—A, B, and C (Table 32.2). Stage A indicates an asymptomatic HIV infection, while Stage B denotes symptoms of HIV infection that have not yet progressed to Stage C. Stage C is identified by the presence of AIDS-defining illnesses, such as *Pneumocystis jirovecii* pneumonia.

Table 32.1 Classification by the Centers for Disease Control and Prevention (CDC)

			A	B	C
AIDS in Europe: C1–C3 AIDS in the United States: A3, B3, and C1–C3			Asymptomatic acute (primary) HIV infection generalized lymphadenopathy	Symptomatic Not A or C	AIDS indicator diseases
CD4+ helper cells	1	>500/ml	A1	B1	C1
	2	200–499/ml	A2	B2	C2
	3	<200/ml	A3	B3	C3

Table 32.2 Clinical classification according to the CDC

Category	Classification	Comments
Category A	Classification only permissible if neither category B nor C occurred previously	– Acute (primary) HIV infection with concomitant disease in the sense of HIV infection a – Symptomatic HIV infection – PGL (persistent generalized lymphadenopathy)
Category B	Symptomatic diseases that do not belong to category C and fulfill at least one of the following categories	Attributed to HIV infection or indicative of impaired cellular immunity and/or whose disease course or treatment is considered to be affected by HIV infection in medical judgment Examples of diseases – General symptoms, unless they can be attributed to a specific disease and persist for more than 1 month, e.g. fever >38.5 – Bacillary angiomatosis (Bartonella) – Fever or diarrhea longer than 1 month – Herpes zoster, at least two episodes or more than one dermatome – Immune thrombocytopenia (idiopathic thrombocytopenic purpura) – Listeriosis – Oral hairy cell leukoplakia – Oropharyngeal or vulvovaginal candidosis (persistent or recurrent) – Pelvic inflammatory disease (PID, tuboovarian abscess) – Peripheral neuropathy – Therapy-refractory Candida infection with oropharyngeal or vaginal localization – Cervical dysplasia (moderate or severe), carcinoma in situ of the cervix

(continued)

Table 32.2 (continued)

Category	Classification	Comments
Category C: AIDS indicator Diseases	Opportunistic infections	
	Bacterial	– Atypical mycobacteria, disseminated (20%) – Recurrent bacterial pneumonia – Recurrent salmonella sepsis (5–10%) – Tuberculosis (pulmonary, extrapulmonary or disseminated) (10%)
	Viral	– CMV infection (disseminated, retinitis, CNS infection, gastrointestinal) (30%) – HSV infection with chronic ulcerations (>1 month) or bronchitis, pneumonia or esophagitis (HSV1: >95%, HSV2: 10–30%) – Progressive multifocal leukoencephalopathy (PML, Papova virus = JC virus) (3%)
	Protozoa	– Intestinal isosporidiosis longer than 1 month – Neurotoxoplasmosis (30%) – Gastrointestinal cryptosporidiosis longer than 1 month (frequent) – Pneumocystis pneumonia (85%, first manifestation in every 2nd patient) – Strongyloidiasis
	Mycosis	– Candida infection (esophageal, tracheobronchial) (local infestation in almost all patients) – Cryptococcosis (disseminated, extrapulmonary, meningoencephalitis) (5%) – Histoplasmosis (disseminated, extrapulmonary, meningoencephalitis) – Coccidomycosis (disseminated, extrapulmonary)
	Opportunistic tumors	– Anal carcinoma – Burkitt's lymphoma (EBV-associated) – Cervical carcinoma – Highly malignant B-cell NHL – Kaposi's sarcoma – Non-Hodgkin's lymphomas – Primary lymphoma of the brain

- **Additionally, there are three CD4 cell count categories:**
  - **Stage 1:** More than 500 cells per microliter
  - **Stage 2:** Between 200 and 499 cells per microliter
  - **Stage 3:** Fewer than 200 cells per microliter
- **Example of clinical classification:**
  - **Stage A1:** An individual is HIV-positive without any symptoms of HIV infection. The CD4 cell count exceeds 500 cells per microliter.
  - **Stage B3:** The individual exhibits symptoms of HIV infection, yet these do not meet the criteria for an AIDS-defining illness. The CD4 cell count is below 200 cells per microliter, qualifying as AIDS per US definitions (but not European).
  - **Stage C2:** The individual develops AIDS-defining conditions, such as Pneumocystis jirovecii pneumonia, and has a CD4 cell count between 200 and 499 cells per microliter. This case is classified as AIDS under both U.S. and European criteria.
- **Alternative staging system:**
  - **Stage I:** Acute HIV infection; within a week to a few months post-infection, about 10% of individuals may develop a mononucleosis-like illness that typically resolves within 4 weeks.
  - **Stage II:** Asymptomatic HIV infection; lasting from 5 to over 12 years.
  - **Stage III:** Lymphadenopathy syndrome, characterized by swollen lymph nodes persisting for more than 3 months without additional symptoms.
  - **Stage IV:** Symptomatic HIV infection.
    - **Stage IVA:** Symptoms include fever, weight loss, diarrhea, night sweats, and reduced performance.
    - **Stage IVB:** Manifestations of full-blown AIDS, including infections caused by opportunistic and obligate pathogens.

In the absence of therapy, the typical interval from the onset of the first AIDS-defining illness to patient death is approximately 2–4 years. Modern antiretroviral therapy allows individuals to manage with a chronic condition effectively.

32.4.3 Pregnancy

Vertical transmission of HIV can occur pre-, peri-, and postnatally, with evidence suggesting that at least half of all vertical transmissions happen directly during the perinatal period.

Maternal risk factors linked to increased vertical transmission:
- **High body viral load, indicated by elevated plasma viral load**
- **Presence of virulent HIV isolates (such as SI variants, rapid/high replication rates, and T-tropism)**
- **Low T-helper cell counts**
- **Lack of TH1 stimulation**

HIV transmission is multifactorial. However, through combined interventions, the risk of transmission can be reduced to less than 2%. Approximately 20–30% of vertically infected fetuses may present with a severe early form characterized by a high viral load at birth, rapid loss of T-helper cells, opportunistic infections, or severe encephalopathy within the first 18 months of life. If untreated, life expectancy in these cases is generally less than 5 years.

32.5 Diagnosis

32.5.1 General

Diagnostic methods for HIV infection include the detection of antibodies and antigens, as well as reverse transcriptase polymerase chain reaction (RT-PCR). The absolute count of T-helper cells in peripheral venous blood serves as a surrogate marker for progressive immune system damage and plays a role in clinical staging.

The two-step diagnostic procedure for HIV detection involves serologic screening utilizing an HIV screening test (Ag-Ab combination test), followed by confirmatory diagnostics with antibody-based tests such as Western blot and/or HIV PCR (Table 32.3). Additionally, HIV resistance tests are conducted to assess the virus's susceptibility to various medications. It is important to note that serologic tests may take 3–12 weeks, or occasionally longer, to yield positive results. Routine laboratory tests encompass the analysis of lymphocyte differentiation, including the absolute CD4 count and CD4/CD8 ratio, as well as other functional parameters (Table 32.4). Testing for opportunistic infections is also carried out as necessary.

If HIV infection is suspected, repeat testing is recommended after an interval of approximately 2–4 weeks.

32.5.2 Pregnancy

The virological and immunological diagnosis of HIV-exposed newborns and infants aims to achieve the following objectives:

Table 32.3 Laboratory diagnostic profiles

Virus detection HIV RNA/ antigen	HIV antibody detection	Infection status
+	–	Acute infection
+	Questionable	Acute infection
+	–	Acute or chronic infection
–	+	Chronic infection (mostly under antiretroviral therapy)

Table 32.4 Suggested laboratory tests (initial and follow-up). The specific recommendations for examinations and their intervals depend on the respective region and country and are determined by local guidelines

Laboratory tests (initial examination)	Follow-up examinations

• CBC and differential blood count
• CRP (or BSG)
• Neopterin
• Electrolytes
  – Calcium, chloride, potassium, magnesium, sodium, phosphate
• Total protein
• Electrophoresis
• IgA, IgG, IgM, IgE
• Liver parameters
  – Transaminases
  – Glutamate dehydrogenase (GLDH)
  – Gamma-GT
  – alkaline phosphatase
  – Bilirubin
• Kidney parameters
  – Urea
  – Creatinine (creatinine clearance)
• B-2-microglobulin
• Lymphocyte differentiation:
  – CD4 absolute count
  – CD4/CD8 ratio
• HIV RNA PCR (quantitative)
• Hepatitis serology (HBV and HCV)
• Syphilis serology
• Cryptococcosis antigen in serum
• CMV serology
	• Intervals
	  – Minor immunodeficiency: every 6 months
	  – Moderate immunodeficiency: every 2–4 months
	  – Severe immunodeficiency: monthly
	Like initial examination
	Without
	• CMV serology
	• Hepatitis serology (HBV and HCV)
	• Syphilis serology
	• Cryptococcosis antigen in serum
	Plus
	• Lymphocyte differentiation
	  – CD4 absolute count
	  – CD4/CD8 ratio
	• If (CD4-positive) T helper cells <100/µl additionally:
	  – CMV PCR
	  – Cryptococcosis antigen
	and
	Possible clarification of opportunistic infections

- Early identification of HIV-infected newborns and infants to initiate appropriate prophylactic measures (such as immunoglobulin substitution and nutritional optimization)
- Detection of HIV-infected patients at high risk for rapid disease progression, identifying candidates for early antiretroviral therapy
- Monitoring for potential side effects of pre- and postnatal prophylaxis with antiretroviral chemotherapeutic agents (e.g., zidovudine), even in non-HIV-infected children

32.5.3 Resistance Testing

Given the risk of infections with zidovudine-resistant HIV strains, genotypic detection of wild-type HIV should be conducted prior to the administration of zidovudine to exclude the presence of genotypic resistance.

Indications for Resistance Testing Include:

- To prevent potential reduction in the effectiveness of antiretroviral prophylaxis or therapy during pregnancy due to pre-existing resistance, it is recommended that all previously untreated pregnant women undergo resistance testing before initiating therapy or prophylaxis.
- Resistance testing is advised for pregnant women on antiretroviral therapy who experience virological failure.
- If the viral load is detectable in the pregnant woman at the end of antiretroviral prophylaxis for HIV transmission (evaluated approximately one week before or at the time of delivery), resistance testing should be performed to document any development of resistance during prophylaxis, which may guide future treatment decisions.
- In cases of ultra-short prophylaxis with nevirapine (administered as a single dose to the mother shortly before delivery), resistance testing is recommended 4 to 6 weeks after the cessation of antiretroviral therapy.

32.5.4 Diagnosis of Opportunistic Infections

Opportunistic infections result from pathogens that typically do not cause serious illness but can pose significant threats to immunocompromised individuals. Common opportunistic infections in HIV include fungal infections (such as candidosis), toxoplasmosis, Pneumocystis pneumonia, various bacterial infections (including mycobacteria and atypical mycobacteria), and viral infections (such as cytomegalovirus [CMV] and herpes simplex virus [HSV]). Effective prevention and treatment of these infections are critical to avoiding complications.

Opportunistic infections can be diagnosed using various tests, including:

- **Serology:** Tests for amoebic dysentery, aspergillosis, coccidioidomycosis, cytomegalovirus (CMV), Epstein–Barr virus (EBV), hepatitis B and C, herpes simplex virus (HSV), histoplasmosis, Legionella, syphilis, toxoplasmosis, and varicella-zoster virus (VZV)
- **Bacteriology:**
  - Sputum and urine analyses for common pathogens and mycobacteria
  - Stool samples for the detection of Salmonella, Shigella, Campylobacter, and Yersinia
- **Direct evidence:**
  - Bronchoalveolar lavage or sputum tests for Aspergillus, *Pneumocystis carinii*, and Legionella
  - Serum and cerebrospinal fluid samples for amoeba and *Cryptococcus neoformans*
  - Stool samples for detecting Candida, cryptosporidia, Isopora, Giardia, and other parasites

32.6 Treatment

32.6.1 Gynecology

The primary objective of treatment is to inhibit HIV replication, aiming for complete suppression of viral replication across all body compartments (serum viral load <50 copies/ml). Before initiating therapy, the initial viral load and CD4 cell count should be assessed. Antiretroviral therapy is indicated when the CD4 cell count falls below 200, while a "gray area" exists for counts between 200 and 350. The viral load also plays a critical role in decision-making. Prophylactic measures against opportunistic infections (such as Pneumocystis carinii pneumonia and CMV retinitis) have proven effective.

Various treatment options, including nucleoside analogs, nonnucleoside analogs, and protease inhibitors, are available and may be used in combination (Table 32.5). Numerous HIV medications have been developed and approved, either as monotherapies or as fixed-dose combinations (Table 32.6). Combination therapy (commonly involving a three-drug regimen) has substantially improved patient prognosis, resulting in an approximately 85% reduction in mortality compared to a lack of therapy.

Initiation of and adjustments to therapy should be conducted in consultation with a specialist. The specific recommendations also depend on the respective region and country and are determined by local guidelines.

Table 32.5 Combination therapy options against HIV infection

Combination	Advantages	Disadvantages
PI(s) plus 2 NRTI	– Very active – Longest documented effectiveness – Proven reduction in mortality/morbidity – Low resistance selection	– Complex therapy – Long-term toxicity
NNRTI plus 2 NRTI	– Very active – Simple therapy regime	– High resistance selection
3 NRTI	– Simple therapy regime – PI + NNRTI options remain	– Long-term toxicity – Unclear effect with high viral load
PI(s) plus NNRTI plus NRTI	– Very active	– Complex therapies – Long-term toxicity – Minimal further follow-up therapy options

NRTI nucleoside reverse transcriptase inhibitor, *NNRTI* nonnucleoside reverse transcriptase inhibitor, *PI* protease inhibitor

Table 32.6 Antiretroviral medications

Designation		Drug (components)	Common/important adverse effects
Fixed combinations — STR (single-tablet regimens)	ABC/3TC/DTG	Abacavir/lamivudine/dolutegravir	Hypersensitivity (abacavir; HLA-B*57:01)—fever, rash; GI upset; insomnia; headache; weight gain; ↑ transaminases
	AZT/ABC/3TC	Azidothymidine (zidovudine)/abacavir/lamivudine	Bone marrow suppression (AZT)—anemia, neutropenia; mitochondrial toxicity; GI symptoms; abacavir hypersensitivity
	FTC/TAF/BIC	Emtricitabine/tenofovir alafenamide/bictegravir	Headache; insomnia; GI upset; weight gain; renal safety better vs TDF; possible dyslipidemia
	FTC/TAF/DRV/c	Emtricitabine/tenofovir alafenamide/darunavir/cobicistat	Diarrhea; nausea; hepatotoxicity; rash; metabolic effects; multiple drug–drug interactions (cobicistat)
	DTG/RPV	Dolutegravir/rilpivirine	Insomnia; headache; depression/psychiatric symptoms (rilpivirine susceptible patients); ↑ transaminases
	DTG/3TC	Dolutegravir/lamivudine	Insomnia; headache; GI upset; weight gain (possible)
	DOR/TDF/3TC	Doravirine/tenofovir disoproxil/lamivudine	Dizziness; headache; GI upset; TDF-associated renal dysfunction and ↓ bone mineral density
	EFV/TDF/FTC	Efavirenz/tenofovir disoproxil/emtricitabine	Neuropsychiatric effects (vivid dreams, mood changes); rash; hepatotoxicity; TDF renal/bone effects
	TDF/FTC/EVG/c	Tenofovir disoproxil/emtricitabine/elvitegravir/cobicistat	GI upset; creatinine rise (cobicistat effect); TDF renal/bone toxicity; drug–drug interactions
	FTC/TAF/EVG/c	Emtricitabine/tenofovir alafenamide/elvitegravir/cobicistat	GI upset; creatinine rise (cobicistat); fewer renal/bone effects vs TDF; weight gain possible
	FTC/TAF/RPV	Emtricitabine/tenofovir alafenamide/rilpivirine	Headache; depressive symptoms; QT prolongation risk (rare); ↑ transaminases
	TDF/FTC	Tenofovir disoproxil/emtricitabine	Renal tubular dysfunction; ↓ bone mineral density; GI upset; headache
	TDF/FTC/RPV	Tenofovir disoproxil/emtricitabine/rilpivirine	As for TDF/FTC; plus rilpivirine-associated depression, QT risk
NRTI—nucleoside/nucleotide RT inhibitors	ABC	Abacavir	Hypersensitivity reaction (HLA-B*57:01); fever; rash; GI upset
	ABC/3TC	Abacavir/lamivudine	As for components; hepatic enzyme elevations possible
	AZT/3TC	Azidothymidine (zidovudine)/lamivudine	AZT: bone marrow suppression, myopathy; GI upset
	AZT/ZDV	Azidothymidine/zidovudine (synonyms)	See AZT/3TC entry
	DDI	Didanosine	Peripheral neuropathy; pancreatitis; lactic acidosis; mitochondrial toxicity
	FTC	Emtricitabine	Generally well tolerated: headache; GI upset; rare hyperpigmentation
	FTC/TAF	Emtricitabine/tenofovir alafenamide	Fewer renal/bone effects vs TDF; headache; GI symptoms
	TDF/FTC	Tenofovir disoproxil/emtricitabine	Renal tubular dysfunction; ↓ bone density; GI upset
	3TC	Lamivudine	Well tolerated; headache; GI upset; risk of HBV flare on discontinuation
	D4T	Stavudine	Peripheral neuropathy; lactic acidosis; lipoatrophy; pancreatitis
	TDF	Tenofovir disoproxil	Renal tubular dysfunction; ↓ bone mineral density; GI upset

(continued)

Table 32.6 (continued)

Designation		Drug (components)	Common/important adverse effects
NNRTI—nonnucleoside RT inhibitors	DOR	Doravirine	Headache; dizziness; nausea; generally fewer CNS effects than efavirenz
	EFV	Efavirenz	Neuropsychiatric symptoms; rash; hepatotoxicity; dyslipidemia
	ETV	Etravirine	Rash (rare SJS/TEN); nausea; hepatotoxicity
	NVP	Nevirapine	Rash (including SJS/TEN); severe hepatotoxicity (monitor LFTs)
	RPV	Rilpivirine	Depression; insomnia; QT prolongation risk; requires administration with food
Protease inhibitors	ATV	Atazanavir	Indirect hyperbilirubinemia (benign); jaundice; nephrolithiasis; PR prolongation
	DRV	Darunavir	Rash; hepatotoxicity; GI upset; metabolic disturbances; drug interactions
	fAPV	Fosamprenavir	Rash; GI upset; hyperlipidemia
	IDV	Indinavir	Nephrolithiasis; hyperbilirubinemia; GI upset
	LPV	Lopinavir/ritonavir	GI intolerance; hyperlipidemia; hepatotoxicity
	NLV	Nelfinavir	Diarrhea; metabolic disturbances
	SQV	Saquinavir	GI upset; PR/QT prolongation; hepatotoxicity
	TPV	Tipranavir	Hepatotoxicity; increased intracranial hemorrhage risk (rare); hyperlipidemia
Booster substances	/c	Cobicistat	CYP3A inhibition; increases drug levels; serum creatinine rise (tubular secretion inhibition); many drug–drug interactions
	/r	Ritonavir	GI intolerance; dyslipidemia; potent CYP3A inhibition—extensive drug–drug interactions
Entry inhibitors	ENF (T-20)	Enfuvirtide	Injection-site reactions (very common); ↑ risk bacterial pneumonia; hypersensitivity (rare)
	MRV	Maraviroc	Hepatotoxicity (rare); cough; orthostatic hypotension; drug interactions (CYP3A)
Integrase inhibitors	DTG	Dolutegravir	Insomnia; headache; weight gain; rare ↑ creatine kinase; historical neural tube defect signal early pregnancy
	EVG (TOE)	Elvitegravir	GI upset; headache; creatinine rise (with cobicistat); drug–drug interactions
	RAL	Raltegravir	↑ creatine kinase; myopathy (rare); insomnia; GI upset

32.6.2 Pregnancy

32.6.2.1 Basic Principles

In addition to inhibiting maternal viral replication, the optimal initial treatment regimen during pregnancy aims to effectively prevent HIV transmission. The treatment criteria defined for adult HIV patients apply to pregnancy, albeit with certain modifications. Treatment is generally administered in combination with medications from three distinct classes that inhibit the function of HIV-specific enzymes at two sites:

- Inhibition of HIV-specific reverse transcriptase through:
  - Nucleoside reverse transcriptase inhibitors (NRTIs)
  - Nonnucleoside reverse transcriptase inhibitors (NNRTIs)
- Inhibition of an HIV protease that cleaves the HIV gag-pol protein into separate proteins (protease inhibitors, PIs) later in the replication cycle.

Once diagnosis is established, referral to an interdisciplinary HIV competence center is essential to ensure close collaboration between the patient and her gynecologist. Effective monitoring can be achieved through strategic scheduling.

At these centers, every HIV-positive pregnant woman should be provided with psychosocial support and connections to women's groups affiliated with AIDS service organizations. Patients will receive comprehensive information regarding the potential risk of maternal–fetal transmission, current options for risk reduction, any residual risks, and the possible short- and long-term effects of antiretroviral therapy on the developing fetus. Risk-adjusted antiretroviral therapy plans should be collaboratively developed with the patient, in accordance with the local guidelines for managing treatment during pregnancy (Table 32.7). Any changes to therapy or the initiation of therapy during pregnancy should be carried out in consultation with a physician or center experienced in antiretroviral therapy.

32.6.2.2 Reduction of Maternal–Fetal Transmission During Pregnancy

Pregnancy in an HIV-infected woman necessitates meticulous monitoring. In addition to antiretroviral therapy, monthly assessments of clinical chemistry, immunological parameters, and virological parameters (including lymphocyte subpopulations and HIV viral load) should be conducted by a qualified laboratory. Mothers presenting with a high viral load and/or low T-helper cell counts are at an increased risk of transmitting HIV to their offspring; hence, successful maternal treatment benefits the child and poses some risks. The long-term implications of intrauterine exposure to combination antiretroviral therapy on the child are not currently fully understood.

Suggested Diagnostic Procedures During Pregnancy in HIV-Infected Patients

The following diagnostic procedures are recommended for pregnant patients with HIV infection. The frequency and timing of these examinations may vary based on local, regional, or national guidelines. These procedures aim to monitor maternal health, reduce the risk of vertical transmission, and address potential complications during pregnancy.

Table 32.7 Antiretroviral medications and their potential uses during pregnancy

Substance	Recommended medication or with most experience	Alternative medication	Medication with little experience	Not recommended medications/ combinations
NRTI	Zidovudine (ZDV) (toxicity: anemia, leukopenia, nausea)	Stavudine (d4T) (toxicity: polyneuropathy, lipid dystrophy) Didanosine (DDI) (toxicity: polyneuropathy, pancreatitis) Abacavir (toxicity: hypersensitivity)	Tenofovir (TNF) (creatinine control) Emtricitabine (FTC)	Zalcitabine (DDC) (teratogenicity) Combination of d4T and DDI due to high mitochondrial toxicity with risk of lactic acidosis
	Lamivudine (3TC) (toxicity: anemia, leukopenia, nausea)			
NNRTI	Nevirapine (NVP) (toxicity: increased risk of liver toxicity with CD4 >250 c/μl; frequent drug exanthema; hypersensitivity)			Efavirenz (EFV) (toxicity: teratogenicity) Delaviridine (DLV) (toxicity: teratogenic, carcinogenic risk)
PI	Nelfinavir (NFV) (no longer recommended as unboosted PI) Saquinavir (SQV) + ritonavir (RTV) Lopinavir/ritonavir (LPV/r)	Indinavir (IDV) + RTV (toxicity: kidney stones, possibly kernicterus in newborns) Amprenavir + RTV	Atazanavir (ATV) + RTV (toxicity: possible kernicterus in newborns) Fosamprenavir (FPV) + RTV	Ritonavir (RTV) is only given as a booster in combination with other PIs
Fusion inhibitor			Enfuvirtide (T20) and others (initial reports show good tolerability, not placental) Salvage therapy	

NRTI nucleoside reverse transcriptase inhibitor, *NNRTI* nonnucleoside reverse transcriptase inhibitor, *PI* protease inhibitor

1. **HIV Antibody Test and Confirmation (if required):**
   - **Timing:** Routinely performed during the first trimester of pregnancy.
   - **Purpose:**
     - To confirm the diagnosis of HIV infection.
     - Early diagnosis is essential for initiating antiretroviral therapy (ART) to reduce the risk of vertical transmission of HIV to the fetus during pregnancy, labor, delivery, or breastfeeding.

2. **CD4 Cell Count and Viral Load Monitoring:**
   - **Timing:** Performed at least every 2 months throughout pregnancy.
   - **Purpose:**
     - To assess the patient's immune status by monitoring CD4 cell counts.
     - To evaluate the effectiveness of ART by measuring the viral load (the amount of HIV RNA in the blood).
     - A suppressed viral load is crucial for minimizing the risk of mother-to-child HIV transmission and improving maternal health outcomes.
3. **Genotypic Resistance Testing:**
   - **Timing:**
     1. Before starting ART for pregnant patients who are treatment-naïve.
     2. In cases of virologic failure (when viral load increases despite ART).
     3. If viral load remains detectable near term or 4–6 weeks after discontinuation of HIV prophylaxis.
   - **Purpose:**
     - To identify any drug-resistant strains of HIV that may limit the effectiveness of ART.
     - To aid in selecting the most effective ART regimen tailored to the patient's specific resistance profile.
     - To document changes in resistance patterns that could impact future treatment options.
4. **Hemoglobin Level Assessment:**
   - **Timing:** Performed monthly throughout pregnancy.
   - **Purpose:**
     - To monitor for anemia, which is common in pregnancy and can be exacerbated by HIV infection or ART.
     - To detect thrombocytopenia (low platelet count), which may occur due to HIV-associated conditions or ART side effects.
     - Early identification and management of these conditions are essential to reduce complications, such as preterm birth or low birth weight.
5. **Lactate Levels, Liver Function, and Kidney Function Testing:**
   - **Timing:**
     - At the start of pregnancy to establish baseline values.
     - Shortly after initiating or adjusting ART/prophylaxis regimens.
     - When clinically indicated (e.g., in cases of suspected toxicity).
     - Monthly during the third trimester when risks of complications are higher.
   - **Purpose:**
     - To detect lactic acidosis, a rare but potentially life-threatening condition associated with some antiretroviral drugs, especially during late pregnancy.
     - To monitor for liver toxicity, which may present as elevated liver enzymes.
     - To assess kidney function and detect nephrotoxicity, which can occur due to certain antiretroviral medications.

6. **Oral Glucose Tolerance Test (OGTT):**
   - **Timing:** Performed between 24 and 28 weeks of gestation.
   - **Purpose:**
     - To screen for gestational diabetes mellitus (GDM), a condition characterized by glucose intolerance during pregnancy.
     - Patients on protease inhibitors—a class of ART—are at a higher risk of developing GDM due to their impact on glucose metabolism.
     - Early detection and management of GDM are critical to preventing complications, such as macrosomia (large-for-gestational-age fetus) and preeclampsia.
7. **Vaginal pH Assessment and Native Microscopy:**
   - **Timing:** Conducted at every antenatal checkup throughout pregnancy.
   - **Purpose:**
     - To identify vaginal infections (e.g., bacterial vaginosis, fungal infections) through pH assessment and microscopy.
     - Untreated vaginal infections can increase the risk of premature rupture of membranes, preterm labor, and vertical transmission of HIV.
     - Early treatment reduces these risks and improves pregnancy outcomes.
8. **Microbiological Cultures:**
   - **Timing:** Conducted at the beginning of pregnancy or when clinically indicated based on symptoms.
   - **Purpose:**
     - To screen for sexually transmitted infections (STIs), such as chlamydia, gonorrhea, trichomoniasis, syphilis, and hepatitis B or C.
     - These infections may coexist with HIV and increase the risk of complications, such as preterm birth, miscarriage, or neonatal infections.
     - Prompt detection allows for appropriate treatment and the prevention of further transmission.
9. **Toxoplasmosis Screening:**
   - **Timing:** Performed at the beginning of pregnancy and repeated during the second and third trimesters.
   - **Purpose:**
     - To diagnose new *Toxoplasma gondii* infections or reactivation of latent toxoplasmosis, which is more likely in immunocompromised patients.
     - Congenital toxoplasmosis can lead to severe fetal complications, such as hydrocephalus, intracranial calcifications, and chorioretinitis.
10. **Colposcopy and Cytological Examination for Dysplasia:**
    - **Timing:** Performed at the start of pregnancy. If abnormalities are found, a colposcopic evaluation and biopsy may be necessary.

  - **Purpose:**
    - To screen for cervical, vaginal, or vulvar dysplasia, conditions that are more common in HIV-infected women due to persistent human papillomavirus (HPV) infection.
    - Early detection allows for timely intervention to prevent progression to invasive cancer.
11. **Sonography (Ultrasound):**
  - **Timing:** Conducted in early pregnancy and during the second trimester.
  - **Purpose:**
    - To confirm gestational age, assess fetal development, and exclude structural anomalies.
    - Includes nuchal translucency measurement in the first trimester as part of screening for chromosomal abnormalities, such as Down syndrome.

Enhanced prophylactic measures are necessary due to the additional risks associated with pregnancy. For obstetric HIV transmission risks, intensified prophylaxis must be implemented in accordance with established guidelines. Adherence to regularly updated recommendations is essential throughout this process.

32.6.2.3 Multiple Pregnancy, Preterm Labor, and Preterm Delivery

In multiple pregnancies, prophylactic zidovudine should be initiated at 29 weeks of gestation due to an elevated risk of preterm delivery. If preterm labor begins and the pregnant woman has not independently received combination therapy, and cesarean delivery is unfeasible due to fetal immaturity, yet there remains potential to halt labor, the immediate initiation of antiretroviral combination therapy is recommended. Suitable regimens may include zidovudine, lamivudine, and nevirapine, or a boosted protease inhibitor.

Extreme prematurity (24–28 weeks of gestation) poses significant challenges as prolonging the pregnancy until at least lung maturation is critical for the child's further development. In such cases, careful consideration must balance the increased risk of HIV transmission against the overall prognosis for the preterm infant.

32.6.2.4 Premature Rupture of Membranes, Chorionamnionitis

In exceptional obstetric cvomplcations like premature rRupture of membranes (PROM) or chorioamnionitis, the risk of HIV transmission is markedly heightened, increasing the vertical transmission rate by approximately 2% per hour. If time allows, the antenatal prophylaxis regimen should be enhanced by the administration of nevirapine (200 mg) in addition to zidovudine monotherapy.

Postnatal transmission prophylaxis for the newborn may include the administration of nevirapine at a dose of 2 mg/kg body weight (one dose should be administered if the mother has received one dose prenatally; if she has not received nevirapine prenatally, two doses should be given within 72 hours) plus combination prophylaxis with zidovudine and lamivudine, which should be intensified. The preferred mode of delivery is cesarean section, which should be conducted immediately after membrane rupture. If more than 4 h have passed since rupture of membranes, cesarean delivery may no longer provide a significant advantage regarding transmission risk. However, the decision should be guided by obstetric considerations.

The extended use of nevirapine beyond ultrashort prophylaxis is not currently recommended due to a lack of sufficient pharmacokinetic and safety data.

32.6.2.5 Reduction of Maternofetal Transmission at Birth

Despite the residual risk of intrauterine infection during the early weeks of pregnancy, focusing medical prophylaxis on the last trimester for a woman not requiring treatment is warranted. To reduce the risk of HIV transmission, the HIV-1 RNA concentration should be lowered to below 500–1000 copies/mm^3.

Known Risk Factors for Perinatal HIV Transmission Include:
- High Maternal Viral Load
- Low CD4 Cell Count
- Maternal AIDS
- Vaginal Delivery
- Premature Rupture of Membranes for More than 4 Hours
- Preterm Birth (Gestation Less than 37 Weeks)
- Breastfeeding

Prophylactic Measures to Reduce Maternal-to-Fetal Transmission:
- Maternal Antiretroviral Therapy (ART)
- Primary Cesarean Section
- Weaning
- Newborn Drug Prophylaxis

32.6.2.6 Drug Treatment of the Mother

In a pregnant woman who has no obstetric risk and does not require antiretroviral treatment, zidovudine can be administered at 32 weeks of gestation, concurrently with a primary cesarean section scheduled between 36 and 37 weeks of gestation, provided there are no contraindications. Additionally, intravenous zidovudine should be administered antepartum and intrapartum, with zidovudine also administered postpartum to the infant.

Timeframe for Zidovudine (ZDV) Administration

- **Antepartum:** Oral administration of ZDV 500 mg daily, starting at 32 weeks of gestation and continuing until delivery.
- **Intrapartum:** Intravenous administration of ZDV beginning 3 h prior to delivery:
  - Initial dose: 2 mg/kg body weight (bw) over the first hour.
  - Maintenance dose: 1 mg/kg body weight (bw) per hour until delivery.
- **Postpartum:** Oral administration of ZDV to the newborn for a duration of 2–4 weeks.

32.6.2.7 Mode of Delivery: Primary Cesarean Section

Pregnant women with HIV who are not eligible for vaginal delivery due to detectable levels of HIV RNA should undergo primary cesarean section by an experienced team from 37 weeks of gestation. In rare cases, a single low HIV RNA measurement may not indicate virological failure, allowing for the consideration of vaginal delivery. Pregnant women are advised to continue their antiretroviral therapy on the day of delivery.

For intrapartum exposure prophylaxis, intravenous zidovudine should begin 3 h prior to the scheduled cesarean section (or at labor onset for rare instances of vaginal delivery). The dosing regimen is 2 mg/kg body weight for the first hour, followed by 1 mg/kg body weight per hour until delivery. Although immediate delivery may be necessary, priority should be given to intrapartum exposure prophylaxis.

When maternal HIV RNA levels are between 50 and 1000 copies/mL at delivery, administering oral zidovudine to the newborn within 6 h of birth for 4 weeks is recommended. Alternatively, intravenous zidovudine may be given for 10 days if oral intake is not feasible. In cases where neonatal anemia occurs, investigation for potential causes, such as blood loss or infection, should be conducted before considering red blood cell transfusion or discontinuation of zidovudine. For neonates experiencing anemia post-exposure prophylaxis after 2 weeks of life, a liberal evaluative approach is advisable.

If maternal HIV RNA exceeds 50 copies/mL at 36 weeks of gestation, an elective cesarean section should be performed at 37 weeks of gestation at the earliest. Both intrapartum exposure prophylaxis and postnatal exposure prophylaxis should be administered. The specific recommendations also depend on the respective region and country and are determined by local guidelines.

32.6.2.8 Mode of Delivery: Vaginal Birth

Vaginal delivery may be considered if maternal HIV RNA levels remain below 50 copies for at least 4 weeks leading up to delivery. Under these optimal conditions (effective ART with viral load undetectable throughout pregnancy, especially near delivery), vaginal delivery is justified.

Practical Recommendations for Vaginal Delivery Include:

- Maintaining the integrity of the amniotic sac for as long as possible
- Avoiding the use of an internal cardiotocography (CTG) line
- Applying restrictive criteria for operative vaginal deliveries and microsurgery
- Allowing more liberal indications for a second cesarean section in cases of abnormal ctg readings, prolonged labor, or suspected amniotic infection syndrome
- Inducing labor in accordance with standard obstetric practices

If HIV RNA is fully suppressed at the time of delivery, administering zidovudine during labor offers no additional benefits; therefore, intrapartum exposure prophylaxis is not recommended in this scenario. Postpartum exposure prophylaxis decisions should hinge on maternal HIV RNA levels during pregnancy. If maternal prepartum HIV RNA is below 50 copies/mL, the risk of transmission is considered very low. For postnatal exposure prophylaxis, zidovudine administration orally to the newborn within 6 h of birth for 2 weeks is recommended. If optimal conditions are present, postnatal exposure prophylaxis may be unnecessary. These optimal conditions are met when an HIV-positive woman has been on ART with a viral load below 50 copies/mL prior to pregnancy and continues this throughout pregnancy and immediately before delivery.

Vaginal delivery should be considered if maternal HIV RNA levels remain below 50 copies/mL for at least 4 weeks before and up to the time of delivery. This approach requires that the pregnant woman is receiving antiretroviral therapy (ART) and exhibits no significant obstetric risks. Intrapartum exposure prophylaxis should be avoided, while postnatal exposure prophylaxis should be implemented. Postpartum exposure prophylaxis may be omitted only when maternal HIV RNA levels have consistently been below 50 copies/mL throughout the pregnancy and before delivery, indicating successful ART initiation prior to pregnancy.

32.6.2.9 No Breastfeeding

Approximately 30–50% of all HIV-infected children worldwide have contract the virus through breastfeeding. According to WHO recommendations, HIV-positive mothers should refrain from breastfeeding in countries where safe and hygienically prepared infant formula is readily available, to mitigate the risk of HIV transmission to their infants. In many African countries, however, this access may not be adequately ensured, making exclusive breastfeeding for the first 6 months advisable to reduce non-HIV-related mortality risks (e.g., severe diarrhea).

32.6.3 Neonatology

32.6.3.1 Evisceration of the Infant/Aspiration of Bloody Amniotic Fluid from the Stomach

If the infant sustains cuts or if bloody amniotic fluid is aspirated from the stomach, percutaneous inoculation or mucosal exposure to HIV-containing bodily fluids should be suspected. In such cases, it is justified to extend the standard neonatal prophylaxis to include a combination of two NRTIs, following adult post-exposure prophylaxis guidelines.

32.6.3.2 Postnatal Transmission Prophylaxis

Postnatal transmission prophylaxis should be initiated within the first 6 h following birth, if feasible. The previous recommendation of oral zidovudine at 2 mg/kg body weight every 6 h has been truncated to 2–4 weeks. A retrospective study in the United States indicated a transmission rate of 9.3% when zidovudine therapy commenced within 48 h after vaginal delivery, compared to 18.4% if administered later (>48 h). In the absence of therapy, 26.6% of infants contracted the virus.

Current data suggest that the acute toxicity of zidovudine during pregnancy and in neonates is tolerable; however, the potential for long-term harm from prenatal exposure to zidovudine remains uncertain.

32.6.3.2.1 Postnatal Prophylaxis for Low-Risk Preterm Infants and Neonates

- For neonates and preterm infants (≥35 weeks of gestation), zidovudine is recommended at a dosage of 4 mg/kg orally twice daily for 4 weeks. Alternatively, intravenous zidovudine may be administered at 3 mg/kg per dose, twice daily.
- For premature infants between 30 weeks and 34 weeks and 6 days gestation, a dosage of 2 mg/kg/dose orally, twice daily, for 4 weeks is advised. From day 15 onward, the dosage may be escalated to 3 mg/kg per dose twice daily orally. Intravenous zidovudine may also be given at 1.5 mg/kg/dose twice daily, increasing to 2.3 mg/kg/dose twice daily after day 15.

- For premature infants born before 30 weeks of gestation, a dosage of 2 mg/kg/dose twice daily orally for 4 weeks is recommended, with intravenous zidovudine as an alternative, particularly if oral administration is intolerable.

32.6.3.2.2 Recommendations for Extended Postnatal Prophylaxis Against HIV Transmission in Premature Infants and Neonates

Postnatal treatment should commence as soon as possible and no later than 6–12 h following birth.

- For zidovudine treatment, a dosage of 4 mg/kg per dose, administered orally twice daily is advised for neonates at ≥35 weeks of gestation, or 3 mg/kg per dose twice daily intravenously over a period of 4–6 weeks. Preterm infants between 30 weeks and 34 weeks and 6 days gestation should receive 2 mg/kg/dose twice daily orally; dosage may be escalated to 3 mg/kg/dose orally from day 15 onward. Alternatively, intravenous zidovudine may be given to preterm infants at a dosing of 1.5 mg/kg/dose, increasing to 2 mg/kg/dose given orally twice daily for those less than 30 weeks gestation.
- Lamivudine should be administered orally at a dosage of 2 mg/kg/dose twice daily for 14 days; specific dosage recommendations for lamivudine in premature infants are currently unavailable.
- Nevirapine dosing should be according to the newborn's weight, either at 8 mg/dose or 12 mg/dose orally. For infants weighing 1500–2000 g, the dose is 8 mg; for those over 2000 g, the dose is 12 mg. Administer the first dose within 48 h of birth, with additional doses after another 48 and 96 h later. If the HIV-positive mother has received nevirapine during pregnancy for more than 3 days, neonatal nevirapine metabolism may be accelerated, warranting careful consideration of its use in the neonate during extended therapy, with potential for double dosing as needed. Strict adherence to dosing guidelines for nevirapine is highly recommended to ensure treatment efficacy and safety.
- Different dosages of raltegravir should be followed for infants born from 37 weeks gestation who weigh over 2000 g; dosages vary depending on weight and should be administered once or twice daily. Adherence to dosing guidelines is critical, particularly during the first 4 weeks post-birth.

32.7 Differential Diagnosis

The differential diagnosis of HIV and AIDS encompasses various diseases and conditions exhibiting symptoms similar to those associated with HIV infection or advanced AIDS. Conditions for differential consideration include infectious diseases such as mononucleosis, hepatitis B and C, syphilis, as well as opportunistic infections like tuberculosis, pneumocystis pneumonia, and cytomegalovirus infections. Autoimmune disorders such as systemic lupus erythematosus and rheumatoid arthritis should also be contemplated. Additionally, malignancies, such as lymphoma and solid tumors, must be included in the differential diagnosis. Given the multitude of potential differential diagnoses, thorough patient history-taking, clinical examination, and laboratory testing are necessary.

The specific recommendations for prophylaxis and treatment can vary, depending on the respective region and country, and are determined by local guidelines.

32.8 Prevention

HIV prevention encompasses a range of measures aimed at obstructing the virus's transmission and minimizing the risk of infection. These measures include educational campaigns promoting safe sex practices, condom use, regular HIV testing, and early treatment for individuals with HIV-positive partners. The availability of antiretroviral therapy, access to clean syringes for individuals who inject drugs, and pre-exposure prophylaxis (PrEP) initiatives targeting those at high infection risk are also vital in HIV prevention. Furthermore, enhancing public awareness, reducing stigma and discrimination against individuals living with HIV/AIDS, and fostering open discussions about sexual health remain fundamental components of HIV prevention.

- **Education:** Education on the sources of HIV infection and protective measures to mitigate transmission is crucial. Instruction for children and adolescents regarding sexually transmitted diseases and hygiene can effectively prevent HIV infection. Utilizing condoms during sexual intercourse is recommended to safeguard against infection.
- **Vaccinations:** Individuals living with HIV should receive vaccinations for influenza, hepatitis A and B, herpes zoster (beginning at age 50), and pneumococcal disease.
- **Pre-exposure Prophylaxis (PrEP):** PrEP is a medical strategy to inhibit infection in high-risk situations. This typically entails taking emtricitabine in conjunction with tenofovir either on a daily basis or intermittently around potential exposure events. Alternatives to PrEP include tenofovir or maraviroc alone. Regular checkups are essential: an HIV-negative test is required before initiating PrEP, which does not protect against other sexually transmitted infections; thus, STD and HIV screenings should be carried out after 3 months.
- **Post-exposure Prophylaxis (PEP):** PEP aims to limit infection risk for healthcare workers following exposures to HIV-infected blood (mostly from needlesticks). Prolonged contact with mucous membranes (e.g., eyes or mouth) or infected bodily fluids, such as semen, vaginal fluid, or blood, may also pose a risk. Protective gear, such as gloves, should be used at all times. Body fluids like saliva, urine, tears, nasal secretions, vomit, or sweat are generally not considered infectious unless visibly contaminated with blood.

Approximately 30% of pregnant women are diagnosed with HIV during the antenatal period, typically in the early stages of pregnancy. These women are not exclusively from high-risk groups; an increasing proportion are heterosexually infected without origin from regions with high HIV prevalence. Several studies have demonstrated that comprehensive HIV screening in pregnant women represents a cost-effective strategy, even within low-prevalence countries, as each infected newborn can impose a significant burden on the healthcare system.

Considering that no vaccine or therapeutic cure exists despite extensive efforts, prophylaxis against exposure remains of utmost importance.

Key Points

- Human immunodeficiency virus types 1 (HIV-1) and 2 (HIV-2) represent two distinct types of the virus.
- The primary target cells are CD4-positive T cells and the monocyte-macrophage system.
- HIV is the causative agent of acquired immune deficiency syndrome (AIDS).
- A global pandemic has led to approximately 35 million individuals becoming infected.
- Prevalence is particularly pronounced in sub-Saharan Africa.
- Acute HIV infection often presents with mononucleosis-like symptoms.
- This is followed by a latency phase during which opportunistic infections may develop (stage B).
- The AIDS stage (stage C) is distinguished by the emergence of severe infections and malignancies.
- Diagnosis relies on detecting antibodies, antigens, and reverse transcriptase polymerase chain reaction (RT-PCR).
- CD4 cell counts are utilized as surrogate markers.
- Pre-therapy resistance testing is recommended, particularly for pregnant women.
- The objective is achieving complete suppression of HIV replication.
- The standard therapeutic regimen typically consists of a combination of nucleoside/nucleotide analogs, nonnucleoside reverse transcriptase inhibitors (NNRTIs), and protease inhibitors.
- Special considerations should be taken for pregnant women to mitigate mother-to-child transmission risks.
- HIV screening during pregnancy has been implemented in many developed countries.
- Prophylaxis against exposure is critical, as a vaccine is currently unavailable.

Human T-Cell Lymphotropic Virus (HTLV) 33

Abstract

Human T-cell lymphotropic virus (HTLV), particularly HTLV-1, is transmitted predominantly through blood transfusions, contaminated needles, sexual intercourse, and breastfeeding. It is most prevalent in Japan, the Caribbean, and Central and South America. HTLV is associated with diseases such as adult T-cell leukemia (ATL) and tropical spastic paraparesis (TSP). Mother-to-child transmission, particularly via breast milk, represents a significant route of infection. Diagnosis is primarily achieved through polymerase chain reaction (PCR) and antibody detection; currently, no cure exists. Preventive measures encompass screening in high-risk areas, discouraging breastfeeding by infected mothers, and utilizing condoms to avert sexually transmitted infections. A minority of infected individuals develop symptoms, while the majority remain asymptomatic.

33.1 Background

Modes of Transmission

- **Transfusion of Cellular Blood Products:** Transmission is most efficient when infected lymphocyte-containing blood components (e.g., whole blood, packed cells, and non-leukoreduced products) are transfused to a susceptible recipient.
- **Parenteral Exposure from Contaminated Injection Equipment:** Transmission occurs via shared or non-sterile syringes and needles, representing a major risk among persons who inject drugs.
- **Sexual Contact:** Infection is transmitted sexually; epidemiological studies indicate higher efficiency of male-to-female transmission compared with female-to-male.
- **Breastfeeding:** Prolonged breastfeeding facilitates mother-to-child transmission because infected maternal lymphocytes are present in breast milk.

I. Mylonas, *Sexually Transmitted Diseases*,
https://doi.org/10.1007/978-3-031-78204-6_33

- **Vertical (Intrauterine and Peripartum) Transmission:** Transplacental or peripartum transfer of infected cells may occur, although rates are lower than those associated with breastfeeding or transfusion.

Risk Groups

- **Residents of Endemic Regions and Their Sexual Contacts:** Persons living in or originating from endemic areas (notably southwestern Japan, the Caribbean Basin, parts of Central and West Africa, and regions of South America) are at increased risk. Sexual partners of HTLV-infected individuals carry elevated risk regardless of geography.
- **Persons with High-Risk Sexual Behavior:** Individuals with multiple sexual partners, inconsistent condom use, or engagement in transactional sex have increased probability of exposure through sexual transmission.
- **People Who Inject Drugs (PWID):** Sharing needles, syringes, or other injection paraphernalia permits direct transfer of infected lymphocytes and substantially increases transmission risk.
- **Recipients of Blood Products or Solid-Organ Transplants in Inadequately Screened Settings:** Transfusion of cellular blood components or transplantation from an infected donor can transmit HTLV when donor screening, leukoreduction, or inactivation procedures are absent or incomplete.
- **Infants Born to or Breastfed by HTLV-Infected Mothers:** Vertical transmission is most commonly mediated by prolonged breastfeeding; offspring of seropositive mothers therefore face a substantially increased risk, with risk magnitude related to duration of breastfeeding.
- **Health-Care Workers with Percutaneous or Mucocutaneous Exposures:** Although less common than other routes, occupational exposures (e.g., needlestick injuries and contaminated mucous membrane contact) can result in transmission if infected cellular material is introduced.
- **Immunocompromised Persons:** Individuals with impaired cellular immunity (e.g., advanced HIV infection and transplant recipients on immunosuppression) may be at greater risk for acquisition and for progression to HTLV-associated disease following infection.
- **Populations with Limited Access to Screening and Preventive Services:** Communities in which antenatal screening, blood-donor testing, harm-reduction programs, or sexual-health services are unavailable or underutilized bear a higher burden of undetected infection and onward transmission.

33.2 Pathogen

HTLV is classified within the retrovirus family and is composed of two primary types: HTLV-1 and HTLV-2. The significance of newer variants, HTLV-3 and HTLV-4, remains uncertain. These viruses are of significant medical concern due to their potential association with certain lymphatic system malignancies.

33.3 Epidemiology

The distribution of HTLV varies across global regions. While the overall incidence of HTLV is sporadic, the viruses are observed worldwide.

- HTLV-1 exhibits high prevalence in nations such as Japan, New Guinea, Central Africa, and the Caribbean, affecting over 10% of the population.
- Conversely, HTLV-2 mostly occurs in the United States.
- In Europe, HTLV-1 is considered rare, with isolated instances reported in countries including Austria, Belgium, Spain, and the United Kingdom.
- In Asia, notably Japan, the prevalence of HTLV-1 is significantly elevated compared to Europe, with certain Indian communities exhibiting rates over 40%.
- Japan is classified as a high-endemic area for HTLV-1, with prevalence rates reaching up to 37% in specific regions.
- Africa represents the largest high-endemic area for HTLV-1, with the highest prevalence reported in West, Central, and Southern Africa, occasionally reaching 10–25% in rural settings.
- HTLV-3 and HTLV-4 strains were first identified in Cameroon in 2005, though the clinical significance of these novel variants is presently unclear.

The incubation period for HTLV is estimated to be 10–20 years, with approximately 20 million individuals worldwide reported as infected.

33.4 Clinical Manifestations

33.4.1 Gynecology

Human T-lymphotropic virus type 1 (HTLV-1) is associated with a defined spectrum of diseases, although the majority of infected persons remain asymptomatic throughout life. Epidemiological data indicate that approximately 2–5% of carriers develop overt clinical disease, with geographic variation and higher incidence in endemic areas such as southwestern Japan, the Caribbean, parts of South America, and West/Central Africa. The two principal disease entities causally linked to HTLV-1 infection are adult T-cell leukemia/lymphoma (ATL) and HTLV-1-associated myelopathy/tropical spastic paraparesis (HAM/TSP); both conditions carry substantial morbidity and, in the case of aggressive ATL subtypes, poor prognosis.

Adult T-cell leukemia/lymphoma is an aggressive malignancy of mature CD4+ T lymphocytes that is classified within non-Hodgkin lymphomas and subdivided into acute, lymphomatous, chronic, and smoldering clinical forms, each with distinct natural history and therapeutic implications. ATL is typically manifested by cutaneous lesions, generalized lymphadenopathy, hepatosplenomegaly, hypercalcemia,

Table 33.1 Etiological associations of HTLV with various diseases

HTLV type	Diseases
HTLV-1	– Adult-type T-cell leukemia (ATL)
	– Tropical spastic paraparesis (TSP): paraparesis, urinary and fecal incontinence, back pain, and possibly psoriasis, uveitis, keratoconjunctivitis sicca, arthritis, and polymyositis
	– HTLV-I-associated myelopathy (HAM)
	– B-cell leukemia
	– Chronic persistent oligoarthritis
	– Lymphocytic uveitis
	– Bronchioalveolar lymphocytosis
HTLV-2	Association probable with:
	– Hairy cell leukemia
	– Tropical spastic paraparesis (TSP)-like clinical picture
	– Mycosis fungoides
	– Cutaneous CD8+ cell lymphoma
	– Chronic lung infections (pneumonia, bronchitis, etc.)
	– COPD
	– Sensory neuropathies
	– Motor symptoms
HTLV-3	Similar diseases to HTLV-1 possible, but not yet proven
HTLV-4	Similar diseases to HTLV-1 possible, but not yet proven

HTLV human T-cell lymphotropic virus, *ATL* adult T-cell leukemia, *TSP* tropical spastic paraparesis, *HAM* HTLV-I-associated myelopathy, *COPD* chronic obstructive pulmonary disease

and recurrent opportunistic infections due to profound immunosuppression. The lifetime risk of ATL among HTLV-1 carriers is estimated at about 2–4%, with earlier recognition and prompt initiation of subtype-appropriate therapy being essential because acute and lymphomatous forms progress rapidly and are associated with limited survival.

HTLV-1-associated myelopathy/tropical spastic paraparesis is a chronic, progressive, immune-mediated demyelinating myelopathy characterized by slowly progressive spastic paraparesis, gait disturbance, lower-limb stiffness and weakness, sensory symptoms, urinary and fecal dysfunction, and chronic back pain; disease progression is usually gradual but can result in significant long-term disability. Additional inflammatory conditions have been linked to HTLV-1, including severe dermatitis and other dermatologic disorders, uveitis and sicca syndromes, HTLV-1-associated arthritis and polymyositis, peripheral neuropathies, and neurogenic bladder secondary to spinal cord involvement. Co-infections such as HIV and *Strongyloides stercoralis* have been associated with accelerated disease progression and poorer outcomes, and associations with other T-cell lymphoproliferative disorders have been reported but remain less well established than the relationships with ATL and HAM/TSP.

HTLV-2 has rarely been associated with disease manifestation, and other factors may be necessary to induce clinical disease. It has been suggested that HTLV-2 may play a role in hairy cell leukemia and is associated with mycosis fungoides, a type of cutaneous T-cell lymphoma (Table 33.1). Symptoms of HTLV-2 infection can include sensory neuropathy and motor dysfunction, with patients potentially experiencing chronic lung infections such as pneumonia or bronchitis, alongside chronic obstructive pulmonary disease (COPD).

The potential for opportunistic and neurological disorders or infections to occur with greater frequency and severity is a plausible concern after HTLV infection.

33.4.2 Pregnancy

Risk factors for mother-to-child transmission of HTLV include prolonged breastfeeding and elevated maternal proviral load; both factors substantially increase infant infection risk. Preconception HTLV screening is recommended, particularly in endemic areas, to enable informed reproductive counseling and risk-reduction planning. In seropositive women, avoidance of breastfeeding is advised because the omission of lactation markedly reduces the probability of vertical transmission.

When breastfeeding is not undertaken, the likelihood of neonatal HTLV acquisition is significantly lowered; nevertheless, intrauterine and peripartum transmission, although less frequent, can still occur. Infants who acquire HTLV remain at lifelong risk for HTLV-associated conditions—notably adult T-cell leukemia/lymphoma (ATLL) and HTLV-1-associated myelopathy/tropical spastic paraparesis (HAM/TSP)—although the absolute lifetime risk for these disorders is influenced by viral, host, and environmental cofactors and is relatively low in most cohorts.

Preventive strategies should be implemented systematically in high-prevalence settings: antenatal HTLV screening, counseling on infant-feeding alternatives, consideration of formula feeding or safe processing of expressed breast milk where feasible, and follow-up serological testing of exposed infants. Assessment of maternal proviral load may be used to stratify transmission risk and to guide counseling; multidisciplinary management involving obstetrics, infectious diseases, and pediatric services is recommended for seropositive pregnancies.

Vertical transmission from mother to fetus is possible but uncommon. Postnatal transmission via breast milk occurs with greater frequency and constitutes a notable risk.

33.5 Diagnosis

The diagnosis of infection with human T-lymphotropic virus (HTLV-1 and HTLV-2) is based upon a staged approach combining screening assays with specific confirmatory testing. Initial screening is most commonly performed by antibody detection methods, typically enzyme-linked immunosorbent assay (ELISA) or particle agglutination assays, which detect host immunoglobulins directed against HTLV structural proteins (envelope and core antigens). Historically, p19 Gag antigen-based assays were utilized for epidemiologic screening; however, antibody-based immunoassays have largely superseded antigen tests in routine use. Specimen selection for screening is standardized as serum or plasma collected under appropriate conditions.

Confirmatory serological testing is required for any reactive screening result because of the potential for false-positive results due to nonspecific antibodies or cross-reactivity with other retroviruses. Western blot and line immunoassays are the principal confirmatory techniques and are used to verify specificity and to assist in discrimination between HTLV-1 and HTLV-2. Diagnostic criteria are based on the demonstration of antibodies to multiple distinct HTLV proteins on confirmatory assays; detection of reactivity to at least two defined HTLV antigens is generally considered supportive of true infection.

Molecular methods, principally polymerase chain reaction (PCR) for proviral DNA, are employed for definitive diagnosis, particularly when serology is indeterminate or when clinical disease requires virologic confirmation. PCR permits high-sensitivity detection of integrated HTLV provirus and enables genotypic discrimination between HTLV-1 and HTLV-2; validated specimen types include EDTA-anticoagulated peripheral blood, bone marrow aspirates, cerebrospinal fluid, skin biopsies, and lymph node tissue as clinically indicated. In the setting of suspected HTLV-associated neurologic or hematologic disease (e.g., HTLV-associated myelopathy/tropical spastic paraparesis or adult T-cell leukemia/lymphoma), molecular testing on the most relevant tissue compartment is recommended.

Limitations of the diagnostic pathway should be acknowledged and addressed in clinical practice. Serologic screening tests are associated with a greater risk of false positives and indeterminate patterns, particularly in early seroconversion or in the immunosuppressed, and cross-reactivity with other flaviviruses and retroviruses has been reported though it is uncommon; repeat serology or PCR for proviral DNA is advised when results are equivocal. Specimen choice, timing relative to symptom onset, and the availability of confirmatory and molecular assays should guide testing algorithms; where available, PCR is regarded as the reference confirmatory method and should be used to resolve indeterminate serology or to provide definitive subtype identification.

HTLV-PCR does not serve as an antibody confirmation test but can be beneficial in cases where antibody findings are ambiguous.

33.6 Differential Diagnosis

A number of diseases must be considered when evaluating symptoms associated with HTLV, including amyotrophic lateral sclerosis (ALS), funicular spinal disorders, and HIV/AIDS. Other factors to consider encompass intoxications, collagenoses, and leukemias such as lymphocytic leukemia (T-cell type) and lymphomas. Multiple sclerosis should also be included in the differential diagnosis.

33.7 Treatment

Antiviral Strategy and Rationale

- **Objective:** The principal objective of antiviral therapy in HTLV-1 infection is reduction of the proviral load, since lower proviral loads correlate with decreased risk of disease progression and reduced secondary transmission.
- **Mechanism and Agents:** Nucleoside reverse transcriptase inhibitors (notably zidovudine [AZT] or lamivudine [3TC]) are commonly combined with immunomodulatory therapy—primarily interferon-alpha (IFN-α)—to suppress viral replication and to limit clonal proliferation of infected T-lymphocytes. This strategy is intended to stabilize clinical disease (particularly adult T-cell leukemia/lymphoma, ATL) and to prevent further hematologic or neurologic deterioration; eradication of integrated provirus is not the expected outcome.

Recommended Regimens and Duration

- **First-Line Regimen:** A combination of AZT or 3TC with IFN-α is recommended, especially for smoldering, chronic, or acute ATL. In selected circumstances, arsenic trioxide has been added to the antiviral/immunotherapeutic regimen.
- **Treatment Duration:** Therapy is customarily prescribed for 6–12 months. Duration should be individualized according to clinical response, serial proviral load measurements, hematologic tolerance, and adverse-effect profile.
- **Monitoring During Therapy:** Complete blood count (CBC), hepatic transaminases and bilirubin, and proviral load quantification should be measured at baseline and at regular intervals during treatment; monitoring frequency should be adapted to treatment phase and toxicity.

Clinical Indications

- **ATL:** Use of AZT/IFN-α is most often indicated in smoldering and chronic ATL and has been applied in acute presentations as part of combined modality management or as a temporizing measure prior to cytotoxic chemotherapy or hematopoietic stem cell transplantation.
- **Other HTLV-1-Associated Disorders:** Evidence for antiviral efficacy in HTLV-1-associated myelopathy/tropical spastic paraparesis (HAM/TSP) and other inflammatory manifestations is limited; management of these conditions is primarily supportive and symptom-directed.

Cytotoxic Chemotherapy for Acute ATL

- **CHOP-Based Therapy:** Acute or lymphoma-type ATL should be treated with systemic combination chemotherapy (for example, CHOP: cyclophosphamide, doxorubicin [hydroxydaunorubicin], vincristine, and prednisone) according to established oncologic protocols. The addition of rituximab is not routinely indicated for T-cell neoplasms unless aberrant B-cell markers are identified.

- **Combination with Antiviral Therapy:** Concurrent or sequential administration of AZT/IFN-α has been reported to confer benefit in certain ATL subtypes; such combinations require rigorous hematologic and infectious surveillance and multidisciplinary coordination.

Management in Pregnancy and Prevention of Perinatal Transmission

- **Evidence Base and Guideline Status:** No universally accepted, evidence-based antenatal antiviral protocol for prevention of HTLV-1 mother-to-child transmission exists. Recommendations are therefore derived from limited cohort data, expert opinion, and extrapolation from other vertically transmitted viruses.
- **Antiviral Use During Pregnancy:** Maternal administration of AZT or 3TC to reduce proviral load has been considered; however, high-quality data on efficacy and fetal-maternal safety specific to HTLV-1 are lacking. Antiviral therapy in pregnancy should be individualized after multidisciplinary consultation (maternal–fetal medicine, infectious diseases, and hematology) and after counseling regarding uncertain benefit and potential risks. Maternal CBC and liver function tests should be monitored if therapy is initiated.
- **Mode of Delivery and Feeding:** Cesarean delivery is not routinely indicated solely for HTLV-1 prevention and should be guided by obstetric indications and individualized risk assessment. Postnatal transmission via breastfeeding is the principal documented route of vertical HTLV-1 transmission; avoidance of breastfeeding or limitation of breastfeeding duration has been associated with reduced transmission in observational studies and should be discussed with the patient. Where breastfeeding avoidance is not feasible, alternatives such as short-term breastfeeding with close follow-up or human-milk pasteurization may be considered after specialist counseling.

Monitoring and Follow-Up

- **Laboratory Surveillance:** Baseline and periodic measurement of proviral load, CBC, and organ function tests is recommended. Interval adjustments should be made according to clinical status and treatment toxicity.
- **Clinical Surveillance:** Patients should be assessed for neurologic deficits suggestive of HAM/TSP, cutaneous lesions, lymphadenopathy, hepatosplenomegaly, and hematologic evidence of leukemic transformation.

The benefits of antiretroviral therapy remain largely undetermined, with the exception of a reduced transmission rate.

33.8 Prevention

Immune Response and Persistence: HTLV infection triggers a durable humoral antibody response that can last for decades. Although only about 5% of infected individuals develop symptoms, the virus integrates permanently into the host's DNA, establishing lifelong infection.

Transmission and Prevention: HTLV spreads mainly through unprotected sexual contact, exposure to infected blood, and mother-to-child transmission via breastfeeding. Male-to-female sexual transmission is more common. Consistent condom use reduces transmission risk significantly. Blood transfusion-related transmission has been nearly eliminated in developed countries due to screening and leukoreduction measures.

Preventing Mother-to-Child Transmission: Most vertical transmissions occur through prolonged breastfeeding. Strategies to reduce risk include exclusive formula feeding, short-term breastfeeding (less than 3 months), freeze-thawing expressed breast milk, and emerging antiretroviral prophylaxis in high-risk pregnancies.

Patient Education and Counseling: HTLV-positive individuals require counseling on preventing transmission—avoiding donation of blood or tissues, consistent condom use, and not sharing needles. Infants should ideally be formula-fed. Education should cover partner testing, pre-conception planning, and the importance of regular follow-up for early detection of HTLV-related diseases. Psychosocial support is also essential to address stigma.

Clinical Management and Public Health: Risk-based management considers proviral load, symptoms, and disease status. High-risk cases may need antiretroviral therapy, elective cesarean delivery, and neonatal prophylaxis. Public health efforts focus on antenatal screening, provider education, community awareness, and culturally appropriate counseling. Special attention is required in resource-limited settings to support safe infant feeding and reduce transmission.

Diagnosis during pregnancy is a critical component of comprehensive prenatal care. In populations or regions with high prevalence or increased risk, routine screening is strongly advised to enable early detection of potential complications. When screening results are positive, prompt counseling and appropriate medical management must be provided to optimize maternal and fetal outcomes.

Enhanced Hygiene Education: HTLV-positive individuals require personalized guidance on hygienic practices to prevent inadvertent viral spread. This includes strict avoidance of sharing personal items such as razors, toothbrushes, or any objects that might be contaminated with blood or other bodily fluids, thereby minimizing the risk of blood-borne transmission.

Permanent Deferral from Donation of Blood, Tissue, and Organs: Persons infected with HTLV must be permanently excluded from donating blood, plasma, tissues, organs, or reproductive materials. This measure is critical to safeguard the integrity of the blood supply and prevent iatrogenic transmission during transfusions, transplants, or assisted reproductive procedures.

Counseling on Safe Sexual Practices: Clear and thorough counseling should be provided regarding sexual transmission risks. Emphasis should be placed on the consistent and correct use of latex condoms during all sexual activities to significantly reduce the risk of HTLV transmission, alongside partner notification and testing to identify infected contacts and enable appropriate management within sexual networks; additionally, preconception counseling is essential to discuss the implications of HTLV infection for conception and pregnancy, including strategies aimed at minimizing vertical transmission.

Infant Feeding Recommendations: To prevent mother-to-child transmission, exclusive formula feeding is strongly advised for infants born to HTLV-infected mothers. Breastfeeding—even briefly—poses a significant risk due to the presence of infected lymphocytes in breast milk, which can facilitate viral transmission.

Ongoing Clinical Monitoring and Psychosocial Support: Regular medical follow-up is essential to identify early signs of HTLV-associated complications such as adult T-cell leukemia/lymphoma (ATLL) or HTLV-associated myelopathy/tropical spastic paraparesis (HAM/TSP). Additionally, providing psychosocial support helps address stigma, psychological distress, and quality-of-life issues related to living with chronic viral infection.

Potential consequences of HTLV infection to infected persons:

- Education on hygiene practices.
- Prohibition of blood and organ donations.
- Information regarding transmission via unprotected sexual intercourse.
- Recommendation for bottle-feeding infants of infected mothers.

Newborns of HTLV-1 infected mothers should not be breastfed.

Key Points

- HTLV-1 and HTLV-2 are the primary types of the human T-cell leukemia virus.
- Transmission occurs via blood transfusions, contaminated needles, sexual contact, and breastfeeding.
- The virus is prevalent in Japan, the Caribbean, and Central and South America.
- HTLV can result in conditions such as adult T-cell leukemia (ATL) and tropical spastic paraparesis (TSP).
- Vertical transmission, particularly through breast milk, is a concern.
- Diagnosis relies on PCR and antibody detection, with no available cure.
- Preventive strategies include screening in at-risk areas, avoiding breastfeeding by infected mothers, and using condoms.
- A small percentage of infected individuals exhibit symptoms.
- HTLV-2 is less frequently associated with clinical conditions.
- Infants born to infected mothers are at an increased risk; therefore, breastfeeding should be avoided.

Zika Virus

34

Abstract

Zika virus (ZIKV), primarily transmitted by Aedes mosquitoes, typically results in mild infections; however, it can cause severe fetal defects such as microcephaly in pregnant women. Symptoms include fever, arthralgia, myalgia, rash, and conjunctivitis, but many infections remain asymptomatic. Diagnosis is made based on clinical symptoms, exposure risk, and confirmed through real-time reverse transcription polymerase chain reaction (rRT-PCR) and antibody detection. No specific therapy exists for Zika virus; supportive measures are recommended. Preventative strategies include reducing mosquito exposure, implementing protective measures for travelers, and recommending temporary abstinence from pregnancy and safe sex after infection. Breastfeeding is advised, despite the potential risk for viral transmission.

34.1 Background

Zika virus (ZIKV) is primarily transmitted by infected mosquitoes of the Aedes genus, with *Aedes aegypti* being the principal vector. Additional modes of transmission include blood transfusion, sexual contact, and vertical transmission.

ZIKV typically causes a mild infection characterized by symptoms including rash, arthralgia, myalgia, conjunctivitis, and fever. If infection occurs during pregnancy, ZIKV can infect the placenta and cross into the fetal brain, damaging neural stem cells and impeding brain growth. A significant complication associated with this infection is congenital microcephaly. The incubation period for ZIKV ranges from 3 to 12 days, with symptom duration typically lasting 2–7 days.

I. Mylonas, *Sexually Transmitted Diseases*,
https://doi.org/10.1007/978-3-031-78204-6_34

34.2 Pathogen

Zika virus (ZIKV) belongs to the Flavivirus genus in the Flaviviridae family and is genetically related to other viruses such as Dengue virus (DENV-1 to DENV-4), West Nile virus (WNV), yellow fever virus (YFV), and Japanese Encephalitis virus (JEV). There are two primary strains of the virus: the African strain and the Asian strain, both capable of causing significant illness in humans, including fever, rash, joint pain, and severe neurological complications such as Guillain–Barré syndrome or congenital malformations in the offspring of infected pregnant women.

Zika virus is an arthropod-borne virus primarily transmitted by the *Aedes aegypti* mosquito and exhibits neurotropic properties, specifically targeting neural progenitor cells. Maternal infection leads to placental infection and damage, followed by viral transmission to the fetal brain. This process results in the destruction of neural progenitor cells and disrupts neuronal proliferation, migration, and differentiation. Consequently, brain growth is hindered, reducing neuronal cell viability.

34.3 Epidemiology

The **Zika virus** (a mosquito-borne flavivirus closely related to dengue, yellow fever, and West Nile virus) was **first identified in April 1947** in the Zika Forest of Uganda. The virus was initially isolated from a febrile rhesus macaque, which had been placed in a tree canopy as part of a yellow fever surveillance study conducted by the Virus Research Institute in Entebbe. Shortly thereafter, Zika virus was also isolated from *Aedes* mosquitoes in the same region.

The **first confirmed human infections** were reported in **1952 in Uganda and the United Republic of Tanzania**, where Zika virus-specific neutralizing antibodies were detected in sera from local populations, establishing that human exposure was occurring in Africa. Throughout the subsequent decades, sporadic cases and serologic evidence of infection were detected across **Africa and Asia**, but no large epidemics were documented, and the disease remained relatively obscure.

A major shift occurred in the **twenty-first century**:

- **2007:** The **first large documented outbreak** occurred on **Yap Island, Micronesia**, in the Pacific. Approximately 75% of the island's population was infected, though most experienced only mild illness.
- **2013–2014:** Subsequent **outbreaks occurred in French Polynesia and other Pacific Islands** (New Caledonia, Cook Islands, and Easter Island), marking the first recognition of an association between Zika virus infection and severe neurological complications, including **Guillain–Barré syndrome (GBS)**.
- **2015:** The virus was identified for the **first time in the Americas**, beginning in **Brazil**, where explosive transmission was accompanied by unprecedented clusters of microcephaly and congenital malformations, leading to recognition of **congenital Zika syndrome (CZS)** as a distinct entity. The outbreak spread rapidly to Central America, Mexico, and the Caribbean.

- **2016:** By the time of the **Rio de Janeiro Olympic Games**, local transmission had been confirmed in more than **60 countries and territories**, particularly in the Americas and Caribbean.
- **2017–2019:** Transmission declined globally, coinciding with population-level immunity and vector-control measures, though clusters continued in **Southeast Asia, India, Africa, and the Pacific Islands**.

Current Global Situation

- As of **2023**, **89 countries and territories** have reported **local vector-borne transmission** of Zika virus since its emergence in 2007. These include nearly all countries of the Americas, with exceptions such as continental **Chile, Uruguay, and Canada** (no autochthonous cases).
- Epidemiological surveillance indicates that the **largest disease burden** was borne by Latin America, especially **Brazil, Colombia, and Venezuela**, which together accounted for the majority of reported cases between 2014 and 2023. In fact, **10 countries were responsible for approximately 89% of all globally recorded cases** during this period.
- **Demographics:** The most affected age group is **15–49 years**, with a higher prevalence in women, reflecting both biological susceptibility and the heightened surveillance of infections during pregnancy.
- **Disease Burden:** While WHO and PAHO confirm declining incidence since 2017, sporadic outbreaks and continued low-level transmission persist in the Americas, Southeast Asia, and parts of Africa. No country has yet been declared Zika-free, as the virus remains part of the **circulating pool of arboviruses sustained by** Aedes aegypti **and** Aedes albopictus **vectors**.

Trends and Incidence

- According to modeled global burden data, between **2011 and 2015**, the **age-standardized incidence rate** increased nearly **73% per year**, peaking in **2015–2016** with >20 cases per 100,000 individuals.
- After 2017, incidence sharply declined, falling to approximately **3–4 cases per 100,000** by **2019**.
- Despite this decline, Zika virus is expected to persist **endemic in many tropical and subtropical regions**, with future outbreaks remaining possible due to climate change, urbanization, and continued vector distribution.

The risk of microcephaly is estimated at approximately 1% if maternal infection occurs during the first trimester. Overall, fetal abnormalities occur in approximately 29% of cases when infection occurs during pregnancy.

34.4 Clinical Manifestations

34.4.1 Gynecology

In up to 80% of cases, Zika virus infection is oligo- or asymptomatic, with symptoms typically lasting between 2 and 7 days. Many patients recover spontaneously during this time. However, the risk of a severe disease trajectory should not be underestimated, particularly in individuals with pre-existing medical conditions.

The clinical diagnosis of Zika virus infection is contingent upon the presence of at least two of the following four main symptoms: fever, skin lesions, arthralgia or arthritis-like symptoms, and non-purulent conjunctivitis. Additional symptoms such as gastrointestinal disturbances, headache, myalgia, and general malaise may also present. Zika virus infection has been associated with various severe medical conditions, including cardiac issues, musculoskeletal disorders, eye conditions, and neurological disorders.

Primary Clinical Features of Zika Virus Infection

- **Fever**
  - **Characteristics:** Typically **low-grade to moderate**, ranging between 37.8 and 38.5 °C (100.0–101.3 °F). Unlike dengue and chikungunya, fever in Zika is **milder and shorter in duration**.
  - **Duration:** Usually **2–3 days**, rarely lasting longer than 1 week.
  - **Frequency:** Present in about **65–75% of symptomatic cases**.
  - **Diagnostic Note:** High-grade fever (>39 °C/102 °F) is **more characteristic of dengue or chikungunya**, not Zika. Thus, absence or mild fever **does not exclude Zika**, especially if rash and conjunctivitis are present.
- **Rash**
  - **Characteristics:** A **generalized maculopapular erythematous rash**, often associated with **intense pruritus**. Typically begins on the face and upper body, then spreads to trunk, upper limbs, distal extremities, and palms.
  - **Prevalence:** Seen in up to **80–90%** of symptomatic Zika cases, making it the **most consistent feature**.
  - **Duration:** Persists for **5–7 days**, occasionally longer.
  - **Diagnostic Clue:** The **early onset and rapid spread** of rash, in combination with conjunctivitis, helps distinguish Zika from dengue (rash appears later in dengue). Differs from measles in being less confluent and less persistent.
- **Arthralgia/Arthritis-Like Symptoms**
  - **Characteristics:** Symmetrical **polyarthralgia and peri-articular pain**, mimicking arthritis. Most commonly involves **hands, wrists, ankles, and knees**.

  - **Duration:** Generally **several days to 2 weeks**; in some cases, pain persists for >1 month.
  - **Prevalence:** Occurs in about **60–70% of patients**.
  - **Differential Diagnosis:** May resemble chikungunya (which causes **more severe, prolonged joint pain and swelling**). In Zika, joint pain is usually **milder and resolves faster**.
- **Non-Purulent Conjunctivitis**
  - **Characteristics:** Acute, bilateral, non-purulent conjunctivitis, often one of the **earliest presenting signs**. Accompanied by conjunctival hyperemia, tearing, irritation, mild pain, and photophobia.
  - **Prevalence:** Reported in **35–55% of cases**.
  - **Duration:** Typically lasts **3–5 days**.
  - **Clinical Relevance:** Absence of mucopurulent discharge helps distinguish it from bacterial conjunctivitis. Presence along with rash strongly suggests Zika in endemic areas.

Additional Symptoms of Zika Virus Infection

- Beyond the characteristic triad of rash, arthralgia, and conjunctivitis, Zika virus infection may present with several additional manifestations. **Gastrointestinal symptoms** such as nausea, vomiting, and diarrhea are not uncommon and can complicate fluid balance, especially in children and pregnant women. These symptoms are generally self-limiting but may contribute to dehydration if not managed appropriately.
- Systemic complaints including **general malaise** are frequently reported. Patients may experience a diffuse sense of illness, fatigue, and loss of appetite. In some instances, **anorexia and painful oral ulcers** occur, further affecting nutritional intake. These nonspecific symptoms often overlap with those of other arboviral infections, underscoring the importance of considering epidemiological exposure when forming a differential diagnosis.
- **Headache and myalgia** are additional common features, with headaches often described as persistent, sometimes retro-orbital, and accompanied by diffuse muscle pain. The severity can vary widely, and while these symptoms are usually mild, they may interfere with daily functioning during the acute illness.
- Neurological symptoms may also appear during acute infection. Patients sometimes report **photophobia**, **dizziness**, and recurrent **vomiting**, which can raise suspicion for central nervous system involvement. Although uncommon in most adults, these neurological features can be more concerning in pregnant individuals and may indicate the need for closer monitoring.

Serious Complications Associated with Zika Virus Infection

- Although most cases are mild, Zika virus has been associated with several serious medical conditions affecting multiple organ systems. **Cardiac complications** such as arrhythmias and, in rare cases, heart failure, have been documented, likely reflecting the virus's capacity to trigger systemic inflammatory or immune responses.

- **Musculoskeletal complications** are most notable in congenital Zika virus syndrome, with **arthrogryposis multiplex congenita** being a key feature. This condition, marked by multiple joint contractures at birth, results from impaired fetal motor neuron function and intrauterine damage to the central nervous system.
- Ocular involvement is increasingly recognized as part of both congenital and postnatal infection. **Chorioretinal atrophy** and **optic neuritis** may present in infants with congenital Zika syndrome, but ocular damage has also been reported in older patients. These complications can lead to significant and sometimes irreversible visual impairment.
- The **neurological complications** of Zika virus infection are among the most serious. Acutely, cases of **myelitis** and **encephalitis** have been described, underlining the virus's neurotropic potential. In adults, **Guillain–Barré syndrome (GBS)** represents the most widely documented post-infectious complication, characterized by rapidly progressive muscle weakness, ascending paralysis, and potentially life-threatening respiratory involvement. In congenital cases, Zika infection disrupts brain development, resulting in severe structural abnormalities such as **lissencephaly** (a smooth brain surface due to defective neuronal migration) and **microcephaly**, which has emerged as the hallmark neonatal outcome with profound long-term neurodevelopmental consequences.

34.4.2 Pregnancy

Zika virus can be transmitted **transplacentally** at any stage of gestation; both **symptomatic** and **asymptomatic** maternal infections have been associated with adverse fetal outcomes. Estimates of the overall risk of **fetal abnormalities** among infants born to mothers infected during pregnancy range approximately from **6% to 42%**, reflecting heterogeneity in study populations, timing of infection, and diagnostic criteria. Maternal infection has been linked with increased risks of **spontaneous abortion**, **stillbirth**, **preterm delivery**, **hydrops fetalis**, and **intrauterine growth restriction (IUGR)**, although definitive causal quantification for some outcomes remains limited.

Microcephaly is the most prominent and recognized manifestation of congenital Zika virus infection and is most strongly associated with **first-trimester** maternal infection when **neurogenesis** and **cortical organization** are highly vulnerable. **Microcephaly** is defined as **head circumference >2 standard deviations below the mean** for sex, gestational age, and postnatal age; **delayed-onset microcephaly** has been documented, whereby infants born with normal head size subsequently develop growth failure and microcephaly in infancy. Population-based estimates suggest an approximate **1–4%** risk of microcephaly among pregnancies with confirmed maternal infection, and **severe microcephaly** is associated with substantial early neonatal mortality in a proportion of cases.

Neuropathology **and** neuroimaging findings characteristic of congenital infection include **ventriculomegaly**, **cortical atrophy**, **subcortical and periventricular calcifications**, **abnormal gyral formation** including **lissencephaly**, and

cerebellar or **brainstem hypoplasia**. These structural abnormalities commonly correlate with long-term **neurodevelopmental impairment**, including **severe motor dysfunction**, **intellectual disability**, **epilepsy**, and **sensory deficits**.

The constellation of anomalies recognized as **congenital Zika syndrome (CZS)** constitutes a specific pattern of malformations: **severe microcephaly** with **partially collapsed skull**, **thin cerebral cortices** with **subcortical calcifications**, **congenital contractures (arthrogryposis)**, **hypertonia** and **spasticity** impairing early motor development, and **visual** and **auditory impairments**. Diagnosis **is based on maternal** exposure history, laboratory confirmation **when possible, and characteristic** clinical **and** imaging findings **in the fetus or neonate.**

Congenital Zika Virus Syndrome (CZS)
WHO and CDC recognize CZS as a distinct pattern of birth defects, characterized by:

- Severe microcephaly and partly collapsed skull
- Thin cerebral cortices with subcortical calcifications
- Congenital contractures (arthrogryposis)
- Hypertonia and spasticity interfering with early motor development
- Visual and auditory impairments

In clinical practice, pregnant persons in endemic areas or with possible exposure should be evaluated for compatible symptoms such as maculopapular pruritic rash, arthralgia (particularly of small joints), nonpurulent conjunctivitis, and low-grade fever. Diagnostic RT-PCR testing on serum and urine is most informative within the first 7–14 days after symptom onset; serology (IgM, IgG) and plaque reduction neutralization testing (PRNT) may supplement diagnosis but are subject to cross-reactivity with other flaviviruses, notably dengue.

Pregnancy management following confirmed or suspected maternal infection requires serial obstetric ultrasound surveillance to monitor fetal growth, head circumference trajectory, intracranial anatomy, and amniotic fluid volume, with consideration of referral to maternal–fetal medicine specialists. Postnatal care for infants with *in utero* exposure should include comprehensive neonatal assessment: measurement of head circumference, cranial ultrasound or MRI when indicated, audiologic and ophthalmologic evaluation, and longitudinal neurodevelopmental follow-up to detect delayed manifestations and to initiate early intervention services as required.

34.5 Diagnosis

Diagnosing Zika virus infection requires consideration of both an individual's clinical symptoms and exposure history, including travel to areas where Zika virus transmission occurs or unprotected sexual contact with an individual meeting these exposure criteria.

It is crucial to understand that antibody responses to other flavivirus infections, such as Dengue virus, West Nile virus, and yellow fever vaccine, can yield cross-reactive results during antigen-antibody testing. Therefore, detecting ZIKV antibodies in populations previously exposed to these diseases may lead to nonspecific results.

To confirm a suspected Zika virus infection, rRT-PCR can be utilized to detect the presence of Zika virus RNA in serum, urine, or whole blood specimens. PCR testing is recommended within 2 weeks of initial suspicion of infection. Nucleic acid testing of whole blood also serves as an effective option for Zika virus detection.

Infections are typically diagnosed following a systematic stepwise approach (Fig. 34.1). Accurate detection of specific antibodies (IgG and IgM) and the virus itself requires timely testing.

- **Antibody Detection**
  - **Timing:** Antibodies (IgG and IgM) become detectable starting from day 7 after symptom onset.
  - **Serologic Testing:**
    - **Day 8–27 After Symptom Onset:** Antibodies can often be detected via serologic testing. Virus detection in urine may occur simultaneously.
    - **From Day 28 Onward:** Antibodies typically remain detectable for extended periods, serving as an indicator of prior infection.
- **Virus Detection**
  - **Sample Types:** Virus detection is possible in blood, urine, saliva, and semen.
  - **Day 1–7:** Viral RNA can be detected in blood and urine.
  - **Day 8–27:** Viral RNA detection in urine can be performed alongside serologic antibody testing.
- **Fetal Monitoring and Diagnostics**
  - **Ultrasound:**
    - **Frequency:** Performed every 3–4 weeks.
    - **Purpose:** To assess fetal infection, identify signs of congenital infection, and monitor fetal growth following maternal Zika virus infection.
  - **Magnetic Resonance Imaging (MRI):**
    - **Purpose:** Recommended for identifying fetal brain abnormalities associated with maternal Zika virus infection.
- **Advanced Diagnostic Considerations**
  - **Abnormal Ultrasound Findings:** May indicate the need for further diagnostic evaluation.
  - **Amniocentesis:**
    - **Consideration:** The decision to perform amniocentesis depends on individual clinical circumstances.
    - **Accuracy:** The reliability of amniotic fluid RT-PCR testing for Zika virus varies based on the timing of testing relative to maternal infection onset. Results should be interpreted with caution.

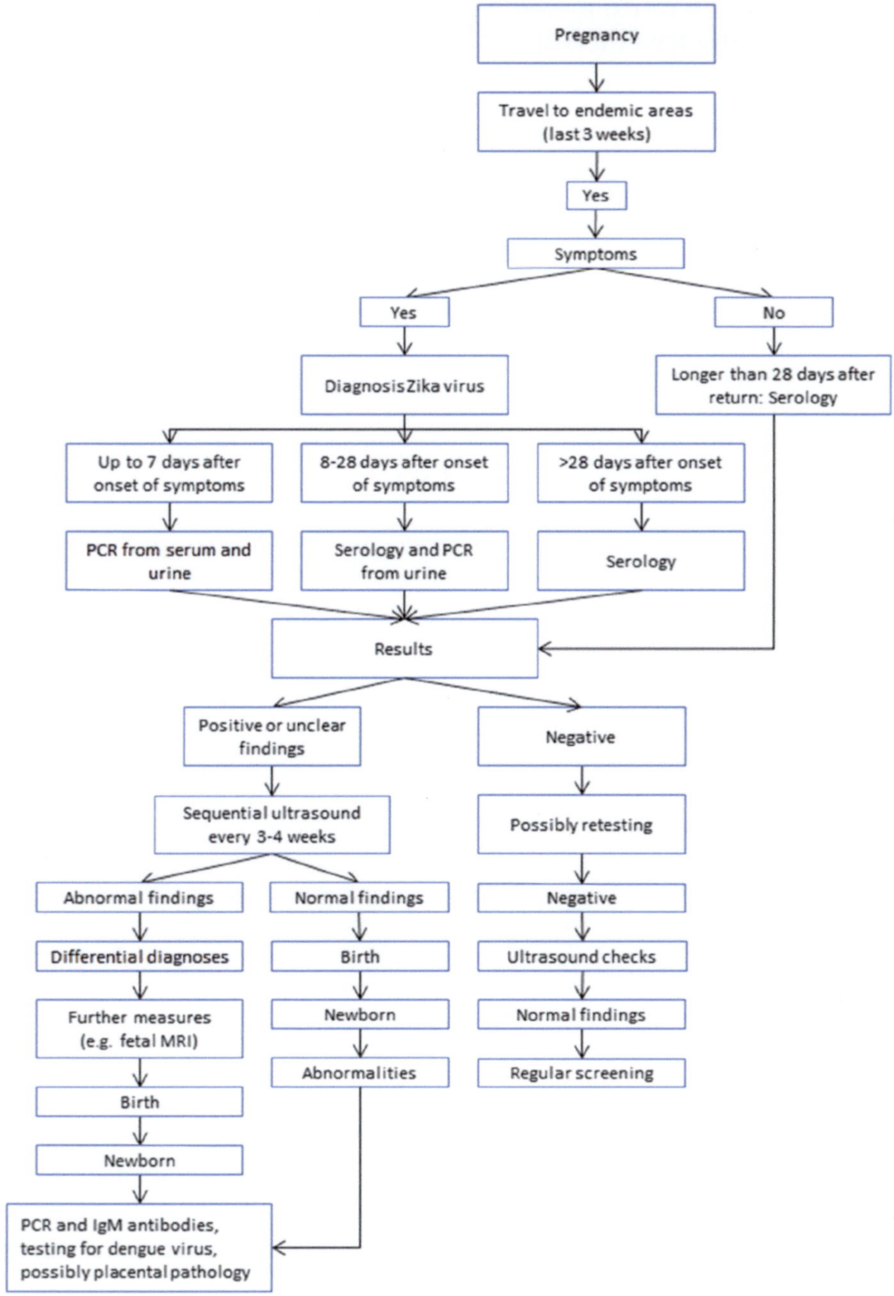

Fig. 34.1 Management protocol for suspected Zika virus infection during pregnancy. (Courtesy of I. Mylonas)

- **Positive RT-PCR Results:** May indicate fetal infection.
- **Negative RT-PCR with Abnormalities:** If RT-PCR results are negative but ultrasound abnormalities are present, alternative causes for fetal abnormalities should be considered.

The duration of rRT-PCR positivity in amniotic fluid remains unknown, indicating that a negative rRT-PCR result does not definitively eliminate the possibility of fetal Zika virus infection.

34.6 Treatment

At present, there is no specific antiviral treatment available for Zika virus disease. Management is primarily supportive and focuses on alleviating symptoms and preventing complications.

WHO and CDC recommend the following supportive measures:

- **Rest and Supportive Care**: Adequate rest and supportive management are essential to promote recovery.
- **Hydration**: Ensure sufficient fluid intake to prevent dehydration, particularly in patients with fever, vomiting, or reduced oral intake.
- **Antipyretics and Analgesics**: Acetaminophen (paracetamol) is recommended for the relief of fever and pain. Non-steroidal anti-inflammatory drugs (NSAIDs) and aspirin should be avoided until dengue virus infection has been excluded, due to the risk of bleeding complications.
- **Monitoring for Complications**: Patients should be observed for possible neurological (e.g., Guillain–Barré syndrome) or ophthalmological manifestations and managed accordingly in a hospital setting if complications develop.
- **Psychosocial Support**: WHO emphasizes the importance of providing emotional and psychosocial support to patients and families, particularly when Zika virus infection occurs during pregnancy. Families dealing with Zika-associated complications, such as congenital Zika syndrome, require long-term multidisciplinary support involving medical, social, and psychological services.

Treatment of Zika virus infection is symptomatic and supportive. Early recognition, appropriate fever management, careful exclusion of dengue before NSAID use, and comprehensive psychosocial support—especially for affected pregnant women and families—represent the core of WHO-recommended management.

34.7 Differential Diagnosis

The infectious differential diagnosis should include adenoviruses, chikungunya virus, dengue fever, and enteroviruses. Other diseases to consider are tick-borne encephalitis (TBE), yellow fever, hepatitis C virus (HCV), and influenza. Possible causes also include leptospirosis, malaria, measles, and parvovirus B19. In addition, infections caused by Rickettsia, rubella, and Group A Streptococcus (GAS) should be evaluated. West Nile virus infection may also need to be taken into account.

When microcephaly or abnormal findings are suspected, several differential diagnoses must be considered. Genetic factors play a significant role, either in the presence of existing clinical symptoms or sporadically. Moreover, infections such as herpes simplex virus (HSV), parvovirus B19, rubella, toxoplasmosis, *Treponema pallidum*, varicella (VZV), and cytomegalovirus (CMV) can contribute to developmental delays. Environmental factors and illnesses must also be considered; for instance, environmental toxins and medications can act as teratogens, while malnutrition and maternal diseases such as hypothyroidism may negatively impact the child's development.

34.8 Prevention

34.8.1 Exposure Prophylaxis

Preventing mosquito bites is essential to reduce the risk of Zika virus infection. Recommended measures include:

- **General Prevention Strategies**
  - **Use of Mosquito Nets:** Sleeping under mosquito nets, especially at night, is one of the simplest and most effective ways to reduce the risk of mosquito bites. This is particularly important in areas where mosquito-borne diseases such as Zika virus are prevalent. Nets treated with insecticide provide additional protection by killing mosquitoes on contact.
  - **Screens and Air Conditioning:** Installing screens on windows and doors helps to prevent mosquitoes from entering indoor spaces. Using air conditioning can further deter mosquitoes, as they are less active in cooler environments. Ensuring that screens are properly maintained and free of holes is crucial for optimal protection.
  - **Protective Clothing:** Wearing long trousers, long-sleeved shirts, and closed shoes reduces exposed skin, making it harder for mosquitoes to bite. Bright or light-colored clothing is recommended, as dark colors can attract mosquitoes. Protective clothing is especially important during the day and evening when *Aedes* mosquitoes, the primary carriers of the Zika virus, are most active.

- **Insect Repellents:**
  - **Application:** Apply mosquito repellents on exposed skin and clothing to repel mosquitoes effectively. Ensure the product chosen is specifically effective against *Aedes* mosquitoes, which are responsible for transmitting Zika virus. Repellents should be reapplied as directed on the label, particularly after swimming or sweating.
  - **Examples of Suitable Repellents:**
    - **Ircadin:** This repellent is considered safe for use throughout pregnancy and provides effective protection against mosquito bites.
    - **Diethyltoluamide (DEET):** While highly effective, DEET is not recommended during the first trimester of pregnancy due to potential risks. It may be used during later stages of pregnancy under medical guidance.
- **Post-Infection Measures**
  - **Preventing Virus Spread:** Individuals diagnosed with active Zika virus infections should take precautions to avoid being bitten by mosquitoes for at least 1 week. This measure helps prevent mosquitoes from acquiring the virus and transmitting it to others, thereby reducing the risk of further spreading the infection within the community.
  - **Post-Travel Precautions:** Travelers returning from regions where Zika virus is endemic should continue to protect themselves from mosquito bites for at least 3 weeks after their return, regardless of whether they exhibit symptoms. Asymptomatic individuals may still carry the virus and contribute to its transmission through mosquito vectors.
- **Recommendations for Couples Planning Pregnancy**
  - **Women:** It is recommended that women wait up to 8 weeks after the onset of Zika virus symptoms before attempting conception. This precaution minimizes the risk of passing the virus to the fetus during early pregnancy.
  - **Men:** Men should wait up to 6 weeks after symptom onset before attempting conception to reduce the risk of transmitting the virus to their partner during conception.
- **Sexual Transmission Risk**
  - **Men with Pregnant Partners:** Men who live in or travel to areas where Zika virus is endemic pose a potential risk of sexually transmitting the virus to their pregnant partner. To prevent this, consistent condom use throughout the duration of pregnancy is strongly recommended. Alternatively, abstaining from sexual activity during pregnancy is an effective way to eliminate this risk entirely.
- **Post-Infection Immunity and Guidelines**
  - **Confirmed Zika Virus Infection:** Current scientific evidence indicates that a confirmed Zika virus infection provides immunity against reinfection. Additionally, there is no increased risk for future pregnancies following

recovery from a Zika virus infection. This information offers reassurance to individuals planning pregnancies after recovering from the illness.
- **Vaccination and Reporting Requirements:** At present, no active or passive immunization is available for Zika virus prevention. In most countries, reporting Zika virus cases is mandatory to enable public health authorities to monitor and control outbreaks effectively.

Current evidence suggests that infection with the Zika virus induces a robust immune response, including the development of neutralizing antibodies. Based on available observational studies, serological follow-up, and analogy with other flaviviruses, Zika virus infection is believed to confer long-lasting—most likely lifelong—protective immunity, thereby preventing subsequent reinfections.

34.8.2 Breastfeeding

Breastfeeding provides optimal nutrition, immunological protection, and supports growth and neurodevelopment, while also reducing maternal risks of breast and ovarian cancer and improving birth spacing.

Based on this balance of evidence, WHO recommends that:

- Initiation of Breastfeeding: All newborns, including those born to mothers with suspected, probable, or confirmed Zika virus infection—or to mothers who have resided in, or returned from, Zika-endemic regions within the previous 2 weeks—should be placed skin-to-skin with their mothers and begin breastfeeding within the first hour after birth.
- Exclusive Breastfeeding: Infants should be exclusively breastfed for the first 6 months of life, with no other food or liquids provided.
- Complementary Feeding: At 6 months of age, appropriate and safe complementary foods should be introduced while breastfeeding continues.
- Prolonged Breastfeeding: Continued breastfeeding is recommended up to 2 years of age or longer, according to maternal preference and cultural context.

Overall, WHO emphasizes that breastfeeding should not be interrupted due to maternal Zika virus infection or exposure history, as the protective effects of breast milk decisively outweigh the unsubstantiated theoretical risks of viral transmission.

Key Points

- Zika virus is primarily transmitted by mosquitoes, specifically within the Aedes genus. The incubation period spans 3–12 days, and symptom duration generally ranges from 2 to 7 days.
- Zika virus falls within the Flavivirus genus and shares genetic relations with other viruses such as dengue virus, West Nile virus, and yellow fever virus. Both African and Asian strains of the virus exist, each capable of inducing severe disease in humans.
- Zika virus infection is often oligo- or asymptomatic but can manifest classic symptoms, including fever, rash, arthralgia, and conjunctivitis.
- Pregnant women face heightened risks of significant complications and fetal defects, with microcephaly being a critical concern. The risk of microcephaly is estimated at approximately 1% for infections occurring during the first trimester.
- Diagnosis is based on clinical symptoms and exposure history, employing antibody and RNA testing for detection of the virus.
- At present, there is no specific treatment for Zika virus infection.
- The differential diagnosis includes other infections, such as dengue fever, chikungunya virus, and enteroviruses.
- Preventative measures emphasize avoiding mosquito bites through the use of bed nets, appropriate clothing, and insect repellent. Those returning from endemic areas should remain protected from mosquito bites.
- Breastfeeding is recommended for infants born to mothers with suspected, probable, or confirmed Zika virus infection.

Part VII

Potential Sexually Transmitted Diseases

Bacterial Vaginosis

35

Abstract

Bacterial vaginosis (BV) is a disorder of the vaginal microbiome that is prevalent among women of childbearing age. It is characterized by an unpleasant odor, thin vaginal discharge, and an elevated vaginal pH. Diagnosis is primarily based on clinical symptoms and microscopic examination. Although BV is associated with a variety of bacterial species, *Gardnerella vaginalis* is recognized as a significant contributor. The condition is known to increase the risk of preterm delivery and warrants treatment during pregnancy. Recommended therapeutic agents include antibiotics such as metronidazole or clindamycin, administered either locally or systemically. Preventive measures for bacterial vaginosis include maintaining good vaginal hygiene, avoiding perfumed products, wearing cotton underwear, and utilizing condoms during sexual intercourse.

35.1 Background

Bacterial vaginosis (BV) is a common, clinically important disorder of the vaginal microenvironment, characterized by a dysbiotic shift in the vaginal microbiota. Although BV has not traditionally been classified as a classical sexually transmitted infection because of its polymicrobial etiology and its occurrence in sexually inactive persons, accumulating epidemiologic and molecular data implicate sexual exposure in acquisition and recurrence. High concordance rates reported in female same-sex partnerships—up to 90%—support a model of mechanical transfer of bacterial communities or biofilm components between sexual partners rather than a solely idiopathic process. Many scientific professional societies therefore increasingly consider BV to be a sexually transmitted disease (STD), although this

I. Mylonas, *Sexually Transmitted Diseases*,
https://doi.org/10.1007/978-3-031-78204-6_35

classification is not consistently confirmed in clinical practice; epidemiological and molecular data support a role for sexual transmission and partner-associated recolonization, while the frequent occurrence of BV in sexually inactive persons, its polymicrobial etiology, and the absence of a single clearly transmissible pathogen indicate that BV does not conform to the strict definition of a STD.

35.2 Pathogen

Bacterial vaginosis (BV) is characterized by a polymicrobial imbalance of the vaginal microbiota. Despite extensive investigation, no single pathogen has been identified as the sole causative agent. Culture-based studies typically reveal a diverse spectrum of bacterial species, although only a subset is integral to the pathogenesis (Table 35.1).

Gardnerella vaginalis is currently recognized as the principal pathogen in BV. This facultative anaerobic, gram-variable, non-motile rod was first described by Gardner and Dukes in 1954. It is detected in approximately 95% of BV cases but may also be present in up to 30% of asymptomatic healthy women. *Gardnerella vaginalis* functions as the primary colonizer initiating biofilm formation on the vaginal mucosa and plays a critical role in establishing dysbiosis.

The characteristic polymicrobial flora in BV includes, in addition to *Gardnerella vaginalis*, several accompanying organisms:

- ***Atopobium vaginae* (Now *Fannyhessea vaginae*):** This gram-positive, strictly anaerobic rod commonly coexists with *Gardnerella vaginalis* within the typical BV biofilm. *Atopobium vaginae* is an essential biofilm constituent and is associated with chronic and recurrent BV due to its production of enzymes that inactivate metronidazole, contributing to resistance against this standard antibiotic.

Table 35.1 Bacteria associated with bacterial vaginosis

Primary species/strongly associated with BV	Common accompanying species (uncertain association)
• *Gardnerella vaginalis* • *Atopobium vaginae* (*Fannyhessea vaginae*) • *Clostridium* spp. • BVAB-1, BVAB-2, BVAB-3 • *Megasphaera* spp. • *Mobiluncus* spp. • *Mycoplasma hominis* • *Peptostreptococcus* spp. • *Prevotella* spp./*Bacteroides* spp. (including *Bacteroides fragilis* group)	• *Leptotrichia* spp., *Sneathia* spp., *Dialister* spp. • *Mageeibacillus indolicus*, *Lachnocurva vaginae* • B-Streptococci (*Streptococcus agalactiae*) • *Enterococcus* spp. • *Escherichia coli* • *Lactobacillus iners* • *Staphylococcus aureus* • *Streptococcus viridans* • *Ureaplasma urealyticum*

Sensitivity to various beta-lactam antibiotics remains preserved. Detection relies primarily on molecular techniques such as polymerase chain reaction (PCR) or 16S rRNA gene sequencing, as conventional culture methods are unreliable. *Atopobium vaginae* is considered a critical marker of persistent or treatment-resistant BV.

- ***Prevotella* spp., *Porphyromonas* spp., *Bacteroides* spp.:** These groups demonstrate the high diversity of obligate anaerobic bacteria in BV. Taxonomic revisions have reclassified some former Bacteroides species under *Prevotella* spp. They commonly form part of the BV polymicrobial spectrum and contribute significantly to biofilm composition. Their prevalence varies with lifestyle, geographic factors, and individual risk profiles. These bacteria produce volatile amines responsible for the characteristic malodor associated with BV.
- ***Mobiluncus* spp.:** These motile, curved, gram-positive (often gram-variable) anaerobes are present in nearly all BV cases but only about 5% of healthy individuals. They adhere strongly to vaginal epithelial cells and exhibit distinctive rotational motility in wet mount preparations. *Mobiluncus* spp. are linked to an elevated risk of ascending infections and preterm birth, likely through induction of inflammatory responses along the genital tract.
- ***Peptostreptococcus* spp., *Ureaplasma urealyticum*, *Mycoplasma hominis*:**
  - *Peptostreptococcus* spp. are gram-positive anaerobic cocci found within BV biofilms.
  - *Ureaplasma urealyticum* and *Mycoplasma hominis*, members of the Mycoplasmataceae family, are small, cell wall-deficient bacteria frequently detected in BV but also part of normal vaginal flora. The clinical-pathogenic association is better established for *M. hominis*, particularly as a cofactor for pregnancy complications. Both species are significant causes of non-gonococcal urethritis, can cause urinary tract and ascending genital infections, and are detectable by molecular diagnostics.
- **BV-Associated Bacteria (BVAB-1, BVAB-2, and BVAB-3):** These species have thus far been identified exclusively by molecular methods, such as PCR and sequencing; they are not cultivable by conventional techniques. BVAB species serve as diagnostic markers for BV forms that exhibit particular treatment resistance or increased risk for ascending infections and recurrence.
- **Additional Accompanying Flora:** Anaerobic organisms including *Megasphaera* spp., *Leptotrichia* spp., *Sneathia* spp., *Dialister* spp., *Mageeibacillus indolicus*, and *Lachnocurva vaginae* are often detectable only through molecular genetic methods. These species indicate highly complex and treatment-refractory BV and have been increasingly documented in recent metagenomic[1] studies. They

[1] Metagenomic analyses have significantly advanced the study of bacterial vaginosis by enabling comprehensive identification and quantification of genomic fragments from vaginal samples. These studies confirm that BV is characterized by a polymicrobial biofilm structure and reveal numerous previously uncultivated BV-associated bacteria such as BVAB-1 to 3, Mageeibacillus indolicus, and *Lachnocurva vaginae*.

may contribute to immunomodulation, biofilm development, and persistence of the infection.

Bacterial vaginosis is marked by disruption of the normal lactobacillus-dominated vaginal flora. While *Lactobacillus iners* is frequently detected during BV episodes, it is not considered a classical pathogen but rather part of a disturbed yet not necessarily pathogenic microbiota.

A key pathogenic feature of BV is biofilm formation. *Gardnerella vaginalis* initiates biofilm development on the vaginal mucosa, with prominent integration of *Atopobium vaginae*. This biofilm structure shields embedded bacteria from host immune defenses and antibiotic therapies, contributing to frequent recurrences. The anaerobic microenvironment within the biofilm promotes proliferation of additional anaerobic companion bacteria.

Modern molecular diagnostic approaches such as PCR have demonstrated that traditional culture methods inadequately capture the full range of pathogens involved in BV. Bacterial vaginosis is associated with an increased risk of gynecological complications, secondary infections, and adverse pregnancy outcomes.

Other bacteria frequently detected in vaginal specimens include enterococci, staphylococci, various streptococci (notably group B Streptococcus), and *Escherichia coli*. However, their pathogenetic roles in BV remain unclear; these organisms are generally regarded as facultative pathogens or commensals.

35.3 Epidemiology

Epidemiology of Bacterial Vaginosis

Bacterial vaginosis represents one of the most prevalent causes of vaginal discharge among women of reproductive age worldwide, exhibiting significant variability in prevalence rates across geographic regions, ethnic populations, and clinical contexts. This complex vaginal dysbiosis syndrome poses considerable public health implications, particularly regarding adverse pregnancy outcomes and reproductive health complications.

Global Prevalence Estimates

The global prevalence of bacterial vaginosis among women of reproductive age ranges from 23% to 29%, based on systematic reviews and meta-analyses incorporating data from diverse populations. Among asymptomatic women aged 15–45 years, prevalence estimates are substantially lower at approximately 5%, indicating that a significant proportion of BV cases remain clinically unrecognized. Overall prevalence varies considerably, ranging from 10% to 38%, reflecting differences in diagnostic criteria, study populations, socioeconomic factors, and regional characteristics.

Regional Prevalence Variations

- **Europe**: European studies demonstrate marked regional heterogeneity, with prevalence rates spanning 5–30%. Eastern and Southern European regions consistently report higher prevalence rates compared to Northern and Western Europe. The United Kingdom exhibits prevalence estimates between 12% and 18%, while Scandinavian countries demonstrate comparatively lower rates, typically ranging in the mid-single digits.
- **North America**: In the United States, BV affects approximately 29.2% of women aged 14–49 years, corresponding to an estimated 21.2 million cases. The prevalence exhibits pronounced racial and ethnic disparities: African American women experience rates as high as 51.6%, Hispanic women approximately 32.1%, and non-Hispanic White women around 23.2%. These disparities reflect complex interactions between socioeconomic factors, genetic predisposition, stress exposure, and healthcare access.
- **Asia**: Asian populations demonstrate prevalence rates predominantly ranging from 10% to 30%, with considerable intraregional variation. Countries such as India, Bangladesh, and China report elevated prevalence rates, while recent studies from Malaysia indicate lower values of approximately 10.1%. These variations likely reflect differences in diagnostic methodologies, population characteristics, and environmental factors.
- **Africa**: sub-Saharan Africa exhibits the highest global BV prevalence rates, frequently exceeding 50%. Within this region, Southern and Eastern Africa demonstrate higher prevalence (33.3%) compared to Western and Central Africa (20.6%). Recent studies from Ethiopia report prevalence rates of 22.3% among pregnant women.
- **Latin America**: Although epidemiological data remain limited for Latin American populations, prevalence estimates range from 10% to 30%, with elevated rates observed in economically disadvantaged regions. The highest documented prevalence of 32.5% was reported among Black women in Rio de Janeiro, Brazil.

Prevalence in Pregnant Women

Bacterial vaginosis prevalence among pregnant women ranges from 23% to 29% globally, with higher rates predominantly observed in developing countries. Recent meta-analyses demonstrate significant trimester-specific variations:

- **First Trimester:** 26.2% (14.3% pooled estimate)
- **Second Trimester:** 14.1%
- **Third Trimester:** 8.9%
- **Symptomatic Pregnant Women:** 24.2%
- **Asymptomatic Pregnant Women:** 11.8%

Regional prevalence among pregnant women exhibits similar patterns to the general population, with Europe reporting 10–20%, the United States approximately 16% (with ethnic disparities persisting), Asia ranging from 5% to over 30%, and Africa exceeding 50% in many sub-Saharan regions.

Association with Adverse Pregnancy Outcomes

Current evidence establishes robust associations between bacterial vaginosis and adverse pregnancy outcomes, with multiple meta-analyses confirming significant relative risks. Key associations include:

- **Preterm Birth**: BV increases preterm delivery risk with odds ratios ranging from 1.4 to 2.9 across studies. Meta-analyses demonstrate a pooled 60% increased risk of preterm delivery in BV-positive women, with particularly elevated risks for delivery before 34 weeks gestation.
- **Premature Rupture of Membranes (PROM)**: The association between BV and PROM is consistently reported, with relative risks ranging from 1.1 to 6.8 across populations. Some studies report relative risks as high as 6.75 for PROM in BV-positive pregnancies.
- **Low Birth Weight**: BV significantly increases low birth weight risk, with relative risks ranging from 1.5 to 3.2. The association appears particularly pronounced in women with concurrent vaginal pathogens, such as *Mycoplasma hominis*.
- **Perinatal Mortality**: Globally, 10–30% of BV-positive pregnant women experience preterm birth, with approximately 70% of these cases associated with increased perinatal mortality. Studies demonstrate that preterm delivery following BV exposure accounts for up to 70% of worldwide perinatal mortality.
- **Neonatal Morbidity**: BV exposure significantly increases neonatal intensive care unit admissions (41.7% vs. 19.0%), respiratory support requirements (29.2% vs. 7.6%), and respiratory distress syndrome (33.3% vs. 9.0%). Histologic chorioamnionitis occurs in over 55% of BV-positive pregnancies, indicating intrauterine inflammatory processes.

- **Bacterial vaginosis is a prevalent condition among women of childbearing age globally, exhibiting significant regional variability.**
- **The highest prevalence rates are typically documented in Africa and parts of Asia, while Europe and North America show moderate prevalence with occasional regional variations.**
- **Pregnant women demonstrate considerable incidence of BV, highlighting the necessity for monitoring and managing this condition to avert potential complications.**

The microorganisms associated with bacterial vaginosis have been shown to suppress or outcompete the normal Lactobacillus-dominated vaginal flora. Several extrinsic and intrinsic factors have been associated with increased susceptibility to BV. Vaginal bleeding during pregnancy, higher frequency of sexual exposure—particularly with multiple partners—and administration of broad-spectrum antibiotics have been implicated; these factors disrupt Lactobacillus function and raise vaginal pH, thereby facilitating overgrowth of anaerobic organisms. Estrogen deficiency, as occurs in the postpartum period, has also been associated with increased risk of BV due to reduced glycogen availability and consequent impairment of Lactobacillus colonization.

In recent years, numerous risk factors have been identified concerning the onset of bacterial vaginosis. However, the relationship between these risk factors and the incidence of bacterial vaginosis is not always clearly delineated. Population studies indicate that women of African American descent are three times more likely to develop bacterial vaginosis compared to their Caucasian counterparts.

Important risk factors include:

- **Frequent Vaginal Douching**: This disrupts the natural vaginal microbiota, encouraging the growth of pathogenic bacteria.
- **Frequent Sexual Activity**: Engaging in regular intercourse, particularly with multiple partners, can alter the vaginal environment, increasing susceptibility to BV.
- **Low Socioeconomic Status**: Reduced access to healthcare, education, and hygiene products correlates with higher BV rates.
- **Physical Stress**: Stress can compromise immune defenses, making individuals more prone to infections such as BV.
- **Use of Vaginal Cosmetics**: Products like sprays and perfumes may irritate the vaginal mucosa and disturb its microbial balance.

35.4 Clinical Manifestations

35.4.1 Gynecology

Bacterial vaginosis (BV) is defined as a disturbance of the vaginal flora characterized by the absence of typical inflammatory signs. The condition features an elevated vaginal pH and the presence of a thin, often creamy, whitish-gray discharge (see Fig. 35.1). This discharge is commonly accompanied by a distinctive "fishy" odor, resulting from anaerobic bacterial metabolites, which patients frequently find distressing.

The primary subjective symptom of bacterial vaginosis is an unpleasant odor originating from vaginal discharge, occurring without clinical indications of vaginitis.

BV typically involves chronic polymicrobial colonization of the vagina by a diverse array of bacterial species with varying morphologies. Once established, this mixed bacterial community proves difficult to eradicate, even with targeted

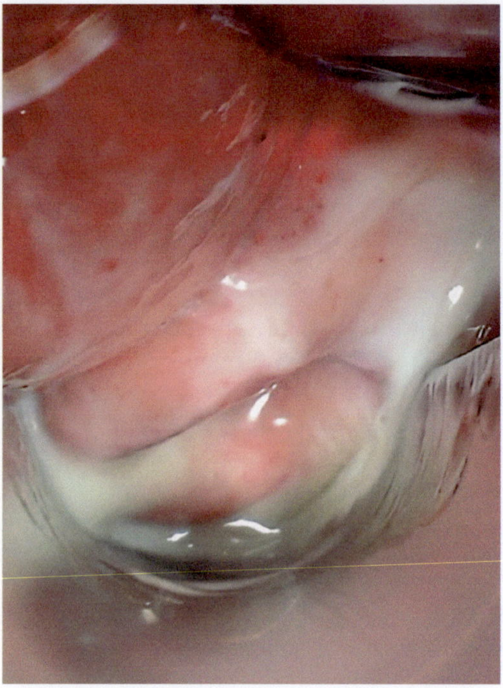

Fig. 35.1 Bacterial vaginosis characterized by thin, creamy, whitish-gray discharge (Mylonas 2025). (Courtesy of I. Mylonas)

antimicrobial therapy, contributing to high rates of recurrence. It is believed that facultative pathogens may interact synergistically, amplifying their pathogenic potential beyond that observed in infections caused by single-species pathogens. Many commensal pathogens possess effective mechanisms to evade the mucosal immune response, thus complicating the complete eradication of BV.

Epidemiologic investigations have consistently demonstrated an association between BV and increased acquisition of STDs. Multiple cohort and case control studies have reported higher incidence rates of *Chlamydia trachomatis*, *Neisseria gonorrhoeae*, *Trichomonas vaginalis*, *Mycoplasma genitalium*, and HIV among women with BV compared with those exhibiting lactobacillus dominant vaginal flora. These findings have been reproduced across heterogeneous populations and study designs, supporting a robust epidemiologic link between BV and susceptibility to STDs.

The magnitude of risk attributable to BV varies by pathogen and has been quantified in meta-analyses and individual studies. Relative risks and odds ratios in the range of approximately 1.8–4.0 have been described, with particularly elevated estimates reported for chlamydial and gonococcal infections. A dose–response relationship has been observed: higher Nugent scores, indicating more pronounced disruption of the vaginal microbiota, have been associated with incrementally greater risk of certain STDs.

Patterns of coinfection further substantiate the clinical relevance of BV. Both single and multiple concurrent STD diagnoses have been identified more frequently in women with BV, indicating a generalized susceptibility to a spectrum of sexually transmitted pathogens rather than an association confined to a solitary organism. This increased burden of coinfection has implications for targeted screening, partner notification, and integrated management strategies.

Patients diagnosed with bacterial vaginosis exhibit an increased risk of transmitting other infectious diseases, including HIV, HSV-2, trichomoniasis, gonorrhea, and *Chlamydia trachomatis* infections.

35.4.2 Pregnancy

Bacterial vaginosis (BV) is established as an important risk factor for preterm birth and other adverse obstetric outcomes, including preterm premature rupture of membranes (PROM) and histologic chorioamnionitis. The pathogenesis is primarily attributable to perturbation of the normal lactobacillus-dominated vaginal microbiota with subsequent overgrowth of anaerobic organisms capable of ascending into the upper genital tract. Ascension is facilitated after membrane rupture and may permit direct microbial access to the amniotic cavity, thereby increasing the likelihood of intra-amniotic infection and chorioamnionitis.

Mechanistically, BV-associated organisms have been shown to provoke inflammatory reactions within the decidua and amnion. Production of proteolytic enzymes (e.g., proteases) and membrane-active phospholipases by these bacteria results in biochemical weakening of fetal membranes and predisposes to rupture. Concurrently, stimulated release of proinflammatory cytokines—including interleukin-6 (IL-6), interleukin-8 (IL-8), and tumor necrosis factor-alpha (TNF-α)—has been implicated in the cascade leading to uterine contractility, cervical remodeling, and membrane rupture, thereby promoting preterm labor.

Histopathological analyses have demonstrated an increased frequency of chorioamnionitis in pregnancies complicated by BV. Epidemiological data correlate BV, particularly when present early in gestation, with higher rates of preterm delivery, low birth weight, and neonatal morbidity. Importantly, the inflammatory response and associated obstetric risk are not confined to symptomatic cases; asymptomatic BV has been associated with similar pathophysiological effects, supporting the rationale for consideration of screening and early management in selected populations.

Overall, BV contributes to preterm birth through ascending infection, enzymatic degradation of fetal membranes, and cytokine-mediated inflammatory pathways that compromise membrane integrity and promote parturition.

Despite conflicting results from various studies involving patients with bacterial vaginosis, this condition is now recognized as one of the most common causes of preterm birth.

Bacterial vaginosis during pregnancy is associated with several serious obstetric complications:

- **Premature Rupture of Membranes (PROM): Early rupture of the amniotic sac, which may lead to infection and preterm birth.**
- **Intrauterine Infection and Chorioamnionitis**: Infection of the fetal membranes, posing significant risks to both the mother and fetus.
- **Spontaneous Abortion**: An increased risk of miscarriage, particularly in early pregnancy.
- **Preterm Delivery**: A major contributor to neonatal morbidity and mortality, with bacterial vaginosis identified as a significant risk factor.
- **Postpartum Endometritis**: Infection of the uterine lining following childbirth, leading to prolonged recovery and increased maternal morbidity.
- **Fetal Growth Retardation**: Impaired fetal growth in utero, resulting in low birth weight and potential long-term developmental challenges.

Diagnosis of BV within the first 16 weeks of gestation has been associated with a markedly increased risk of miscarriage and preterm delivery, with effect sizes of up to fivefold reported and independent of other covariates, such as prior preterm birth. Meta-analyses indicate that BV identified before 16–20 weeks' gestation confers the greatest risk: pooled odds ratios for preterm delivery have been reported between 4.2 and 7.5 and for spontaneous abortion up to 9.9.

The prevalence of BV is higher among women with a history of preterm birth (approximately 25%) compared with women whose prior deliveries were at term (≈11%). In this high-risk subgroup, screening and antimicrobial treatment—most consistently with clindamycin when initiated in the second trimester—have been demonstrated to reduce preterm delivery rates in several studies, indicating a protective effect. By contrast, in low-risk populations routine antibiotic treatment for BV has not been shown to reduce the incidence of late miscarriage or preterm birth.

Pregnant women with subclinical or asymptomatic BV are more often found to have a history of sexually transmitted infections and increased vaginal colonization with Mobiluncus species. Reported stress levels are frequently lower in asymptomatic patients compared with symptomatic ones. Crucially, symptom status has not been correlated reliably with adverse pregnancy outcomes, underscoring the importance of detecting and managing asymptomatic BV to mitigate the risk of poor obstetric outcomes.

In summary, early detection and targeted therapy of BV—particularly in women with a prior preterm delivery—are recommended to reduce the risks of miscarriage and preterm birth. Asymptomatic BV is common and clinically relevant; therefore, it should be considered in risk assessment and management algorithms even in the absence of symptoms.

Because bacterial vaginosis is easily detectable, requires no complex diagnostic procedures, and has well-established treatment protocols, it is recommended that all pregnant women undergo screening for this condition. Such screening can lead to significant reductions in preterm births at low cost and with minimal time investment.

35.5 Diagnosis

35.5.1 Wet Mount Microscopy

Diagnosis is established through clinical symptoms and microscopic examination of vaginal specimens (Sect. 3.4.5), along with pH measurement if necessary. A phase contrast microscope with 400× magnification should be utilized when possible.

Diagnosis of Bacterial Vaginosis—Amsel Criteria:
Bacterial vaginosis is diagnosed when three of the following four criteria are met:

- Gray-white, homogeneous vaginal discharge
- pH $\geq$ 4.4 (normal range is approximately 3.8–4.4)
- Positive amine test (odor intensification following the addition of 10% KOH solution — whiff test)
- Detection of clue cells in at least 20% of epithelial cells.

However, it is now accepted that the detection of only two of the four criteria is sufficient for diagnosing bacterial vaginosis:

- pH > 4.4
- One of the other three criteria

Characteristic of bacterial vaginosis are the so-called clue cells, observed in native preparations, 0.1% methylene blue, or Gram-stained specimens. Clue cells are epithelial cells heavily colonized with *Gardnerella vaginalis* and anaerobes, rendering their borders indistinguishable (Fig. 35.2).

The amine odor test (whiff test), in which a 10% KOH solution is applied to a microscope slide containing vaginal secretions, aids in diagnosis by intensifying the fishy odor. The presence of clue cells is associated with a sensitivity of 43.1% and a

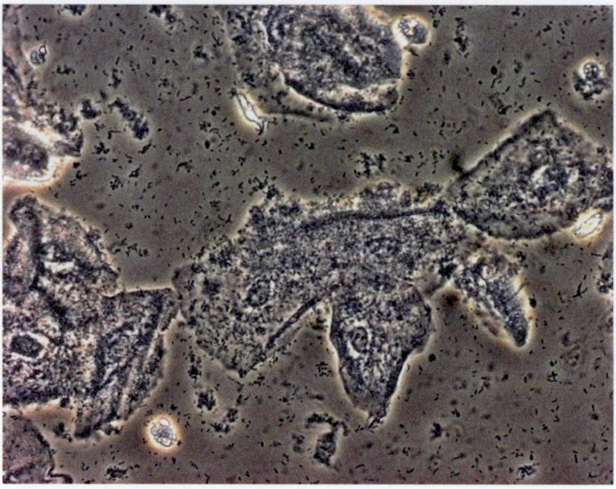

Fig. 35.2 Phase-contrast microscopy of bacterial vaginosis demonstrating absence of lactobacilli and presence of characteristic clue cells (Mylonas 2025). (Courtesy of I. Mylonas)

specificity of 99.6% for diagnosing bacterial vaginosis, while a positive whiff test alone displays only a sensitivity of 6.58% and a specificity of 73.6%.

Bacterial vaginosis is diagnosed in the outpatient clinic by microscopic examination of a wet-mount (native) preparation of vaginal secretions at 400× magnification, combined with assessment of vaginal pH using a test strip. Routine bacteriological culture is of limited clinical value in this context and may prompt unnecessary treatment of laboratory findings, with potential harm to the patient.

35.5.2 Nugent Score for Diagnosing Bacterial Vaginosis

The Nugent score utilizes a standardized approach based on the microscopic examination of Gram-stained vaginal swabs to diagnose bacterial vaginosis. This scoring system provides an objective and reproducible method for evaluating vaginal microbiota (Table 35.2).

Advantages of the Nugent score:

- **Objective and Reproducible:** Supplies a consistent and standardized method for diagnosing bacterial vaginosis.
- **Severity Grading:** Enables assessment of severity based on Gram-staining results of vaginal swabs (Fig. 35.3).
- **Risk Assessment:** May assist in evaluating the potential risks for complications such as preterm delivery or postoperative infection.

Table 35.2 Nugent score for Gram-stained vaginal smears. The average number of morphotypes counted per field of view at 1000× magnification is given. Rating: 0–3 points = Normal, 4–6 points = Intermediate, unclear, 7–10 points = Bacterial vaginosis

Score	Gram-positive rods[a]	Gram-negative/Gram-variable rods[b]	Gram-variable curved rods[c]
0	≥30 per field	0 (none)	0 (none)
1	5–30 per field	<1 per field	<1 per field
2	1–4 per field	1–4 per field	1–4 per field
3	<1 per field	5–30 per field	5–30 per field
4	0 (none)	≥30 per field	≥30 per field

[a]Gram-positive rods (*Lactobacillus* spp.)—large, uniformly stained Gram-positive bacilli that predominate in healthy vaginal flora

[b]Gram-negative/Gram-variable rods (*Gardnerella* spp., *Prevotella* spp., and *Porphyromonas* spp.)—small to pleomorphic rods with reduced or inconsistent Gram staining; increased numbers are associated with dysbiosis

[c]Gram-variable curved rods (*Mobiluncus* spp.)—slender, curved bacilli showing variable Gram staining and typically present in elevated counts in bacterial vaginosis

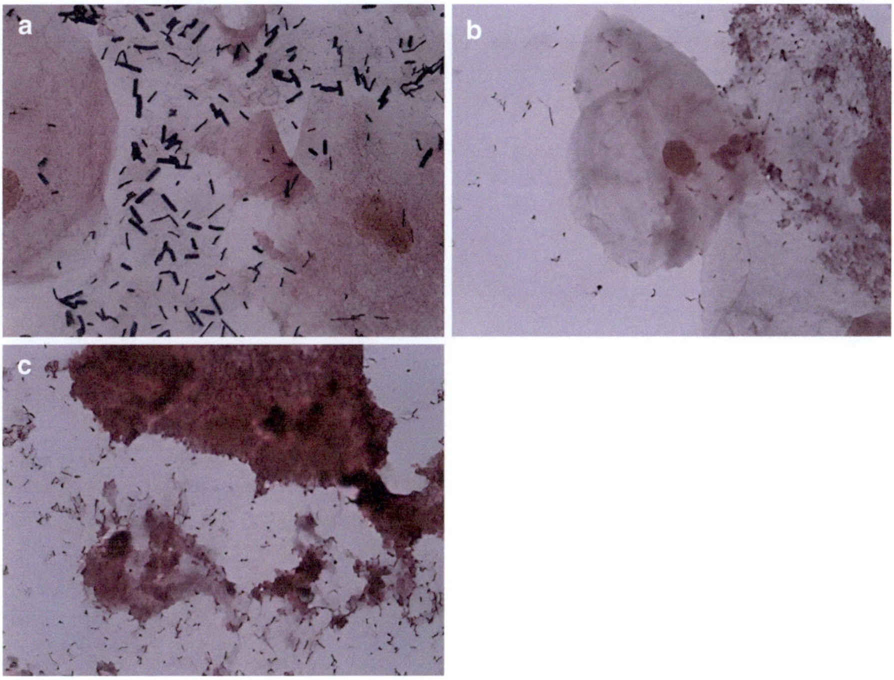

Fig. 35.3 Bacterial vaginosis and Gram stain (Nugent Score) (Mendling 2006). (**a**) Normal vaginal flora (Nugent score: 0); (**b**) Intermediate flora (Nugent score: 6); (**c**) Bacterial vaginosis with abundant Mobiluncus (Nugent score: 10)

Disadvantages of the Nugent Score:

- **Equipment Requirements:** Necessitates specific laboratory equipment for Gram staining.

- **Expertise Needed:** Requires specialized knowledge for appropriate application and interpretation. The method distinguishes between different types of bacteria, not all of which are pertinent to bacterial vaginosis.
- **Reliability Issues:** May exhibit lower reliability in specific populations, such as pregnant or postmenopausal women.
- **Limited Scope:** Does not incorporate all relevant aspects of bacterial vaginosis, including clinical symptoms or the pH of vaginal secretions.
- **Additional Testing:** May necessitate further tests or examinations to confirm the diagnosis.
- **Potential for Misdiagnosis:** External factors, such as antibiotic therapy or menstrual bleeding, may influence results, leading to potential misdiagnosis.
- **Interpretation Challenges:** Interpretation may present ambiguities, especially between varying severity levels.

While the Nugent score offers advantages, including objective assessment and graded severity, its application requires specific equipment and expertise. Additionally, it may lack reliability in certain populations. Furthermore, the Nugent score does not encompass all relevant clinical aspects, often necessitating additional tests for confirmation.

The Nugent score is not routinely employed in many countries.

35.6 Treatment

Clinically equivalent preparations, including metronidazole and clindamycin, are available for the medical treatment of bacterial vaginosis, both prior to and during pregnancy. However, these medications produce different antibiotic resistance profiles in anaerobic bacteria. Clindamycin, in particular, is commonly utilized to treat antibiotic-resistant anaerobes.

A multitude of regimens and combinations has been investigated for the treatment of bacterial vaginosis. Variations in dosages and routes of administration have demonstrated therapeutic efficacy. However, oral therapy is typically *preferable* to topical applications, offering slightly improved cure rates. Single-dose therapies exhibit lower response rates compared to continuous antibiotic administration over a seven-day period. Therefore, single-dose therapy should only be reserved for exceptional situations (e.g., noncompliance).

Oral antibiotic therapy should be prioritized over intravaginal formulations to optimize treatment outcomes. Single-day or single-dose regimens are reserved for exceptional circumstances (e.g., anticipated nonadherence) and frequently require repeat administration within 1 week.

Systemic Therapy

- Metronidazole 500 mg orally twice daily for 7 days. In patients with increased volume of distribution (e.g., obesity), metronidazole 500 mg orally three times daily for 7 days may be considered.
- Metronidazole 250 mg orally three times daily for 7 days.
- Metronidazole 2000 mg orally as a single dose. Single-dose therapy is less effective than multi-day regimens and should be reserved for exceptional circumstances (e.g., anticipated nonadherence).
- Clindamycin 300 mg orally twice daily for 7 days. In patients with increased volume of distribution (e.g., obesity), clindamycin 300 mg orally three times daily for 7 days may be considered.
- Amoxicillin 750 mg orally three times daily for 7 days. In patients with increased volume of distribution (e.g., obesity), amoxicillin 1 g, orally three times daily for 7 days may be considered.
- Novel Option: Secnidazole 2 g as an oral granule given as a single dose; the granules are typically sprinkled onto a small amount of applesauce, yogurt, or pudding and swallowed immediately without chewing or mixing with liquids. Availability is limited in some countries.[2]

Local (Vaginal) Therapy: Availability of specific topical formulations varies by country. Vaginal applicators should be prescribed separately for individual treatments if they are not available.

- Metronidazole Cream 5%: Apply intravaginally 2–3 times daily for 7 days.
- Clindamycin Cream 2%: Apply intravaginally once daily for 7 days.
- Tetracycline/Amphotericin B Vaginal Ovules: Insert 1–2 ovules daily for 5–10 days.
- Tetracycline/Amphotericin B Cream: Fill 1–2 applicator volumes daily for 5–10 days.

Adjunctive or Post-Treatment Local Options (Controversial): The evidence supporting these options is heterogeneous; formulation availability differs by region.

- Dequalinium Chloride Vaginal Tablets: 1–2 tablets daily for 6 days.
- Vaginal Lactobacilli Preparations (Suppositories/Ovules): Insert one suppository nightly for 6 days.
- Octenidine Dihydrochloride Vaginal Preparation: Apply once daily for 7 days.
- Acidification with Lactic Acid Preparations: Apply 1–2 times daily or use 1–2 suppositories daily for 4–8 days.

[2] Secnidazole is approved by the FDA in the United States for the treatment of bacterial vaginosis in adult women and in females aged 12 years and older. The recommended single oral dose is 2 g (granules). Common adverse effects reported include headache, nausea, vomiting, diarrhea, and metallic taste; less commonly reported events include vaginal odor, abnormal vaginal discharge, and vaginal pruritus. Secnidazole is contraindicated in suspected pregnancy and should be avoided during breastfeeding; it is contraindicated in individuals with hypersensitivity to nitroimidazoles (e.g., metronidazole and tinidazole). Availability and approved indications vary by country.

Table 35.3 Treatment strategies for bacterial vaginosis during pregnancy

Therapy	Medication	Dosage	Duration
Local therapy (1st trimester)	2% clindamycin cream	Once daily	7 days
Local therapy (2nd to 3rd trimester)	5% metronidazole cream	2–3 times daily	7 days
	2% clindamycin cream	Once daily	7 days
Systemic therapy (2nd to 3rd trimester)	Metronidazole	500 mg orally twice daily	7 days
	Metronidazole	250 mg orally three times daily	7 days
	Metronidazole	2000 mg orally, as a single dose	–
	Clindamycin	300 mg orally twice daily	7 days

While topical antiseptics may be employed, their therapeutic efficacy is generally inferior to that of antibiotic regimens. Post-treatment administration of lactobacilli or lactic acid preparations is frequently undertaken; however, the clinical effectiveness of these interventions remains disputed, including when used prophylactically. Because bacterial vaginosis has been associated with an increased risk of preterm delivery, treatment is indicated when the condition is diagnosed during pregnancy. Irrespective of gestational age, intravaginal clindamycin administered for 7 days is recommended. Intravaginal metronidazole may be administered beginning in the second trimester (Table 35.3).[3]

Beginning in the second trimester, systemic therapy is preferred, regardless of the antibiotic employed.

The efficacy of treating bacterial vaginosis with lactobacilli preparations, both outside of and during pregnancy, cannot be conclusively established; however, it is probable that such treatments may bolster local defenses by contributing to a lower pH environment.

35.7 Differential Diagnosis

In the differential diagnosis of bacterial vaginosis, other infectious forms of vaginitis must be considered. These include gonorrhea, genital herpes, lichen planus mucosae, lichen sclerosus et atrophicus, streptococcal vaginitis, Trichomonas vaginitis, vulvodynia, and vulvovaginal candidosis.

[3]Metronidazole has been authorized for first-trimester use in several countries.

35.8 Prevention

Due to the current limited and inconclusive evidence concerning specific sexual and nonsexual risk factors for BV, definitive prophylactic guidelines cannot be established at this time. The multifactorial etiology of this disease, together with individual variability in susceptibility, complicates the identification of clear preventive measures. Nevertheless, practical guidance regarding appropriate vaginal hygiene and lifestyle modifications should be provided to minimize disturbance of the natural vaginal ecosystem.

Patient education should emphasize the avoidance of practices that disrupt the vaginal microbiota, such as vaginal douching or the internal use of cleansing devices and substances. These interventions have been shown to alter vaginal pH and microbial balance, facilitating the overgrowth of anaerobic bacteria implicated in BV. Additionally, certain behaviors and lifestyle factors—such as having multiple or new sexual partners—have been epidemiologically associated with an increased risk of BV development. Although causality remains unproven, raising awareness of these risks and encouraging behavioral modification where appropriate is advisable.

Preventive strategies aimed at preserving or restoring a balanced vaginal microbiota are recommended to reduce the incidence and recurrence of BV. The following key approaches should be highlighted during patient counseling:

- **Avoid Excessive Personal Hygiene:** The vagina possesses a natural self-cleaning mechanism maintained by lactobacilli and mucosal secretions. Aggressive cleansing with harsh soaps or irritants can disrupt this defense system.
- **Refrain from Using Perfumed Products in the Genital Area:** Fragranced soaps, sprays, powders, and shower gels may disturb the delicate microbial environment and cause mucosal irritation, increasing susceptibility to dysbiosis.
- **Use mild, Unscented Soaps Exclusively for External Cleansing:** These products effectively maintain perineal hygiene without negatively impacting vaginal flora or mucosal integrity.
- **Choose Cotton Underwear:** Cotton's breathable properties promote ventilation and reduce moisture retention in the genital area, thereby preventing conditions conducive to bacterial overgrowth.
- **Avoid Tight-Fitting Clothing:** Restrictive garments limit airflow and increase humidity in the vulvovaginal region, facilitating proliferation of pathogenic bacteria.
- **Limit Unnecessary Antibiotic Use:** Antibiotics can indiscriminately eradicate beneficial lactobacilli, contributing to microbial imbalance. Antibiotic therapy should be reserved for clinically justified indications under medical supervision.
- **Consistently Use Condoms During Sexual Activity:** Barrier protection reduces transmission of STD that may predispose to BV by altering the vaginal flora or inducing mucosal inflammation.

- **Adopt a holistic approach to vaginal health, including:**
  - Balanced intimate hygiene practices that support mucosal health without causing irritation or disruption;
  - A nutritious diet rich in vitamins, minerals, and probiotics to enhance systemic immunity and maintain a healthy vaginal microbiome;
  - Stress management techniques and smoking cessation, as both stress and tobacco use have been implicated in microbial dysbiosis and impaired mucosal defenses;
  - Identification and management of individual risk factors such as frequent changes in sexual partners to mitigate susceptibility to BV.

Partner therapy is not presently recommended due to limited efficacy in preventing recurrence.

Given the well-established association between bacterial vaginosis (BV) and preterm birth, vaginal pH measurement and microscopic examination of vaginal secretions should be included in the initial gynecological assessment. During pregnancy, these evaluations are recommended in the first trimester, with subsequent screenings once per trimester as part of routine prenatal care.

Furthermore, pregnant patients should receive counseling about the increased risk of acquiring and transmitting other sexually transmitted infections (STIs), including HIV, herpes simplex virus type 2 (HSV-2), trichomoniasis, gonorrhea, and *Chlamydia trachomatis*. Comprehensive patient education regarding these risks is important to promote awareness and facilitate timely preventive measures and interventions.

Key Points

- Bacterial vaginosis is a disorder of the vaginal environment.
- It is not classified as a sexually transmitted disease, although sexual transmission is possible.
- A well-documented association exists between bacterial vaginosis and preterm birth, as well as other obstetric complications.
- Prophylaxis and treatment remain significant challenges.
- Pathogens implicated in bacterial vaginosis include *Gardnerella vaginalis*, Prevotella spp., Porphyromonas spp., Bacteroides spp., Mobiluncus spp., Peptostreptococcus spp., *Ureaplasma urealyticum*, *Mycoplasma hominis*, and *Atopobium vaginae*.
- Symptoms include grayish-white homogeneous discharge, elevated vaginal pH, and a fishy odor.

(continued)

- Diagnosis is based on the Amsel criteria, including vaginal discharge, pH measurement, the amine test, and identification of clue cells.
- Treatment options include metronidazole or clindamycin, administered either locally or systemically.
- Prevention strategies involve proper vaginal hygiene, avoiding excessive antibiotic use, and employing condoms during sexual intercourse.
- Diagnosis and treatment during pregnancy are particularly critical.
- Patients should be informed about the increased risk of other infectious diseases.
- Measurement of pH and evaluation of native preparations in pregnant women are essential.

Vulvovaginal Candidosis

36

Abstract

Vulvovaginal candidosis is an infection caused by fungi of the genus Candida, primarily affecting the external genitalia, vagina, intercrural region, and perianal area. Approximately 85–95% of cases are attributed to *Candida albicans*. Symptoms typically include pruritus, erythema, burning sensations, dyspareunia, dysuria, and vaginal discharge. Diagnosis relies upon patient medical history, clinical manifestations, and microscopic identification of the organism. Treatment often involves local and systemic antifungal agents. Non-albicans species, such as *Candida glabrata*, *Candida tropicalis*, and *Candida parapsilosis*, present therapeutic challenges. Intermittent antifungal therapy may be advocated for patients experiencing recurrent candidosis. Vaginal antifungal treatments are generally considered safe during pregnancy. Preventive strategies encompass hygienic practices and management of underlying conditions.

36.1 Background

Vulvovaginal candidosis (VVC), often also known as vulvovaginal candidiasis, is a common infection of the estrogenized vagina and vestibule caused by *Candida* spp., most frequently *Candida albicans*, although non-albicans species such as *C. glabrata*, *C. tropicalis*, and *C. krusei* are encountered. Candida organisms are commensal constituents of the lower female genital tract and may colonize the external genitalia, introitus, intercrural folds, and perianal region without producing symptoms.

Under conditions that alter the local environment or host defenses—for example, elevated estrogen states, antibiotic exposure, pregnancy, diabetes mellitus, or systemic immunosuppression—*Candida* spp. may proliferate and invade the vaginal epithelium. Symptomatic infection is typically manifested by pruritus, burning, erythema, and a thick, curd-like (white) vaginal discharge.

I. Mylonas, *Sexually Transmitted Diseases*,
https://doi.org/10.1007/978-3-031-78204-6_36

Although the term "candidiasis" is widely employed in clinical practice, the alternative nomenclature "candidosis" is also used; both terms are accepted interchangeably in the medical literature.

Vulvovaginal candidosis is frequently classified as a sexually transmitted infection in many English-speaking countries. Although an association with sexual activity has been observed, the condition's high recurrence rates—even when sexual contact is absent—and the presence of multiple additional risk factors indicate that transmission cannot be attributed exclusively to sexual intercourse.

36.2 Pathogens

Fungal taxonomy has historically been based on macroscopic and microscopic morphological features; however, genomic and molecular methods are increasingly integrated to refine taxonomic resolution and to clarify phylogenetic relationships.

Clinically, fungal infections are commonly categorized into three principal groups that correspond to the D-H-S classification (Dermatophyte–Yeast–Mold):

- Dermatophyte Infections: Keratin-targeting fungi producing tinea corporis, tinea pedis, onychomycosis (e.g., *Trichophyton rubrum*, *Microsporum canis*, and *Epidermophyton floccosum*).
- Yeast Infections: Mucocutaneous and vulvovaginal infections predominantly caused by *Candida* spp. (e.g., *Candida albicans*, *C. glabrata*, *C. tropicalis*, and *C. krusei*).
- Mold Infections: Infections caused by filamentous fungi that may involve skin, soft tissue, sinopulmonary sites, or become invasive in immunocompromised hosts (e.g., *Aspergillus fumigatus* causing invasive aspergillosis or cutaneous aspergillosis; *Fusarium* spp. producing keratitis and disseminated infection; Mucorales such as *Rhizopus* spp. causing mucormycosis).

Within gynecology, most mycotic disease is attributable to facultatively pathogenic yeasts of the *Candida* genus, particularly *C. albicans*; non-albicans Candida species (*C. glabrata*, *C. tropicalis*, and *C. krusei*) have been increasingly implicated in clinical disease and may demonstrate differing antifungal susceptibility patterns. *Candida* spp. are commensal members of the lower genital tract but are able to cause symptomatic infection when host or environmental factors are altered (e.g., antibiotic exposure, immunosuppression, or hormonal changes).

While morphological classification retains clinical utility, the incorporation of molecular and genomic data has improved diagnostic accuracy, informed epidemiology, and directed therapeutic decision-making—particularly for Candida-related gynecologic infections where species identification and susceptibility profiling influence management.

- **General Characteristics**: Although most *Candida* species are considered apathogenic, fewer than 20 are recognized as facultative pathogens.
- **Candida albicans**: Accounts for 85–95% of vaginal colonization in premenopausal, pregnant, and asymptomatic women, and is prevalent among those experiencing acute vaginal candidosis.
- **Non-albicans species**:
  - *Candida glabrata* (newer phylogenetic classification: *Nakaseomyces glabrata*): More frequently isolated from postmenopausal and immunocompromised women; the second most common yeast in candidosis post-*C. albicans*.
  - *Candida tropicalis*: The third most common species implicated in candidosis, following *C. glabrata*.
  - *Candida parapsilosis*: Often observed in catheter-associated infections; capable of causing vulvovaginitis.
  - *Candida krusei*, *Candida guilliermondii*, and other species: These can produce vulvovaginitis with classic symptoms, though they are less prevalent.
  - *Saccharomyces cerevisiae*: Rarely linked to vaginal discomfort, identified in 1–2% of vaginal cultures.

In gynecological practice, *Candida* species remain the primary etiological agents of mycoses. *Candida albicans* predominates, accounting for the majority of vaginal infections, while the incidence of non-albicans species, particularly *Candida glabrata*, is rising, especially among postmenopausal and immunocompromised populations.

Facultative Pathogenic Candida Species:
Common: *Candida albicans, Candida glabrata, Candida tropicalis, Candida parapsilosis*
Isolated: *Candida guilliermondii, Candida krusei, Candida kefyr, Candida lusitaniae, Candida veswanathii*
Rare: *Candida africana, Candida catenulata, Candida dubliniensis, Candida famata, Candida haemulonii, Candida holmii, Candida inconspicua, Candida intermedia, Candida lusitania, Candida norvegensis, Candida ceylanoides, Candida rugosa, Candida utilis*

C. albicans is a highly polymorphic yeast capable of transitioning among four morphological forms—oval blastospores (budding yeast), elongated pseudohyphae, true septate hyphae, and thick-walled chlamydospores—each of which contributes to its pathogenicity and tissue invasiveness. In contrast, *C. glabrata* exists almost exclusively in the budding-yeast (blastosporic) form and lacks both pseudohyphal and true-hyphal stages, which influences its interaction with host tissues and antifungal susceptibility.

In the genital tract, pseudohyphal formation by Candida species correlates with colonization potential, yet most colonizing isolates remain in the budding-yeast morphology. Among women with vulvovaginal candidosis, *C. albicans* accounts for 80–95% of all episodes, making it by far the most prevalent causative species. *C. glabrata* is the second most commonly isolated pathogen, particularly in older or diabetic patients and in those with recurrent or refractory infections.

Molecular typing studies have revealed extensive genetic heterogeneity among *C. albicans* isolates. Multiple genotypes can be recovered from both asymptomatic carriers and symptomatic women with acute or chronic recurrent vulvovaginal candidosis, indicating that host factors—such as immune status, vaginal microbiome composition, and local estrogen levels—play a critical role in determining whether colonization progresses to symptomatic infection. Genotypic variation also influences virulence traits, including adhesin expression, biofilm formation, and secretion of hydrolytic enzymes (e.g., secreted aspartyl proteinases), which contribute to disease persistence and recurrence.

36.3 Epidemiology

The incidence of vulvovaginal candidosis (VVC) is modulated by estrogen-dependent factors within the vaginal microenvironment, including glycogen availability and resultant glucose concentration, and by the expression of estrogen-responsive pathways in *Candida albicans*. Consequently, children and postmenopausal women are susceptible to VVC predominantly when additional predisposing conditions (e.g., exogenous estrogen exposure, diabetes mellitus, or local mucosal compromise) are present.

VVC is widespread worldwide; the annual global incidence has been estimated at approximately 372 million cases. Substantial geographic variation in prevalence has been reported among women of reproductive age, with point or period prevalence estimates ranging from approximately 5–75% depending on region and study methodology. European prevalence has been estimated at roughly 20–30%, whereas lifetime prevalence estimates in the United States approach 75%. Asian prevalence is heterogeneous, with reported rates between ~10% and >50%; higher frequencies have been observed in parts of South and Southeast Asia. Prevalence in Africa generally exceeds global averages, particularly in sub-Saharan populations. The United Kingdom and Scandinavian countries demonstrate intermediate rates within the European range, whereas socioeconomically disadvantaged areas in Latin America tend to report higher prevalence figures.

Regional estimates are influenced by differences in study design, diagnostic criteria (clinical versus mycological confirmation), sampling frames, and population risk factors (e.g., contraceptive use, pregnancy, diabetes, HIV prevalence, and antibiotic exposure). Therefore, caution is warranted when comparing prevalence figures across studies and regions.

The epidemiological data on VVC during pregnancy demonstrate considerable regional differences. Global estimates suggest prevalence rates of 10–30%. Specific regional prevalence rates include:

- **Europe**: 20–40%, though some countries may report elevated figures.
- **United States**: Approximately 15–25%.
- **Asia**: Estimates range from 10% to 25%.
- **Africa**: Prevalence varies significantly, estimated at 15–30%.
- **UK, Scandinavia, Latin America**: Comparable rates to those observed in Europe, from 20% to 40%.

Yeast colonization of the vagina depends on the presence of estrogen and the associated estrogen receptors linked to *Candida albicans*. Young girls prior to menarche and menopausal women typically demonstrate lower vaginal colonization, resulting in a decreased likelihood of developing Candida vaginitis. Healthy, non-pregnant, premenopausal women show a 20–30% rate of vaginal yeast colonization, which increases to at least 30% during the third trimester of pregnancy and in women with known immunocompromised diseases. *Candida albicans* is the most frequently isolated species during pregnancy.

The transition from asymptomatic vaginal colonization to clinically manifest vulvovaginal candidosis (VVC) is multifactorial and remains incompletely elucidated. Epidemiological data indicate that approximately 70–75% of otherwise healthy women will experience at least one episode of VVC during their lifetime, whereas about 5–10% will develop recurrent VVC (RVVC), conventionally defined as ≥4 symptomatic episodes within 12 months.

Asymptomatic colonization with *Candida* spp. is common; colonization rates of 20% to over 60% have been reported depending on the study population and detection methods. Progression from colonization to symptomatic infection does not occur in all carriers, indicating that additional host, microbial, and environmental determinants are required. Principal contributory factors are outlined below.

- Host Factors: Genetic predisposition and innate and adaptive immune responses have been implicated. Alterations in mucosal immunity (e.g., impaired neutrophil function) and polymorphisms in immune-related genes (e.g., MBL2, IL12, NLRP3, and TLR2) have been associated with increased susceptibility to RVVC. NLRP3 inflammasome activation and related cytokine responses have been implicated in mucosal inflammation in VVC.
- Hormonal Milieu: Estrogenic states (such as pregnancy, combined oral contraceptive use, or exogenous hormone therapy) increase vaginal glycogen content and local epithelial susceptibility, thereby promoting Candida proliferation and symptomatic disease.
- Microbiota and Behavioral Determinants: Disruption of the Lactobacillus-dominant vaginal microbiota—secondary to broad-spectrum antibiotic exposure, uncontrolled diabetes mellitus, or other dysbiotic states—facilitates Candida overgrowth. Additional behavioral or local factors (e.g.,

occlusive clothing, non-cotton underwear, and certain hygiene practices) may further alter the local microenvironment and predispose to infection.

– Candida Virulence Attributes: Transition from yeast to filamentous (hyphal) morphologies, secretion of proteolytic enzymes and the pore-forming peptide candidalysin, and biofilm formation have been shown to enhance epithelial adherence, tissue invasion, and mucosal inflammation, thereby promoting symptomatic disease and recurrence.

The pathogenesis of symptomatic VVC is therefore best understood as the consequence of interactions between host susceptibility, hormonal and microbiotal conditions, and Candida virulence mechanisms.

Approximately 10% of affected women go on to develop chronic-recurrent vulvovaginal candidosis, defined as four or more distinct symptomatic episodes within a single year. This subgroup often requires tailored management strategies—including long-term suppressive antifungal therapy and assessment for predisposing factors such as uncontrolled diabetes or immunosuppression.

Neonatal candidosis represents a notable cause of early superficial fungal disease in the newborn, with manifestations that can range from localized mucocutaneous infections to, rarely, invasive disease in high-risk infants. Risk of transmission is greatest with maternal vaginal colonization at the time of delivery and when peripartum risk factors (prolonged rupture of membranes and maternal broad-spectrum antibiotic use) are present. Neonates delivered vaginally may develop oropharyngeal candidosis (oral thrush) and/or Candida-associated diaper dermatitis secondary to intrapartum exposure to *Candida albicans*. Consequently, prophylactic measures aimed at reducing maternal asymptomatic vaginal Candida colonization in the late third trimester are often advised to decrease the risk of neonatal colonization and early postnatal infection.

Women with diabetes mellitus, particularly those with poorly controlled hyperglycemia, face a significantly elevated risk of developing vulvovaginal candidosis (VVC). Hyperglycemia promotes Candida adherence and growth by increasing vaginal glycogen content and impairs neutrophil function and cell-mediated immunity. Standard single-episode antifungal regimens often fail unless serum glucose levels are optimized; achieving and maintaining euglycemia is therefore essential for treatment success and relapse prevention.

Moreover, infections due to *Candida glabrata* have become increasingly prevalent in women with type 2 diabetes mellitus. *C. glabrata*'s intrinsic reduced susceptibility to azoles often necessitates alternative therapies—such as intravaginal boric acid or topical nystatin—and underscores the need for species-specific identification prior to treatment.

Additional factors, such as parity, age, nationality, and preeclampsia, do not seem to affect susceptibility to fungal infections.

36.4 Clinical Manifestations

36.4.1 Gynecology

Patients typically report symptoms of vaginal pruritus and erythema, accompanied by marked discomfort, burning sensations, dyspareunia, and dysuria. Labial edema may be observed, and fissures, known as rhagades, especially occur in atopic women.

Itching of the introitus occurs in approximately 90% of fungal infection cases.

Vulvar pruritus is the most frequently reported symptom of vulvovaginal candidosis (VVC); however, it lacks diagnostic specificity. Only approximately 35–40% of women presenting with genital pruritus are ultimately found to have VVC, whereas alternative etiologies such as bacterial vaginosis, trichomoniasis, contact dermatitis, or other dermatoses are commonly identified. Associated symptoms of VVC include burning, vulvovaginal soreness, external dysuria, dyspareunia, and erythema of the vulva and vestibule.

Vaginal discharge is a frequent clinical finding but demonstrates variable appearance. In early or mild VVC, the discharge may be serous or thin, whereas established infection characteristically produces a thick, white, curd-like ("cottage-cheese") discharge that is typically odorless; this feature can assist in distinguishing VVC from bacterial vaginosis, in which a malodorous, fishy discharge is more common.

Neither pruritus nor abnormal discharge is sufficiently specific to confirm VVC. Therefore, clinical assessment should be corroborated by laboratory evaluation—for example, wet-mount microscopy with saline and 10% KOH to identify budding yeasts, pseudohyphae or hyphae, or by culture/speciation when indicated (recurrent, refractory, or non-albicans infections)—to establish the diagnosis and guide appropriate therapy.

Clinical features and diagnostic relevance:

- Vulvar Pruritus: Most common symptom; low specificity (≈35 to 40% attributable to VVC)
- Vaginal Discharge: Often thick, white, curd-like, and odorless in VVC; moderate diagnostic value

– Burning, Soreness, Erythema, Dyspareunia, and External Dysuria: Supportive clinical signs but not pathognomonic

Appropriate laboratory confirmation is recommended before initiating antifungal therapy when diagnostic uncertainty exists, in recurrent disease, or when non-albicans species are suspected (Fig. 36.1).

Symptomatic vulvovaginal candidosis manifests in various forms, complicating clinical diagnosis:

Vesicopustular form:

- Characterized by vesicular lesions.
- Begins with isolated yellowish vesicles, which may later coalesce into larger clusters.

Eczematoid form:

- Exhibits diffuse swelling, erythema, and scaling at the introitus.
- Resembles eczematous dermatitis with significant inflammation.

Follicular form:

- Involves the hair follicles of the pubic region.
- Presents as pustules and papules surrounding hair follicles, indicating localized infection.

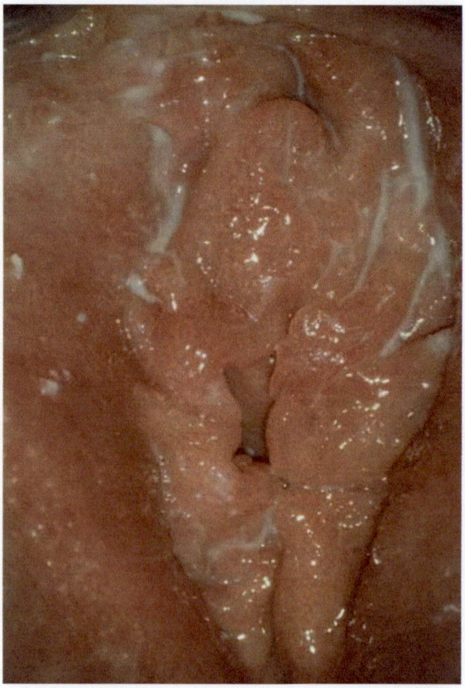

Fig. 36.1 Vulvovaginal candidosis presentation (Mylonas and Petersen 2009)

Extension of vulvovaginal candidosis beyond the vulva to involve the perianal region is uncommon but has been documented. Perianal erythema and irritation are more likely when intestinal colonization with Candida species is concurrent and have been reported in severe or persistent infections, particularly in patients with predisposing conditions such as diabetes mellitus or in those treated with sodium-glucose cotransporter-2 (SGLT2) inhibitors.

Cutaneous hypersensitivity reactions to Candida antigens may present at distant sites as papules, erythema, or pustules. These lesions are generally immunologically mediated rather than resulting from direct fungal invasion of the skin.

Urinary tract involvement by Candida may occur, with urethral colonization or ascending infection of the bladder reported in selected cases. Fungal cystitis is rare and is most frequently observed in the presence of additional risk factors—uncontrolled diabetes, prolonged indwelling urinary catheterization, systemic immunosuppression, or other significant comorbidities. The propensity of *Candida* spp. to form biofilms on indwelling devices (e.g., urinary catheters) increases the likelihood of persistent or device-associated infection.

Rare manifestations and clinical context

- Perianal Involvement: Perianal erythema/irritation associated with intestinal colonization or severe disease; risk factors include diabetes and SGLT2 inhibitor therapy.
- Allergic Cutaneous Reactions: Papular, erythematous, or pustular eruptions occurring via hypersensitivity to Candida antigens rather than by direct cutaneous colonization.
- Fungal Cystitis/Urinary Tract Infection: Uncommon; typically associated with diabetes, prolonged catheter use, or immunosuppression; biofilm formation on devices contributes to pathogenesis.

When atypical or disseminated manifestations are suspected, microbiological confirmation and assessment for underlying predisposing conditions are recommended to guide targeted management.

36.4.2 Pregnancy

Vertical transmission of *Candida* spp. from mother to neonate is frequent. Studies have reported acquisition rates of up to 45% (80% in some studies) among infants delivered vaginally to colonized mothers. Colonization is more likely after vaginal delivery than cesarean section, and *Candida albicans* is the species most commonly transmitted. In healthy, term neonates, colonization typically presents as oropharyngeal candidiasis (oral thrush) or Candida-associated diaper dermatitis, most often within the first year of life.

Invasive candidosis (including candidemia and disseminated infection) represents a substantially more severe complication and predominantly affects preterm and very low birth weight (VLBW) infants. The risk of invasive disease increases as gestational age and birth weight decrease; reported incidences in the absence of prophylaxis range from approximately 4–5% in infants >1500 g to as high as ~10%

in those <1000 g. These infections are associated with considerable morbidity and mortality.

Both vertical (intrapartum) and horizontal (nosocomial) routes contribute to neonatal Candida acquisition. In neonatal intensive care units, environmental reservoirs and transmission via healthcare workers' hands and indwelling devices are important contributors to colonization and subsequent infection.

Preventive measures have been shown to decrease early neonatal colonization and superficial disease. Treatment of maternal vulvovaginal candidosis with topical azoles in late pregnancy reduces neonatal acquisition rates. In high-risk neonates, antifungal prophylaxis and strict infection-control practices (hand hygiene, catheter care, and minimization of broad-spectrum antibiotics) have been associated with substantial reductions in oral thrush and diaper dermatitis incidence—reported reductions from approximately 10% to about 2% by the fourth postnatal week in some settings.

- **Congenital (Fetal) Candidosis:** Congenital or fetal candidosis is caused by in utero infection with *Candida* spp., most commonly via ascending infection from the maternal genital tract; hematogenous (transplacental) dissemination is less frequent. Neonatal clinical presentation may include erythematous, desquamative cutaneous lesions, respiratory distress, signs of systemic inflammatory response or sepsis, pneumonia, meningitis, and multi-organ dysfunction. Preterm and low-birth-weight neonates are at increased risk. The clinical syndrome may be indistinguishable from bacterial neonatal sepsis; therefore, prompt recognition and initiation of antifungal therapy are required, as delayed treatment has been associated with higher mortality and adverse neurodevelopmental outcomes.
- **Candida Amnionitis (Chorioamnionitis):** Candida amnionitis denotes infection of the amniotic fluid and fetal membranes by *Candida* spp. Although uncommon, it has been associated with adverse obstetric outcomes, including preterm labor, fetal infection, and neonatal sepsis. Predisposing factors that have been reported include prolonged rupture of membranes, use of intrauterine devices, cervical cerclage, and assisted reproductive techniques such as in vitro fertilization. Candida albicans is the species most frequently isolated; other species (e.g., *C. glabrata* and *C. kefyr*) have also been described. Diagnosis may be suggested by clinical features and amniotic fluid analysis and is confirmed by culture and/or histopathology of the membranes. Therapeutic data are limited and no universally accepted treatment guideline exists; systemic antifungal agents (e.g., fluconazole or amphotericin B) have been administered in selected cases, with variable outcomes.
- **Congenital Candida Sepsis with Intact Amniotic Sac:** Rarely, systemic fetal candidosis and congenital Candida sepsis have been documented in the presence of an intact amniotic sac. In such instances, infection is

thought to result from hematogenous spread or transplacental transmission, producing disseminated fetal disease that can present with sepsis, multi-organ dysfunction, or intrauterine fetal demise. Case reports and histologic studies have demonstrated that Candida organisms are capable of traversing intact membranes; maternal symptoms or overt vulvovaginal candidosis may be absent.

36.5 Diagnosis

The clinical manifestations of vulvovaginal mycosis can sometimes be ambiguous, particularly during pregnancy. The diagnosis is contingent upon a thorough assessment that includes obtaining the patient's history, recognizing clinical signs and symptoms, and detecting yeast fungi, typically through microscopic evaluation of a native vaginal fluid sample. Staining techniques may be employed; however, they do not significantly enhance diagnostic reliability.

The microscopic examination of vaginal fluid using either saline or a 10% KOH solution at 400× magnification via a phase-contrast microscope represents the most straightforward and rapid diagnostic approach in clinical practice. Experienced examiners can easily identify blastospores, pseudomycelia, or true mycelia (Fig. 36.2). Additionally, a moderate proliferation of leukocytes may be noted in the native specimen, although this finding is often subtle or absent.

A vaginal secretion pH measurement may be performed; however, vulvovaginal candidosis alone does not typically produce an alkaline shift. pH alteration is usually observed only when the lactobacillary flora is substantially disturbed or replaced.

In contemporary clinical practice, microbiological culture has been largely replaced by microscopic detection of yeast for the diagnosis of acute vulvovaginal candidosis. However, in asymptomatic pregnant patients, microscopic identification of yeast is achieved in only approximately 50–60% of cases. When blastospores or pseudohyphae are not visualized, culture with species-level identification is required—particularly for chronic, recurrent vulvovaginal candidosis or for presentations that are diagnostically challenging.

A yeast culture with species identification is indicated in cases of diagnostic uncertainty, recurrence, or complication, including:

- *Candida albicans*: >90% of cases
- *Candida glabrata*: approximately 2%

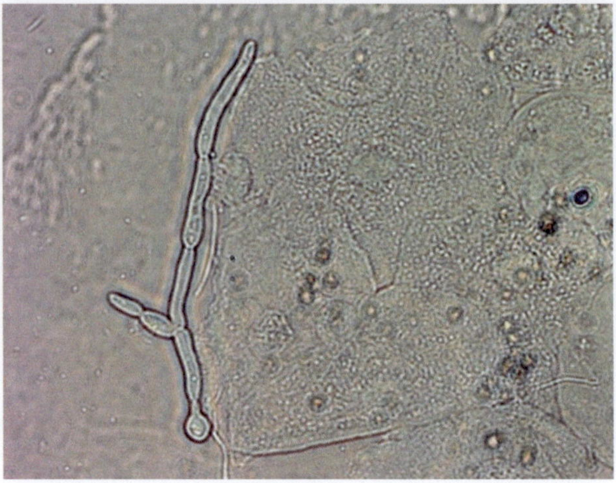

Fig. 36.2 Wet mount microscopy revealing fungal hyphae in symptomatic vulvovaginal candidosis (×400) (Mylonas 2025). (Courtesy of I. Mylonas)

- *Candida krusei*, *Candida parapsilosis*, *Candida guilliermondii*, *Candida tropicalis*, *Candida pseudotropicalis*, and others: each approximately 1%

Despite the availability of alternative and equally sensitive culture media, such as Chroma agar and Microstix-Candida, Sabouraud glucose agar remains the most commonly utilized medium for the culture-based detection of *Candida* infections. Although vaginal isolates of *Candida albicans* with higher minimum inhibitory concentrations to fluconazole have been reported, azole resistance remains a rare exception in gynecologic practice. Consequently, routine resistance testing is generally not recommended.

Superficial vulvovaginal candidosis does not lead to elevated antibody levels, making serologic testing ineffective for diagnosis. The polymerase chain reaction (PCR) represents a highly sensitive method for identifying fungal infections; however, a lack of conclusive studies and no standardized, simple lab methods means PCR is infrequently utilized in the routine diagnosis of *Candida* infections.

Serologic antibody titers are not recommended for superficial vulvovaginal candidosis.

36.6 Treatment

36.6.1 Gynecology

General

Vulvovaginal candidosis is treated with antifungals chosen by clinical category (uncomplicated vs complicated/recurrent), Candida species, and patient factors. Uncomplicated cases (usually *C. albicans*) are managed with short topical azoles or a single 150 mg oral fluconazole dose; complicated or recurrent disease requires prolonged or systemic therapy guided by species identification and susceptibility testing. Patient-specific issues (pregnancy, liver function, drug interactions, diabetes, immunosuppression, and adherence) and adjunctive measures (glycemic control, removal of local irritants, and education) must be considered.

Treatment of asymptomatic sexual partners does not confer additional benefit to the index patient and is therefore not routinely recommended. When partner treatment is considered (e.g., persistent recurrent infections despite appropriate therapy, symptomatic partners, or specific epidemiologic concerns), it should be guided by clinical findings and culture results.

A variety of medications in different dosage and application forms are available for the treatment of acute vulvovaginal candidosis. Treatment options typically include polyenes, imidazoles, or ciclopiroxolamine delivered in various preparations such as vaginal tablets, vaginal suppositories, and vaginal creams, with treatment duration typically spanning from one day to one week. Oral triazoles may also be used for 1-day therapies, accompanied by skin creams for vulvar application (Table 36.1). Comparative studies have indicated that all treatment regimens yield comparably effective clinical and mycological outcomes.

Asymptomatic colonization does not necessitate treatment, provided that there is no underlying immunosuppression, comorbidities, or chronic recurrent vulvovaginal candidosis.

Vulvovaginal Candidosis

Vaginal antifungal treatments are generally well tolerated. Topical azoles (e.g., clotrimazole, miconazole, and econazole) are associated mainly with localized adverse effects; transient burning, stinging, or irritation is reported in approximately 1–10% of users and is usually mild. True allergic contact reactions are uncommon but possible and may present as contact dermatitis; systemic allergic reactions are rare. Systemic adverse effects such as headache, nausea, or gastrointestinal symptoms are uncommon with vaginal formulations and occur more frequently with oral antifungals (e.g., fluconazole).

Efficacy of vaginal antifungals is high for uncomplicated vulvovaginal candidosis. Clinical and mycological cure rates of topical agents are reported in the order of 85–90% within 1–2 weeks after appropriate treatment. At follow-up intervals of 4–6 weeks, sustained cure rates fall modestly (approximately 75–80%), reflecting early recurrence or reinfection in a minority of patients. For uncomplicated

Table 36.1 Antifungal therapy for initial or recurrent vaginal candidosis

Medication	Application form	Dosage	Duration
Clotrimazole	Cream/vaginal ovules (combo pack)	Apply externally two to three times daily: one vaginal ovule or vaginal tablets 200 mg twice daily	3–6 days
Miconazole	2% cream	Apply 5 g once daily	14 days
	Vaginal ovules	Insert 100 mg once daily	7 days
		100 mg single dose	
Tioconazole	Cream	Apply 100 mg once daily	7 days
Fenticonazole nitrate[a]	Vaginal ovules	Insert 600 mg single dose	
Isoconazole	Vaginal tablets	Take 100 mg once daily	7 days
	Vaginal ovules	Insert 600 mg single dose vaginal suppository	
Econazole[a]	1% cream	Apply 5 g intravaginally once daily	14 days
	Vaginal ovules	Insert 150 mg once daily for 3 days, then 150 mg twice daily for 1–3 days	
Nystatin 100,000 IU	Cream	Apply one to two times daily	10–14 days
Ciclopiroxolamine[b]	Cream	Fill applicator twice daily	3–7 days
Tetracycline/	Vaginal ovules	Insert one to two times daily	7–10 days
amphotericin B[b]	Cream	Fill one to two applicators per day	7–10 days

Before any medication is prescribed, availability should be ensured. Vaginal applicators may need to be separately prescribed for most treatments

[a] May damage condoms

[b] Recommended for difficult cases. Not available in every country

infections, topical and single-dose oral regimens have broadly comparable effectiveness; the choice between them is often guided by patient preference, convenience, contraindications, pregnancy status, and concern for systemic exposure.

Practical considerations include interactions with barrier contraceptives and relapse prevention. Some topical azole formulations may weaken latex condoms and diaphragms while present in the vagina; patients should be advised to avoid unprotected intercourse or to use alternative contraception during treatment. Recurrent or refractory infections warrant evaluation for predisposing factors (e.g., diabetes, immunosuppression, and antibiotic use), confirmation of fungal species and susceptibility where appropriate, and consideration of longer suppressive regimens or specialist referral.

In cases of vulvovaginal candidosis, simultaneous treatment of both vaginal and vulvar areas is recommended.

Recurrent Vulvovaginal Candidosis (RVVC)

For recurrent vulvovaginal candidosis, and in the absence of targeted immunotherapeutic interventions, suppressive intermittent antifungal therapy with an oral triazole is recommended for several months. Fluconazole regimens have yielded the most consistent favorable outcomes in trials and observational studies when administered in weekly or intermittent schedules (see Fig. 36.3 and Table 36.2).

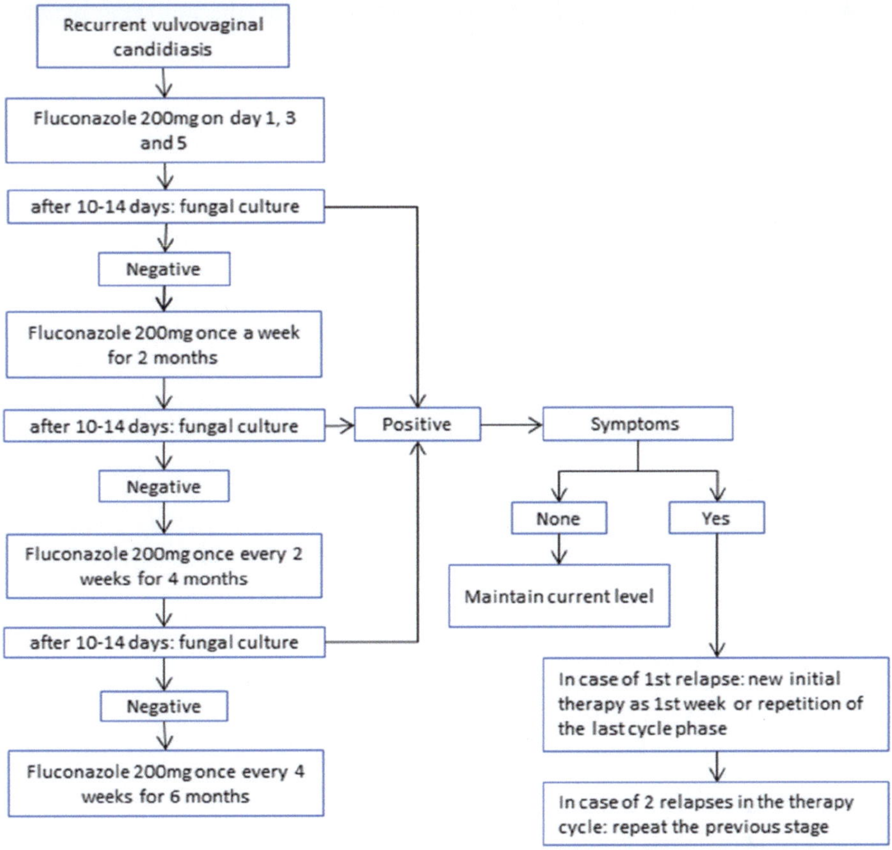

Fig. 36.3 Recommended therapeutic approach for recurrent vulvovaginal candidosis. (Courtesy of I. Mylonas)

Table 36.2 Therapeutic recommendations for chronic recurrent *Candida albicans* vaginitis

Time/duration	Procedure
First week	200 mg fluconazole each on 3 days
14 days later	Fungal culture; if negative, then:
For 2 months	200 mg fluconazole once weekly
14 days later	Fungal culture; if negative, then:
For 4 months	200 mg fluconazole once every 2 weeks
14 days later	Fungal culture; if negative, then:
For 6 months	200 mg fluconazole once monthly

In case of first relapse: new initial therapy as in the first week or repetition of the last cycle level
If there are two relapses in the therapy cycle: repeat the previous level

When itraconazole is employed (less commonly used), the following regimen has been suggested:
- Loading Dose: 200 mg orally twice on day 1
- Consolidation: 200 mg orally twice weekly for 4–6 weeks
- Reduction Phase 1: 200 mg orally twice every 2 weeks for 4–6 weeks
- Reduction Phase 2: 200 mg orally twice every 4 weeks for 4–6 weeks

Itraconazole should be taken with food to enhance absorption. Baseline hepatic function tests are recommended prior to initiation and should be monitored during therapy. Itraconazole is contraindicated in significant hepatic impairment and in patients receiving concomitant medications with clinically significant CYP3A4 interactions; pregnancy, cardiomyopathy, and congestive heart failure represent additional contraindications.

Predisposing factors must be corrected before candidosis can be treated effectively. For example, hyperglycemia in diabetes mellitus should be optimized to achieve adequate glycemic control prior to, or concurrently with, antifungal therapy.

Candida glabrata

Vaginitis caused by *Candida glabrata* is relatively uncommon and often occurs in the form of asymptomatic colonization. Conventional vaginal or oral therapies frequently fail to achieve effective treatment outcomes. The following treatment options are recommended for *Candida glabrata* vaginitis:

Fluconazole:

- **Dosage**: 800 mg/day orally for 2–3 weeks.
- **Efficacy**: Often insufficient for achieving a cure.

Severe or resistant cases:

- **Posaconazole suspension**:
  - **Dosage options**:
    - 400 mg (10 ml) orally daily
    - 4 × 200 mg (5 ml) orally daily
  - **Duration**: 3–14 days
  - **Note**: Posaconazole vaginal tablets have been withdrawn from several markets due to high costs and lack of prescription coverage.
- **Posaconazole tablets**:
  - **Initial Dose**: 300 mg orally twice on the first day
  - **Maintenance Dose**: 300 mg orally once daily from the second day on
  - **Duration**: 3–14 days

- **Voriconazole (for individuals over 40 kg)**:
  - **Loading Dose**: 2 × 6 mg/kg body weight per day on the first day
  - **Maintenance Dose**: 4 mg/kg body weight twice daily from the second day
  - **Duration**: 3 days

Alternative treatments:

- **Amphotericin B Vaginal Treatment**: Demonstrated effectiveness and can serve as an alternative when indicated. However, not available in every country.

Summary:
- **Fluconazole**: Frequently used but often ineffective for *Candida glabrata* vaginitis.
- **Posaconazole**: Available in both suspension and tablet forms for severe or resistant cases with specific dosage guidelines.
- **Voriconazole**: Recommended for individuals over 40 kg, with distinct loading and maintenance dosing strategies.
- **Amphotericin B**: Effective for vaginal treatment and should be considered when other options are inadequate.

In conclusion, *Candida glabrata* vaginitis often necessitates specialized treatment strategies due to resistance to conventional therapies. Posaconazole and voriconazole present effective alternatives for severe or resistant cases, while amphotericin B may serve as a supplementary option.

Candida krusei

Treatment of *Candida krusei* vulvovaginitis requires agents active against this inherently azole-resistant species. First-line therapy consists of intravaginal clotrimazole 100 mg once daily for 6 days. An alternative regimen is topical ciclopirox olamine 1% applied intravaginally for 6–7 days. For patients who cannot tolerate or fail azole-based topical therapy, intravaginal amphotericin B (100 mg in a gelatin capsule inserted daily for 7 days) has demonstrated efficacy and may be used as a salvage option.

36.6.2 Pregnancy

Imidazole derivatives are recognized as safe for topical treatment of fungal skin infections during pregnancy. Suitable polyenes (e.g., nystatin) and azoles (e.g., clotrimazole) may be used for intravaginal therapy. Some studies indicate slight superiority of imidazoles over nystatin in terms of both cure and recurrence rates, making once-daily imidazole therapy preferable for improved compliance.

Topical applications of clotrimazole, bifonazole, butoconazole, econazole, and fenticonazole during early pregnancy are highly unlikely to contribute to miscarriage. Due to rapid hepatic metabolism, drug levels in the blood post-vaginal absorption remain extremely low, and there is currently no established risk to the fetus.

All azole vaginal antifungals have received approval for use throughout pregnancy, including during the first trimester.

Intravaginal treatment should occur if yeasts are identified, regardless of accompanying clinical symptoms. Local vaginal treatment with imidazoles is feasible throughout gestation and is not anticipated to pose risks to the embryo or fetus, particularly if undertaken for short durations and restricted to small application areas.

Oral imidazole derivatives such as fluconazole, itraconazole, and ketoconazole have shown embryotoxic and teratogenic effects in animal studies. Despite the limited research available, high-dose fluconazole (400 mg/day) in the first trimester appears to be teratogenic, and patients requiring this treatment should be informed of potential fetal harm.

Short-term systemic use of imidazole derivatives has not demonstrated an increased risk of malformations. A prospective study involving 175 newborns following first-trimester exposure revealed no accumulation of fetal defects. The lower doses typically used for vaginal mycosis suggest a reduced risk of fetal harm; however, unless absolutely necessary, systemic administration should be avoided. It is advisable to confirm the absence of pregnancy prior to initiating treatment or to ensure effective contraception during the treatment period, lasting up to seven days post-therapy.

Furthermore, ketoconazole has exhibited embryotoxic and teratogenic effects in animal studies at doses equivalent to the maximum human recommended dosage. Accordingly, the oral application of ketoconazole is not advised, despite no observable malformations in a study of 20 newborns following first-trimester exposure.

Dose-dependent toxicity and teratogenicity have also been reported for itraconazole in animal studies; however, currently available data do not suggest a significantly increased risk of malformations with its use during pregnancy. Due to its similarity to fluconazole, itraconazole should be avoided whenever possible, given its potential adverse effects.

Amphotericin B possesses the longest clinical experience among antifungal agents; however, data remain insufficient to permit reliable risk assessment in pregnancy. Vaginal administration may be considered only for strict indications and should be employed when the anticipated maternal benefit outweighs potential fetal risk.

Oral azole antifungals (fluconazole, itraconazole, and ketoconazole) produced embryotoxic and teratogenic findings in animal studies; however, no consistent increase in major fetal malformations has been demonstrated in humans after inadvertent single-dose or short-course exposure in early pregnancy or immediately before conception. Despite this, systemic azole therapy—particularly during the first trimester—is generally avoided when alternatives (topical azoles) are appropriate because of theoretical teratogenic risk. Unintended exposure to these agents prior to pregnancy recognition is not an indication for termination of pregnancy.

36.7 Differential Diagnosis

Differential diagnoses to consider in cases of vulvovaginal candidosis include bacterial vaginosis, trichomoniasis, allergic reactions, atrophic vaginitis, genital herpes, cytolytic vaginosis, lichen sclerosus, and sexually transmitted diseases such as gonorrhea and chlamydia (Table 36.3).

Table 36.3 Differential diagnoses of vulvovaginal candidiasis

Differential diagnosis	Pathophysiology	Clinical features	Investigations
Allergic contact dermatitis	Type IV hypersensitivity or irritant contact reaction to topical agents (detergents, soaps, fragrances, preservatives, and latex)	Well-demarcated erythema; vesiculation and oozing in acute stages; chronic lichenification, fissuring, and persistent pruritus	Directed exposure history; patch testing for suspected allergens
Atrophic vaginitis (genitourinary syndrome of menopause)	Estrogen deficiency with thinning and decreased elasticity of the vulvovaginal epithelium	Vaginal dryness, dyspareunia, vulvovaginal irritation, urinary frequency/urgency; vaginal pH typically >4.5	Clinical assessment; vaginal pH measurement; cytology if indicated
Bacterial vaginosis (BV)	Dysbiosis with loss of lactobacilli and anaerobic overgrowth (e.g., Gardnerella and Atopobium)	Thin, homogeneous gray discharge; fishy odor on KOH (positive Whiff); clue cells on microscopy; vaginal pH >4.5	Amsel criteria or Nugent scoring on Gram stain; NAAT as adjunct

(continued)

Table 36.3 (continued)

Differential diagnosis	Pathophysiology	Clinical features	Investigations
Contact dermatitis (irritant)	Nonimmunologic chemical or physical damage from soaps, cleansers, friction, or occlusion	Localized erythema, dryness, scaling, fissuring, burning	Exposure history and improvement after cessation of suspected irritant; patch testing less useful
Genital herpes (HSV infection)	HSV-1 or HSV-2 infection causing mucocutaneous lesions	Clustered vesicles progressing to painful ulcers; prodromal burning or neuralgia; possible systemic symptoms	PCR from lesion swab (preferred); viral culture; type-specific serology when indicated
Lichen planus (vulvar)	Immune-mediated mucocutaneous disorder with interface dermatitis	Erosive, hypertrophic, or papulosquamous vulvar lesions; severe pruritus, painful erosions, dyspareunia; possible adhesions	Biopsy for histopathology (lichenoid infiltrate, basal layer changes)
Lichen sclerosus	Chronic inflammatory dermatosis producing atrophic, sclerotic vulvar changes	Porcelain-white atrophic plaques, fissures, labial fusion, introital narrowing; intense pruritus and dyspareunia	Clinical diagnosis; biopsy if atypical or suspicion of malignancy
Other sexually transmitted diseases (STD)	Diverse bacterial and spirochetal pathogens (*Neisseria gonorrhoeae*, *Chlamydia trachomatis*, *Mycoplasma genitalium*, *Treponema pallidum*)	Purulent or abnormal discharge, pelvic pain, cervicitis, systemic signs in some infections	NAATs for urogenital and extra-genital sites; Gram stain/culture where appropriate; syphilis serology; baseline HIV/HBV/HCV testing per guidelines
Psoriasis (genital)	Chronic immune-mediated dermatosis of skin and occasionally mucosa	Well-demarcated erythematous plaques in intertriginous/genital areas with minimal scale; associated nail or scalp disease	Clinical assessment; biopsy if diagnosis uncertain
Trichomoniasis	Protozoal infection with *Trichomonas vaginalis*	Frothy yellow-green malodorous discharge, vulvovaginal pruritus, dysuria; "strawberry" cervix in some cases	NAAT (preferred); wet mount microscopy or antigen tests
Vulvitis (nonspecific)	Inflammation of the vulva secondary to infectious, irritant, dermatologic, hormonal, or systemic causes	Erythema, edema, burning, pruritus, or pain	Focused history and examination; targeted swabs/NAATs/cultures as indicated; consider biopsy for persistent or atypical lesions

36.8 Prevention

Effective prevention of vulvovaginal candidosis hinges on a comprehensive approach that encompasses proper hygiene, a balanced diet, lifestyle modifications, and management of individual risk factors. Key strategies for preventing vulvovaginal candidosis include:

Optimizing Glycemic Control: In patients with diabetes mellitus, stringent glycemic management is essential to reduce the risk of vulvovaginal candidosis. Targeting a hemoglobin A1c of <7.0% minimizes fluctuations in blood glucose, thereby reducing the deposition of vaginal epithelial glycogen that serves as a nutrient source for Candida. Stable euglycemia also preserves neutrophil chemotaxis, phagocytosis, and oxidative burst activity, reinforcing innate immune defenses against fungal overgrowth. Regular monitoring, personalized insulin or oral hypoglycemic regimens, and patient education on carbohydrate counting and glycemic variability are critical components of this strategy.

Judicious Antibiotic Use: Broad-spectrum antibiotics indiscriminately eradicate commensal *Lactobacillus* spp., disrupting vaginal pH homeostasis and diminishing lactic acid production—conditions that favor Candida proliferation. Antibiotics should be prescribed only for well-defined bacterial infections, with narrowest-spectrum agents and shortest effective durations. Upon completion of antibiotic therapy, adjunctive probiotic supplementation may facilitate restoration of a protective vaginal microbiome.

Safe Sexual Practices: Barrier contraception—such as male and female condoms, dental dams, and polyurethane diaphragms—reduces the mechanical transfer of Candida cells and other microorganisms between sexual partners. Consistent condom use also preserves the integrity of the vaginal mucosa by preventing microabrasions and maintaining physiological pH. Counseling on genital hygiene before and after intercourse further minimizes residual moisture and microbial transfer.

Genital Hygiene: Daily cleansing of the external vulvovaginal area with a pH-balanced, fragrance-free cleanser removes excess secretions without stripping protective lipids or altering pH. Thorough but gentle drying—preferably by air-drying or patting with a soft, absorbent towel—prevents retention of moisture. Patients should avoid tight-fitting, non–breathable garments (e.g., synthetic underwear and leggings) and remove damp swimwear or workout attire promptly to reduce local temperature and humidity that promote yeast proliferation.

Irritant Avoidance: Perfumed soaps, sprays, douches, and feminine hygiene products can disrupt mucosal integrity, induce microabrasions, and elevate local pH, all of which facilitate Candida adherence and invasion. Patients should use only plain water or specialized mild cleansers for genital hygiene and avoid topical irritants in the vulvar area.

Dietary Considerations: Diets high in refined carbohydrates and added sugars provide fermentable substrates that encourage Candida growth and biofilm formation. Reducing intake of simple sugars and processed grains while emphasizing complex carbohydrates, lean proteins, healthy fats, and dietary fiber supports stable blood glucose levels, systemic metabolic health, and a balanced gut–vaginal microbial axis.

Weight Management: Adiposity contributes to skinfold moisture, friction, and local heat retention in the genital region, creating an ecological niche favorable to yeast overgrowth. Achieving and maintaining a healthy body mass index through calorie-appropriate nutrition and regular aerobic and resistance exercise reduces these risk factors. Weight loss interventions should be individualized, with behavioral counseling, structured exercise programs, and nutritional guidance to ensure sustainable outcomes.

Stress Management: Chronic psychological stress activates the hypothalamic–pituitary–adrenal axis, increasing circulating cortisol and inducing relative immunosuppression that raises susceptibility to opportunistic infections, including vulvovaginal candidosis. Evidence-based interventions—mindfulness-based stress reduction, progressive muscle relaxation, yoga, cognitive-behavioral therapy, and maintenance of adequate sleep hygiene (7–9 h nightly)—should be incorporated into comprehensive care to enhance immune resilience and help reduce recurrence.

Personal Hygiene Practices: Items that contact the genital or perianal area (towels, washcloths, underwear, razors, and intimate grooming devices) should not be shared between household members or sexual partners. Such fomites may permit mechanical transfer of *Candida* spp. and other pathogens and increase infection risk; laundering at high temperatures and avoiding damp storage of textiles are advised.

Alcohol Consumption Guidelines: Excessive alcohol intake (>1 standard drink per day for women) impairs innate and adaptive immune responses and may increase susceptibility to infections. Although moderate alcohol consumption has not been shown to directly alter vaginal microbiota composition, limiting intake to recommended levels supports immune function and is advised as part of risk-reduction counseling for patients with recurrent vulvovaginal candidosis.

Integrated prevention of vulvovaginal candidosis includes several measures: optimal control of underlying conditions (especially diabetes and immunosuppression), judicious and targeted use of antibiotics, avoidance of local irritants (no douching and no scented products), maintenance of perineal dryness (change wet clothing promptly, wear breathable cotton underwear, and avoid tight synthetic garments), safe sexual practices, and not sharing personal items. Weight management, stress reduction, and a balanced low-sugar diet may reduce recurrences. Probiotics are not routinely recommended.

Given that prophylaxis during pregnancy does not incur greater costs than postnatal therapy, a focus on adequate preventive strategies is recommended:

- **Vaginal Yeast Culture**: Initiation of vaginal yeast cultures is suggested starting at 34 weeks of gestation, although this has yet to be universally adopted as standard practice.
- **Intravaginal Therapy**: Should yeasts be detected, intravaginal therapy must commence irrespective of the presence of clinical symptoms.
- **Treatment Efficacy**: Imidazoles demonstrate significantly greater effectiveness than polyenes in treating yeast infections during pregnancy.
- **Risk of Preterm Delivery**: If preterm delivery is a concern, antifungal cultures should be obtained, and appropriate treatment should continue.

While vulvovaginal candidosis is not typically associated with preterm delivery or rupture of membranes, studies indicate a reduction in preterm delivery following vaginal treatment with cotrimoxazole during the first trimester. The implications of these findings remain largely unclear.

Key Points

- Vulvovaginal candidosis (VVC) is an infection affecting the estrogenized vagina and vestibule, caused by fungi of the genus *Candida*.
- VVC can manifest on the external genitalia, in the vagina, intercrural region, and perianal region, with *Candida albicans* responsible for 85–95% of vaginal colonization.
- Non-albicans species, including *Candida glabrata*, *Candida tropicalis*, and *Candida parapsilosis*, can also contribute to vulvovaginitis.
- Common symptoms of vulvovaginal candidosis include itching, erythema, burning sensations, dyspareunia, dysuria, and vaginal discharge.
- The diagnosis is established through a comprehensive medical history, clinical assessment, and microscopic evidence of yeast.
- Treatment options encompass both vaginal and oral antifungal agents, with the selection of therapy dependent on the infection's severity.
- Treatment of *Candida glabrata*, *Candida tropicalis*, and *Candida parapsilosis* infection may prove more challenging.
- Suppressive intermittent antifungal therapy with oral triazoles may be employed.
- Vaginal antifungal therapy is deemed safe during pregnancy, while systemic therapies should generally be avoided.
- Preventive measures include practicing good hygiene and managing underlying conditions.
- Educating patients about prevention and monitoring for potential treatment needs is essential.

Literature

Figures Sources

Abeck D (2005) Andere venerische Erkrankungen. In: Braun-Falco O, Plewig G, Wolff HH et al. (eds) Dermatologie und Venerologie. Springer, Berlin, pp 246–253. https://doi.org/10.1007/3-540-26624-0_18

Allen DH (2014) How mechanics shaped the modern world. Springer, Cham. https://doi.org/10.1007/978-3-319-01701-3

Boutellier R, Heinzen M (2014) Growth through innovation. Springer, Cham. https://doi.org/10.1007/978-3-319-04016-5

Buder S, Lautenschlager S (2022) Gonorrhea and urethritis. In: Plewig G, French L, Ruzicka T et al (eds) Braun-Falco's dermatology. Springer, Berlin, pp 293–310. https://doi.org/10.1007/978-3-662-63709-8_18

Caspary WF, Kist M, Stein J (2006) Infektiologie des Gastrointestinaltraktes. Springer, Berlin. https://doi.org/10.1007/3-540-37211-3

Friese K, Schäfer A, Hof H (2003) Infektionskrankheiten in Gynäkologie und Geburtshilfe. Springer, Berlin. https://doi.org/10.1007/978-3-642-55586-2

Geusau A (2022) Syphilis. In: Plewig G, French L, Ruzicka T et al (eds) Braun-Falco's dermatology. Springer, Berlin, pp 311–334. https://doi.org/10.1007/978-3-662-63709-8_19

Harms D (2008) Rudolf Virchowals Politiker. Mit Hinweis auf die Gesamtausgabe seiner Werke (Rudolf Virchow as a politician. With reference to the complete edition of his works). Pathologe 29:165–167. https://doi.org/10.1007/s00292-008-0991-5

Hatzinger M, Hatzinger J (2009) Giacomo Casanova (1725-1798): Ein Leben mit Aphrodisiaka (Giacomo Casanova (1725-1798): a life with aphrodisiacs). Der Urologe Ausg A 48:415–418. https://doi.org/10.1007/s00120-009-1937-0

Kagan K, Mylonas I, Enders M et al (2011) Intrauterine Zytomegalievirusinfektion: Neues zur Pränataldiagnostik und Hyperimmunglobulinbehandlung. Gynakologe 44:601–609. https://doi.org/10.1007/s00129-011-2776-9

Kost BP, Mylonas I, Kästner R et al (2007) Congenital cytomegalovirus infection in pregnancy: a case report of fetal death in a CMV-infected woman. Arch Gynecol Obstet 276:265–268. https://doi.org/10.1007/s00404-007-0327-3

Leal Passos MR, De Almeida L, Filho G, Castelo Branco Coêlho I et al (2018) Atlas of sexually transmitted diseases: clinical aspects and differential diagnosis. Springer, Cham. https://doi.org/10.1007/978-3-319-57470-7

Mendling W (2006) Vaginose, Vaginitis, Zervizitis und Salpingitis. Springer, Berlin. https://doi.org/10.1007/978-3-540-30096-0

Mylonas I (2010) Infektionserkrankungen der Vulva und Vagina. Gynäkologe 43:429–440. https://doi.org/10.1007/s00129-010-2570-0

I. Mylonas, *Sexually Transmitted Diseases*,
https://doi.org/10.1007/978-3-031-78204-6

Mylonas I (2011) Herpes genitalis in der Schwangerschaft. Gynäkologe 44:623–629. https://doi.org/10.1007/s00129-011-2771-1

Mylonas I (2013) Vaginale infektiologische Diagnostik. In: Friese K, Mylonas I, Schulze A (eds) Infektionserkrankungen der Schwangeren und des Neugeborenen. Springer, Berlin, pp 53–58. https://doi.org/10.1007/978-3-540-78325-1_6

Mylonas I (2016) Sexuell übertragbare Erkrankungen: Ein Leitfaden für Frauenärzte. Springer, Berlin. https://doi.org/10.1007/978-3-642-37928-4

Mylonas I (2025) Sexuell übertragbare Erkrankungen: Ein Leitfaden für Frauenärztinnen und Frauenärzte, 2nd edn. Springer, Berlin

Mylonas I, Friese K (2009) Adnexitis - eine klinische Herausforderung. Gynäkologe 42:786–792. https://doi.org/10.1007/s00129-009-2352-8

Mylonas I, Petersen EE (2009) Infektionserkrankungen der Vulva. Gynäkologe 42:247–255. https://doi.org/10.1007/s00129-008-2302-x

Seiler C (2009) Collateral circulation of the heart. Springer, London. https://doi.org/10.1007/978-1-84882-342-6

Vormbaum T, Bohlander M (2014) The twentieth century. In: Vormbaum T, Bohlander M (eds) A modern history of German criminal law. Springer, Berlin, pp 127–249. https://doi.org/10.1007/978-3-642-37273-5_5

Weissenbacher ER (2013) Trichomoniasis. In: Friese K, Mylonas I, Schulze A (eds) Infektionserkrankungen der Schwangeren und des Neugeborenen. Springer, Berlin, pp 501–506. https://doi.org/10.1007/978-3-540-78325-1_38

Wintergerst U, Hübener C, Strauss A et al (2006) Schwere kongenitale CMV-Infektion trotz maternem CMV-Durchseuchungstiter. Monatsschr Kinderheilkd 154:558–564. https://doi.org/10.1007/s00112-004-1030-0

Zangerle R, Fritsch P, Schwarz T (2018) Venerologie. In: Fritsch P, Schwarz T (eds) Dermatologie Venerologie: Grundlagen Klinik. Atlas. Springer, Berlin, pp 1045–1115. https://doi.org/10.1007/978-3-662-53647-6_23

Further Reading

Allan-Blitz L-T, Fifer H, Klausner JD (2024) Managing treatment failure in Neisseria gonorrhoeae infection: current guidelines and future directions. Lancet Infect Dis 24(8):e532–e538. https://doi.org/10.1016/S1473-3099(24)00001-X

Amaral E, Money D, Jamieson D, Pasupathy D, Aronoff D, Jacobsson B, Lizcano EIO (2023) Vaccination during pregnancy: a golden opportunity to embrace. Int J Gynaecol Obstet 163(2):476–483. https://doi.org/10.1002/ijgo.14981

Bachmann LH, Barbee LA, Chan P, Reno H, Workowski KA, Hoover K et al (2024) CDC clinical guidelines on the use of doxycycline postexposure prophylaxis for bacterial sexually transmitted infection prevention, United States, 2024. MMWR Recomm Rep 73(2):1–8. https://doi.org/10.15585/mmwr.rr7302a1

Bennett JE, Dolin R, Blaser MJ (eds) (2020) Mandell, Douglas, and Bennett's principles and practice of infectious diseases. Elsevier, Philadelphia

Benson J, Pierre C, Joseph NT (2024) Updates in the management of HIV during pregnancy. Clin Obstet Gynecol 67(3):644–651. https://doi.org/10.1097/GRF.0000000000000887

Braun-Falco O, Plewig G, Wolff HH, Burgdorf WHC, Landthaler M (2005) Dermatologie und Venerologie. Springer, Berlin

Brodt H-R, Hörauf A, Kresken M, Solbach W, Welte T (2024) Infektionstherapie: Antibiotika, Virostatika, Antimykotika, Antiparasitäre Wirkstoffe, 13th edn. Thieme, London

Brook G, Church H, Evans C, Jenkinson N, McClean H, Mohammed H et al (2020) 2019 UK National Guideline for consultations requiring sexual history taking: Clinical Effectiveness Group British Association for sexual health and HIV. Int J STD AIDS 31(10):920–938. https://doi.org/10.1177/0956462420941708

Carvalho NS, Palú G, Witkin SS (2020) Mycoplasma genitalium, a stealth female reproductive tract. Eur J Clin Microbiol Infect Dis 39(2):229–234. https://doi.org/10.1007/s10096-019-03707-8
Caspary WF, Kist M, Stein J (2006) Infektiologie des Gastrointestinaltraktes. Springer, Berlin
Cohen J, Powderly WG, Opal SM (2017) Infectious diseases. Elsevier, London
D'Alberti E, Rizzo G, Khalil A, Mappa I, Pietrolucci ME, Capannolo G et al (2024) Counseling in fetal medicine: congenital cytomegalovirus infection. Eur J Obstet Gynecol Reprod Biol 295:8–17. https://doi.org/10.1016/j.ejogrb.2024.01.037
Dionne-Odom J, Cozzi GD, Franco RA, Njei B, Tita AT (2022) Treatment and prevention of viral hepatitis in pregnancy. Am J Obstet Gynecol 226(3):335–346. https://doi.org/10.1016/j.ajog.2021.09.002
Dutra K, Lazenby G (2023) An update on gonorrhea and chlamydia. Obstet Gynecol Clin N Am 50(2):299–310. https://doi.org/10.1016/j.ogc.2023.02.004
Enders G, Mylonas I, Schulze A, Friese K (2013) Zytomegalie. In: Friese K, Mylonas I, Schulze A (eds) Infektionserkrankungen der Schwangeren und des Neugeborenen. Springer, Berlin, pp 243–267. https://doi.org/10.1007/978-3-540-78325-1_19
Espinal M, Yee LM, Fisher SA (2024) Advances in HIV management during pregnancy and infant feeding. Infect Dis Clin N Am 38(3):423–452. https://doi.org/10.1016/j.idc.2024.06.005
Farr A, Swidsinski S, Surbek D, Tirri BF, Willinger B, Hoyme U et al (2023) Bacterial vaginosis: guideline of the DGGG, OEGGG and SGGG (S2k-level, AWMF Registry No. 015/028, June 2023). Geburtshilfe Frauenheilkunde 83(11):1331–1349. https://doi.org/10.1055/a-2169-8539
Farrar J, Hotez PJ, Junghanss T, Kang G, Lalloo DG, White NJ, García PJ (2024) Manson's tropical diseases, 24th edn. Elsevier, Philadelphia
Fehm T, Janni W, Stickeler E, Tempfer C, Prieske K, Wölber L (eds) (2020) Gynäkologie - differenzialdiagnostik und differenzialtherapie: klug entscheiden - gut behandeln, 1st edn. Elsevier, München
Fehm T, Rody A, Hadji P, Solomayer E-F (2021) Referenz gynäkologie. Thieme, Stuttgart
Feige A, Rath W, Schmidt S (2022) Kreißsaal-Kompendium: das Praxisbuch für die Geburtshilfe, 3rd edn. Thieme, Stuttgart
Friese K, Schäfer A, Hof H (2003) Infektionskrankheiten in Gynäkologie und Geburtshilfe. Springer, Berlin
Fritsch P, Schwarz T (2018) Dermatologie Venerologie. Springer, Berlin
Gaspar PC, Barreto JOM, Bigolin A, Miranda AE, Aires Júnior LF, Bazzo ML et al (2023) Brazilian clinical practice guidelines for sexually transmitted infections that cause urethral discharge: assessment according to the AGREE II and critical analysis based on the WHO recommendations. Sex Transm Dis 50(12):804–809. https://doi.org/10.1097/OLQ.0000000000001873
Gesellschaft für Virologie (2014) S2k-Leitlinie - Labordiagnostik schwangerschaftsrelevanter Virusinfektionen. Springer, Berlin
Gilbert RK, Petersen LR, Honein MA, Moore CA, Rasmussen SA (2023) Zika virus as a cause of birth defects: were the teratogenic effects of Zika virus missed for decades? Birth Defects Res 115(3):265–274. https://doi.org/10.1002/bdr2.2134
Grant JS, Chico RM, Lee AC, Low N, Medina-Marino A, Molina RL et al (2020) Sexually transmitted infections in pregnancy: a narrative review of the global research gaps, challenges, and opportunities. Sex Transm Dis 47(12):779–789. https://doi.org/10.1097/OLQ.0000000000001258
Gross G (2011) Sexually transmitted infections and sexually transmitted diseases. Springer, Berlin
Handsfield HH (2011) Color atlas & synopsis of sexually transmitted diseases, 3rd edn. McGraw-Hill Medical, New York
Hill DR, Ryan ET, Aronson N, Solomon T, Endy TP (eds) (2020) Hunter's tropical medicine and emerging infectious diseases. Elsevier, Edinburgh
Holmes K, Sparling P, Stamm W, Piot P, Wasserheit J, Corey L et al (2008) Sexually transmitted diseases, 4th edn. McGraw-Hill, New York
Hufstetler K, Llata E, Miele K, Quilter LAS (2024) Clinical updates in sexually transmitted infections. J Women's Health 33(6):827–837. https://doi.org/10.1089/jwh.2024.0367
Janni W, Hancke K, Fehm T, Scholz C, Rack BK (2021) Facharztwissen Gynäkologie, 3rd edn. Elsevier, München

Jückstock J, Blankenstein T, Mahner S, Mylonas I (2016) Entzündliche Erkrankungen des Uterus und der Adnexe. Gynäkologe 49:189–200. https://doi.org/10.1007/s00129-016-3840-2

Kainer F (2021) Facharztwissen Geburtsmedizin, 4th edn. Elsevier, München

Khanna N (2019) Illustrated synopsis of dermatology & sexually transmitted diseases. Elsevier, New Delhi

Kim WB, Lee S-J, Bae S, Ku JY, Oh TH, Oh MM et al (2024) Korean sexually transmitted infection guidelines 2023 revision, guideline update of viral infections: genital herpes and anogenital warts. Invest Clin Urol 65(1):9–15. https://doi.org/10.4111/icu.20230275

Kissinger PJ, Gaydos CA, Seña AC, Scott McClelland R, Soper D, Secor WE et al (2022) Diagnosis and management of trichomonas vaginalis: summary of evidence reviewed for the 2021 Centers for Disease Control and Prevention sexually transmitted infections treatment guidelines. Clin Infect Dis 74(Suppl_2):S152–S161. https://doi.org/10.1093/cid/ciac030

Kost BP, Mylonas I, Kästner R, Rack B, Gingelmaier A, Friese K (2007) Congenital cytomegalovirus infection in pregnancy: a case report of fetal death in a CMV-infected woman. Arch Gynecol Obstet 276(3):265–268. https://doi.org/10.1007/s00404-007-0327-3

Kreienberg R, Ludwig H (2010) 125 Jahre Deutsche Gesellschaft für Gynäkologie und Geburtshilfe - Werte, Wissen, Wandel. Springer, Heidelberg

Leal Passos MR, De Almeida L, Filho G, Castelo Branco Coêlho I, Moreira LC, Pellegrini Nah Jurior E, Eleutério J (2018) Atlas of sexually transmitted diseases: clinical aspects and differential diagnosis. Springer, Cham

Lin Y-P, Chen W-C, Cheng C-M, Shen C-J (2021) Vaginal pH value for clinical diagnosis and treatment of common vaginitis. Diagnostics 11:1996. https://doi.org/10.3390/diagnostics11111996

Maldonado YA, Nizet V, Barnett ED, Edwards KM, Malley R, Remington JS, Klein JO (2025) Remington and Klein's infectious diseases of the fetus and newborn infant. Elsevier, Philadelphia

Maliyar K, Mufti A, Syed M, Selk A, Dutil M, Bunce PE, Alavi A (2019) Genital ulcer disease: a review of pathogenesis and clinical features. J Cutan Med Surg 23(6):624–634. https://doi.org/10.1177/1203475419858955

Marre R, Mertens T, Trautmann M, Zimmerli W (eds) (2008) Klinische Infektiologie – Infektionskrankheiten erkennen und behandeln. Elsevier, München

Mendling W (2006) Vaginose, Vaginitis, Zervizitis und Salpingitis. Springer, Berlin

Mendling W, Mylonas I, Schulze A, Hilgendorff A (2013) Pilzinfektionen. In: Friese K, Mylonas I, Schulze A (eds) Infektionserkrankungen der Schwangeren und des Neugeborenen. Springer, Berlin, pp 421–442. https://doi.org/10.1007/978-3-540-78325-1_33

Monif GR, Baker DA (2019) Infectious diseases in obstetrics and gynecology. CRC Press, Boca Raton

Morse SA, Holmes KK, Ballard RC (2010) Atlas of sexually transmitted diseases and AIDS, 4th edn. Elsevier, London

Mylonas I (2010) Infektionserkrankungen der Vulva und Vagina. Gynäkologe 43:429–440. https://doi.org/10.1007/s00129-010-2570-0

Mylonas I (2011a) Antibiotic chemotherapy during pregnancy and lactation period: aspects for consideration. Arch Gynecol Obstet 283(1):7–18. https://doi.org/10.1007/s00404-010-1646-3

Mylonas I (2011b) Herpes genitalis in der Schwangerschaft. Gynakologe 44(8):623–629. https://doi.org/10.1007/s00129-011-2771-1

Mylonas I (2011c) Sexuell übertragene erkrankungen - Teil I: "Klassische" sexuell übertragene Erkrankungen (STD). Gynakologe 44(2):133–142

Mylonas I (2011d) Sexuell übertragene Erkrankungen - Teil II: andere sexuell übertragene Erkrankungen. Gynäkologe 44(3):213–226

Mylonas I (2013) Vaginale infektiologische Diagnostik. In: Friese K, Mylonas I, Schulze A (eds) Infektionserkrankungen der Schwangeren und des Neugeborenen. Springer, Berlin, pp 53–58. https://doi.org/10.1007/978-3-540-78325-1_6

Mylonas I (2016) Sexuell übertragbare Erkrankungen: Ein Leitfaden für Frauenärzte. Springer, Berlin

Mylonas I (2019) Infektionen. In: Feige A, Rath W, Schmidt S (eds) Kreißsaalkompendium: Das Praxisbuch für die Geburtshilfe, 2nd edn. Thieme, Stuttgart. https://doi.org/10.1055/b-0038-163881
Mylonas I (2024a) Infektionen in Gynäkologie und Geburtshilfe, 2nd edn. Elsevier, Mün chen
Mylonas I (2024b) Praxis der gynäkologischen Infektiologie. De Gruyter, Berlin
Mylonas I (2025) Sexuell übertragbare Erkrankungen: ein Leitfaden für Frauenärztinnen und Frauenärzte, 2nd edn. Springer, Berlin
Mylonas I, Bergauer F (2011) Diagnosis of vaginal discharge by wet mount microscopy: a simple and underrated method. Obstet Gynecol Surv 66(6):359–368
Mylonas I, Friese K (2005a) Infektionsbedingte fetale Schädigungen. In: Ganten D, Ruckpaul K (eds) Molekularmedizinische Grundlagen von fetalen und neonatalen Erkrankungen. Springer, Heidelberg, pp 265–323
Mylonas I, Friese K (2005b) Zytomegalie-Infektion in der Schwangerschaft: Von der Forschung zur Klinik. Geburtshilfe Frauenheilkd 65(5):465–473
Mylonas I, Friese K (2007) Fluor vaginalis. MMW Fortschr Med 149(35-36):42–46
Mylonas I, Friese K (2009) Adnexitis - eine klinische Herausforderung. Gynäkologe 42(10):786–792. https://doi.org/10.1007/s00129-009-2352-8
Mylonas I, Friese K (2010) Pregnancy and herpes genitalis – a diagnostic and therapeutic challenge. Arch Hellenic Med 27(6):871–878
Mylonas I, Friese K (2012) Infektionen und Frühgeburt. Gynäkologe 45:520–526. https://doi.org/10.1007/s00129-011-2934-0
Mylonas I, Mendling W (2013) Bakterielle Vaginose. In: Friese K, Mylonas I, Schulze A (eds) Infektionserkrankungen der Schwangeren und des Neugeborenen. Springer, Berlin, pp 271–283. https://doi.org/10.1007/978-3-540-78325-1_20
Mylonas I, Petersen EE (2009) Infektionserkrankungen der Vulva. Gynäkologe 42(4):247–255. https://doi.org/10.1007/s00129-008-2302-x
Mylonas I, Wirth S (2013) Hepatitisviren. In: Friese K, Mylonas I, Schulze A (eds) Infektionserkrankungen der Schwangeren und des Neugeborenen. Springer, Berlin, pp 129–161. https://doi.org/10.1007/978-3-540-78325-1_12
Mylonas I, Dian D, Friese K (2005) Antibiotikatherapie in der Schwangerschaft. Gynäkologe 38(9):761–770
Mylonas I, Gingelmaier A, Friese K (2006) Systemische Infektionen in der Geburtshilfe. Gynäkologe 39(3):223–232
Mylonas I, Bolz M, Spellerberg B, Kühn J, Friese K (2008a) Weibliche Geschlechtsorgane. In: Marre R, Mertens T, Trautmann M, Zimmerli W (eds) Klinische Infektiologie – Infektionskrankheiten erkennen und behandeln. Elsevier, München, pp 559–578
Mylonas I, Bredt W, Doerr HW, Friese K (2008b) Infektionen in der Schwangerschaft. In: Marre R, Mertens T, Trautmann M, Zimmerli W (eds) Klinische Infektiologie – Infektionskrankheiten erkennen und behandeln. Elsevier, München, pp 987–1016
Mylonas I, Bruning A, Kainer F, Friese K (2010) HTLV infection and its implication in gynaecology and obstetrics. Arch Gynecol Obstet 282(5):493–501. https://doi.org/10.1007/s00404-010-1559-1
Mylonas I, Friese K, Grabein B (2013a) Ulcus molle. In: Friese K, Mylonas I, Schulze A (eds) Infektionserkrankungen der Schwangeren und des Neugeborenen. Springer, Berlin, pp 399–403. https://doi.org/10.1007/978-3-540-78325-1_31
Mylonas I, Friese K, Hiedl S (2013b) Gonorrhöe. Infektionserkrankungen der Schwangeren und des Neugeborenen. Springer, Berlin, pp 309–318. https://doi.org/10.1007/978-3-540-78325-1_23
Mylonas I, Hoyme U, Flemmer AW (2013c) Chlamydiainfektionen. In: Friese K, Mylonas I, Schulze A (eds) Infektionserkrankungen der Schwangeren und des Neugeborenen. Springer, Berlin, pp 297–307. https://doi.org/10.1007/978-3-540-78325-1_22
Nabarro L, Morris-Jones S, Moore DA (2019) Peters' atlas of tropical medicine and parasitology. Elsevier, Amsterdam
National Institute for Health and Care Excellence (NICE) (2022) Reducing sexually transmitted infections. NICE, London

Neumann G, Schäfer A, Mendling W (2014) Phasenkontrastmikroskopie in der Frauenarztpraxis. Springer, Berlin

Ngalame AN, Mubiana-Mbewe M, Dionne JA (2022) Genital tract infections in women, pregnancy and neonates. Obstet Gynecol Clin N Am 49(4):751–769. https://doi.org/10.1016/j.ogc.2022.07.004

Nyirjesy P, Brookhart C, Lazenby G, Schwebke J, Sobel JD (2022) Vulvovaginal candidiasis: a review of the evidence for the 2021 Centers for Disease Control and Prevention of sexually transmitted infections treatment guidelines. Clin Infect Dis 74(Suppl_2):S162–S168. https://doi.org/10.1093/cid/ciab1057

Olaleye AO, Babah OA, Osuagwu CS, Ogunsola FT, Afolabi BB (2020) Sexually transmitted infections in pregnancy - an update on Chlamydia trachomatis and Neisseria gonorrhoeae. Eur J Obstet Gynecol Reprod Biol 255:1–12. https://doi.org/10.1016/j.ejogrb.2020.10.002

Paparini S, Whelan I, Mwendera C, Hayes R, Maatouk I, Lewis R et al (2024) Prevention of sexual transmission of mpox: a systematic review and qualitative evidence synthesis of approaches. Infect Dis 56(8):589–605. https://doi.org/10.1080/23744235.2024.2364801

Petersen EE (2011) Infektionen in Gynäkologie und Geburtshilfe: Lehrbuch und Atlas, 5th edn. Thieme, Stuttgart

Plewig G, French L, Ruzicka T, Kaufmann R, Hertl M (2022) Braun-Falco's dermatology. Springer, Berlin

Pontes KF, Nardozza LM, Peixoto AB, Werner H, Tonni G, Granese R, Araujo E (2024) Cytomegalovirus and pregnancy: a narrative review. J Clin Med 13(2):640. https://doi.org/10.3390/jcm13020640

Powell A, Goje O, Nyirjesy P (2024) A comparison of newer and traditional approaches to diagnosing vaginal infections. Obstet Gynecol 143(4):491–498. https://doi.org/10.1097/AOG.0000000000005529

Rath W, Strauss A (2018) Komplikationen in der Geburtshilfe: Aus Fällen lernen. Springer, Berlin

Rath W, Gembruch U, Schmidt S (2022) Referenz Geburtshilfe und Perinatalmedizin. Thieme, Stuttgart Rietze

Rietze K, Jaeger S, Mylonas I (2016) Parasitäre Erkrankungen in der Schwangerschaft: Würmer, Läuse, Flöhe Der Gynäkologe. https://doi.org/10.1007/s00129-016-3921-2

Rogstad KE (2011) ABC of sexually transmitted infections, 6th edn. Wiley, Hoboken

Rybak-Krzyszkowska M, Górecka J, Huras H, Massalska-Wolska M, Staśkiewicz M, Gach A et al (2023) Cytomegalovirus infection in pregnancy prevention and treatment options: a systematic review and meta-analysis. Viruses. https://doi.org/10.3390/v15112142

Saavedra AP, Roh E, Mikailov A (2023) Fitzpatrick's color atlas and synopsis of clinical dermatology. McGraw-Hill, New York

Schindlbeck C, Mylonas I (2012) Vorgehen bei Adnexitis: gundsätzlich operative Diagnostik? Gynäkol Praxis 36(4):663

Schneider H, Husslein P, Schneider K (2016) Die Geburtshilfe, 5th edn. Springer, Berlin. https://doi.org/10.1007/978-3-662-45064-2_25

Skolnik NS (2013) Sexually transmitted diseases: a practical guide for primary care, 2nd edn. Humana Press, Totowa

Spinner CD, Lang GF, Boesecke C, Jessen H, Schewe K (2019) Summary of German-Austrian HIV PrEP guideline. HIV Med 20(6):368–376. https://doi.org/10.1111/hiv.12724

Stafford IA, Workowski KA, Bachmann LH (2024) Syphilis complicating pregnancy and congenital syphilis. N Engl J Med 390(3):242–253. https://doi.org/10.1056/NEJMra2202762

Stanberry LR (2013) Sexually transmitted diseases: vaccines, prevention, and control, 2nd edn. Elsevier, Amsterdam

Strauss A, Janni W, Maass N (eds) (2009) Klinikmanual Gynäkologie und Geburtshilfe. Springer, Heidelberg

Truglio J (2022) Sexual and reproductive health: a practical guide for primary care, 1st edn. Springer, Cham

Vo C, Zomorodi R, Silvera R, Bartram L, Lugo LA, Kojic E et al (2023) Clinical characteristics and outcomes of patients with Mpox who received tecovirimat in a New York City health system. Open Forum Infect Dis 10(11):ofad552. https://doi.org/10.1093/ofid/ofad552

Wang Y, Liu Z, Chen T (2024) Vaginal microbiota: potential targets for vulvovaginal candidiasis infection. Heliyon 10(5):e27239. https://doi.org/10.1016/j.heliyon.2024.e27239

Weissenbacher E-R, Wirth M, Mylonas I, Ledger WJ, Witkin SS (2016) Immunology of the female genital tract, 1st edn. Springer, Berlin

Wiesenfeld HC, Manhart LE (2017) Mycoplasma genitalium in women: current knowledge and research priorities for this recently emerged pathogen. J Infect Dis 216(suppl_2):S389–S395. https://doi.org/10.1093/infdis/jix198

Wihlfahrt K, Günther V, Mendling W, Westermann A, Willer D, Gitas G et al (2023) Sexually transmitted diseases-an update and overview of current research. Diagnostics. https://doi.org/10.3390/diagnostics13091656

Workowski KA, Bachmann LH, Chan PA, Johnston CM, Muzny CA, Park I et al (2021) Sexually transmitted infections treatment guidelines, 2021. MMWR Recomm Rep 70(4):1–187. https://doi.org/10.15585/mmwr.rr7004a1

World Health Organization (2021) Guidelines for the management of symptomatic sexually transmitted infections. World Health Organization, Geneva

World Health Organization (2022) Consolidated guidelines on HIV, viral hepatitis and STI prevention, diagnosis, treatment and care for key populations. World Health Organization, Geneva

World Health Organization (2024a) Consolidated guidelines on differentiated HIV testing services. World Health Organization, Geneva

World Health Organization (2024b) Recommendations for the treatment of Trichomonas vaginalis, Mycoplasma genitalium, Candida albicans, bacterial vaginosis and human papillomavirus (anogenital warts). World Health Organization, Geneva

World Health Organization (2024c) Updated recommendations for the treatment of Neisseria gonorrhoeae, Chlamydia trachomatis and Treponema pallidum (syphilis), and new recommendations on syphilis testing and partner services. World Health Organization, Geneva

Yazdy GM, Mitchell C, Sobel JD, Tuddenham S (2024) Recurrent infectious vaginitis: a practical approach for the primary care clinician. Med Clin North Am 108(2):373–392. https://doi.org/10.1016/j.mcna.2023.08.017

MIX
Papier aus verantwortungsvollen Quellen
Paper from responsible sources
FSC® C105338

If you have any concerns about our products,
you can contact us on
ProductSafety@springernature.com

In case Publisher is established outside the EU,
the EU authorized representative is:
Springer Nature Customer Service Center GmbH
Europaplatz 3, 69115 Heidelberg, Germany

Printed by Libri Plureos GmbH
in Hamburg, Germany